The OSCE Revision Guide
For Medical Students

First edition

CHRISTOPHER MANSBRIDGE

MBCHB (HONS) MRES (DIST) MRCP (UK)

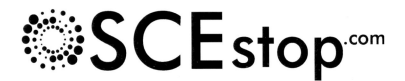

First edition published 2018

ISBN – 978-1-9997198-0-7

A catalogue record for this book is available from the British Library.

Important note: every effort was made to try to ensure the information provided in this book was accurate and up to date at the time of publication. However, unfortunately, it is still possible there may be errors in the text. The author accepts no legal liability or responsibility for any errors or the use of any information in this book. Furthermore, guidelines and legislation change frequently and readers are advised to check information with up to date sources.

Website: **www.OSCEstop.com**

Contact/feedback: **contact@OSCEstop.com**

CONTENTS

PREFACE

The Objective Structured Clinical Examination (OSCE) is central to the assessment of clinical competence at medical school and beyond. It is also the exam that many candidates fear the most. To do well, you need to combine your knowledge with a wide range of practical and communication skills. You also need to be able to function under pressure. The key to OSCE preparation will always be practice and no book will ever remove the need for that. But what I have tried to do here is summarise the basic knowledge you require and integrate it with a practical guide to all the various essential skills.

The book is divided into nine chapters, each focusing on a major part of the OSCE. History-taking is covered first in **Chapter 1** because this usually forms the start of the patient encounter. The diagnosis can be made from the history in around 80% of cases. The history is then supplemented by clinical examination, which is covered in **Chapter 2**.

Many OSCE stations will also include a *viva* about the condition, and I have aimed to provide the key information for all of the common subjects examined in this way in **Chapter 3**. Observation alone can reveal important clinical signs and so I also provide advice on *spotter skills* that are often tested.

All doctors must be able to assess and manage acutely unwell patients. This differs from other clinical scenarios because treatment must be administered quickly in order to stabilise the patient. **Chapter 4** covers the major emergencies you are likely to encounter as a junior doctor.

There are several clinical procedures that a junior doctor must be competent to perform for the purpose of patient investigation and management. These are covered in **Chapter 5**. After performing investigations, you need to be able to interpret the results. This is covered in **Chapter 6**. Treatment will often involve medication and you must learn to prescribe safely to ensure you *do no harm* – part of The Hippocratic Oath. I try to equip you with the basic principles of safe prescribing in **Chapter 7**.

Patient-centred care is paramount both in exams and, more importantly, in real life. You must treat every patient as an individual and be alert to the fact that you may be encountering them at the worst moment of their life. Good communication, undertaken with respect and sensitivity, is essential. You must find your own way to do this but there are some basic principles that should be taken on board. These are outlined in **Chapter 8**.

Chapter 9 aims to bring everything together and put it in context. I hope this will help you start your journey as a new junior doctor.

I wish you the best of luck and hope this book serves you well, both at medical school and when you begin to practice. Though you may not always feel it, medicine is one of the most rewarding careers that exists and one in which you have the opportunity to have a profound and positive impact on the lives of others every day.

Christopher Mansbridge

CONTRIBUTORS

Dr Annabel Freeborough
General practitioner

Dr Alexander Suebsaeng
Junior doctor

Mr Declan McDonnell
Surgical registrar

Dr Frederick Speyer
Paediatric registrar

Dr Kellie Bateman
Junior doctor

Dr Nicholas Farmer
Core surgical trainee

Dr Joanna Higgins
Orthopaedic registrar

Mrs Abigail Mezzullo
Pharmacist

Dr Hannah Sinclair
Cardiology registrar

Mr Derek Mansbridge
Lay reviewer

Dr Nazera Dodia
Trainee general practitioner

ATTRIBUTIONS

Scoring systems

Apgar score: Apgar V (1953). A proposal for a new method of evaluation of the newborn infant. Current Researches in Anesthesia & Analgesia. 32: 260-267.

DVT Wells score: Wells PS, Anderson DR, Rodger M et al. (2003). Evaluation of D-dimer in the diagnosis of suspected deep-vein thrombosis. New England Journal of Medicine. 349: 1227-1235.

Glasgow-Blatchford score: Blatchford O, Murray WR, Blatchford M (2000). A risk score to predict need for treatment for uppergastrointestinal haemorrhage. The Lancet. 356: 1318-1321.

GRACE score: Eagle KA, Lim MJ, Dabbous OH et al. (2004). A validated prediction model for all forms of acute coronary syndrome: estimating the risk of 6-month postdischarge death in an international registry. JAMA. 261: 2727-2733.

Malnutrition Universal Screening Tool: Elia M, Russell C, Stratton R et al. (2003). Malnutrition Universal Screening Tool. British Association for Parenteral and Enteral Nutrition. Online [http://www.bapen.org.uk/].

PE Wells score: Wells PS, Anderson DR, Rodger M et al. (2001). Excluding pulmonary embolism at the bedside without diagnostic imaging: management of patients with suspected pulmonary embolism presenting to the emergency department by using a simple clinical model and d-dimer. Annals of Internal Medicine. 135: 98-107.

Rockall score: Rockall TA, Logan RF, Devlin HB et al. (1996). Risk assessment after acute upper gastrointestinal haemorrhage. Gut. 38: 316-321.

ROSIER scale: Nor AM, Davis J, Sen B et al. (2005). The Recognition of Stroke in the Emergency Room (ROSIER) scale: development and validation of a stroke recognition instrument. Lancet Neurology. 4: 727-734.

Guidelines

The below organisations have not checked the use of their content in this book to confirm that it accurately reflects the publications from which the information is taken.

British Thoracic Society guidelines: British Thoracic Society. Online [www.brit-thoracic.org.uk].
Life support guidelines: Resuscitation Council (UK). Online [www.resus.org.uk/resuscitation-guidelines].
NICE guidelines: National Institute for Health and Care Excellence. Online [www.nice.org.uk].
Scottish Intercollegiate Guidelines Network guidelines: Scottish Intercollegiate Guidelines Network. Online [http://www.sign.ac.uk/].

Protocols
SPIKES protocol: Baile WF, Buckman R, Lenzi R et al. (2000). SPIKES—A Six-Step Protocol for Delivering Bad News: Application to the Patient with Cancer. The Oncologist. 5: 302-311.

Algorithms
Algorithms for management of tachycardia, bradycardia and adult basic and advanced life support: reproduced with the kind permission of the Resuscitation Council (UK).

Image attributions		
Page	Image	Copyright ©
Cover	Cover image	Used with kind permission from floralset © 123RF.com (www.123rf.com/profile_floralset)
47	Peripheral cyanosis	2011 James Heilman, licensed under the Creative Commons Attribution-Share Alike 3.0 Unported license
	Digital clubbing	2009 Desherinka, licensed under the Creative Commons Attribution-Share Alike 4.0 International, 3.0 Unported, 2.5 Generic, 2.0 Generic and 1.0 Generic license and GNU Free Documentation licence 1.2
	Splinter haemorrhages	2010 Splarka, in public domain
	Osler's nodes	2010 Robert J Galindo, licensed under the Creative Commons Attribution-Share Alike 4.0 International, 3.0 Unported, 2.5 Generic, 2.0 Generic and 1.0 Generic license and GNU Free Documentation licence 1.2
	Janeway lesions	2015 Warfieldian; licensed under the Creative Commons Attribution-Share Alike 4.0 International license
	Corneal arcus	2008 Loren A Zech Jr and Jeffery M Hoeg, licensed under the Creative Commons Attribution 2.0 Generic license, edited
	Pectus excavatum	2006 Ahellwig, licensed under the Creative Commons Attribution-Share Alike 3.0 Unported license and GNU Free Documentation licence 1.2
	Pitting oedema	James Heilman, licensed under the Creative Commons Attribution-Share Alike 3.0 Unported license
	Varicose veins	2010 Lakeland1999, in public domain
	Pectus carinatum	2010 Tolson411, licensed under the Creative Commons Attribution-Share Alike 3.0 Unported license, edited
	Tar-stained fingers	James Heilman, licensed under the Creative Commons Attribution-Share Alike 3.0 Unported license
	Horner's syndrome	2010 Tolson411, licensed under the Creative Commons Attribution-Share Alike 3.0 Unported license, edited
48	Xanthelasma	2007 Bobtheowl2 at the English language Wikipedia, licensed under the Creative Commons Attribution-Share Alike 3.0 Unported license and GNU Free Documentation licence 1.2
	Gynaecomastia	Licensed under the Creative Commons Attribution-Share Alike 3.0 Unported license and GNU Free Documentation licence 1.2
	Dupuytren's Contracture	2006 Frank C. Müller, Creative Commons Attribution-Share Alike 4.0 International license
	Massive ascites	2011 James Heilman, licensed under the Creative Commons Attribution-Share Alike 3.0 Unported license
	Inguinal hernia	James Heilman, licensed under the Creative Commons Attribution-Share Alike 3.0 Unported license
	Spider nevus	2008 Herbert L. Fred, MD and Hendrik A. van Dijk, licensed under the Creative Commons Attribution 2.0 Generic license, edited
	Glossitis	2011 Grook Da Oger, licensed under the Creative Commons Attribution-Share Alike 3.0 Unported license
63	Heberden's nodes	2006 Drahreg01, licensed under the Creative Commons Attribution-Share Alike 3.0 Unported license and GNU Free Documentation licence 1.2
	Boutonnière deformity	2013 Alborz Fallah, licensed under the Creative Commons Attribution-Share Alike 3.0 Unported license
	Ganglion	Cieslaw, licensed under the Creative Commons Attribution-Share Alike 3.0 Unported license and GNU Free Documentation licence 1.2
	Carpal tunnel release scar	2009 HenrykGerlach, licensed under the Creative Commons Attribution-Share Alike 3.0 Unported license
	Rheumatoid arthritis	National Library of Medicine (http://nihseniorhealth.gov/arthritis/toc.html), in public domain
	Gouty tophi	2006 NickGorton, licensed under the Creative Commons Attribution-Share Alike 3.0 Unported license and GNU Free Documentation licence 1.2
64	Acromegaly images	2008 Chanson and Salenave (Acromegaly. Orphanet Journal of Rare Diseases 3:17), licensed under the Creative Commons Attribution 2.0 Generic license
136	Varicose veins	2010 Lakeland1999, in public domain
	Rheumatoid hand	James Heilman, licensed under the Creative Commons Attribution-Share Alike 3.0 Unported license
	Wrist sign	2013 Staufenbiel et al. (Periodontal conditions in patients with Marfan syndrome - a multicenter case control study. BMC Oral Health 13:59), licensed under the Creative Commons Attribution 2.0 Generic license
	Goitre	2007 Drahreg01, licensed under the Creative Commons Attribution-Share Alike 3.0 Unported, 2.5 Generic, 2.0 Generic and 1.0 Generic license and GNU Free Documentation licence 1.2
	Dupuytren's Contracture	2006 Frank C. Müller, Creative Commons Attribution-Share Alike 4.0 International license
144	Bamboo spine	Stevenfruitsmaak, licensed under the Creative Commons Attribution-Share Alike 3.0 Unported license
	Rheumatoid arthritis on X-Ray	Bernd Brägelmann Braegel Mit freundlicher Genehmigung von Dr. Martin Steinhoff, licensed under the Creative Commons Attribution 3.0 Unported license and GNU Free Documentation licence 1.2, edited
	Osteoarthritis on X-Ray	James Heilman, licensed under the Creative Commons Attribution-Share Alike 3.0 Unported license
155	Onycholysis	2013 Alborz Fallah, licensed under the Creative Commons Attribution-Share Alike 3.0 Unported license
	Basal cell carcinoma (top)	2007 Watplay, licensed under the Creative Commons Attribution 3.0 Unported license
	Guttate psoriasis	2010 Bobjgalindo, licensed under the Creative Commons Attribution-Share Alike 4.0 International, 3.0 Unported, 2.5 Generic, 2.0 Generic and 1.0 Generic license and GNU Free Documentation licence 1.2
	Plaque psoriasis	2004 Marnanel, licensed under the Creative Commons Attribution-Share Alike 3.0 Unported license and GNU Free Documentation licence 1.2
	Basal cell carcinoma (bottom)	2006 John Hendrix, in public domain
156	Vitiligo	Produnis, licensed under the Creative Commons Attribution-Share Alike 3.0 Unported license and GNU Free Documentation licence 1.2
	Seborrhoeic keratosis	James Heilman, licensed under the Creative Commons Attribution-Share Alike 3.0 Unported license
	Neurofibromatosis type 1	2008 Almazi, in public domain
	Clubbing	2009 Desherinka, licensed under the Creative Commons Attribution-Share Alike 4.0 International, 3.0 Unported, 2.5 Generic, 2.0 Generic and 1.0 Generic license and GNU Free Documentation licence 1.2
216	Suturing techniques	Reproduced and adapted with kind permission from Serag-Wiessner (www.serag-wiessner.de)
237	Nasopharyngeal airway	2007 Pflegewiki-User Würfel, licensed under the Creative Commons Attribution-Share Alike 3.0 Unported license and GNU Free Documentation licence 1.2
	Supraglottic airway (iGel)	2007 Qqq1, licensed under the Creative Commons Attribution-Share Alike 3.0 Unported license and GNU Free Documentation licence 1.2
	Supraglottic airway (LMA)	2006 ignis, licensed under the Creative Commons Attribution-Share Alike 3.0 Unported license and GNU Free Documentation licence 1.2
	Tracheostomy	2008 Klaus D. Peter, Wiehl, Germany, licensed under the Creative Commons Attribution 2.0 Germany license
	Endotracheal tube	2007 bigomar2, licensed under the Creative Commons Attribution-Share Alike 3.0 Unported license and GNU Free Documentation licence 1.2

Creative Commons Attribution-Share Alike licence links: 1.0 www.creativecommons.org/licenses/by-sa/1.0, 2.0 www.creativecommons.org/licenses/by-sa/2.0, 2.5 www.creativecommons.org/licenses/by-sa/2.5, 3.0 www.creativecommons.org/licenses/by-sa/3.0, 4.0 www.creativecommons.org/licenses/by-sa/4.0; Creative Commons Attribution licence links: 2.0 www.creativecommons.org/licenses/by/2.0, 2.0 Germany www.creativecommons.org/licenses/by/2.0/de, 2.5 www.creativecommons.org/licenses/by/2.5, 3.0 www.creativecommons.org/licenses/by/3.0; GNU Free Documentation licence link: 1.2 www.gnu.org/licenses/old-licenses/fdl-1.2.en.html

ABBREVIATIONS

-ve	negative	CKD	chronic kidney disease
+ve	positive	CMV	*Cytomegalovirus*
ΔΔ	differential diagnosis	CN	cranial nerve
1°	primary	COCP	combined oral contraceptive pill
2°	secondary	COPD	chronic obstructive pulmonary disease
AAA	abdominal aortic aneurysm		
ABCDE	airway, breathing, circulation, disability, everything else	CPAP	continuous positive airway pressure
ABG	arterial blood gas	CPR	cardiopulmonary resuscitation
ABPI	ankle-brachial pressure index	CRP	C-reactive protein
ACE	angiotensin converting enzyme	CT	computerised tomography
ACS	acute coronary syndrome	CTPA	computerised tomography pulmonary angiogram
ACTH	adrenocorticotropic hormone		
AF	atrial fibrillation	CVD	cardiovascular disease
AKI	acute kidney injury	CXR	chest X-ray
ALP	alkaline phosphatase	DC	direct current
ALS	advanced life support	DHx	drug history
ALT	alanine aminotransferase	DIP	distal interphalangeal
APTT	activated partial thromboplastin time	DKA	diabetic ketoacidosis
		DM	diabetes mellitus
AR	aortic regurgitation	DMARD	disease-modifying antirheumatic drug
AS	aortic stenosis		
ASAP	as soon as possible	DOAC	direct oral anticoagulant
ASIS	anterior superior iliac spine	DOB	date of birth
AST	aspartate aminotransferase	DPP4	dipeptidyl peptidase-4
ATP	adenosine triphosphate	DTP	diphtheria tetanus polio
AV fistula	arteriovenous fistula	DVLA	Driver and Vehicle Licensing Agency (organisation responsible for drivers in the UK)
AV node	atrioventricular node		
AVPU	alert, voice, pain, unresponsive		
AXR	abdominal X-ray	DVT	deep vein thrombosis
BBB	bundle branch block	EBV	*Epstein–Barr* virus
BD	twice daily	ECG	electrocardiogram
BE	base excess	echo	echocardiogram
BiPAP	Bi-level Positive Airway Pressure	eGFR	estimated glomerular filtration rate
BMI	body mass index		
BNF	British National Formulary (UK pharmaceutical reference book)	ENT	ear, nose and throat
		ERCP	endoscopic retrograde cholangiopancreatography
BP	blood pressure		
CABG	coronary artery bypass grafting	ESR	erythrocyte sedimentation rate
CF	cystic fibrosis		

ESWL	extracorporeal shock wave lithotripsy	KCO	transfer coefficient
FBC	full blood count	KUB	kidneys, ureter and bladder
FEV1	forced expiratory volume in 1 second	LBBB	left bundle branch block
		LDL	low-density lipoprotein
FFP	fresh frozen plasma	LFT	liver function test
FHx	family history	LIF	left iliac fossa
FiO$_2$	fraction of inspired oxygen	LLQ	left lower quadrant
FVC	forced vital capacity	LMA	laryngeal mask airway
G&S	group and save	LMN	lower motor neuron
GCS	Glasgow Coma Scale	LMWH	low molecular weight heparin
GFR	glomerular filtration rate	LOC	loss of consciousness
GI	gastrointestinal	LRTI	lower respiratory tract infection
GLP-1	glucagon-like peptide 1	LV	left ventricle
GP	general practitioner (family doctor)	LVF	left ventricular failure
		MC&S	microscopy, culture and sensitivity
GT	glutamyl transpeptidase	MCP	metacarpophalangeal
GTN	glyceryl trinitrate	MHA	mental health act
Hb	haemoglobin	MI	myocardial infarction
HCG	human chorionic gonadotropin	MMR	measles, mumps, and rubella
HDL	high-density lipoprotein	MR	mitral regurgitation
Hib	*Haemophilus influenzae* type B	MRI	magnetic resonance imaging
HIT	heparin-induced thrombocytopenia	MS	mitral stenosis (in cardiovascular sections) or multiple sclerosis (in neurological sections)
HIV	human immunodeficiency virus		
HLA	human leukocyte antigen	MSU	mid-stream urine
HPC	history of presenting complaint	MTP	metatarsophalangeal
HPV	human papillomavirus	Mx	management
HR	heart rate	N	normal
HRT	hormone replacement therapy	N/A	not applicable
HUS	haemolytic uraemic syndrome	NBM	nil by mouth
Hx	history	NEB	nebulised
IBD	inflammatory bowel disease	NG	nasogastric
IBS	irritable bowel syndrome	NHS	National Health Service (UK public health service)
ICD	implantable cardioverter defibrillator	NICE	National Institute for Health and Care Excellence (UK department of health organisation that produces healthcare guidelines)
ICE	ideas, concerns and expectations		
ICU	intensive care unit		
IE	infective endocarditis		
Ig	immunoglobulin	NJ	nasojejunal
IHD	ischaemic heart disease	NSAID	non-steroidal anti-inflammatory drug
IM	intramuscular		
INR	international normalised ratio	NSTEMI	non-ST-elevation myocardial infarction
IP	interphalangeal		
ITP	idiopathic thrombocytopenic purpura	OD	once daily
		OGD	oesophago-gastro-duodenoscopy
IUD	intrauterine device	OSCE	obstructive structured clinical examination
IUS	intrauterine system		
IV	intravenous	OSM	osmolality
Ix	investigation	p	page
JVP	jugular venous pressure		

P2	second heart sound produced by closure of the pulmonary valve	SIADH	syndrome of inappropriate antidiuretic hormone
Pa	partial pressure (arterial)	SLE	systemic lupus erythematosus
PC	presenting complaint	SOB	short of breath
PCI	percutaneous coronary intervention	SOCRATES	site, onset, character, radiation, associated symptoms, timing, exacerbating factors, severity
PCNL	percutaneous nephrolithotomy		
PCOS	polycystic ovary syndrome	SOL	space occupying lesion
PCR	polymerase chain reaction	SSRI	selective serotonin uptake inhibitor
PE	pulmonary embolism		
PEA	pulseless electrical activity	STAT	given immediately
PEFR	peak expiratory flow rate	STEMI	ST-elevation myocardial infarction
PET	positron emission tomography		
PID	pelvic inflammatory disease	STI	sexually transmitted infection
PIP	proximal interphalangeal	SVT	supraventricular tachycardia
PMHx	past medical history	Sx	symptoms
PO	*per os* (by mouth)	TB	tuberculosis
PPARγ	peroxisome proliferator-activated receptor gamma	TCA	tricyclic antidepressant
		TDS	three times daily
PPI	proton pump inhibitor	TFT	thyroid function test
PR	*per rectum* (rectal)	TIA	transient ischaemic attack
PRN	as required	TNF	tumour necrosis factor
PS	pulmonary stenosis	TSH	thyroid-stimulating hormone
PSA	prostate specific antigen	TWOC	trial without catheter
PT	prothrombin time	Tx	treatment
PTH	parathyroid hormone	U&Es	urea and electrolytes
PTSD	post-traumatic stress disorder	UC	ulcerative colitis
PV	*per vaginam* (by vagina)	UMN	upper motor neuron
QDS	four times daily	UO	urine output
RA	rheumatoid arthritis	URTI	upper respiratory tract infection
RBBB	right bundle branch block	USS	ultrasound scan
Rh	rheumatic	UTI	urinary tract infection
RIF	right iliac fossa	VBG	venous blood gas
RLQ	right lower quadrant	VC	vital capacity
RR	respiratory rate	VF	ventricular fibrillation
RUQ	right upper quadrant	VT	ventricular tachycardia
RV	right ventricle	VTE	venous thromboembolism
RVF	right ventricular failure	V/Q	ventilation-perfusion
S1	first heart sound	WCC	white cell count
S2	second heart sound		
S3	third heart sound		
S4	fourth heart sound		
SA	sinoatrial		
sats	saturations		
SBO	small bowel obstruction		
SBP	systolic blood pressure		
S/C	subcutaneous		
SE	side effect		
SGLT2	sodium-glucose co-transporter 2		
SHx	social history		

Units

Weight: kg kilograms, **g** grams, **mg** milligrams, **mcg** micrograms
Volumes: L litre, **ml** millilitre
Moles: mol moles, **mmol** millimoles
Calories: kcal kilocalories
Energy: J joules
Distances: m metre, **cm** centimetre, **mm** millimetre

Chemical formulas

Na^+ sodium, K^+ potassium, Mg^{2+} magnesium,
Ca^{2+} calcium, PO_4^{3-} phosphate, Cl^- chloride,
HCO_3^- bicarbonate, H_2O water, O_2 oxygen, CO_2 carbon dioxide

CHAPTER 1: HISTORY TAKING

TAKING A HISTORY

SPECIFIC HISTORIES

DIFFERENTIAL DIAGNOSIS OF COMMON PRESENTING COMPLAINTS

HISTORY-TAKING SKILLS

THE MEDICAL HISTORY

INTRODUCTION
- <u>W</u>ash hands; <u>I</u>ntroduce self; ask <u>P</u>atient's name, DOB and what they like to be called; <u>E</u>xplain and obtain consent

PRESENTING COMPLAINT
- Determine symptoms which brought patient in

HISTORY OF PRESENTING COMPLAINT
- **Explore each symptom** (including further symptoms you elicit in system reviews)
  - ○ Timeframe
    - ▪ Duration
    - ▪ Onset (sudden or gradual)
    - ▪ Progression
    - ▪ Timing (intermittent or continuous)
  - ○ Symptom-specific questions, e.g. SOCRATES for pain (*see notes on exploring symptoms p3*)
- **Relevant system reviews** to determine presence/absence of possible associated symptoms (*see notes on systems review p7*)

PAST MEDICAL/SURGICAL HISTORY
- Ask generally about medical conditions and past operations
- Ask specifically about conditions/risk factors <u>relevant</u> to differentials (e.g. hypertension, diabetes etc. for cardiac chest pain)
- For relevant conditions, find out when diagnosed, what treatment, control of condition etc.

DRUG HISTORY
- **Allergies** (including reactions)
- **Medications** (with doses and frequencies) – *include over-the-counter medications and natural remedies*

FAMILY HISTORY
- Ask family history of conditions <u>relevant</u> to differentials

SOCIAL HISTORY

- **Living situation**: house/flat/nursing home, who's at home, carers, who does activities of daily living, mobility aids
- **Occupation** ± occupational history if relevant
- **Smoking and alcohol:** smoking (calculate pack years*), alcohol (calculate weekly units*), recreational drugs (if relevant)
- **Travel**/pets/hobbies/sexual history if relevant

*Pack years = (number of cigarettes smoked per day/20) × years smoked
*Rough alcohol units: medium wine glass 2, beer can 2, beer pint 3,
wine bottle 9-10, 35cl spirit bottle 15, 70cl spirit bottle 30

OTHER POINTS
- **Ideas, concerns and expectations:** this is a vital part of the history and should be integrated throughout
  - ○ Ask ideas and concerns about condition
  - ○ Ask expectations from consultation
- Remember to pick up on **cues** throughout history
- Some specialties have **specific histories** with additional parts (*see section on specific histories from p8*)
- Finish by **summarising** and ask the patient if they have any questions

EXPLORING SYMPTOMS

For every symptom you elicit (whether it's the presenting complaint or not), you must ask a series of further, symptom-specific questions – this is called *exploring* the symptom. After this, you must also ask relevant system review questions to determine the presence/absence of any significant associated features (*see notes on systems review p7*).

FOR ALL SYMPTOMS ALSO REVIEW THE TIMEFRAME

- **Timeframe**
    - **Duration**
    - **Onset:** sudden or gradual (if sudden, what were they doing at the time?)
    - **Progression**
    - **Timing:** intermittent or continuous (if intermittent, are there any triggers/associations?)

PAIN

- **Pain**

S	**S**ite
O	**O**nset
C	**C**haracter (e.g. sharp, stabbing, pressure, ache, burning)
R	**R**adiation
A	**A**ssociated symptoms (*see notes on systems review p7*)
T	**T**iming (intermittent or continuous)
E	**E**xacerbating/relieving factors
S	**S**everity

GENERALISED SYMPTOMS

- **Tiredness**
    - What they mean by tiredness: what, constant or episodic, onset, duration
    - Sleep: hours, quality, snoring/apnoeic episodes
    - How it affects the patient
    - Associated symptoms (*see notes on systems review p7*)
        - Anaemia symptoms: breathlessness on exertion, dizziness/headache
        - Hypothyroidism symptoms: constipation, weight gain, cold intolerance, menorrhagia
        - Depression symptoms: mood, early morning waking
        - Diabetes symptoms: polydipsia, polyuria

CEREBRAL SYMPTOMS

- **Headache**
    - Explore as pain
    - Meningism symptoms: rash, fever, neck stiffness, photophobia
    - Temporal arteritis symptoms: visual problems, jaw claudication, scalp tenderness (e.g. when brushing hair)
    - Glaucoma symptoms: visual blurring, red eye, halos around lights
    - Associated neurological symptoms (*see notes on systems review p7*)

> **HEADACHE RED FLAGS: intracranial bleed** (*thunderclap headache, recent trauma*), **raised intracranial pressure** (*posture/Valsalva-related*), **SOL** (*immunosuppression, malignancy, focal neurology, onset >50 years*), **meningitis** (*rash, fever, neck stiffness, photophobia*), **temporal arteritis** (*visual problems, jaw claudication, scalp tenderness*), **glaucoma** (*visual blurring, red eye, halos*)

- **Weakness**
    - Pattern of weakness
    - Characterise weakness (*e.g. fatigable in myasthenia gravis*)
    - Associated neurological symptoms (*see notes on systems review p7*)
- **Fit/fall/syncope** (get corroboration!)
    - **Before:** warning, circumstance
    - **During:** duration, LOC, movements (floppy/stiff/jerking), incontinence/tongue biting, complexion
    - **After:** amnesia, muscle pain, confusion/sleepiness, injuries from fall
    - Background to attacks: previous episodes, frequency, impact on life
    - Associated cardiorespiratory/neurological symptoms (*see notes on systems review p7*)
    - *! Check if patient drives – there may be driving restrictions*

CHEST SYMPTOMS

- **SOB**
  - Current vs. normal exercise tolerance (what makes them stop?)
  - Orthopnoea
  - Paroxysmal nocturnal dyspnoea
  - Diurnal/seasonal variation *if chronic*
  - Associated cardiorespiratory symptoms (*see notes on systems review p7*)
- **Cough**
  - Productive or non-productive
  - Triggers
  - Nocturnal
  - Associated cardiorespiratory symptoms (*see notes on systems review p7*)
- **Sputum**
  - How much, how often
  - Colour, consistency
  - Any blood
- **Haemoptysis**
  - Volume and frequency
  - Fresh or altered blood
  - Nature of associated sputum if any? Mixed in?
- **Palpitations**
  - Fast or slow
  - Regular or irregular (ask patient to tap out palpitation on table)
  - Any dizziness, LOC, nausea, sweating/clamminess, dyspnoea
  - Associated cardiorespiratory symptoms (*see notes on systems review p7*)

ABDOMINAL SYMPTOMS

- **Diarrhoea/constipation/vomiting**
  - How much, how often, any at night
  - Colour, consistency and contents (mucus, blood *if diarrhoea*; blood, bile *if vomiting*)
  - Weight loss, appetite/intake
  - Associated gastrointestinal symptoms (*see notes on systems review p7*)
- **Dysphagia**
  - Solids/liquids/both, which came first
  - Constant/intermittent, progressive/non-progressive
  - Odynophagia
  - Weight loss, food intake
  - Associated gastrointestinal and neurological symptoms (*see notes on systems review p7*)
- **Dyspepsia/reflux**
  - Explore as pain
  - Associated gastrointestinal symptoms (*see notes on systems review p7*)

> **DYSPEPSIA/REFLUX RED FLAGS – ALARMS:** *A*naemia, *L*oss of weight, *A*norexia, *R*ecent onset progressive symptoms, *M*elaena/haematemesis, *S*wallowing difficulty; also: >55 years old, >4 weeks/relapsing symptoms, persistent vomiting

GYNAECOLOGICAL SYMPTOMS

- **Vaginal discharge**
  - Quantity
  - Colour (including blood), odour, itching
  - Associated gynaecological symptoms (*see notes on systems review p7*)
- **Abnormal PV bleeding**
  - Type: menorrhagia, intermenstrual, post-coital, post-menopausal
  - Quantity of loss: number of sanitary towels/tampons, passage of clots/flooding
  - Pain with blood loss
  - Anaemia symptoms: tiredness, breathlessness on exertion
  - Thyroid symptoms
  - Chance of pregnancy
  - Associated gynaecological symptoms (*see notes on systems review p7*)
- **Secondary amenorrhoea (work down the body)**
  - General: weight loss, stress, exercise, diet
  - Head: visual problems, headaches
  - Thyroid: heat intolerance, tremor, palpitations, diarrhoea
  - Torso: hirsutism, acne
  - Abdomen: possibility of pregnancy

Remember in all gynaecological histories you also need to ask about **Menstrual, Obstetric, Sexual** *and* **Contraception/Cervical smear** *history (MOSC) – see notes on gynaecological history p13*

ORTHOPAEDIC AND RHEUMATOLOGICAL SYMPTOMS

- **Back pain**
    - Explore as pain
    - Early morning stiffness
    - Sciatica
    - Urinary incontinence/retention, faecal incontinence/constipation
    - Associated neurological symptoms of lower limbs (*see notes on systems review p7*)

> ***BACK PAIN RED FLAGS: cauda equina*** *(urinary incontinence/retention, faecal incontinence/constipation, bilateral leg pain, severe/progressive neurological deficit, decreased anal tone/saddle anaesthesia),* ***infection or cancer*** *(age <20 or >55 years at onset, weight loss, fever/night sweats, recent infection, cancer history, injecting drugs, immunosuppression),* ***fracture*** *(trauma, severe central spinal pain, structural spine deformity, spinal tenderness),* ***spondyloarthropathy*** *(early morning stiffness, night pain, worse with rest)*

- **Joint pain/stiffness/swelling**
    - Worse in morning?, how long for (>30 minutes suggests inflammatory cause)
    - Better with exercise (inflammatory) or worse after exercise (osteoarthritis)
    - Sleep disturbance
    - Loss of function
    - Associated rheumatological symptoms (*see notes on systems review p7*)
- **Bone/tissue/joint injury**
    - Explore as pain
    - Stiffness/swelling
    - Movement restriction/ability to weight-bear
    - Mechanical symptoms: locking, giving way
    - Neurological symptoms distally: weakness, numbness, paraesthesia

PSYCHIATRIC SYMPTOMS

NB: you must assess <u>RISK</u> in every psychiatric history (see p10).

- **Depression**
    - **Core**: mood, anhedonia
    - **Biological**: sleep, energy, appetite
    - **Future** (including risk): hopelessness, suicidal thoughts/plans for suicide
    - Others: history of mania/hypomania
- **Anxiety**
    - Timing: onset and duration, episodic/constant, triggers, effect on life, frequency
    - Somatic symptoms: palpitations, breathlessness, chest tightness, sweating, dizziness
    - Associated psychological symptoms: depression screen, stress, worry, avoidance
    - Psychiatric differential questions: obsessions, compulsions, post-traumatic stress disorder symptoms (psychological trauma, flashbacks, nightmares, hyperarousal)
    - Organic differential questions: e.g. hyperthyroidism symptoms, ACS symptoms
- **Auditory hallucinations**
    - Voice detail: male/female, familiar/unfamiliar, always same/different, when heard etc.
    - Real/pseudo: out/inside of head
    - $2^{nd}/3^{rd}$ person: to you/about you, comments
    - What they say (including <u>commands</u>)
    - Risk to self/others
    - Associated psychiatric symptoms (*see notes on psychiatric history p10*)
- **Delusions**
    - Expand and challenge the delusion
    - Risk to self/others
    - Associated psychiatric symptoms (*see notes on psychiatric history p10*)
- **Memory loss** (get a collateral history)
    - Short/long-term
    - Insight and concerns
    - Functional levels (washing, dressing etc.)
    - Perform a cognitive assessment (e.g. mini mental state examination)
    - Risk to self/others
- **Eating disorder**
    - BMI: weight, height
    - Symptoms: avoidance of weight gain/need to lose weight, preoccupation with appearance, efforts to purge (vomiting, laxatives, exercise), any binge eating/fasting
    - Food diary: what they eat each day
    - Results: menstrual cycle disturbance, poor dental hygiene
    - Screen for depression (including risk to self), diabetes and thyroid problems

PAEDIATRIC SYMPTOMS

Most symptoms are explored as you normally would for adults but some are specific. *See p8 for full paediatric history.*

- **Diarrhoea and vomiting**
  - As normal, but include hydration questions (wet nappies, fluid intake, drowsiness)
- **Soiling/enuresis**
  - Primary or secondary
  - Full account of toilet training
  - School toilet behaviour
  - Protest behaviour: stressful/chaotic life
  - If soiling: faeces consistency (diarrhoea/constipation – *use Bristol Stool Chart*) and any painful anal conditions
  - If enuresis: have they ever had a dry night?
  - If secondary: urinary/GI infection symptoms, spinal cord compression symptoms (*see notes on neurological system review p7*)
- **Failure to thrive/weight loss**
  - Ask to see growth chart
  - **Input**: detailed dietary history, feeding history, hunger
  - **Use**: energy, activity level
  - **Output**: wet nappies, stools
  - Others: chronic cough (*CF*), recurrent infections (*CF, primary ciliary dyskinesia, immunological*), sweating/breathless when feeding (*cardiac*), behaviour, general health, happiness, parents' health
  - Associated gastrointestinal symptoms (*see notes on systems review p7*)
- **Weight gain**
  - *As for failure to thrive:* see growth chart; input, use and output questions
  - Hypothyroidism symptoms: growth impairment, delayed puberty, mental slowness, constipation, cold intolerance
  - Cushing's syndrome symptoms: growth impairment, proximal weakness, central obesity
  - Syndromic features, e.g. Laurence-Moon (extra digits, intellectual impairment), Prader-Willi (poor muscle tone, distinct facial features, lack of eye co-ordination)
- **Walking/sitting delay**
  - Ages of milestones (*see examination notes on child developmental assessment p98*)
  - Mobility
  - Hand dominance
  - Balance problems
  - Behavioural problems
  - Associated neurological symptoms (*see notes on systems review p7*)
- **Speech delay**
  - Ages of milestones (*see examination notes on child developmental assessment p98*)
  - Senses: vocals, hearing, vision
  - Communication: comprehension (follows commands, responds to voice), non-verbal communication (pointing, gestures, facies), social responses (how acts in new situations, tantrums, playing, gestures)
- **Early puberty/late puberty/primary amenorrhoea/short stature**
  - Pubertal development review: testes, breast development, menarche, pubic/axillary hair, height, acne, mood changes
  - Intracranial pressure symptoms: visual problems, headaches
  - Family pubertal/stature history
  - Symptoms of other systemic diseases (*CF, thyroid disorder, anorexia, Crohn's disease*)
- **Behavioural disorder**
  - Attention deficit hyperactivity disorder symptoms: poor concentration, hyperactivity
  - Conduct disorder symptoms: hostile, aggressive, cruel
  - Autism symptoms: poor social interaction, reciprocal communication behaviour, restricted interests, repetitive behaviours, difficulties recognising/responding to emotions
- **Allergies**
  - Pattern, frequency, duration, persistent/intermittent
  - Reaction: wheeze, rash, sneezing/itchy eyes, abdominal pain/diarrhoea, swelling of eyes/eye-lids/tongue
  - Specifically ask about anaphylaxis symptoms
  - Triggers/associations: pollen/season, chemicals, pets, latex, dust, foods (milk/eggs/wheat/peanuts/fish/shellfish)
  - Ask about atopy in child and family (asthma, eczema, hay fever) and about food allergies
  - Ensure you ask about home (heating, dampness, pets) and social (smokers in family, exposure to pollutants)

OTHER SYMPTOMS

- **Rash**
  - Duration, progression, frequency
  - Sites, size and shape
  - Description: what does it look like? Any blisters or raised areas? What colour is it? Does it blanch?
  - Secondary features: itchy/painful, crusting
  - Exacerbating/relieving factors, e.g. heat, sunlight, cold, treatment, allergies
  - Associated rheumatological symptoms (*see notes on systems review p7*)

SYSTEMS REVIEW

A full systems review is not necessary for every patient. You should only review systems <u>relevant</u> to the presenting complaint with the aim of identifying/excluding significant associated features. For example, for left iliac fossa pain, a complete history will include questions about gastrointestinal, urological and, if female, obstetric and gynaecological systems. You must also go on to ask further symptom-specific questions for each positive symptom (*see notes on exploring symptoms p3*).

GENERAL

- Fever/rigors/night sweats, weight loss, fatigue, skin rashes/bruising

NEUROLOGICAL

- **General**: fits/falls/LOC, headache, dizziness, vision/hearing, memory loss, neck stiffness/photophobia
- **Motor**: weakness/wasting, incontinence
- **Sensory**: pain, numbness, tingling

ENT

- **Ear:** hearing loss, tinnitus, otalgia
- **Nose:** rhinorrhoea, epistaxis
- **Throat:** sore throat, odynophagia

CARDIORESPIRATORY

- Chest pain, palpitations, SOB/wheeze, cough, sputum, haemoptysis, leg swelling

GASTROINTESTINAL

- **Weight:** weight loss, appetite change
- **Work down body:** dysphagia, nausea/vomiting, indigestion/heartburn, abdominal pain, bowel habit, tenesmus, blood/mucus in stool, flatus

UROLOGICAL

- **Storage:** frequency, volume, urgency, nocturia, incontinence (overflow/stress/urge)
- **Infection:** dysuria, haematuria, odour
- **Prostatic/voiding (if male):** hesitancy, poor flow/dribbling, feeling of incomplete emptying

OBSTETRIC AND GYNAECOLOGICAL (THE 4 P'S)

- **PV Bleeding:** menorrhagia, intermenstrual, post-coital, post-menopausal
- **PV Discharge**
- **Pain:** pelvic, dysmenorrhoea, dyspareunia
- **Pregnancy:**
  - Chance of pregnancy
  - If pregnant: fetal movements, contractions/tightening, PV loss, pre-eclampsia symptoms (headache, visual disturbance, epigastric pain, oedema)

> *Remember in all gynaecological histories you also need to ask about **Menstrual, Obstetric, Sexual** and **Contraception/Cervical smear** history (MOSC) – see notes on gynaecological history p13*

RHEUMATOLOGICAL

- **Joints:** pain, stiffness, swelling
- **Work down body**: skin (rashes, ulcers, Raynaud's), hair loss, eyes (redness, dryness), mouth (dryness), chest (breathlessness, SOB), GI (IBD symptoms), genitourinary (discharge)

ORTHOPAEDIC

- **Joints/bone/soft tissue:** pain, stiffness, swelling, movement restriction/ability to weight-bear
- **Mechanical symptoms:** locking, giving way
- **Neurological symptoms distally:** weakness, numbness, paraesthesia

PRESENTING COMPLAINT

- Determine symptoms which brought patient in

Definitions	
Neonate	<28 days
Infant	1-12 months
Child	1-12 years
Adolescent	>12 years

HISTORY OF PRESENTING COMPLAINT

- **Explore each symptom** (including further symptoms you elicit in system reviews)
  - Timeframe
    - Duration
    - Onset (sudden or gradual)
    - Progression
    - Timing (intermittent or continuous)
  - Symptom-specific questions, e.g. SOCRATES for pain (*see notes on exploring symptoms p3*)
- **Paediatric systems review** (*similar to adults but slightly different*)
  - General: fever, behaviour, activity/apathy/alertness, rashes, growth and weight
  - Cardiorespiratory: cough, noisy breathing (stridor, croup, wheeze), dyspnoea, cyanosis
  - Gastrointestinal: vomiting, abdominal pain, diarrhoea/constipation
  - Genitourinary: wetting nappies/toilet trained, dysuria, frequency
  - Neuromuscular: seizures/fits, headaches, abnormal movements
  - ENT: sore throat, snoring, noisy breathing, earache

BIRTH

- **Pregnancy:** scan results (dating and anomaly; if had extra scans – why?), any problems (e.g. maternal illness/alcohol/drug use)
- **Birth history**
  - Location, mode of delivery, gestation (term = 38-42 weeks) and birth weight (normal = 2.5-4.5kg)
  - Birth complications, e.g. resuscitation required, birth injury, maternal/fetal compromise, risk factors for sepsis (group B *Streptococcus*, maternal fever, prolonged rupture of membranes), any meconium?
  - Neonatal problems, e.g. jaundice, fits, fevers, bleeding, feeding problems, admissions to neonatal unit/neonatal ICU

FEEDING

- **Diet and appetite** – *ascertain what the child normally feeds and compare against current feeding*
  - Breast/bottle milk (usually <12 months): type (breast, standard formula, modified formula e.g. hydrolysed, high energy etc.), volume and frequency, feeding difficulties (e.g. latching difficulties, reflux symptoms, SOB)
  - Weaning (usually from 6 months): starts with pureed jars, then mashed up food, then solids gradually added
  - Solid meals and cow's milk (usually >12 months)
- **Toileting**
  - Toilet training (between 2-4 years; dry by day at 2 years; dry by night at 3-4 years)
  - Frequency: wet nappies? (usually ~5 soaking wet nappies per day and 3 yellow stools)

GROWTH

- **Weights:** ask to see *The Red Book* (personal child health record) – used from birth to 5 years
- **Puberty** if older child/adolescent (on average, starts at 11 years for girls, 12 years for boys)

DEVELOPMENT

- Any **concerns**
- **School** progress and attendance
- **Developmental screen** if <5 years
  - Smiling by 6 weeks
  - Turns to sounds by 6 months
  - Sitting by 9 months
  - First words by 18 months
  - Walking by 18 months
  - Short sentences by 3 years

Normal developmental milestones				
	Gross motor	**Fine motor and vision**	**Hearing and language**	**Social**
Neonate	Moves all limbs	Looks, startles	Startles to noise	Cries Smiles (6 weeks)
3 months	Head control	Reaches for objects Fixes and follows	Cries, laughs, vocalises (4 months)	Laughs
6 months	Rolls over Pushes up	Co-ordination Transfers	Localises sound Babbles	Alert and interested Starts solids
9 months	Sits alone Crawls	Pincer grip	Inappropriate sounds	Stranger anxiety
12 months	Stands alone		Babbles Understands simple commands Says mamma/dadda	Socially responsive Wave bye
18 months	Walks alone	Uses spoon	Uses words	Stranger shyness Tantrums
2 years	Runs Stairs	Circular scribbles and lines	2 word phrases	Knows identity Parallel play
3-4 years	Stand on one foot	Builds bridge with bricks	Short sentences Knows colours	Interactive play
5 years	Skips/hops	Full drawings	Fluent speech	Dresses self

PAST MEDICAL HISTORY

- Medical problems
- Previous illness, accidents, surgery
- Previous hospital/emergency department visits

DRUG HISTORY

- **Immunisations:** up to date? – *see schedule below*
- Current medication (including creams etc.): include dose, route, compliance
- Relevant recent medication, e.g. course of corticosteroids for asthma
- Allergies: drugs, foods, others

FAMILY HISTORY

- Anything relevant to HPC
- Anyone else ill?
- 'Anything in the family that affects newborn babies or children?'

SOCIAL HISTORY

- Family unit: parents, siblings, who lives at home – *draw family tree of who's at home*
- Does anyone smoke in the family (inside or outside)?
- Housing situation
- Social services involvement (child, parents or siblings) or any other safeguarding concerns
- Playgroup (2-5 years), nursery school (3-4 years) or school (5-16 years) – performing well?
- Other, e.g. hobbies, travel, pets

IDEAS, CONCERNS AND EXPECTATIONS

- How has the illness affected the family?
- Have the symptoms kept the child from **attending** nursery/school?
- What are the parents'/child's concerns, beliefs, hopes etc.?

Immunisation schedule	
2 months:	6 in 1, rotavirus, pneumococcal, meningitis B
3 months:	6 in 1, rotavirus
4 months:	6 in 1, pneumococcal, meningitis B
1 year:	MMR, pneumococcal, meningitis B, *Haemophilus influenzae* type B/meningitis C
Preschool (3 years 4 months):	MMR, 4 in 1 (diphtheria, polio, tetanus, pertussis)
Girls 12-13 years:	HPV (two injections 6-12 months apart)
Teens:	3 in 1 (diphtheria, tetanus, polio), meningitis ACWY

***6 in 1** = diphtheria, tetanus, polio, pertussis, Haemophilus influenzae type B, hepatitis B*
***MMR** = measles, mumps, rubella*

NB: influenza annual nasal vaccine is also offered to 2-7 year olds

INTRODUCTION

- **W**ash hands; **I**ntroduce self; ask **P**atient's name, DOB and what they like to be called; **E**xplain and obtain consent

PRESENTING COMPLAINT

- Determine symptoms which brought patient in
- Did they come voluntarily or were they detained
- Who prompted it (patient, family, friend)

HISTORY OF PRESENTING COMPLAINT

- **Explore every symptom**
  - Timeframes – *any triggers?*
  - Symptom-specific questions (*see notes on exploring symptoms p3*)
- **Psychiatric system review**
  - **Psychosis screen (first rank symptoms):** 3rd person auditory hallucinations, running commentary auditory hallucinations, delusions of thought/control/perception
  - **Depression screen:** core (mood, anhedonia), biological (sleep, energy), future (hopelessness, suicidal thoughts)
  - **Other:** memory loss, anxiety, insight
  - **RISK:** to self (suicide/self-harm), to others

PAST MEDICAL HISTORY

- Past **psychiatric history**
  - Diagnoses
  - First and last episodes
  - How many episodes and admissions (check if voluntary or involuntary and if any to psychiatric intensive care)
  - Previous self-harm/suicide attempts
  - Mental health worker/care co-ordinator
- Past **medical history**

DRUG HISTORY

- As usual
- Check **compliance**

FAMILY HISTORY

- **Family psychiatric history**
- Family history of suicide

SOCIAL HISTORY

- **Alcohol and drug use** (VERY IMPORTANT!)
- **Social circumstances**
  - Current situation
  - Relationships
  - Dependants and contact with children – *determine if their children are safe (who are they with?)*
  - Home (support, home state)
  - Finances (benefits, debts)
  - Education/work
  - Coping with activities of daily living
- **Forensic history** (especially important if there may be any risk to others): e.g. ever been arrested or in prison? Types of crimes? Longest prison sentence? Any domestic abuse?
- **Personal upbringing history:** include if any child abuse
- **Pre-morbid personality**

NEVER FORGET RISK!

ALCOHOL HISTORY

INTRODUCTION
- Wash hands; Introduce self; ask Patient's name, DOB and what they like to be called; Explain and obtain consent

ALCOHOL USE
- Current use
  - **What**: how much (units = %abv. x litres volume), type of alcohol
  - **When**: times of day, days of week, continuous/binge
  - **Where**: pub, home alone, work
  - **Why**: social, underlying issues (family, relationships, depression etc.), availability, stress, psychiatric problems
- Past (alcohol timeline)
  - 5 year intervals – any personal correlations?
  - Ever tried to cut down – what happened?
  - Treatments and detoxes and how they went
  - Relapse reasons

SOCIAL EFFECTS
- Effect on self (e.g. injuries, medical conditions)
- Effect on family/friends
- Effect on work
- Effect on finances
- Any trouble with police related to alcohol
- Driving

DEPENDENCE
- **Physical dependence**
  - Tolerance
  - Autonomic withdrawal symptoms: tremor, sweating, nausea/vomiting, palpitations
  - Neurological withdrawal symptoms: agitation, headache, hallucinations, seizures, insomnia
- **Psychological dependence**
  - Compulsion/persistent desire to drink
  - Lots of time spent drinking
  - Given up activities/hobbies or spending less time with family/friends

MOOD AND RISK
- Effect on mood
- Assess risk of self harm/suicide

REST OF HISTORY
- **Past psychiatric history:** any disorders including anxiety and depression
- **PMHx:** physical health problems due to alcohol/drugs (e.g. peptic ulcer disease, liver disease, upper GI bleeding, memory loss)
- **DHx**
- **FHx:** family alcohol use
- **SHx:** recreational drug use, smoking, family/living/working situation

Help available
- Groups/charities, e.g. Alcoholics Anonymous
- Community alcohol team
- Detox options
  - Gradual reduction over time
  - Community detox – chlordiazepoxide weaning regimen
  - Hospital detox – if previous delirium tremens, poor response, or lack of support
- Help with reducing relapses
  - Acamprosate (reduces cravings)
  - Disulfiram (creates unpleasant reaction in response to alcohol)
  - Naltrexone/nalmefene (block effects of alcohol)
- Vitamin B supplements (important for all)

Rough alcohol units	
Medium wine glass	2
Beer can	2
Beer pint	3
Wine bottle	9-10
35cl spirit bottle	15
70cl spirit bottle	30

ATTEMPTED SUICIDE HISTORY

INTRODUCTION

- **W**ash hands; **I**ntroduce self; ask **P**atient's name, DOB and what they like to be called; **E**xplain and obtain consent

THE EVENT

BEFORE

- **Events** leading up to suicide attempt
  - Life events
  - Depression
- **Planning** (e.g. 'How long was there between thinking of overdosing and doing it?')
- Suicide **note**/did they tell anybody?
- **Precautions** taken to avoid being detected (e.g. locking doors, ensuring nobody would be around)

DURING

- Their **intention** – did they intend to commit suicide or was it a cry for help?
- **When** and **where**
- Alcohol/drug **intoxication**
- Exactly **how** they did it
  - If overdose: what, how many, where they got them, what they thought would happen
  - If self-harm lacerations: where, quantity, depth, how they felt while doing it, what they thought would happen
- How were they **discovered** and how did they get here? Who called for help?

AFTER

- **Feelings** now
- **Angry/regretful**?
- Current **mood**

THE FUTURE

- **Protective factors**
  - Any positive things or things they want to live for
  - What might stop them committing suicide?
- **Future feelings**
  - How they feel about the future
  - e.g. 'If you were to go home now, what would happen?'
  - If they've changed their mind, what changed?
  - Are they going back to the same situation?
- **Future plans**
  - Any future suicidal plans
  - Any positive plans, e.g. find job, get married, holidays

FURTHER QUESTIONS TO HELP ASSESS RISK

- **Depression symptoms screen**: core symptoms (low mood, anhedonia), biological (sleep, energy), future (hopelessness, suicidal thoughts)
- **Psychosis symptoms screen**: auditory hallucinations, running commentary, delusions of thought/control/perception
- **Past medical history**
  - Past medical history (including any psychiatric diagnoses)
  - Past suicide attempts/self harm (find out about the methods used and help sought)
- **Drug history**
- **Family history** of self-harm/suicide and psychiatric conditions
- **Social history**
  - Drug/alcohol use
  - Social stresses (including financial)
  - Relationships and support network (family nearby?)
  - Jobs
  - Living situation (living alone?)
  - Hobbies

Suicide risk factors

- **Demographics**
  - Male
  - Old or young
- **Current situation**
  - Unemployed
  - Homeless
  - Depressed
  - Lack of social support
  - Significant life events
- **History**
  - Chronic illness
  - Psychiatric disorder
  - Previous attempts
  - Alcohol/drug abuse

GYNAECOLOGICAL HISTORY

INTRODUCTION

- Wash hands; Introduce self; ask Patient's name, DOB and what they like to be called; Explain and obtain consent

PRESENTING COMPLAINT

- Determine symptoms which brought patient in

HISTORY OF PRESENTING COMPLAINT

- **Explore every symptom**
  - Timeframes
  - Symptom-specific questions (*see notes on exploring symptoms p3*)
- **Relevant systems reviews** (*see notes on systems review p7*)
  - General
  - Gynaecological (The 4 P's)
    - **P** PV bleeding: menorrhagia, intermenstrual, post-coital, post-menopausal
    - **P** PV discharge
    - **P** Pain: pelvic, dysmenorrhoea, dyspareunia
    - **P** Pregnancy (chance of pregnancy)
  - Gastrointestinal (ΔΔ IBS, malignancy, appendicitis, diverticulitis etc.)
  - Urological (ΔΔ UTI, incontinence etc.)

MENSTRUAL HISTORY

- 1st day of **last menstrual period**
- **Menarche** (usually 12-13 years) ± **menopause** (usually 48-55 years)
- **Regularity** and **cycle length** (range from 21-35 days)
- **Duration** of periods (range from 3-7 days) and **character** (heaviness, number of pads per day, flooding, pain)

OBSTETRIC HISTORY

- **Gravida and para** (gravida/gravidity = pregnancies; para/parity = birth of fetuses over 24 weeks, regardless if born alive or not)
- **Miscarriages, ectopic pregnancies and terminations:** stage, treatment, complications
- **Children (living):** number, ages, birth-weights, type of deliveries, previous problems during pregnancy/delivery

SEXUAL HISTORY

- **Partners:** current partner (male/female, relationship duration), previous partners (last three or all in last 6 months), high-risk encounters
- **Intercourse:** type, pain/discomfort, contraception used
- **Subfertility**

CONTRACEPTION AND CERVICAL SMEAR HISTORY

- **Contraception:** current use, previous methods
- **Cervical smears:** date of last smear, results

NB: some parts of MOSC are more or less important depending on the presenting complaint – adapt as necessary.

REST OF HISTORY AS NORMAL

- **PMHx:** including previous abdominal surgery
- **DHx:** including HRT/hormones, over-the-counter remedies, allergies
- **FHx:** breast/bowel/ovarian cancer
- **SHx**

Extra bits: MOSC

OBSTETRIC HISTORY

INTRODUCTION
- **W**ash hands; **I**ntroduce self; ask **P**atient's name, DOB and what they like to be called; **E**xplain and obtain consent

PRESENTING COMPLAINT
- Determine symptoms which brought patient in

HISTORY OF PRESENTING COMPLAINT
- **Explore every symptom**
  - Timeframes
  - Symptom-specific questions (*see notes on exploring symptoms p3*)
- **Relevant systems reviews** (*see notes on systems review p7*)
  - General
  - Obstetric and gynaecological systems review (**The 4 P's**):
    - **P** PV bleeding
    - **P** PV discharge
    - **P** Pain
    - **P** Pregnancy
      - Fetal movements (if over 16-20 weeks)
      - Contractions/tightening
      - PV blood loss
      - Pre-eclampsia symptoms (headache, visual disturbance, epigastric pain, oedema)
  - Gastrointestinal (ΔΔ IBS, malignancy, appendicitis, diverticulitis etc.)
  - Urological (ΔΔ UTI, incontinence etc.)

CURRENT PREGNANCY
- 1st day of **last menstrual period** (gestation = time since then) and when +ve pregnancy test
- **Scans** so far (intra-uterine? Any abnormalities?)
- **Investigations** (especially Rhesus group, Down's syndrome risk, mid-trimester scan)
- **Problems/admissions** this pregnancy
- Vomiting/hydration

OBSTETRIC HISTORY
- **G** **Gravida and para** (gravida/gravidity = pregnancies; para/parity = birth of fetuses over 24 weeks, regardless if born alive or not)
- **M** **Miscarriages, ectopic pregnancies and terminations:** stage, treatment, complications
- **C** **Children (living):** number, ages, birth-weights, type of deliveries, previous problems during pregnancy/delivery

REST OF HISTORY AS NORMAL
- **PMHx**
- **DHx**
- **FHx**
- **SHx:** including drugs, alcohol and smoking

SEXUAL HISTORY

INTRODUCTION

- **W**ash hands; **I**ntroduce self; ask **P**atient's name, DOB and what they like to be called; **E**xplain and obtain consent
- Explain that some of the questions you will need to ask will be sensitive in nature and you may need to ask details about sex and sexual partners
- Stress confidentiality
- Check the reason for attendance: check-up or any symptoms (e.g. pain, discharge, ulcers, lumps)

HISTORY OF PRESENTING COMPLAINT

- **Explore every symptom**
  - Timeframes
  - Symptom-specific questions (*see notes on exploring symptoms p3*)
- **Sexual health systems review**
  - Discharge (urethral/vaginal/rectal)
  - Dysuria
  - Swellings/growths/ulcers
  - Pain (anogenital, pelvic, dyspareunia)
  - PV bleeding (if female)

PARTNERS

- **Current partner and recent partners** (all partners in last 3 months)
  - Dates
  - Male/female
  - Condom use
  - Contact type (oral/vaginal/anal)
- **High risk encounters**
  - Sex with men (if male)
  - Partners from abroad
  - Bisexual partners
  - Sex with sex workers

FEMALES

- **Menstrual history** (including last menstrual period)
- Current **contraceptives** and adherence

PAST MEDICAL HISTORY

- Previous STIs and tests
- HIV and hepatitis B/C status
- Vaccines (hepatitis B)

DRUG HISTORY

- As usual. Ask specifically about PrEP use if male (pre-exposure prophylaxis for HIV).

SOCIAL HISTORY

- Alcohol use
- Recreational drug use (including ChemSex and needle sharing)

INTRODUCTION

- **W**ash hands; **I**ntroduce self; ask **P**atient's name, DOB and what they like to be called; **E**xplain and obtain consent

GENERAL

- How long been trying
- Any previous investigations/medical treatments/in vitro fertilisation

COITUS

- Coitus frequency
- Difficulties
- Relation to fertile days
- Pain

THE PARTNERS

Consider each separately:
- Age
- Occupation
- Body mass index
- Previous children (same or different partner?)
- Smoking and alcohol use
- Current medications
- PMHx

WOMAN'S GYNAECOLOGICAL HEALTH

- Current symptoms/problems
  - **Gynaecological system review:** discharge, pain, abnormal PV bleeding
  - **PCOS symptoms:** hirsutism, greasy skin, obesity
  - **Prolactinoma symptoms:** galactorrhoea
- Gynaecological history (**MOSC**)
  - **M**enstrual history
  - **O**bstetric history
  - **S**exual history
  - **C**ervical smears and contraception history
  - PMHx (especially abdominal/pelvic operations, past STIs/PID, previous subfertility Ix/Tx), DHx, FHx, SHx

Causes of infertility

Coital difficulty	**Abnormal spermatogenesis**	**Ovulatory failure**
• Mechanical	• Hypogonadotropic hypogonadism (e.g. pituitary disease, Kallmann's, idiopathic, syndromic, anabolic steroids, functional e.g. weight loss/exercise)	• Hypogonadotropic hypogonadism (e.g. pituitary disease, Kallmann's, idiopathic, syndromic, anabolic steroids, functional e.g. weight loss/exercise)
• Erectile dysfunction	• Hypergonadotropic hypogonadism (e.g. Klinefelter, gonadal damage)	• Hypergonadotropic hypogonadism (i.e. premature ovarian failure)
• Periods of separation	• Varicocele	• Hyperprolactinaemia
• Timing of intercourse	• Anti-sperm antibodies	• PCOS
• Ejaculation problems		
	Passage problems	**Passage problems**
	• Absence/blockage of Vas deferens	• Tubal damage
	• Anatomical defects	• Pelvic inflammatory disease
		• Endometriosis
		• Congenital malformations
		• Polyps/fibroids

COLLATERAL HISTORY FOR DELIRIUM/DEMENTIA

INTRODUCTION

- **W**ash hands; **I**ntroduce self; ask **P**atient's and relative's names; **E**xplain the need for a collateral history
- Establish their relation to the patient

PRESENTING COMPLAINT

- Confusion/memory loss

HISTORY OF PRESENTING COMPLAINT

- **Onset:** acute/chronic/acute-on-chronic (establish baseline function and cognition)
- **Progression:** slowly progressive (*Alzheimer's*), step-like (*vascular*)
- **Triggers:** infection, stress
- **Associated symptoms**
    - Depression
    - Psychiatric symptoms: hallucinations/delusions
    - Behavioural change: agitation, aggression, wandering, disinhibition, calling out
    - Sleeping pattern: awake at night (*Alzheimer's*), early morning waking (*depression*), fluctuating consciousness (*delirium*)
    - Cognitive disturbances: aphasia, apraxia, agnosia, difficulty planning/organising

PAST MEDICAL HISTORY

- Ask about: Parkinson's disease, vascular disease/diabetes, head injuries, recent infections
- Psychiatric history

DRUG HISTORY

- Blood pressure/diabetes medication
- Parkinson's drugs
- Alzheimer's drugs: galantamine, donepezil, rivastigmine
- New medications
- Allergies

FAMILY HISTORY

- Related conditions, e.g. dementia, vascular disease, depression

SOCIAL HISTORY

- **Living** situation, carer/home support
- **Mobility**/walking aids
- Effect on function/coping with **activities of daily living**: washing, dressing, cooking, cleaning
- **Working/driving**
- **Smoking, alcohol** and other cardiovascular risk factors
- RISK
    - **To self:** wandering, leaving gas on, abuse, neglect by self or others
    - **To others:** aggression, risky behaviour
- **Carer's needs:** empathise with the demands; ask about stress, coping, and support

ENDING

- **ICE (Ideas, Concerns, Expectations):** how does the relative/carer expect you to help? What are they worried about?
- **Summarise** situation and patient needs. Thank relative.

Causes of dementia

- **Alzheimer's:** most common; prevalence increases with age; some genetic association. Slowly progressive. Presents with memory/cognitive impairment (**5A's**: Anomia, Apraxia, Agnosia, Amnesia, Aphasia). Due to generalised atrophy of cortex with amyloid plaques and neurofibrillary tangles.
- **Vascular Dementia:** stepwise deterioration. Often have multiple cardiovascular risk factors. May have focal neurology. CT head may show areas of ischemia or small vessel disease.
- **Lewy-Body Dementia:** progressive dementia with daily fluctuations of awareness due to Lewy bodies in the cerebral cortex. Parkinsonian features (e.g. bradykinesia, tremor, rigidity) and psychiatric symptoms (e.g. hallucinations) are common.
- **Other causes/differentials:** frontotemporal lobe dementia, Creutzfeldt-Jakob disease, depression ('pseudodementia'), HIV, Huntington's disease, normal pressure hydrocephalus, space-occupying lesion, nutritional deficiencies (thiamine, nicotinic acid, B12), alcohol abuse, neurosyphilis, hypothyroidism, autoimmune/paraneoplastic

Presenting complaint	Exploring symptom	Relevant system reviews	Differential diagnoses		Clues to differential
			Grouping	**Differentials**	
Weight loss	•How much •Over how long •Associated symptoms	Gastrointestinal •**Weight:** appetite change •**Work down body:** dysphagia, nausea/vomiting, indigestion/heartburn, abdominal pain, bowel habit change, tenesmus, blood/mucus in stool Full systems review Consider full systems review if diagnosis unclear	Malignancy	Any malignancy	•Symptoms of tumour, e.g. breast lump, haemoptysis (lung), prostatic symptoms, change in bowel habit (bowel), haematuria (TCC), jaundice (head of pancreas), post-menopausal bleed (uterine) etc.
			Gastrointestinal	Colon cancer	•Elderly •Blood/melaena PR •Change in bowel habit
				Inflammatory bowel disease	•Diarrhoea with blood/mucus •Abdominal pain
				Coeliac disease	•Diarrhoea, steatorrhoea •Anaemia symptoms, e.g. SOB, tiredness •Abdominal discomfort
			Endocrinological	Thyrotoxicosis	•Diarrhoea •Heat intolerance •Irritability/restlessness •Tremor •Oligomenorrhoea/amenorrhoea
			Psychological	Anorexia/bulimia nervosa	•BMI <17.5 in anorexia •Binge eating in bulimia •Effort to lose weight (gym, vomiting, laxatives) •Menstrual cycle disturbance
				Depression	•Core: low mood, anhedonia •Biological: poor sleep, lack of energy •Future: hopelessness, suicidal thoughts
				Stress	•Organic stress
			Other differentials	Diet changes/malnutrition Substance misuse End organ failure Diabetes mellitus type 1 Chronic inflammatory diseases Chronic infection (e.g. TB) HIV/AIDS	

Presenting complaint	Exploring symptom	Relevant system reviews	Differential diagnoses		Clues to differential
			Grouping	**Differentials**	
Tiredness	Timeframe •Duration •Onset (sudden or gradual) •Progression •Timing (intermittent or continuous) Tiredness •What they mean by tiredness •Sleep pattern/quality •How it affects patient Associated symptoms •**Anaemia symptoms:** breathlessness on exertion •**Hypothyroidism symptoms:** constipation, weight gain, cold intolerance etc. •**Depression symptoms:** mood •**Diabetes symptoms:** polydipsia, polyuria	Full systems review Consider full systems review if diagnosis unclear	Haematological	Anaemia	•Breathlessness on exertion •Weakness •May get palpitations, worsening angina, worsening claudication
			Endocrine	Hypothyroidism	•Constipation •Cold intolerance •Weight gain
				Diabetes	•Polydipsia/thirst •Polyuria •Weight loss •Visual disturbance
			Psychological	Depression	•Core: low mood, anhedonia •Biological: poor sleep, lack of energy •Future: hopelessness, suicidal thoughts
			Respiratory	Sleep apnoea	•Loud snoring •Night time breathing interrupted by apnoeas/gasping/snorting •Excessive daytime sleepiness •Obesity is a risk factor
			Other differentials	Stress Post-viral fatigue Organ failure Drugs (e.g. recreational, β-blockers, diuretics) Malignancy Chronic inflammatory diseases (e.g. connective tissue diseases) Chronic infection (e.g. TB) Addison's disease	

COMMON CEREBRAL HISTORIES

Presenting complaint	Exploring symptom	Relevant system reviews	Differential diagnoses		Clues to differential
			Grouping	**Differentials**	
Headache	Pain Site Onset Character Radiation Associated symptoms Timing Exacerbating/relieving factors Severity Red flags •**Intracranial bleed:** thunderclap headache, recent trauma •**Raised intracranial pressure:** posture/Valsalva-related •**SOL:** immunosuppression, malignancy, focal neurology, onset >50 years •**Meningitis:** rash, fever, neck stiffness, photophobia •**Temporal arteritis:** visual problems, jaw claudication, scalp tenderness •**Glaucoma:** visual blurring, red eye, halos	General Fever, skin rashes/bruising Neurological •**General:** fits/falls/LOC, dizziness, vision/hearing, memory loss, neck stiffness/photophobia •**Motor:** weakness/wasting, incontinence •**Sensory:** pain, numbness, tingling	Primary	Tension headache	•Bilateral tight band sensation •Recurrent •Occurs late in day •Association with stress
			Primary	Cluster headache	•Short painful attacks around one eye •Last between 30 minutes – 3 hours •Occur once/twice a day for 1-3 months •May have lacrimation and flushing
			Primary	Migraine	•Unilateral pulsating headache in trigeminal nerve distribution •Last between few hours – days •May have aura (usually visual) •Need to lie down in dark room (photophobia)
			Primary	Trigeminal neuralgia	•2 second paroxysms of stabbing pain in unilateral trigeminal nerve distribution •Face screws up with pain
			Secondary – intracranial	Meningitis	•Photophobia •Neck stiffness •Systemic symptoms, e.g. fever, non-blanching rash
			Secondary – intracranial	Temporal arteritis	•Unilateral throbbing pain •Scalp tenderness and jaw claudication •>55 years •May have visual involvement
			Secondary – intracranial	Subarachnoid haemorrhage	•Very sudden onset severe headache •'Like someone hit me with a brick over the head' •Meningism
			Secondary – intracranial	Raised intracranial pressure (e.g. tumour, benign intracranial hypertension)	•Worse in morning and with coughing and bending •Vomiting and reduced GCS •May have neurological symptoms/seizures •History of malignancy/immunocompromise
			Secondary – extracranial	Glaucoma	•Pain around one eye •Swollen red eye •Visual blurring and halos
			Secondary – extracranial	Sinusitis	•Facial pain exacerbated by leaning head forward •Rhinorrhoea
			Other differentials	Intracranial venous thrombosis Intracranial haemorrhages (intracerebral, subarachnoid, subdural) Infections (abscess, encephalitis, meningitis) Malignant hypertension Hypoxia/hypercapnia Viraemia Cervical spondylosis Pre-eclampsia Drugs (e.g. nitrates, PPI, caffeine, analgesia overuse, hormones)	
Vertigo	Timeframe •Duration •Onset (sudden or gradual) •Progression •Timing (intermittent or continuous) Background to attacks e.g. Previous attacks, frequency, impact on life	General Fever ENT •**Ear:** hearing loss, tinnitus, otalgia •**Nose:** rhinorrhoea, epistaxis •**Throat:** sore throat, odynophagia Neurological •**General:** fits/falls/LOC, headache, dizziness, vision/hearing, memory loss, neck stiffness/photophobia •**Motor:** weakness/wasting, incontinence •**Sensory:** pain, numbness, tingling	Peripheral (vestibular)	Benign positional vertigo	•Attacks of sudden rotational vertigo •Evoked by head turning •Lasts ~30 seconds
			Peripheral (vestibular)	Vestibular neuritis (e.g. Herpes virus)	•Often preceded by URTI •Sudden rotational vertigo and vomiting •Lasts several days but imbalance may persist •May re-occur several times per year
			Peripheral (vestibular)	Viral labyrinthitis	•Often preceded by URTI •Severe vertigo and hearing disturbance •May have tinnitus, otalgia, nausea, fever
			Peripheral (vestibular)	Ménière's disease	•TRIAD: vertigo + tinnitus + hearing loss •Attacks last minutes-hours
			Central	Vertebrobasilar insufficiency	•Momentary vertigo attacks precipitated by neck extension •Elderly with cervical osteoarthritis
			Other differentials	Peripheral Acoustic neuroma (vestibular schwannoma) Chronic otitis media Eustachian tube dysfunction Ramsay-Hunt syndrome (vertigo, facial palsy, otalgia, zoster rash) Cholesteatoma Central Vertebrobasilar stroke Cerebellar stroke Neurological conditions (e.g. MS, epilepsy, brain tumour, migraine) Head injury Drugs e.g. alcohol, salicylates, quinine, aminoglycosides, metronidazole, co-trimoxazole, diuretics	

Presenting complaint	Exploring symptom	Relevant system reviews	Differential diagnoses		Clues to differential
			Grouping	**Differentials**	
Fit/Fall/ Syncope	Attack •**Before:** warning, circumstance •**During:** duration, LOC, movements (floppy/stiff/jerking), incontinence/tongue biting, complexion (get corroboration) •**After:** amnesia, muscle pain, confusion/sleepiness, injuries from fall Background to attacks e.g. Previous attacks, frequency, impact on life	General Fever Cardiorespiratory Chest pain, palpitations, SOB/wheeze, leg swelling Neurological •**General:** fits/falls/LOC, headache, dizziness, vision/hearing, memory loss, neck stiffness/photophobia •**Motor:** weakness/wasting, incontinence •**Sensory:** pain, numbness, tingling	Cardiovascular	Postural hypotension	•Dizziness ± LOC on standing from lying •Recently medication changes (e.g. antihypertensives)
				Arrhythmia	•Fall after transient arrhythmia •May have had palpitations or felt strange before collapse •Cardiac history or family history of sudden death •May have occurred during exercise or when supine
				Aortic stenosis	•Collapse on exertion •SOB worse on exertion
			Neurological	Seizure	Partial •**Simple partial:** focal motor seizure, no LOC •**Complex partial (e.g. temporal lobe epilepsy):** strange actions with impaired awareness Generalised •**Tonic-clonic (grand mal):** sudden LOC, limbs stiff then jerk, may become incontinent, bite tongue, feel awful with myalgia and confusion afterwards •**Absence (petit mal):** unresponsively stare into space for ~5 seconds (in childhood) •**Atonic:** all muscles relax and drop to floor •**Tonic:** all muscles become rigid •**Myoclonic:** involuntary flexion
				Parkinson's disease	•TETRAD = rigidity + tremor + bradykinesia + postural instability
				TIA/stroke	•Neurological symptoms, e.g. limb/face weakness, slurred speech, hemianopia •LOC/syncope very uncommon
				Vasovagal	•Occurs in response to stimuli, e.g. emotion/pain/fear/prolonged standing •Preceding nausea, pallor, sweat, closing visual fields •Then LOC for ~2 minutes
			Other differentials	Mechanical Mechanical fall/postural instability Cardiovascular Structural e.g. hypertrophic obstructive cardiomyopathy, arrhythmogenic right ventricular dysplasia Situation syncope (e.g. cough syncope, effort syncope, micturition syncope) Carotid sinus hypersensitivity (precipitated by head turning/shaving) Vertebrobasilar insufficiency (elderly with cervical osteoarthritis) PE Neurological Neuropathy e.g. MS Intracranial haemorrhage (extradural, subarachnoid, subdural) Drop attack (sudden leg weakness without warning/LOC/confusion) Alcohol/drugs use Alcohol excess Polypharmacy Recreational drugs Abdominal Ectopic pregnancy Ruptured AAA Miscellaneous Delirium (secondary to infection) Any cause of vertigo above Anaemia Hypoglycaemia Eyesight problems Arthritis	

Presenting complaint	Exploring symptom	Relevant system reviews	Differential diagnoses		Clues to differential
			Grouping	**Differentials**	
Chest pain	**S**ite **O**nset **C**haracter **R**adiation **A**ssociated symptoms **T**iming **E**xacerbating/relieving factors **S**everity	General Fever, sweats Cardiorespiratory Palpitations, SOB/wheeze, cough, sputum, haemoptysis, leg swelling	Cardiac	Myocardial infarction	•Crushing central chest pain •Radiates to neck/left arm •Associated nausea/SOB/sweatiness •Cardiovascular risk factors
				Angina	•Cardiac-type chest pain •Associated with exertion •Relieved by rest
				Aortic dissection	•Tearing chest pain of <u>very</u> sudden onset •Radiates to back •Pain in other sites, e.g. arms, legs, neck, head
				Pericarditis	•Retrosternal/precordial pleuritic chest pain •Relieved by sitting forward •May radiate to trapezius ridge/neck/shoulder
			Respiratory	Pulmonary embolism	•Pleuritic chest pain •SOB ± haemoptysis •Risk factors (e.g. long haul flight, recent surgery, immobility, malignancy)
				Pneumothorax	•Sudden onset pleuritic chest pain •SOB if large enough •Risk factors, e.g. tall/thin, Marfan syndrome, COPD/asthma
			Non-cardiorespiratory	Gastro-oesophageal reflux disease	•Retrosternal burning chest pain •Related to meals, lying, straining •Water brash
				Anxiety/panic attack	•Tight chest pain, SOB, sweating, dizziness, palpitations, feeling of impending doom •Anxious personality and other symptoms of generalised anxiety disorder •Recurrent episodes triggered by a stimulus (e.g. crowds)
				Musculoskeletal	•Sharp chest pain •Exacerbated by movement and inspiration •Can point to where it is worst •Exacerbated by pressure over area
			Other differentials	Costochondritis and Tietze's syndrome (sharp pleuritic sternal pain with tenderness) Pleurisy (sharp unilateral pleuritic chest pain) Gastritis Myocarditis	

Presenting complaint	Exploring symptom	Relevant system reviews	Differential diagnoses		Clues to differential
Breathlessness	Timeframe •Duration •Onset (sudden or gradual) •Progression •Timing (intermittent or continuous) Breathlessness •Normal vs. current exercise tolerance (what makes them stop?) •Orthopnoea •Paroxysmal nocturnal dyspnoea •Diurnal/seasonal variation	General Fever, sweats Cardiorespiratory Chest pain, palpitations, cough, sputum, haemoptysis, leg swelling	Cardiac	Myocardial infarction	•Acute onset SOB, often wakes them •Associated nausea/sweatiness •May have crushing central chest pain •Cardiovascular risk factors
				Heart failure	•SOB, orthopnoea, paroxysmal nocturnal dyspnoea •Pink frothy sputum if acute LVF •Peripheral oedema •Cardiac history
			Respiratory	LRTI/pneumonia	•Acute SOB, cough and sputum •Systemic symptoms, e.g. fever
				Asthma	•Intermittent wheeze •Diurnal variation •Nocturnal cough •Exacerbating factors, e.g. exercise, pets
				COPD	•Chronic SOB •Significant smoking history •Chronic sputum production
				Pneumothorax	•Sudden onset pleuritic chest pain •Risk factors, e.g. tall/thin, Marfan syndrome, COPD/asthma
				Pulmonary embolism	•Pleuritic chest pain •Haemoptysis •Risk factors (e.g. long haul flight, recent surgery, immobility, malignancy)
				Pulmonary fibrosis	•Progressive SOB over long period •Dry cough
			Other differentials	Anaemia Hyperventilation in anxiety Pleural effusion DKA Lobar collapse Bronchiectasis Aortic stenosis Neuromuscular causes Sarcoidosis/TB/extrinsic allergic alveolitis	

Presenting complaint	Exploring symptom	Relevant system reviews	Differential diagnoses		Clues to differential
			Grouping	Differentials	
Cough	Timeframe •Duration •Progression •Timing (intermittent or continuous) Cough •Productive or non-productive •Triggers, nocturnal Sputum (if present) •How much, how often •Colour, consistency •Any blood Haemoptysis (if present) •Volume •Fresh or altered blood •Frequency •Nature of associated sputum. Mixed in?	General Fever, sweats, weight loss Cardiorespiratory Chest pain, palpitations, SOB/wheeze, leg swelling	Respiratory	URTI/LRTI/ pneumonia	•Acute productive cough •May have associated SOB •Systemic symptoms, e.g. fever
				Asthma	•Nocturnal cough •Intermittent wheeze •Diurnal variation •Exacerbating factors, e.g. exercise, pets
				Post-nasal drip	•Chronic rhinitis/sinusitis •Chronic cough to clear throat
				COPD	•Chronic productive cough •Chronic SOB •Significant smoking history
				Lung tumour	•Haemoptysis •Weight loss •Significant smoking history
			Other differentials	GORD Smoking LVF Drugs (e.g. ACE inhibitor) Bronchiectasis Interstitial lung disease Sarcoidosis/TB Cystic fibrosis	
Haemoptysis	Timeframe •Duration •Progression •Timing (intermittent or continuous) Cough •Productive or non-productive •Triggers, nocturnal Haemoptysis •Volume •Fresh or altered blood •Frequency •Nature of associated sputum. Mixed in? Sputum (if present) •How much, how often •Colour, consistency	General Fever, sweats, weight loss Cardiorespiratory Chest pain, palpitations, SOB/wheeze, leg swelling	Respiratory	Pneumonia	•Acute productive cough •May have associated SOB •Systemic symptoms, e.g. fever
				Pulmonary embolism	•Pleuritic chest pain and SOB •Risk factors (e.g. long haul flight, recent surgery, immobility, malignancy)
				Lung tumour	•Weight loss •Significant smoking history
				Bronchiectasis	•Chronic productive cough •Recurrent chest infections •Cause e.g. CF, childhood respiratory illness, TB, immunosuppression
			Other differentials	Prolonged coughing Pulmonary oedema Mitral stenosis TB Laryngeal carcinoma Polyarteritis nodosa Goodpasture's syndrome Aspergillosis	

COMMON ABDOMINAL HISTORIES

Presenting complaint	Exploring symptom	Relevant system reviews	Differential diagnoses Grouping	Differentials	Clues to differential
Abdominal pain	**S**ite **O**nset **C**haracter **R**adiation **A**ssociated symptoms **T**iming **E**xacerbating/relieving factors **S**everity	General •Fever, sweats Gastrointestinal •**Weight:** loss, appetite change •**Work down body:** dysphagia, nausea/vomiting, indigestion/heartburn, bowel habit change, tenesmus, blood/mucus in stool Urological •**Storage:** frequency, volume, urgency, nocturia, incontinence •**Infection:** dysuria, haematuria, odour Gynaecological •**PV bleeding:** menorrhagia, intermenstrual, post-coital, post-menopausal •**PV discharge** •**Pain:** pelvic, dysmenorrhoea, dyspareunia •**Pregnancy risk**	Gastrointestinal	Appendicitis	•Most commonly young patient •Periumbilical pain •Moves to RIF •Anorexia
				Gallstones	Biliary colic •Intermittent severe RUQ/epigastric pain •Exacerbated by fatty food (after 30-60 minutes) Cholecystitis •Continuous RUQ/epigastric pain CBD stones •Jaundice •RUQ pain Cholangitis – *Charcot's triad* •Jaundice •Fever/rigors •RUQ pain
				Pancreatitis	Acute pancreatitis •Severe epigastric/central pain •Radiating to back •Relieved by sitting forwards •Vomiting
				Gastritis/peptic ulcer	•Epigastric pain related to meals •Risk factors, e.g. NSAIDs, alcohol, spicy food
				Diverticulitis	•Elderly •LIF pain •Pyrexia
				Bowel obstruction	•Vomiting + abdominal distension + no bowel motions •Colicky pain
			Urological	Renal colic	•Spasms of loin to groin pain (excruciating) •Nausea and vomiting •Cannot lie still
			Gynaecological	Ectopic pregnancy	•Increasing iliac fossa/pelvic pain •4-12 weeks gestation/not using contraception/recent period of amenorrhoea •May have spotting
			Other differentials	Ruptured AAA Gastroenteritis Volvulus Pyelonephritis IBD Mesenteric ischaemia/ischaemic colitis Pelvic inflammatory disease Endometriosis Constipation Non-abdominal (MI, pneumonia, DKA)	

Presenting complaint	Exploring symptom	Relevant system reviews	Differential diagnoses Grouping	Differentials	Clues to differential
Change in bowel habit	Timeframe •Duration •Progression Stool •How much, how often •Consistency, colour and contents (mucus, blood)	Gastrointestinal •**Weight:** loss, appetite change •**Work down body:** dysphagia, nausea/vomiting, indigestion/heartburn, abdominal pain, tenesmus, blood/mucus in stool, flatus	Gastrointestinal	Colon cancer	•Elderly •Blood in stool/melaena •Weight loss + anaemia Sx (SOB, tiredness)
				Gastroenteritis	•Acute diarrhoea •Nausea and vomiting
				Inflammatory bowel disease	•Blood/mucus in stool •Abdominal pain •Weight loss
				Irritable bowel syndrome	•Fluctuate between diarrhoea/constipation •Anxious personality/associated with stress •Crampy abdominal pain and bloating
				Coeliac disease	•Diarrhoea, steatorrhoea •Anaemia symptoms •Abdominal discomfort
			Endocrinological	Thyrotoxicosis	•Diarrhoea •Heat intolerance •Irritability/restlessness •Tremor •Oligomenorrhoea/amenorrhoea
				Hypothyroidism	•Constipation •Cold intolerance •Lethargy/tiredness •Menorrhagia
			Other differentials	Bowel obstruction (not passing flatus) Diet and lifestyle changes Perianal conditions (haemorrhoids, fissure) Drugs (e.g. opiates, iron, antacids, antibiotics) Diverticulitis Overflow constipation Lactose intolerance Chronic infection	

Presenting complaint	Exploring symptom	Relevant system reviews	Differential diagnoses		Clues to differential
			Grouping	Differentials	
Rectal bleeding	Timeframe •Duration •Onset (sudden or gradual) •Progression – how often? •Timing (intermittent or continuous) Rectal bleeding •Blood: fresh/altered/ melaena •On tissue or mixed in stool •When does it occur Stool •Any mucus •How much, how often, consistency	Gastrointestinal •**Weight:** loss, appetite change •**Work down body:** dysphagia, nausea/vomiting, indigestion/heartburn, abdominal pain, bowel habit change, mucus in stool	Fresh blood (distal) ↑ ↓ Melaena (proximal)	Anal fissure	•Bleeding on defecation •Bright red on tissue paper •Intense anal pain •Constipation history
				Haemorrhoids	•Bleeding on defecation •Bright red on tissue paper •Constipation history •Anal pruritus
				Diverticular haemorrhage	•Sudden painless rectal bleeding •Elderly
				Distal polyp/ malignancy	•Alternating bowel habit •Weight loss •Urgency/tenesmus •Anal discomfort/pruritus
				Inflammatory bowel disease	•Blood mixed with stool •Mucus •Diarrhoea •Abdominal pain •Weight loss
				Haemorrhagic infective gastroenteritis	•Acute diarrhoea and vomiting •History of high risk food intake
				Angiodysplasia	•Elderly •Painless •May be subtle
				Proximal polyp/ malignancy	•Weight loss •Anaemia symptoms
				Haemorrhagic peptic ulcer/ gastritis	•Gastritis symptoms •Haematemesis •Risk factors, e.g. NSAIDs, alcohol, spicy food
				Oesophageal varices	•History of liver disease/alcoholism •May have encephalopathy or alcohol withdrawal •Haematemesis
Haematemesis	Timeframe •Duration •Progression •Timing (intermittent or continuous) Vomit •How much, how often, •Consistency, colour and contents (blood)	Gastrointestinal •**Weight:** loss, appetite change •**Work down body:** dysphagia, indigestion/heartburn, abdominal pain, bowel habit change, blood in stool/melaena	Gastrointestinal	Oesophageal varices	•History of liver disease/alcoholism •May have encephalopathy or alcohol withdrawal
				Mallory-Weiss tear	•Multiple vomits before haematemesis •Commonly after binge drinking
				Peptic ulcer haemorrhage /haemorrhagic gastritis/ oesophagitis	•Previous gastritis symptoms •Risk factors, e.g. NSAIDs, alcohol, spicy food

COMMON URINARY HISTORIES

Presenting complaint	Exploring symptom	Relevant system reviews	Differential diagnoses		Clues to differential
			Grouping	Differentials	
Frequency/ dysuria/ nocturia	Timeframe •Duration •Onset (sudden or gradual) •Progression •Timing (intermittent or continuous) Urination •Try to quantify urinary volume and frequency •Any catheter	General •Fever, sweats, rigors Urological •**Storage:** frequency, volume, urgency, nocturia, incontinence •**Infection:** dysuria, haematuria, odour •**Prostatic/voiding (if male):** hesitancy, poor flow/dribbling, feeling of incomplete emptying	Urological	Cystitis	•Dysuria ('burning pain on urination') •Frequency and urgency
				Urethritis	•Dysuria •Purulent urethral discharge
				Pyelonephritis	•Dysuria and loin pain •Fever/chills/rigors •Vomiting
				Benign prostatic hyperplasia	•Poor flow and terminal dribbling •Hesitancy •Overflow incontinence •Elderly male
			Other differentials	Anxiety Detrusor instability Bladder/lower urethral calculus Prostatitis Pregnancy Drugs (e.g. diuretics, excess caffeine)	

Presenting complaint	Exploring symptom	Relevant system reviews	Differential diagnoses		Clues to differential
			Grouping	**Differentials**	
Haematuria	Timeframe •Duration •Onset (sudden or gradual) •Progression •Timing (intermittent or continuous) Haematuria •Try to quantify bleeding •Thick blood or discoloured urine •Any clots? – *increase risk of urinary retention* •Catheterised? •Anaemia symptoms (tiredness, breathlessness on exertion)	General •Fever, sweats, weight loss, rashes, joint pain/swelling Urological •**Storage:** frequency, volume, urgency, nocturia, incontinence •**Infection:** dysuria •**Prostatic/voiding (if male):** hesitancy, poor flow/dribbling, feeling of incomplete emptying	Urological	Bladder transitional cell carcinoma	•Painless haematuria •History of aromatic amine exposure (e.g. dye washers, painters, decorators)
				Renal cell carcinoma	•Flank pain/mass •May have fever/hypertension/weight loss
				Urethral trauma, e.g. by catheter	•History of catheter use or trauma
				UTI	•Frequency/dysuria/urgency
				Urethritis	•Dysuria •Purulent urethral discharge
				Calculi	•Loin to groin pain
			Other differentials	Urological Glomerulonephritis Benign prostatic hyperplasia/prostate cancer Polycystic kidney disease Schistosomiasis Urinary tract TB Miscellaneous Haematological e.g. anticoagulation, sickle cell, coagulopathy Strenuous exercise Infective endocarditis Drugs (e.g. sulphonamides, cyclophosphamide, NSAIDs) Menstruation Rhabdomyolysis	
Polyuria	Timeframe •Duration •Onset (sudden or gradual) •Progression •Timing (intermittent or continuous) Polyuria •Try to quantify urinary volume and frequency •Try to quantify fluid intake •Other symptoms	General •Fever, sweats, weight loss, malaise, rashes, joint pain/swelling Urological •**Storage:** urgency, nocturia •**Infection:** dysuria, haematuria, odour •**Prostatic/voiding (if male):** hesitancy, poor flow/dribbling, feeling of incomplete emptying	Endocrine	Diabetes mellitus	•Polydipsia/thirst and polyuria •Weight loss and tiredness •Visual disturbance
				Diabetes insipidus	•Polydipsia/thirst and polyuria
			Urological	Chronic kidney disease	•Non-specific symptoms, e.g. fatigue, weakness, pruritus, dyspnoea
			Other differentials	UTI Cushing's syndrome Psychogenic polydipsia Drugs (e.g. diuretics, alcohol, lithium, tetracyclines) Postobstructive diuresis (life-threatening complication of relieving urinary obstruction)	
Incontinence	Timeframe •Duration •Onset (sudden or gradual) •Progression •Timing (intermittent or continuous) Incontinence •Pattern of incontinence, e.g. loss with effort or no control at all •Can they feel when they need to urinate •Try to quantify urinary volume and frequency •Bowel habit (any constipation?)	Urological •**Storage:** frequency, volume, urgency, nocturia •**Infection:** dysuria, haematuria, odour •**Prostatic/voiding (if male):** hesitancy, poor flow/dribbling, feeling of incomplete emptying	Stress incontinence	•Incompetent sphincter	•Small losses with effort, e.g. coughing, bending, exertion •Risk factors: multiple pregnancies, post-menopause, pelvic floor trauma
			Urge incontinence	•Detrusor instability •Spinal cord pathology (e.g. cord compression, cord injury, MS)	•Urge to pass urine followed by uncontrollable bladder emptying
			Overflow incontinence	•Prostatic hypertrophy •Stricture or stone •Spinal cord pathology	•Dribbling and poor stream •Hesitancy •Elderly male or history of obstruction
			Mixed incontinence		•Mix of above types
			True incontinence	•Vesicovaginal or ureterovaginal fistula	•Continuous urine leak
			Other differentials	Post-prostatectomy or other pelvic surgery Bladder stone/tumour Fistula Psychogenic	
Retention	Timeframe •Duration •Onset (sudden or gradual) •Progression •Timing (intermittent or continuous) Retention •Any constipation •Previous catheterisation	Urological •**Storage:** frequency, volume, urgency, nocturia, incontinence •**Infection:** dysuria, haematuria, odour •**Prostatic/voiding (if male):** hesitancy, poor flow/dribbling, feeling of incomplete emptying	Urological	Prostatic hypertrophy	•History of hesitancy, poor flow and terminal dribbling •Elderly male
				Urethral stricture	•History of trauma or recurrent catheterisation
				Bladder neck obstruction (e.g. tumour, calculus)	•May have haematuria
				UTI	•Dysuria
			Other differentials	Urinary Constipation (common) Prostatitis Pelvic mass Genital Herpes Clot retention (after bleed, e.g. from tumour) Phimosis Neurological MS Spinal cord injury/compression Drugs Anticholinergic drugs	

COMMON GYNAECOLOGICAL HISTORIES

Remember history taking in gynaecology requires you to ask extra questions on the **M**enstrual history, **O**bstetric history, **S**exual history and **C**ontraception/Cervical smear history (**MOSC**) – *see notes on the gynaecological history p13.*

Presenting complaint	Exploring symptom	Relevant system reviews	Differential diagnoses		Clues to differential
			Grouping	**Differentials**	
Pelvic pain	**S**ite **O**nset **C**haracter **R**adiation **A**ssociated symptoms **T**iming (relation to period) **E**xacerbating/relieving factors **S**everity	General •Fever, sweats Gynaecological •**PV bleeding:** menorrhagia, intermenstrual, post-coital, post-menopausal •**PV discharge** •**Pain:** dysmenorrhoea, dyspareunia •**Pregnancy risk** Urological •**Storage:** frequency, volume, urgency, nocturia, incontinence •**Infection:** dysuria, haematuria, odour Gastrointestinal •**Weight:** loss, appetite change •Nausea/vomiting, bowel habit change, tenesmus, blood/mucus in stool	Gynaecological	PID/acute salpingitis	•Bilateral pelvic pain •Vaginal discharge •Dyspareunia and dysmenorrhoea •Fever •May have post-coital or intermenstrual bleeding
				Ectopic pregnancy	•Recent period of amenorrhoea •Trying to get pregnant or unprotected sex (usually occurs 4-12 weeks gestation) •May have some vaginal spotting •In tubal rupture, collapse and shoulder tip pain
				Ovarian cyst torsion/rupture/ haemorrhage	•Sudden unilateral pelvic pain •May have fever/vomiting
				Endometriosis	•Cyclical pelvic pain •Dysmenorrhoea •Deep dyspareunia •Menstrual disturbance
			Urological	Pyelonephritis	•Fever/chills/rigors •Loin pain •Urinary frequency and dysuria
			Gastrointestinal	Appendicitis	•Young patient •Periumbilical pain •Moves to RIF •Anorexia
				Diverticulitis	•Elderly •LIF pain •Pyrexia
				IBS/IBD	•Lower abdominal pain •Associated change in bowel habit •May pass blood/mucus in IBD
			Other differentials	Mittelschmerz (ovulation pain) Fibroid degeneration Renal colic Bowel obstruction	

Presenting complaint	Exploring symptom	Relevant system reviews	Differential diagnoses		
PV bleeding	Type •Menorrhagia •Intermenstrual •Post-coital •Post-menopausal Timeframe •Duration •Onset (sudden or gradual) •Progression •Timing (intermittent or continuous) Bleeding •**Pattern:** regular/irregular •**Quantify loss:** number of sanitary towels/tampons, passage of clots, flooding •**Pain** with blood loss, vaginal dryness and itching if post-menopausal •**Anaemia symptoms:** tiredness, breathlessness on exertion •**Thyroid symptoms:** cold intolerance, constipation etc.	General •Fever, sweats Gynaecological •**PV discharge** •**Pain:** pelvic, dysmenorrhoea, dyspareunia •**Pregnancy risk**	**Menorrhagia**	**Dysfunctional uterine bleeding** (most common) **Fibroids** **Endometriosis** Pelvic inflammatory disease IUD Endometrial/cervical polyps Endometrial carcinoma (if >45 years) Contraception **NON-GYNAE:** blood dyscrasia (e.g. von Willebrand), hypothyroidism	
			Intermenstrual	Mid-cycle fall in oestrogen production around ovulation Endometrial/cervical polyps Ectropion Endometrial carcinoma (if >40 years) Cervicitis/vaginitis Hormonal contraception (spotting) IUD Pregnancy related Pelvic inflammatory disease	
			Post-coital	**Cervical trauma** **Cervical polyps** **Cervical carcinoma** Vaginal carcinoma Cervicitis/vaginitis Pelvic inflammatory disease	
			Post-menopausal	**Endometrial carcinoma** (until proven otherwise!) **Atrophic vaginitis** (90%) Foreign bodies, e.g. prolapse shelf Cervical/vulva carcinoma Cervical/endometrial polyps Oestrogen withdrawal	

Presenting complaint	Exploring symptom	Relevant system reviews	Differential diagnoses		Clues to differential
			Grouping	**Differentials**	
Secondary amenorrhoea	Timing •Duration •Triggers Clues to cause (work down body) •**General:** weight loss, stress, exercise, diet •**Head:** visual problems, headaches •**Thyroid:** symptoms •**Torso:** galactorrhoea, hirsutism, acne •**Abdomen:** possibility of pregnancy	Gynaecological •**PV discharge** •**Pain:** pelvic, dysmenorrhoea, dyspareunia •**Pregnancy risk** *Ensure you take a sexual and contraception history*	Gynaecological	Pregnancy	•Trying to get pregnant or unprotected sex
				PCOS	•Acne, hirsutism, obesity
				Menopause/premature ovarian failure	•Menopausal symptoms, e.g. sweats/flushes, aches and pains, previous erratic menstrual cycles, emotional changes etc.
			Endocrine	Hypothalamic amenorrhoea (e.g. anorexia, stress, athletes)	•Extreme anxiety, stress or exertion •Poor diet •Excessive weight loss •Low BMI
				Cushing's syndrome	•Steroid use •Thin skin/bruising •Central obesity and fat redistribution
				Hyperprolactinaemia	•Use of anti-psychotics is one cause •Visual symptoms if tumour •Galactorrhoea •Infertility
			Other differentials	Hyper/hypothyroidism Severe systemic illness Hypopituitarism/pituitary failure Certain contraception methods Post-pill amenorrhoea Cervical stenosis Drugs, e.g. hormonal treatments/contraception, chemotherapy, antipsychotics	

Presenting complaint	Exploring symptom	Relevant system reviews	Differential diagnoses		Clues to differential
Subfertility	General •When started trying Coitus •Frequency •Difficulties •Relation to fertile days •Pain Partners (consider each separately) •Age •Occupation •Body mass index •Previous children (same or different partner?) •Smoking and alcohol •Current medications •Man's PMHx Woman's gynaecological health •**Gynaecological systems review:** discharge, pain, PV bleeding •**PCOS symptoms:** hirsutism, greasy skin, obesity •**Prolactinoma symptoms:** galactorrhoea •**PMHx** including STIs and pelvic operations		Gynaecological	PCOS	•Acne, hirsutism, obesity
				Fallopian tube damage (e.g. 2° to PID or surgery)	•History of STIs, PID or pelvic surgery
				Endometriosis	•Cyclical pelvic pain •Dysmenorrhoea •Deep dyspareunia •Menstrual disturbance
				Cervical barrier e.g. cervical stenosis, hostile mucus, polyp, inflammation	•Previous cervical surgery •Current STI symptoms
				Hyperprolactinaemia	•Use of anti-psychotics is one cause •Visual symptoms if tumour •Galactorrhoea
				Hypothalamic disturbance (e.g. anorexia, stress, athletes)	•Extreme anxiety, stress or exertion •Poor diet •Extreme efforts to lose weight/weight loss •Low BMI
			Other differentials	Other female causes Hypogonadotropic hypogonadism (e.g. pituitary disease) Hypergonadotropic hypogonadism (e.g. premature ovarian failure) Congenital uterine/vaginal malformation Male causes Hypogonadotropic hypogonadism (e.g. pituitary disease) Hypergonadotropic hypogonadism (e.g. Klinefelter, gonadal damage) Varicocele Anti-sperm antibodies Absence/blockage of vas deferens Anatomical defects Coital difficulty Mechanical Erectile dysfunction Timing	

Remember history taking in obstetrics requires you to ask extra questions on the current pregnancy and obstetric history – *see notes on the obstetric history p14.*

Presenting complaint	Exploring symptom	Relevant system reviews	Differential diagnoses		Clues to differential
			Grouping	**Differentials**	
Abdominal pain	Site Onset Character Radiation Associated symptoms Timing Exacerbating/relieving factors Severity	General •Fever, sweats Obstetric •Fetal movements •Contractions/tightening •PV loss •Pre-eclampsia symptoms Gynaecological •PV discharge •PV bleeding Urological •**Storage:** frequency, volume, urgency, nocturia, incontinence •**Infection:** dysuria, haematuria, odour Gastrointestinal •**Weight:** loss, appetite change •**Work down body:** dysphagia, nausea/vomiting, indigestion/heartburn, bowel habit change, tenesmus, blood/mucus in stool	Obstetric	Ectopic	•Unilateral pain + bleeding •Usually between 4-12 weeks gestation
				Miscarriage	•<24 weeks gestation •Associated PV bleeding •May pass clots or products of conception
				Braxton Hicks contractions	•Late pregnancy •Infrequent, irregular contractions
				Labour	•>24 weeks gestation (*premature* if <37 weeks) •Painful regular rhythmic contractions
			Gynaecological	Fibroids (red degeneration or torsion)	•Severe abdominal pain •May have fever/vomiting
				Pelvic inflammatory disease	•PV discharge •Bilateral pelvic pain •Dyspareunia •Fever •May have post-coital bleeding •Unprotected intercourse with new/multiple partners
				Ovarian torsion/haemorrhage /rupture	•Severe unilateral pain •May have fever/vomiting
			General surgical	Any cause of acute abdominal pain in non-pregnant patients (*see notes on common abdominal histories p23*)	
			Other differentials	Placental abruption Pre-eclampsia Uterine rupture Chorioamnionitis Acute fatty liver of pregnancy Round ligament pain Symphysis pubis dysfunction	

Presenting complaint	Exploring symptom	Relevant system reviews	Differential diagnoses		Clues to differential
			Grouping	**Differentials**	
PV bleeding	Timeframe •Duration •Onset (sudden or gradual) •Progression •Timing (intermittent or continuous) Bleeding •Pattern (regular/irregular) •Amount of loss •Pain with blood loss •Anaemia symptoms (tiredness, breathlessness on exertion)	General •Fever, sweats Obstetric •Fetal movements •Contractions/tightening Gynaecological •PV discharge •Pain	Early	Implantation	•Light short-lived bleeding/spotting •Dark with pink/brown tint •6-12 days after conception (near when next menstrual period is expected)
				Ectopic	•Unilateral pelvic pain •Usually between 4-12 weeks gestation
				Miscarriage	•<24 weeks gestation •Pelvic pain •May pass clots or products of conception
			Late	Labour	•>24 weeks gestation (*premature* if <37 weeks) •Painful regular rhythmic contractions
				Placental abruption	•Antepartum haemorrhage •Continuous abdominal pain •Uterine contractions
				Placenta praevia	•Painless bleeding >28 weeks •Sudden profuse intermittent PV bleeding
				Vasa praevia	•Painless bleeding after membrane rupture •Fetal bradycardia/death
			Any time	Cervical pathology (polyps/cancer/trauma/ ectropion)	•Commonly post-coital (contact) bleeding •May have PV discharge
				Other differentials	Cervicitis Vaginitis Pelvic inflammatory disease

Presenting complaint	Exploring symptom	Relevant system reviews	Differential diagnoses		Clues to differential
			Grouping	**Differentials**	
Lower back pain	Pain **S**ite **O**nset **C**haracter **R**adiation **A**ssociated symptoms **T**iming **E**xacerbating/relieving factors **S**everity Associations Sciatica, stiffness/deformity, incontinence, neurological symptoms Red flags •**Cauda equina:** urinary incontinence/retention, faecal incontinence/constipation, bilateral leg pain, severe/progressive neurological deficit, saddle anaesthesia, sexual dysfunction •**Infection or cancer:** age <20 or >55 years at onset, cancer Hx, night pain, weight loss, fever, night sweats, injecting drugs, immunosuppression •**Fracture:** trauma, severe central spinal pain •**Spondyloarthropathy:** early morning stiffness, worse with rest	General Fever, night sweats, weight loss Neuro (lower limbs) •**Motor:** weakness/wasting, incontinence •**Sensory:** pain, numbness, tingling	Orthopaedic	Muscular	•Acute onset lower back pain •Paraspinal muscles affected, not central
				Lumbar spondylosis and facet joint syndrome (lumbar arthritis)	•Chronic episodic mechanical lower back pain •Backache related to standing/walking a lot/sitting in one place •Progressive stiffening
				Lumbar disc prolapse	•Acute onset while lifting/bending/sneezing/coughing •Severe pain •Sciatica, leg pain often worse than back pain •Neurological symptoms, e.g. weakness, numbness (usually L4/L5/S1 distribution)
				Discitis	•Fever and systemic upset •Risk factors, e.g. injecting drug user
				Spinal fracture	•History of trauma •Sudden onset
				Cauda equina syndrome	•Urinary incontinence/retention •Faecal incontinence/constipation •Saddle anaesthesia or paraesthesia •Bilateral leg pain and weakness
			Rheumatological	Ankylosing spondylitis	•Morning stiffness >30 minutes •Pain worse on rest
			Other differentials	Myeloma bone lesions Bony metastasis Paget's disease Spondylolisthesis Osteoporotic vertebral collapse Non-orthopaedic/rheumatological Pyelonephritis PID Pancreatitis AAA	
Joint pain/ stiffness/ swelling	Pain **S**ite(s) **O**nset **C**haracter **R**adiation **A**ssociated symptoms **T**iming **E**xacerbating/relieving factors **S**everity Stiffness/swelling •Worse in morning?, how long for (*>30 mins = inflammatory; <30 mins = osteoarthritis*) •Better or worse after exercise •Sleep disturbance •Loss of function	General Fever, rashes, weight loss Rheumatological •**Joints:** pain, stiffness, swelling •**Work down body:** skin (rashes, ulcers, Raynaud's), hair loss, eyes (redness, dryness), mouth (dryness), chest (breathlessness, SOB), GI (IBD symptoms), genitourinary (discharge)	Rheumatological	Rheumatoid arthritis	•Slowly progressive symmetrical polyarthropathy •Small joints (commonly of hand) •Deforming •Early morning stiffness
				Gout	•First MTP joint most commonly affected •Isolated swollen, hot, painful joint •Hyperuricaemia risk factors, e.g. diuretics, alcohol excess (esp. beer), renal disease
				Psoriatic arthritis	•Associated skin plaques and nail changes •Early morning stiffness •Many patterns of joint involvement
				SLE	•Systemic illness with intermittent fevers •Photosensitive rash •Generalised myalgia and arthralgia •Other systemic symptoms (e.g. psychiatric, pleurisy, ulcers)
				Enteropathic arthritis	•Symmetrical arthritis of lower limb joints and sacroiliac joints •Early morning stiffness •Symptoms/diagnosis of Crohn's or UC
			Orthopaedic	Osteoarthritis	•Elderly •Worse on movement (rest helps) and at end of day, night pain common
				Septic arthritis	•Isolated hot, red, swollen joint •Agonizingly painful •Systemically unwell with fever
			Other differentials	Single joint Traumatic (dislocation/fracture/ligament injury) Haemophilia (haemarthrosis) Pseudogout Joint specific problems (e.g. knee – chondromalacia patellae, Osgood-Schlatter's disease, patellar tendonitis; hip – avascular necrosis) Adhesive capsulitis Transient synovitis Bursitis Reiter's syndrome Multiple joints Viral polyarthritis (e.g. flu, HIV, hepatitis, rubella) Other connective tissue disorders (e.g. systemic sclerosis, polymyositis, polyarteritis nodosa) Other spondyloarthropathies (e.g. ankylosing spondylitis, Reiter's syndrome, Behçet's disease, juvenile chronic arthritis, rheumatic fever)	

Presenting complaint	Exploring symptom	Relevant system reviews	Differential diagnoses		Clues to differential
			Grouping	**Differentials**	
Anxiety	Attack detail •**Timing:** duration, onset, episodic/constant, triggers, effect on life, frequency, avoidance •**Somatic symptoms:** palpitations, breathlessness, tight chest, sweating, dizziness Background to attacks e.g. Previous attacks, frequency, impact on life Associated symptoms •**Associated psychological symptoms:** depression screen, stress, worry, avoidance •**Psychiatric differential questions:** obsessions, compulsions, PTSD symptoms (psychological trauma, flashbacks, nightmares, hyperarousal) •**Organic differential questions:** e.g. hyperthyroidism, ACS	Psych •**Depression screen:** core (mood, anhedonia), biological (sleep, energy), future (hopelessness, suicidal thoughts) •**RISK:** to self, to others	Psychiatric	Generalised anxiety disorder	•Anxiety and worry on most days •Generalised (about everything) •Long-term
				Panic disorder	•Panic attacks (palpitations, sweating, SOB, chest pain etc.) •Unpredictable but certain situations may predispose (e.g. busy places)
				Phobic disorder	•Intense fear triggered by predictable stimulus •Common examples: agoraphobia, isolated phobia (e.g. snakes, flying), social phobia
				Post-traumatic stress disorder	•Caused by stressful life event •Intense anxiety with flashbacks, insomnia, nightmares, avoidance, emotional detachment
				Obsessive compulsive disorder	•Obsessive thoughts •Constant need to check everything •Only relieved by acting on compulsions, e.g. cleaning hands, checking lights or locks
				Depression	•Positive depression screen
			Other differentials	Organic Acute coronary syndrome Arrhythmia Hyperthyroidism Phaeochromocytoma	
Psychosis	Auditory hallucinations •**Voice detail:** male/female, recognisable, always the same?, when heard •**Real/pseudo:** outside/inside head •**2nd/3rd person:** to you/about you •**What they say** (including commands) Delusions •Explore •Challenge the delusion •Assess risk others/self	Psych •**Schizophrenia first rank symptoms:** 1. 3rd person auditory hallucinations 2. Running commentary auditory hallucinations 3. Delusions of thought 4. Delusions of control 5. Delusional perception •**Depression screen:** core (mood, anhedonia), biological (sleep, energy), future (hopelessness, suicidal thoughts) •**Other:** insight •**RISK:** to self, to others	Psychiatric	Schizophrenia	•Schizophrenia first rank symptoms •Other positive symptoms: bizarre delusions, odd behaviour, somatic hallucinations •Negative symptoms: apathy, anhedonia, asociality, lack of motivation
				Delusional disorders	•Non-bizarre delusions •Absence of other psychiatric symptoms
				Bipolar disorder	•Normal mood interspersed with depressive and manic episodes •Manic episodes: irritable, elevated mood, fast speech, flight of ideas, grandiosity, excessive spending/drinking, insomnia, auditory hallucinations, delusions of wealth/power/religion
				Schizoaffective disorder	•Features of bipolar disorder and schizophrenia in same episode
				Psychotic depression	•Depression associated with psychotic symptoms, e.g. delusions or hallucinations
				Puerperal psychosis	•Severe mental illness days/weeks after childbirth
				Delirium	•Elderly patient with current/recent infection •Reduced level of consciousness •Fluctuating •Inversion of day/night cycle
				Dementia (esp. Lewy body)	•Long history of progressive memory loss •Related cognitive deficits (comprehension, orientation, inhibition etc.)
			Other differentials	Organic Drugs (e.g. recreational drugs, corticosteroids, levodopa, antimalarials) Alcohol/drug withdrawal Extreme fatigue Temporal lobe epilepsy Space occupying lesion Hypoxia Huntington's SLE Neurosyphilis Autoimmune/paraneoplastic HIV	

Presenting complaint	Exploring symptom	Relevant system reviews	Differential diagnoses		Clues to differential
			Grouping	**Differentials**	
Low mood	Depression screen •**Core:** mood, anhedonia •**Biological:** sleep, energy •**Future (including risk):** hopelessness, suicidal thoughts Background •Hx of mania/hypomania •Previous episodes and triggers	Psych •**Psychosis symptoms:** hallucinations, delusions •**RISK:** to self, to others	Psychiatric	Depression	•Positive depression screen
				Bipolar disorder	•Normal mood interspersed with depressive and manic episodes •Manic episodes: irritable, elevated mood, fast speech, flight of ideas, grandiosity, excessive spending/drinking, insomnia, auditory hallucinations, delusions of wealth/power/religion
				Adjustment disorder	•Triggered by stressful life event •Stress, upset, anxiety, hopelessness •Reaction greater than expected for the event
				Psychotic depression	•Depression associated with psychotic symptoms, e.g. delusions or hallucinations
				Postnatal depression	•Depression days/weeks after childbirth •Often recurrent
			Other differentials	Organic Hypothyroidism Drug side effects Intracranial lesion Grief reaction	
Memory loss	Memory loss •Onset •Short/long-term •Insight and concerns •Functional levels (washing, dressing etc.) •Risk assessment (e.g. turning off gas stove) •Mini mental state examination	General Any evidence of infection, e.g. fever, urinary symptoms Psych •**Psychosis symptoms:** hallucinations, delusions •**Depression screen:** core (mood, anhedonia), biological (sleep, energy), future (hopelessness, suicidal thoughts) •**Other:** insight •**RISK:** to self, to others	Dementia	Alzheimer's disease	•Relentlessly progressive decline •Disinhibition •Dysphasia and dyspraxia
				Vascular dementia	•Stepwise decline •Cardiovascular risk factors •Preserved insight
				Lewy body dementia	•Fluctuating dementia •Visual hallucinations •Parkinsonism •Delirium like phases
				Other rarer types	Fronto-temporal dementia (Pick's disease) Creutzfeldt-Jakob disease
			Psychiatric	Depression (pseudodementia)	•Positive depression screen
				Delirium	•Reduced level of consciousness •Fluctuating •Inversion of day/night cycle •Evidence of infection
			Other differentials	Degenerative neurological diseases (e.g. Huntington's, MS) Drugs and alcohol Vitamin deficiency (B_{12}, thiamine, folate, nicotinic acid) Electrolyte imbalances/uraemia Organ failure Endocrinopathies Space occupying lesion Neurosyphilis Encephalitis Autoimmune/paraneoplastic HIV	
Eating disorder	•**BMI** •**Symptoms:** avoidance of weight gain/need to lose weight/look in mirror a lot, efforts to lose weight (vomiting, laxatives, exercise), binge eating/fasting •**Food diary:** what they eat each day •**Consequences:** menstrual cycle disturbance •**Self harm** and depression symptoms	Psych •**Depression screen:** core (mood, anhedonia), biological (sleep, energy), future (hopelessness, suicidal thoughts) •**RISK:** to self	Psychiatric	Anorexia nervosa	•BMI <17.5 •Fear of weight gain •Feel fat when thin •Efforts to lose weight: diuretics/laxatives, vomiting, excessive exercise •Consequential symptoms: amenorrhoea, developmental delay, myopathy, poor sleep, GI symptoms
				Bulimia nervosa	•BMI >17.5 •Regular binge eating •Preoccupation with body weight control •Means of avoiding weight gain e.g. starvation, vomiting, laxatives, exercise

Presenting complaint	Exploring symptom	Relevant system reviews	Differential diagnoses		Clues to differential
			Grouping	**Differentials**	
Failure to thrive	•Ask to see growth chart and determine age of onset •**Input:** detailed dietary history, feeding history (including time of weaning), hunger •**Use:** energy, activity level, exercise, anorexic? •**Output:** wet nappies, stools and GI symptoms •**Others:** behaviour, general health, happiness, parents' health	<u>General</u> •Fever, behaviour, activity/apathy/alertness, cough <u>Gastrointestinal</u> •**Work down body:** dysphagia, reflux/vomiting, abdominal pain/colic, diarrhoea/constipation, stools (blood/mucus/pale)	Gastrointestinal	Coeliac disease	•Presents any age after weaning •Diarrhoea (pale stools) •Bloating
				Dietary protein intolerance (e.g. cow's milk protein allergy)	•Cow's milk protein allergy usually presents in first few months •Diarrhoea after being fed with formula milk for a few months •Reflux
				Carbohydrate intolerance (e.g. lactose intolerance)	•Flatulence, diarrhoea, bloating and cramps within a few hours of consuming lactose •May be congenital (rare) or develop after gastroenteritis (transient)
				Pyloric stenosis	•Projectile non-bilious vomiting after feeding •Starts around 3-6 weeks of age
				GORD/oesophagitis	•Effortless regurgitation •Crying during feeding •Cough/hoarseness
				Cystic fibrosis	•Recurrent chest infections •Pale stools that float
				Inflammatory bowel disease	•Older child (e.g. teenager) •Abdominal pain •Diarrhoea with blood/mucus
			Non-gastrointestinal	Not enough food being offered or taken	•Commonest cause
				Nutritional neglect	•Not offered enough food •Hungry, food seeking/hoarding
				Emotional neglect	•Poor interaction between child and parent •Withdrawn, fearful, anxious
				Eating disorder	•Adolescent girls •Fear of weight gain •Feel fat when thin •Efforts to lose weight: diuretics/laxatives, vomiting, excessive exercise •Consequential symptoms: amenorrhoea, developmental delay, myopathy, poor sleep, GI symptoms, poor dental hygiene
			Other differentials	<u>Prenatal</u> Prematurity Intrauterine growth restriction Chromosomal abnormalities Toxins (alcohol, smoking, drugs) <u>Others</u> Poor feeding Inborn errors of metabolism (e.g. abetalipoproteinaemia) Chronic infections (including HIV) Chronic illness Malignancy	

Presenting complaint	Exploring symptom	Relevant system reviews	Differential diagnoses		Clues to differential
Weight increase	•Ask to see growth chart and determine age of onset •**Input:** detailed dietary history, feeding history (including time of weaning), hunger •**Use:** energy, activity level, exercise •**Others:** behaviour, general health, happiness, parents' health and BMI	<u>General</u> •Fever, behaviour, activity/apathy/alertness, cold intolerance <u>Top to toe</u> •Stature (short/normal) •Changes in appearance (skin/hair/acne) •Hirsutism •Fat distribution •Bowel habit •Pubertal changes (including menses)	Endocrine	Hypothyroidism	•Delayed growth/puberty •Fatigue, cold intolerance •Dry skin, coarse hair
				Cushing's syndrome	•Delayed growth/puberty •Central obesity •Easy bruising •Cushingoid facial features •Intrascapular and supraclavicular fat pads
				PCOS	•Adolescent female •Oligo/amenorrhoea •Hirsutism, acne
			Non-endocrine	Simple obesity	•Snacking •Lack of exercise
				Familial	•Parents with high BMI
			Other differentials	Oedema (cardiac or renal) Steroid use Genetic syndromes (e.g. Turner's syndrome, Prader-Willi syndrome) Hepatosplenomegaly (e.g. in leukaemia)	

Presenting complaint	Exploring symptom	Relevant system reviews	Differential diagnoses		Clues to differential
			Grouping	Differentials	

Developmental delay	<u>Development</u>
	•Current developmental stage in each category (*see notes on paediatric history p8*)
	  -Gross motor
	  -Fine motor and vision
	  -Hearing and language
	  -Social
	•Ages of key milestones in each
	
	<u>If motor problem</u>
	•How mobile?
	•Hand dominance
	•Balance problems
	•Behavioural problem
	
	<u>If language/social problem</u>
	•**Senses:** hearing, vision
	•**Vocalisation**/articulation
	•**Comprehension:** follows commands, responds to voice
	•**Non-verbal communication:** pointing, gestures, facies
	•**Social responsiveness:** reaction to new situations, tantrums, playing, gestures
	
	<u>As part of history</u>
	•Prenatal problems (e.g. alcohol/drugs in pregnancy, maternal infections)
	•Perinatal problems (e.g. prolonged/difficulties in labour)
	•Postnatal problems (e.g. meningitis/encephalitis)
	
	The key is in a thorough history!
		<u>General</u>
		•Fever, behaviour, activity/apathy/alertness
		
		<u>Neurological</u>
		•**General:** fits/LOC, headache, dizziness, vision/hearing
		•**Motor:** weakness/wasting
			Generalised delay
			
			(*can also cause any of the specific delays below*)
			
			Prenatal
				Chromosomal/genetic disorders, e.g. Downs	•Dysmorphic features

				Alcohol/drugs in pregnancy	•History of mother taking alcohol or drugs in pregnancy
				TORCH infections in pregnancy	•History of Toxoplasmosis/rubella/CMV/Herpes
			Perinatal	Extreme prematurity	•Born very premature
				Hypoxic brain injury	•Perinatal hypoxic insult, e.g. prolonged/difficult labour
				Hypoglycaemia	•Period of neonatal hypoglycaemia
				Intracerebral haemorrhage	•Risks = abnormal labour, prematurity •Usually diagnosed within first few days
			Postnatal	Meningitis/encephalitis	•Onset after episode of meningitis/encephalitis
				Head injury or hypoxic/hypoglycaemic episode	•Delay subsequent to episode
			Motor delay	Cerebral palsy	•Muscle stiffness/weakness/floppiness •Spasm or dyskinetic or ataxic •Caused by prenatal/perinatal/postnatal insult (<3 years)
				Duchenne muscular dystrophy (or other muscular disorders)	•Progressive muscle weakness (beginning proximally) •Onset 2-3 years
				Hip dysplasia	•Usually identified at birth but may present later with a limp
			Language delay	Deafness	•e.g. due to chronic otitis media
				Articulation problem	•Birth defects (e.g. cleft palate)
				Familial	•Similar history in family
				Lack of stimulus	•Poor interaction with parents •May show signs of neglect
				Autism	•Imposition of routines •Doesn't seek friendships, prefers own company •Limited gestures and expressions
			Social delay	ADHD	•Hyperactivity, inattentiveness

Presenting complaint	Exploring symptom	Relevant system reviews	Differential diagnoses		Clues to differential
Precocious puberty (*boys <9 years, girls <8 years*)	<u>Puberty staging and order</u> **Order for boys:** •Testicular enlargement •Pubic hair •Penis enlargement •Height spurt **Order for girls:** •Breast development •Pubic/axillary hair •Height spurt •Menarche <u>Other development</u> •Previous growth and development •Height •Weight and nutrition •Behavioural changes <u>Family history</u> •Parents' pubertal ages, heights and maternal menarche	<u>General</u> •Fever, behaviour, activity/apathy/alertness, general health <u>Neurological</u> •**General:** fits/LOC, headache, dizziness, vision/hearing •**Motor:** weakness/wasting	Gonadotrophin dependent (*central*)	Familial/idiopathic	•Majority of girls
				Central nervous system abnormalities, e.g. hydrocephalus, hypoxic brain injury	•Relevant history
				Intracranial tumour	•Associated neurological symptoms
			Gonadotrophin independent (*peripheral*) *i.e. sex hormones not under pituitary control*	Adrenal tumour/hyperplasia	•Excessive pubic hair, penis/clitoris enlargement •Weight gain
				Ovarian/testicular tumour	•Ovarian: bloating, menorrhagia, pelvic pain •Testicular: painless lump
			Other differentials	Premature thelarche (breasts only) Premature pubarche (pubic hair only) External sex hormones	

Presenting complaint	Exploring symptom	Relevant system reviews	Differential diagnoses		Clues to differential
Delayed puberty (*boys >15 years, girls >14 years*)	<u>Puberty staging and order</u> **Order for boys:** •Testicular enlargement •Penis enlargement •Pubic hair •Height spurt **Order for girls:** •Breast development •Pubic/axillary hair •Height spurt •Menarche <u>Other development</u> •Previous growth and development •Height •Weight and nutrition •Behavioural changes <u>Family history</u> •Parents' pubertal ages, heights and maternal menarche	<u>General</u> •Fever, behaviour, activity/apathy/alertness, general health •Symptoms of other systemic diseases (*CF, thyroid disorder, anorexia, Crohn's*) <u>Neurological</u> •**General:** fits/LOC, headache, dizziness, vision/hearing •**Motor:** weakness/wasting	Familial	Constitutional	•Majority of cases
			Hypogonadotropic hypogonadism	Systemic disease (e.g. IBD, CF, anorexia)	•Symptoms of underlying disease
				Hypothyroidism	•Delayed growth •Fatigue, cold intolerance •Dry skin, coarse hair
			Hypergonadotropic hypogonadism	Klinefelter/Turner syndrome	•Turner (female): short stature, amenorrhoea •Klinefelter (male): small testes, gynaecomastia, tall and thin
				PCOS	•Oligo/amenorrhoea •Hirsutism, acne
			Other differentials	<u>Hypogonadotropic</u> Kallmann syndrome Intracranial tumour Panhypopituitarism Syndromal <u>Hypergonadotropic</u> Steroid hormone enzyme deficiency Acquired gonadal damage	

Presenting complaint	Exploring symptom	Relevant system reviews	Differential diagnoses		Clues to differential
			Grouping	Differentials	
Behavioural problems	•Expand on nature of problems •Ask about specific symptoms of each described disorders *Get history from school and at home*		Psychiatric	Attention deficit hyperactivity disorder	•Hyperactivity •Inattentiveness
				Conduct disorder	•Bullies/threatens/intimidates •Aggressive •Cruel to people/animals
				Oppositional defiant disorder	•Loses temper •Argues with adults and defies requests •Deliberately annoys others
				Obsessive compulsive disorder	•Intrusive thoughts (obsessions) •Repetitive behaviours (compulsions) •Excessive washing/cleaning/checking
				Autism	•Speech/language delay •Imposition of routines •Doesn't seek friendships, prefers own company •Limited gestures and expressions
			Other differentials	Anxiety disorders Attachment disorder Schizophrenia Depression Bipolar disorder	
Childhood bruising	Bruising •Onset and progression •Pattern •Mechanism of injury •Associated symptoms *Have a low threshold for raising safeguarding concerns*	General •Fever, behaviour, activity/apathy/alertness	Injury related	Non-accidental injury	•Bruises on soft tissues (ears/neck/ chest/abdomen/buttocks/ calves/thighs) •Story inconsistent with injury
				Accidental injury	•Bruising overlying bony prominences (forehead, shins, hips etc.) •Story consistent with injury
			Non-injury related	Henoch-Schönlein purpura	•Symmetrical rash on back of legs and buttocks; purpuric and slightly raised •May have abdominal/joint pain •May have evidence of nephritis
				Idiopathic Thrombocytopenic Purpura	•Spontaneous purpura and petechiae •Usually post-infection
				Meningococcal septicaemia	•Non-blanching rash •Neck pain/stiffness •Photophobia •Fever
			Other differentials	Acute lymphoblastic leukaemia Traumatic petechiae (e.g. due to forceful coughing) Coagulation disorders (e.g. haemophilia)	
Faint/fit/ funny turn	Attack •**Before:** warning, circumstance •**During:** duration, LOC, movements (floppy/stiff/jerking), incontinence/tongue biting, complexion •**After:** amnesia, muscle pain, confusion/sleepiness, injuries from fall Background to attacks e.g. Previous attacks, frequency, impact on life	General •Fever, behaviour, activity/apathy/alertness Neurological •**General:** fits/falls/LOC, headache, dizziness, vision/hearing, memory loss, neck stiffness/ photophobia •**Motor:** weakness/ wasting, incontinence •**Sensory:** pain, numbness, tingling Cardiorespiratory •Dyspnoea, cyanosis, chest pain/palpitations	Neurological	Febrile convulsion	•Short, self-limiting generalised seizure •Early in infection when fever is rising
				Seizure	Types include: •Absence seizure •Focal seizure •Generalised tonic-clonic seizure (suggested by loss of bladder/bowel control, tongue biting)
				Paediatric epileptic syndromes	•Characteristic features of epileptic syndromes, e.g. trunk spasms, trunk flexion, myoclonus, eye deviation, language impairment etc.
				Reflex anoxic seizure	•Often precipitated by a bump on head, emotion (e.g. fear, surprise), crying or fever •Stops breathing, loses consciousness and falls to floor •Very pale
			Non-neurological	Vasovagal syncope	•Faint after prolonged standing/emotion/pain
				Pseudoseizure	•Atypical seizures
				Breath holding spell	•Child holds breath and goes blue •Usually when upset
			Other differentials	Simple faint Narcolepsy Arrhythmia Hypertrophic cardiomyopathy	

HISTORY COMMUNICATION SKILLS

START

W Wash hands

I Introduce self (full name, grade/role)

P Patient's name, DOB and what they like to be called

E Explain why you are there

- Briefly mention **confidentiality**
- Start with an open question (e.g. 'OK Tim, what brought you in today?')
- During the first 60 seconds ('the golden minute'), <u>do not interrupt</u>, just facilitate disclosure (e.g. by head nodding, saying 'yes', 'uhum' etc.)

DURING

- Start with **open questions** and then move to closed questions
- Try to build a **rapport** with the patient (e.g. postpartum patient – 'How was the birth?')
- Use **signposting**: refer back to what you've just covered and link it to what you want to move on to (e.g. 'So you've told me about your recent cough. Next I'd like to ask about other medical problems you've had in the past.')
- Show **empathy**
- Respond to **cues**. It is really important to engage with what the patient says instead of just planning your next question.
  - Cues may be verbal or body language
  - Comment on it, e.g. 'You look worried.'
  - After you hear a cue, repeat it back to the patient and then ask more about it (e.g. 'You mentioned that sometimes you feel down. Can you tell me more about that?')

END

- **Summarise** what you have talked about to the patient
- Ask if they have any **questions** for you
- Explain the next steps

INTEGRATE IDEAS, CONCERNS AND EXPECTATIONS

- **ICE** should be integrated throughout the history
  - Ask about ideas and concerns (e.g. 'What do you think is going on?' 'It has been going on for a while now. Is it worrying you?')
  - Ask about expectations from consultation (e.g. 'Was there anything else you wanted to address today?')

OTHER TIPS

- **Things to AVOID**
  - Leading questions (e.g. 'You haven't missed any doses of the medication, have you?')
  - Asking multiple questions in one go
  - Giving too much information at once
- **Other techniques**

Reflection	Reflect the heat back to the patient, e.g. 'Do you have any ideas about what's causing this?'
Clarification	e.g. 'What do you feel when you get depressed?'
Normalise	e.g. 'Some people think about hurting themselves or even about suicide in these situations. Have you ever had thoughts like that?'
Summarise	If your mind goes blank, summarise the recent part of the history

- Don't be afraid of **pauses**, but don't fill them with 'ummmmm' or 'errrrrrr'

BACKGROUND

- Patient's name, age, relevant chronic conditions
- Where and when they were seen

'Mr Blogs is a 44 year old male with a background of COPD who self-presented to A&E one hour ago.'

HISTORY

- PC and HPC

'He presented with a cough, which started three days ago. It is productive of a moderate amount of thick green sputum – he has produced about a table-spoon full today.'

- Other positive findings and <u>important</u> negative findings from relevant systems review

'He has also been feverish and experiences shortness of breath on walking 50 yards. His normal exercise tolerance is 200 yards. He has not had any haemoptysis, chest pain or leg swelling.'

- PMHx

'Mr Blogs' past medical history includes COPD and hypertension. His COPD was diagnosed two years ago and is currently well controlled with inhalers. He has never been admitted to hospital for his COPD.'

- DHx

'Mr Blogs takes tiotropium 18mcg inhaled once daily and salbutamol 100-200mcg inhaled as required for COPD. He also takes ramipril 2.5mg orally once daily for hypertension. He has no drug allergies.'

- FHx

'He has no significant family history.'

- SHx

'In terms of social history, Mr Blogs is a farmer and currently smokes 20 cigarettes daily with a 40 pack year history. He has never drunk alcohol. He lives at home with his wife and is normally fully independent and mobile.'

EXAMINATION

- Observations

'I examined Mr Blogs and he was hypoxic, with oxygen saturations of 87% on room air. He had a respiratory rate of 22. He was pyrexial at 38°. Heart rate and blood pressure were normal.'

- General state

'Clinically, Mr Blogs appeared well but was slightly short of breath when speaking sentences. He was alert and orientated.'

- General inspection

'On general inspection, there was evidence of accessory muscle use and breathing through pursed lips. There was about 2mls of green sputum in the sputum pot.'

- Major findings from relevant system examination

'Examination of the respiratory system revealed a capillary refill time of 3 seconds, cool peripheries and conjunctival pallor but no peripheral or central cyanosis. The trachea was not deviated and there was no cervical lymphadenopathy. On examination of the chest, there were no scars or chest deformities. Chest expansion was normal. The lungs were resonant to percussion. On auscultation, there were normal vesicular breath sounds with a mild wheeze throughout but no other added sounds. Vocal resonance was normal. The calves were not swollen or tender.'

- Findings from other system examinations

'On examination of the cardiovascular system, the apex beat was non-displaced and there were no heaves or thrills over the precordium. Heart sounds one and two were present with no added sounds. There was no evidence of pulmonary or peripheral oedema. On examination of the abdomen, it was soft and non-tender with no organomegaly. Bowel sounds were normal.'

SUMMARY, IMPRESSIONS AND PLAN

- Summary

'In summary, Mr Blogs is a 44 year old male with COPD who presented with a three day history of a green productive cough and fever. He is currently stable but did have an audible wheeze on examination.'

- Impressions and differentials

'My impression is that this is an infective exacerbation of COPD. However, a differential is community-acquired pneumonia.'

- Investigations and plan

'I would like to take bloods including a full blood count, U&Es, LFTs and a C-reactive protein. I would like to obtain an arterial blood gas sample to more accurately assess his type and degree of respiratory failure and guide oxygen therapy. I would also like to send sputum for MC&S to guide antimicrobial therapy, and get a chest radiograph. I would like to admit Mr Blogs and start him on controlled oxygen therapy, IV amoxicillin, oral clarithromycin and oral prednisolone to treat an infective exacerbation of COPD. In view of his wheeze, I would also like to prescribe nebulised salbutamol and ipratropium.'

In association with

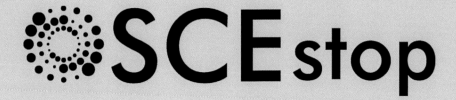

For the latest notes and resources visit

www.OSCEstop.com

Feedback or questions

Contact@OSCEstop.com

STANDARD EXAMINATIONS

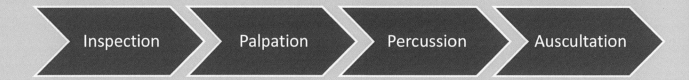

NEUROLOGICAL LIMB EXAMINATIONS

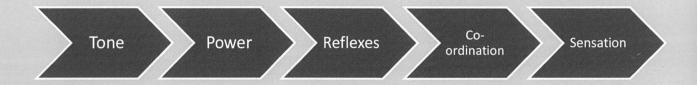

MUSCULOSKELETAL EXAMINATIONS

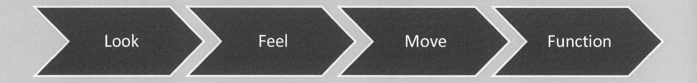

CHAPTER 2: CLINICAL EXAMINATIONS

CARDIAC EXAMINATION

INTRODUCTION

- **W**ash hands; **I**ntroduce self; ask **P**atient's name, DOB and what they like to be called; **E**xplain examination and obtain consent
- Expose and **sit patient at 45°**

GENERAL INSPECTION

- **Patient:** well/unwell, comfortable, alert, breathless, pallor, cyanosis, obvious scars on precordium, pacemaker/devices, audible metallic heart valve sound, age (gives clues to pathology), syndromic features (*e.g. Marfan syndrome associated with AR/MR/mitral prolapse; Turner syndrome associated with AS; Down's syndrome associated with congenital heart disease*)
- **Around the bed:** oxygen, medication, IV infusions

HANDS

- **Perfusion:** temperature, capillary refill (*>2 seconds in hypoperfusion*), peripheral cyanosis
- **Nails:** clubbing (*cyanotic congenital heart disease, IE*), splinter haemorrhages (*IE*), Quincke's sign (visible pulsations; *AR*)
- **Dorsum:** extensor tendon xanthomata (irregular nodules overlying tendons; *hyperlipidaemia*)
- **Palms:** Osler's nodes (**p**ainful **p**urple **p**apules on **p**ulps; *IE*), Janeway lesions (erythematous macules on palms; *IE*)

ARMS

- Inspect for bruising (*anticoagulation*)
- **Radial pulse:** <u>rate</u> (*tachycardia >100, bradycardia <60*), <u>rhythm</u> (*irregularly irregular = AF/ectopics/flutter with variable block; regularly irregular = 2nd degree heart block*), radio-radial delay (*aortic dissection/aneurysm or proximal coarctation*), offer to test for radio-femoral delay (*aortic coarctation*)
- **Collapsing pulse:** first ensure the patient has no shoulder pain. Hold their extended elbow with your left hand and wrap your right hand around their wrist. Start with their arm downwards and release the pressure from around their wrist until you can only just feel their radial pulse. Then quickly lift their arm upwards with your left hand. In a collapsing pulse, you will feel a strong tapping when the arm is elevated. (*Classically a sign of AR, but other causes include patent ductus arteriosus; high-output states e.g. anaemia, thyrotoxicosis; and physiological states e.g. pregnancy, fever.*)
- **Blood pressure** (*wide pulse pressure = AR; narrow pulse pressure = AS*)

HEAD AND NECK

- **Face:** malar flush (*MS*)
- **Eyes:** conjunctival pallor (*anaemia*)/haemorrhages (*IE*), corneal arcus, xanthelasma (periorbital yellow plaques; *hyperlipidaemia*)
- **Mouth:** central cyanosis under tongue (*hypoxia*), petechial haemorrhages (*IE*), poor dental hygiene (*IE risk*), high-arched palate (*Marfan syndrome*)
- **Neck**
  - **JVP:** turn head slightly and look for double pulsation of internal jugular vein – up to 3cm above sternal angle is normal (*raised JVP =* **PQRST**: ***P**ulmonary hypertension/PE/PS/pericardial effusion, **Q**uantity of fluid i.e. overload, **R**VF, **S**VC obstruction, **T**amponade/TR*)
  - **Hepatojugular reflux test:** apply pressure over RUQ while observing JVP (*transient rise = normal; sustained rise = RVF*)
  - **Carotid pulse** <u>character and volume</u> (*slow-rising low volume = AS; bounding/collapsing = AR or patent ductus arteriosus*)
- **Others:** Corrigan's sign (visible carotid pulsation; *AR*), de Musset's sign (head bobbing in time with pulse; *AR*)

CHEST

- **Inspection:** chest deformities (pectus excavatum/carinatum), scars – ask them to lift up arms ± breasts (*see p115*), devices (*pacemaker, ICD, loop recorder*), visible apex beat, distended veins over precordium (*superior vena cava obstruction*)
- **Palpation**
  - **Apex beat position:** palpate with whole hand, then localise to a finger. Count down intercostal spaces with the other hand (*impalpable =* **DOPE**: ***D**extrocardia, **O**bese, **P**ericardial effusion, **E**mphysema; displaced = LV dilation (e.g. due to MR or AR), cardiomegaly, or displacement due to RV enlargement or mediastinal shift*)
  - **Apex beat character** (*heaving = high pressure pulsation in left ventricular hypertrophy, e.g. due to AS or systemic hypertension; thrusting = large area pulsation in volume overload, e.g. due to MR or AR; tapping = palpable S1 in MS*) *NB: if you cannot feel the it, roll patient into left lateral position and palpate during expiration to determine character.*
  - **Parasternal heave:** place the heel of your right hand over the patient's left lower parasternal edge with a straight elbow (*parasternal heave = RV hypertrophy, e.g. due to pulmonary hypertension or PS*)
  - **Thrills** and palpable heart sounds: palpate over valve areas with the pads of the fingers (*AS thrill most common; palpable S2 over pulmonary area = pulmonary hypertension*)

- **Auscultation:** auscultate all heart valves, using the stethoscope diaphragm unless otherwise stated. Simultaneously palpate the carotid pulse. Note S1 and S2 intensity and any splitting, S3/S4, clicks/snaps, rubs, and murmurs. If you hear a murmur, note: site heard loudest, pulse timing, character, volume and radiation.
  - **Mitral valve:** with patient lying at 45°, feel apex beat then place stethoscope over it. **Then** listen in the left axilla for radiation (*MR*). **Then** roll patient onto their left side and listen with the bell over the apex on <u>expiration</u> (*accentuates MS low tones*).
  - **Tricuspid valve**
  - **Pulmonary valve** + specifically listen for loud S2 in this position (*loud pulmonary S2 = pulmonary hypertension*)
  - **Aortic valve:** listen with patient lying at 45°. **Then** listen over right carotid artery with breath held for radiation (*AS*). **Then** sit patient forward and listen at Erb's point (3rd intercostal space, left sternal edge) on <u>expiration</u> (*accentuates AR*).

Murmurs: right valves heard better at full <u>i</u>nspiration, <u>l</u>eft valves at full <u>e</u>xpiration. Never put stethoscope on top of breast – listen in inframammary fold. Systolic murmurs (e.g. MR and AS) radiate. Diastolic murmurs (e.g. MS and AR) are quiet and need a manoeuvre to accentuate them.

FINALLY

- **Pulmonary oedema:** auscultate lung bases for fine crepitations while patient is still sitting (*LVF*)
- **Peripheral oedema:** push over the sacrum for 10 seconds, then run finger over feeling for indent (*RVF, hypoalbuminaemia*); do the same on the tibia (note how far it extends); also look for a vein grafting scar on the legs if the patient had a midline sternotomy scar (*CABG*)

TO COMPLETE

- Thank patient and restore clothing
- 'To complete my examination, I would examine for peripheral pulses, feel for hepatomegaly (*RVF*), look at observation charts and dipstick the urine (*haematuria in IE*).'
- Summarise and suggest further investigations you would consider after a full history

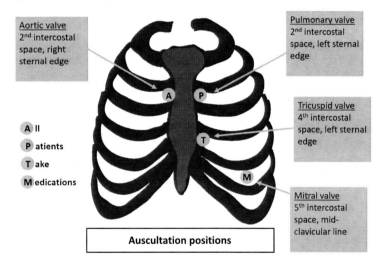

Auscultation positions

Aortic valve — 2nd intercostal space, right sternal edge
Pulmonary valve — 2nd intercostal space, left sternal edge
Tricuspid valve — 4th intercostal space, left sternal edge
Mitral valve — 5th intercostal space, mid-clavicular line

All **P**atients **T**ake **M**edications

Added/split heart sounds			
Sound		**Pathophysiology**	**Causes**
S4/atrial gallop (*before S1*)		Pressure overload: atrial contraction into stiff <u>hypertrophied</u> ventricle	• Left ventricular hypertrophy, hypertension, AS
S1 (AV valves close)	Soft S1	AV valves close with reduced velocity	• Reduced contraction pressure (severe heart failure) • Valves which don't close properly (MR) • Valves already partially closed at the end of diastole because atrial relaxation occurs before LV contraction (prolonged PR interval)
	Loud S1	AV valves close with higher velocity because they are wide open at end of diastole	• High atrial pressure (MS, AF) • Short diastole (short PR interval, tachycardia)
	Split S1	Asynchronous AV valve closure	• Can be normal but wide split may indicate RBBB or atrial septal defect
S2 (aortic/ pulmonary valves close)	Soft S2	Reduced aortic/pulmonary valve mobility	• AS, PS
	Loud S2	Valves close with higher velocity due to high upstream pressure	• Pulmonary hypertension (loud pulmonary valve closure) • Systemic hypertension (loud aortic valve closure)
	Split S2 on inspiration	Physiological: the aortic valve closes first because the pulmonary valve closure is slightly delayed by increased blood return to the right heart due to negative intrathoracic pressure	• Normal
	Wide split S2	Exaggerated split, which increases during inspiration (aortic valve closes before pulmonary valve)	• RBBB • Increased resistance to RV ejection, e.g. pulmonary hypertension/ PS
	Reverse split S2	Split which increases during expiration (pulmonary valve closes before aortic valve)	• LBBB • Increased resistance to LV ejection, e.g. systemic hypertension/AS
	Fixed split S2	No change with respiration	• Atrial septal defect
S3/ventricular gallop (*after S2*)		Volume overload: high volume of blood from atrium rapidly fills ventricle during passive filling phase of cardiac cycle	• LVF • Hyperdynamic states, e.g. athlete, anaemia, fever, thyrotoxicosis

CARDIAC MURMURS

Valve disease	Murmur character	Best heard (→ radiation)	Pathology	Symptoms	Signs	Causes
Systolic (radiate)						
Aortic stenosis (S1 — S2)	Ejection systolic (*differentiate from MR by separate S2*)	Upper right sternal edge (→ carotids and apex) *Loudest on expiration*	Increased resistance between left ventricle and systemic circulation → Limited cardiac output → LV hypertrophy	Exertional dyspnoea Syncope Angina (coronary perfusion impaired) May be signs of LVF (S3, pulmonary oedema)	Slow-rising pulse Narrow pulse pressure Heaving apex beat (pressure-loaded) Soft or absent S2 (depending on AS severity)	**ABCs** Age (senile calcification; most) Bicuspid aortic valve (e.g. Turner's syndrome) Congenital Strep-associated (rheumatic heart disease)
Aortic sclerosis (S1 — S2)	Ejection systolic	Upper right sternal edge (does not radiate)	Valve hard and inflexible (thickened NOT narrowed) → Turbulence → Local sound only	None	No abnormal signs (*differentiate from AS by normal pulse, apex and S2*)	Senile calcification (most)
Mitral regurgitation (S1 — S2)	Pansystolic	Upper left sternal edge *Loudest on expiration*	Backflow of blood from left ventricle to left atrium during systole → LV and left atrial dilation → Pulmonary hypertension	AF Dyspnoea Orthopnoea Paroxysmal nocturnal dyspnoea Fatigue Palpitations May be signs of LVF (S3, pulmonary oedema)	Displaced thrusting apex (volume-loaded) Soft S1 Signs of pulmonary hypertension (RV heave, loud P2)	Papillary muscle dysfunction (post-MI) Dilated cardiomyopathy Rheumatic heart disease Infective endocarditis Congenital Connective tissue disorders (e.g. Marfan's)
Mitral valve prolapse (S1 — CLICK — S2)	Mid-systolic click and/or late systolic murmur (*differentiate from MR by normal S1 then gap before murmur*)	Apex (→ left axilla and back) *Loudest on expiration*	In ventricular systole, a mitral valve leaflet prolapses to left atrium	Atypical chest pain	Murmur only Can develop significant MR	Associations: primary congenital, Marfan's, polycystic kidney disease, congenital heart disease, congestive cardiomyopathy, hypertrophic obstructive cardiomyopathy, myocarditis, Ehlers–Danlos, osteogenesis imperfecta, SLE, muscular dystrophy
Ventricular septal defect (S1 — S2)	Pansystolic loud machinery-like murmur	Lower left sternal edge (loud → whole precordium)	During systole some blood from left ventricle leaks into right ventricle	Often none if small	Signs of pulmonary hypertension (RV heave, loud P2) If acute, may cause cardiogenic shock	Congenital Complication of acute MI
Tricuspid regurgitation (S1 — S2)	Pansystolic (*differentiate from MR by seeing if louder on inspiration because it's on the right + giant JVP + non-displaced apex*)	Lower left sternal edge *Loudest on inspiration*	Backflow of blood from right ventricle to right atrium during systole → Increased right atrial and venous pressure	Fatigue Hepatic pain on exertion Ascites Peripheral oedema	Giant 'v' waves in JVP (*giant JVP waves without RV heave = TR*) Backflow signs (peripheral oedema, ascites, pulsatile hepatomegaly) Signs of lung disease and pulmonary hypertension (RV heave, loud P2) if that is the cause	Most commonly due to RV dilation in pulmonary hypertension (e.g. in chronic lung disease or left heart/valve disease) Rheumatic heart disease Infective endocarditis (IV drug user) Ebstein's anomaly (if split S1 and S2)
Diastolic (need to be accentuated)						
Mitral stenosis (S2 — OS — S1)	Low rumbling mid-diastolic with opening snap	Apex in left lateral position *Loudest on expiration using bell of stethoscope*	Increased resistance between left atrium and left ventricle → High left atrial pressure → Pulmonary hypertension	Dyspnoea Fatigue Haemoptysis Chest pain	Malar flush (due to low cardiac output) AF Tapping apex (palpable S1) Loud S1 Signs of pulmonary hypertension (RV heave, loud P2)	Rheumatic heart disease Others causes rare (e.g. congenital, carcinoid)
Aortic regurgitation (S2 — S1)	Early diastolic (Sounds like a breath)	Upper right sternal edge, or lower left sternal edge sitting forwards *Loudest on expiration*	Regurgitation of blood from aorta back into left ventricle during diastole → Increased left ventricular end-diastolic volume	Fatigue SOB Palpitations	Collapsing pulse Wide pulse pressure Very displaced thrusting apex (volume-loaded) Backflow signs: -Corrigan's (visible carotid pulsation) -de Musset's (head-nodding pulse) -Quincke's (red-coloured pulsation in nails) ±Austin Flint murmur (apical diastolic rumble)	**Acute causes** Infective endocarditis Aortic dissection **Chronic causes** Connective tissue disorders (e.g. Marfan syndrome, ankylosing spondylitis) Rheumatic heart disease Luetic heart disease (syphilis) Congenital/bicuspid aortic valve Longstanding hypertension

LV hypertrophy (e.g. due to stenosis on left side) = non-displaced heaving apex beat **vs.** *LV dilation (e.g. due to regurgitation on left side) = displaced thrusting apex beat*

CARDIAC CONDITION SIGNS

VALVULAR LESIONS

- *See notes on murmurs on previous page*

Assess for severity: e.g. severe **AS:** slow-rising pulse, narrow pulse pressure, S2 intensity; **AR:** collapsing pulse, wide pulse pressure, backflow signs, displaced apex, short early diastolic murmur; **MR:** AF, displaced apex, loud P2/RV heave (pulmonary hypertension); **MS:** AF, short gap between S2 and opening snap, loud P2/RV heave (pulmonary hypertension)
Assess for signs of cardiac decompensation: signs of heart failure
Assess for signs of infective endocarditis: splinter haemorrhages, Osler's nodes/Janeway lesions

VALVE REPLACEMENT

- *See viva notes on valve replacements p117*
- Midline sternotomy
- Abnormal S1 = mitral
- Abnormal S2 = aortic

Assess for valve function: signs of regurgitation or stenosis of replaced valve
Assess for signs of cardiac decompensation: signs of heart failure
Assess for signs of infective endocarditis: splinter haemorrhages, Osler's nodes/Janeway lesions
Assess for complications of over-anticoagulation: bruising, pale conjunctiva
Assess for haemolysis: jaundice, pale conjunctiva

HEART FAILURE

- Tachypnoea/tachycardia
- Cool peripheries
- Raised JVP
- Displaced apex
- S3 (ventricular gallop)
- Bi-basal fine crepitations
- Peripheral oedema

ATRIAL SEPTAL DEFECT

- Soft ejection systolic flow murmur (pulmonary area)
- Fixed, widely split S2
- RV heave

Signs of associations: low set ears/prominent epicanthic folds/flat nasal bridge (*Down's syndrome*), hypoplastic triphalangeal thumb/radial hypoplasia (*Holt-Oram syndrome*)
Signs of complications: loud P2 (*pulmonary hypertension*), peripheral oedema (*right heart failure*); cyanosis (*Eisenmenger's syndrome – late reversal of shunt*)

VENTRICULAR SEPTAL DEFECT

- Pansystolic murmur (loudest at left lower sternal edge)
- Associated thrill
- RV heave/loud P2

Signs of complications: raised JVP/peripheral oedema (*right heart failure*)

COR PULMONALE

- Plethoric facial appearance
- Central cyanosis
- Raised JVP (large 'a' waves)
- Giant V waves + pansystolic murmur (if secondary TR)
- Right ventricular heave
- Palpable/loud S2
- Ankle oedema

Signs of aetiology: end-inspiratory crepitations (*pulmonary fibrosis*), clubbing (*idiopathic pulmonary fibrosis*), signs of COPD

HYPERTROPHIC OBSTRUCTIVE CARDIOMYOPATHY

- Pacemaker/implantable cardioverter defibrillator
- Jerky pulse/pulsus bisferiens
- Double apex beat
- Ejection systolic murmur (left lower sternal edge)
- S4

Signs of complications: signs of heart failure

TETRALOGY OF FALLOT REPAIR

- Sternotomy scar (from repair)
- Lateral thoracotomy scar (if had Blalock-Taussig shunt)
- Left pulse weaker (if had Blalock-Taussig shunt)
- Clubbing
- Loud pulmonary stenosis

Signs of associations: syndromic features
Signs of complications: aortic regurgitation, raised JVP/peripheral oedema (*right heart failure*)

COARCTATION OF AORTA

Pre-repair
- Radio-femoral delay
- Weak left radial pulse (if stenosis proximal to left subclavian artery)
- Systolic vascular murmur over region of stenosis (most commonly left interscapular or left infraclavicular)
- Severe hypertension

Post-repair
- Left lateral thoracotomy scar

Signs of associations: short/webbed neck/short 4th metacarpals (*Turner syndrome*)
Signs of complications: splinter haemorrhages/Osler's nodes/Janeway lesions (*infective endocarditis*), severe hypertension, signs of heart failure

---

Characteristics of the JVP pulsation that help differentiate it from the carotid pulsation

- JVP has a double waveform
- JVP is not palpable
- JVP changes with position and descends with inspiration
- Abdominal pressure increases the JVP (hepatojugular reflux)

43

RESPIRATORY EXAMINATION

INTRODUCTION
- **W**ash hands; **I**ntroduce self; ask **P**atient's name, DOB and what they like to be called; **E**xplain examination and obtain consent
- Expose and **sit patient at 45°**

GENERAL INSPECTION
- **Patient wellbeing:** well/unwell, alert, comfortable, breathless, cachexic (*malignancy, emphysema*), cushingoid (*steroid use*)
- **General breathing:** use of accessory muscles (*COPD, pleural effusion, pneumothorax, severe asthma*), pursed-lip breathing (*prevents bronchial wall collapse by keeping airway pressure high in severe airway obstruction/emphysema*)
- **Noises:** speech abnormalities (*e.g. in recurrent laryngeal nerve palsy*), stridor (*large airway obstruction e.g. mediastinal masses, bronchial carcinoma, retrosternal thyroid*), wheeze, cough (dry/productive/bovine), prolonged expiratory phase (*asthma, COPD*), clicks (*bronchiectasis*), gurgling (*airway secretions*)
- **Around the bed:** oxygen, medication (e.g. inhalers, nebulisers), sputum pots (look at sputum), cigarettes

HANDS
- **Tremors**
  - **Fine tremor:** patient should hold arms out straight, with their fingers spread (*β2 agonists*)
  - **Flapping tremor:** patient should hold their arms out straight, with their wrists 'cocked back' (*flap = CO_2 retention*)
- **Perfusion:** peripheral cyanosis (*hypoxia or hypoperfusion*), capillary refill (*>2 seconds in hypoperfusion*), sweaty/warm/clammy (*CO_2 retention*), small muscle wasting (*Pancoast tumour*)
- **Nails:** clubbing (*idiopathic pulmonary fibrosis, lung cancer, CF, bronchiectasis*), tar-stained fingers (*smoker*)

PULSE AND RESPIRATORY RATE
- **Pulse:** rate and rhythm (*tachycardia may indicate: hypoxia in severe asthma or COPD, PE or infection*), bounding pulse (i.e. increased up-stroke and down-stroke; *CO_2 retention*)
- **Count respiratory rate** (while patient still thinks you are feeling pulse): tachypnoea (*lung disease, infection, hyperventilation, fever, PE*), bradypnoea (*central nervous system depression*)

HEAD AND NECK
- **Face:** cushingoid (*steroid use*), plethoric (*secondary polycythaemia; Cushing's syndrome; superior vena cava obstruction if facial swelling*), telangiectasia/microstomia (*systemic sclerosis*), butterfly rash (*SLE*), lupus pernio (*sarcoid*), lupus vulgaris (*TB*)
- **Eyes:** conjunctival pallor (*anaemia of chronic disease*), Horner's syndrome (ptosis, miosis, anhidrosis; *Pancoast tumour*)
- **Mouth:** central cyanosis under tongue (*hypoxia*)
- **Neck**
  - **JVP height** (*raised in cor pulmonale*)
  - **Tracheal deviation:** place your right hand's index and ring fingers on each clavicle head. Roll your middle finger over the trachea in the sternal notch. (*Pneumothorax pushes to contralateral side; collapsed lung pulls to ipsilateral side.*)
  - **Cricosternal distance and tracheal tug:** place your right hand's index on the inferior border of the cricoid. Now place subsequent fingers in the midline until you reach the sternal notch (*<3 fingers = lung hyperinflation*). Note reduction in inspiration (*'tracheal tug'*).

CHEST
You should examine the front first and repeat everything on the back afterwards.
- **Inspection**
  - **Chest wall:** scars (look under arms as well as on back; *see p115*), skin changes, trauma, deformities (*pectus carinatum may be related to childhood respiratory disease; pectus excavatum may be related to connective tissue disease; barrel chest in emphysema or COPD*), kyphosis/scoliosis (*restrict chest movements*), radiotherapy tattoos
  - **Chest wall movements:** mainly upwards (*emphysema*), asymmetrical (*fibrosis, collapsed lung, pneumonectomy, pleural effusion, pneumothorax*)
  - **Breathing:** in-drawing of intercostal muscles (*generalised = hyperinflation; localised = bronchial obstruction*), powerful expirations (*asthma, COPD*), hyperexpanded chest (*COPD*)
- **Palpation**
  - **Supramammary and inframammary chest wall expansion:** grip very hard around rib cage with thumbs in the air almost touching in expiration. Watch thumbs move away from each other during inspiration (normally ≥5cm).
  - Feel for RV heave (*pulmonary hypertension*)

- **Percussion:** compare left with right – start above clavicles and progress down to axilla (normally resonant; *dull = consolidation or collapse; stony dull = pleural effusion; hyperresonant = increased air space, e.g. in pneumothorax or emphysema*)

  NB: the liver starts at the 5th intercostal space on the right.

- **Auscultation**
  - **Standard auscultation:** ask patient to breathe in and out deeply. Compare sides in turn, starting in supraclavicular area and ending in axillae.
  - **Vocal resonance:** listen in all areas again while the patient repeats 'ninety-nine' (*increased resonance = consolidation; decreased resonance = effusion/pneumothorax*)
  - Listen for loud S2 over pulmonary valve area (*loud pulmonary S2 = pulmonary hypertension*)

- **Repeat all on back:** now ask patient to sit over bedside with crossed arms and percuss, auscultate and assess vocal resonance again on the back

Decreased air entry	Emphysema, pneumothorax, pleural effusion, collapse
Wheeze	Asthma, COPD
Coarse crepitations	Bronchiectasis, consolidation
Fine inspiratory crepitations	Pulmonary oedema
Fine end-inspiratory crepitations (like Velcro)	Pulmonary fibrosis
Bronchial breathing (harsh breath sounds)	Consolidation
Pleural rub (grating sound)	Pleurisy, pulmonary infarction, pneumonia, pleural malignancy

FINALLY

- **Cervical lymph nodes:** examine for lymphadenopathy from posteriorly while patient still sitting (*infection, carcinoma, lymphoma, sarcoidosis*)
- **Legs:** peripheral oedema (*cor pulmonale*), feel calves (*swollen/tender = DVT*)

TO COMPLETE

- Thank patient and restore clothing
- 'To complete my examination, I would like to review the observations chart (*particularly to see oxygen saturations*), and measure peak flow (*if asthmatic*).'
- Summarise and suggest further investigations you would consider after a full history

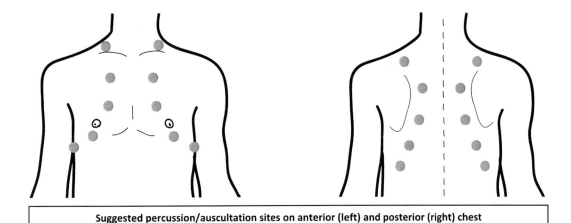

Suggested percussion/auscultation sites on anterior (left) and posterior (right) chest

Examination findings in common respiratory conditions				
	Pneumothorax	**Pneumonia**	**Pleural effusion**	**Collapse**
Tracheal displacement	Away	None	Away (if large)	Towards collapse
Expansion	All reduced ipsilaterally			
Percussion resonance	Increased	Decreased	Stony-dull	Decreased
Breath sounds	Reduced/absent	Bronchial breathing + coarse crepitations	Reduced/absent	Reduced/absent

NB: signs are on side of lesion unless otherwise stated.

PULMONARY FIBROSIS

- Oxygen therapy
- Dry cough
- Tachypnoea
- Reduced expansion
- Fine end-inspiratory crepitations

Signs of aetiology: hand deformity (*RA*), clubbing (*idiopathic pulmonary fibrosis*), sclerodactyly/telangiectasia/microstomia (*systemic sclerosis*), butterfly rash (*SLE*), lupus pernio (*sarcoid*), radiation burns, kyphosis (*ankylosing spondylitis*)
Signs of complications: cushingoid/bruising (*steroid use*), loud P2/RV heave (*pulmonary hypertension*)

COPD

- Bedside inhalers/nebulisers
- Accessory muscle use
- Tar-stained fingers
- Tachypnoea
- Lip pursing
- Reduced cricosternal distance (<3 fingers)
- Tracheal tug
- Indrawing of lower intercostal muscles on inspiration
- Hyper-resonance (with obliterated cardiac and hepatic dullness)
- Quiet breath sounds/wheeze/prolonged expiratory phase

Signs of complications: cushingoid/bruising (*steroid use*), loud P2/RV heave (*pulmonary hypertension*)

PNEUMONECTOMY

- Unilateral chest flattening
- Thoracotomy scar
- Tracheal deviation (towards)
- Reduced expansion
- Dull percussion note
- Reduced breath sounds
- Bronchial breathing in upper zone (due to deviated trachea

Signs of aetiology: cachexia/clubbed/tar-stained fingers (*lung cancer*)

LOBECTOMY

- Thoracotomy scar
- May be no other signs due to compensatory hyperexpansion of the remaining lobes
- May be some reduced expansion, dullness to percussion and reduced air entry

Signs of aetiology: cachexia/clubbed/tar-stained fingers (*lung cancer*), wet cough/clubbed/coarse crepitations (*bronchiectasis*), signs of COPD (*bullectomy*)

PLEURAL EFFUSION

- Reduced expansion
- Stony dull percussion note
- Reduced breath sounds
- Reduced tactile fremitus and vocal resonance

Signs of aetiology: hand deformity (*RA*), clubbing/radiation marks (*mesothelioma/lung malignancy*), butterfly rash (*SLE*), lymphadenopathy (*malignancy*), signs of chronic liver disease (*cirrhosis*), pulmonary/peripheral oedema (*heart failure*)

BRONCHIECTASIS

- Productive cough
- Inspiratory clicks
- Clubbing
- Coarse, late expiratory crepitations

Signs of aetiology: young and thin (*CF*), curved yellow nails and lymphoedema (*yellow nail syndrome*), lymphadenopathy (*malignancy*), dextrocardia (*Kartagener's syndrome*)

KYPHOSCOLIOSIS

- Increased thoracic forward curvature *or* lateral curvature of the spine
- Reduced spine flexion/extension
- Rib hump
- Reduced chest expansion

LUNG CANCER

- Cachexia
- Clubbing
- Tar-stained fingers
- Hard irregular lymphadenopathy
- Radiation burns

Signs of complications: pain and swelling of wrists (*hypertrophic pulmonary arthropathy*), ptosis/meiosis/anhidrosis (*Horner's syndrome*)

LUNG TRANSPLANT

- Mid-sternotomy/bilateral thoracotomy scar

Signs of aetiology: signs of COPD, clubbing (*CF/idiopathic pulmonary fibrosis*)
Signs of complications: cushingoid/bruising (*steroid use*)

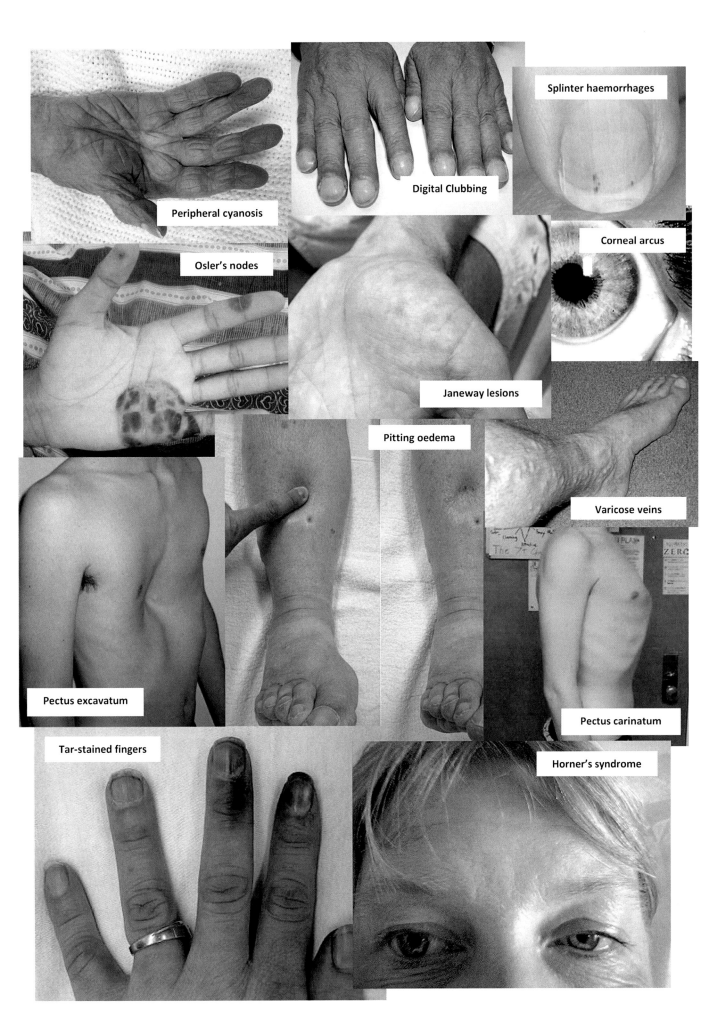

Peripheral cyanosis

Digital Clubbing

Splinter haemorrhages

Osler's nodes

Corneal arcus

Janeway lesions

Pitting oedema

Varicose veins

Pectus excavatum

Pectus carinatum

Tar-stained fingers

Horner's syndrome

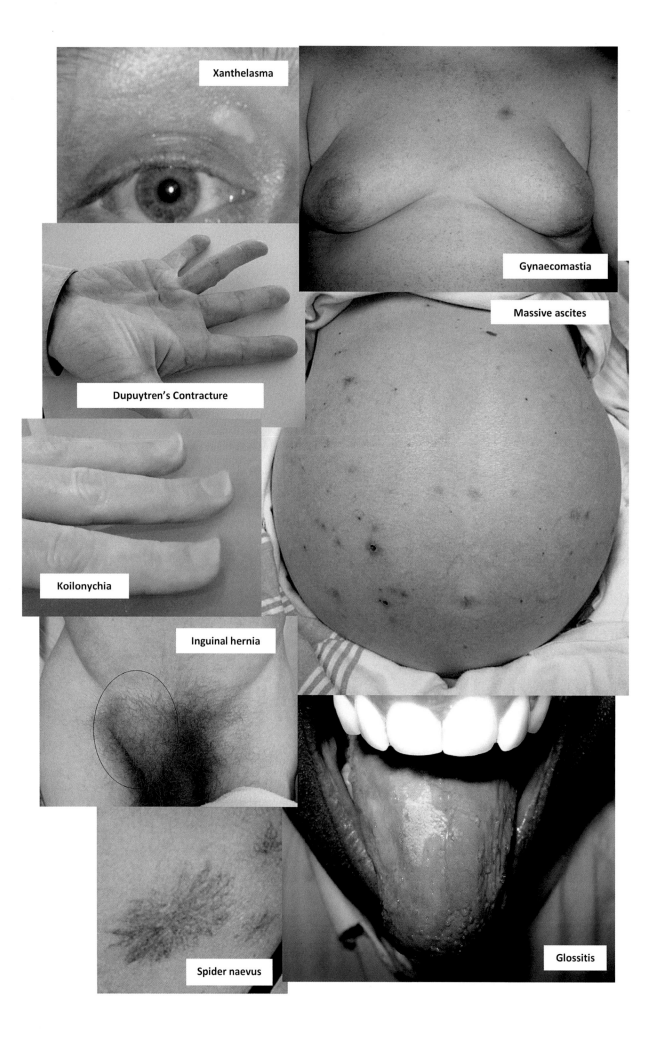

PERIPHERAL ARTERIAL EXAMINATION

You may be asked to focus on the lower limbs – if so, do this after general inspection.

Anatomical landmarks of peripheral pulses

• **Femoral:** midpoint between the ASIS and pubic symphysis (the 'mid-inguinal point')
• **Popliteal:** bimanually palpated with knee slightly flexed, thumbs on tibial tuberosity and finders deep in popliteal fossa
• **Posterior tibial:** halfway between medial malleolus and Achilles tendon
• **Dorsalis pedis:** between first and second metatarsals, lateral to extensor hallucis longus tendon

INTRODUCTION

- **W**ash hands; **I**ntroduce self; ask **P**atient's name, DOB and what they like to be called; **E**xplain examination and obtain consent
- **Lie patient flat** and expose legs

GENERAL INSPECTION

- **Patient:** well/unwell, pain/discomfort, any amputations
- **Risk factors:** age, body habitus
- **Around bed:** oxygen, mobility aids, medications (e.g. insulin), cigarettes, capillary glucose monitor

UPPER LIMBS

- **Inspection:** skin colour changes (pink, pale, mottled), ischaemic changes (e.g. gangrene), tar-stained fingers, tendon xanthomata, capillary glucose testing marks
- **Palpation:**
  1. Temperature (*cool = reduced peripheral perfusion*)
  2. Capillary refill (should be <2 seconds)
  3. Pulses: radial pulse; radio-radial delay (*aortic dissection/aneurysm or proximal coarctation*); offer to test for radio-femoral delay (*aortic coarctation*); brachial pulse; and blood pressure in both arms (*>10mmHg difference = significant and suggests aortic dissection, proximal coarctation or subclavian artery stenosis*)

FACE

- **Eyes:** corneal arcus, xanthelasma (*hyperlipidaemia*)
- **Mouth:** central cyanosis
- **Carotid pulse:** feel character (*see cardiac exam p40*), auscultate for bruits (*carotid artery stenosis*)

ABDOMEN

- **Inspection:** body habitus, scars, visible aortic pulsation
- **Aortic and femoral pulses:** palpate pulses, auscultate for bruits (*'machinery' aortic bruit = AAA*)
NB: to palpate the aorta, press down with finger tips (one hand each side) in the horizontal plane midway between the umbilicus and xiphoid process, starting laterally and moving medially. The ulnar borders of your hands should be parallel with the costal margins. (Pulsatile mass, i.e. upward movement, can be normal; expansile mass, i.e. outward movement, suggests AAA.)

LOWER LIMBS (MAIN PART)

Check for pain in legs. Examine with patient standing and then lying supine.
- **Inspection** (especially feet)
  - Skin colour changes (pink, pale, mottled)
  - Ischaemic changes: especially between toes and heels – don't miss toe amputations!
  - Trophic changes (shiny skin, hair loss, thin skin, ulcers – *types of ulcers described p159*)
  - Muscle wasting
  - Ankle oedema
  - Scars – ensure you also expose the femoral region (*e.g. bypass operations, venous grafting*)
- **Palpation**
  1. Temperature: along length of leg (*cool = reduced peripheral perfusion*)
  2. Capillary refill (should be <2 seconds)
  3. Pulses: feel pulses starting proximally (femoral, popliteal, posterior tibial, dorsalis pedis); squeeze calves (*tenderness may suggest critical ischaemia or DVT*); check peripheral sensation
- **Buerger's angle** and filling/reperfusion time
  - Check for any pain in leg
  - With patient lying supine, lift their leg until heel becomes pale then hold for 30 seconds (if it does not become pale, test is normal; if it becomes pale, the degree of hip flexion is Buerger's angle)
  - Now ask patient to sit up and hang their legs over the edge of the bed
  - Watch their feet for 2-3 minutes
  - Pallor followed by reactive hyperaemia (rubor) on dependency is a positive test and implies significant peripheral arterial disease

TO COMPLETE

- Thank patient and restore clothing
- 'To complete my examination, I would perform a full cardiovascular examination, test sensation, and use Doppler ultrasound to further assess pulses.'
- Summarise and suggest further investigations you would consider after a full history (e.g. ABPI, duplex USS, MR or CT angiography, catheter angiography, bloods, ulcer swabs, ECG, HbA1C etc.)

Vascular bypass procedures				
Procedure	Details	Indication	Signs on examination	Scars
Aortobifemoral	Aorta to both femoral arteries (*open operation*)	Aortoiliac occlusive disease *Axillofemoral used for patients who are unable to tolerate aortobifemoral (often elderly patients or patients with significant comorbidities)*	•Midline laparotomy scar •Bilateral groin scars	
Axillofemoral/ axillobifemoral	Axillary artery to one/both femoral arteries (*graft tunnelled subcutaneously*)		•Axillary scar •Unilateral/bilateral groin scars •Graft may be palpable	
Femorofemoral	Femoral artery to femoral artery (*graft tunnelled subcutaneously or in pre-peritoneal space*)	Unilateral iliac disease	•Bilateral groin scars •Graft may be palpable	
Iliofemoral	Iliac artery to femoral artery (*iliac artery on ipsilateral or contralateral side may be used*)		•Two groin scars (may be on the same or opposite sides depending on operation)	
Femoropopliteal Femorotibial Femorodistal	Femoral artery to popliteal artery, a tibial artery or distally (*graft may be tunnelled subcutaneously or anatomically*)	Femoropopliteal disease	•Groin scar •Medial lower leg scar •Graft may be palpable	

NB: graft is usually a patient's vein, but a synthetic graft may also be used.

Specific conditions

- Intermittent claudication: calf pain on exertion that is relieved by rest; ABPI <0.9
- Acute ischaemic limb: **6 P's** **P**ale, **P**ulseless, **P**araesthesia, **P**aralysis, **P**ain, **P**erishingly cold
- Critical ischaemia: tissue loss + chronic rest pain + ABPI <0.3
- Abdominal aortic aneurysm
- Carotid artery stenosis
- Femoral artery aneurysm
- Cholesterol embolism ('trash foot')
- Post-bypass peripheral arterial disease

Measuring ABPI using Doppler USS

- Measure the brachial SBP of both arms (place the Doppler probe at 45° over the brachial artery, inflate the cuff over the upper arm until the Doppler signal stops, then gradually deflate it – the SBP is the cuff pressure at which the Doppler signal returns)
- Measure the ankle SBP of both legs (repeat the above procedure but with the cuff around the lower shin and the Doppler probe over the dorsalis pedis or posterior tibial artery)
- Right ABPI = right ankle SBP / highest brachial SBP from either arm
- Left ABPI = left ankle SBP / highest brachial SBP from either arm

DVT EXAMINATION

INTRODUCTION
- **W**ash hands; **I**ntroduce self; ask **P**atient's name, DOB and what they like to be called; **E**xplain examination and obtain consent
- Expose the patient's legs. Check for any pain in legs.

GENERAL INSPECTION
- **Patient:** well/unwell, breathless, pain/discomfort
- **DVT risks:** signs of malignancy (e.g. cachexia), signs of immobility (e.g. walking aids), signs of recent surgery or trauma, pregnancy
- **Around bed:** medicines etc.

LEG INSPECTION
Inspect with the patient standing.
- **Skin:** colour changes
- **Ankle/leg swelling** (*unilateral may indicate DVT; bilateral may indicate oedema, e.g. in heart failure*)
- **Venous insufficiency signs**
  1. Venous eczema and haemosiderin deposits (red-brown patches)
  2. Lipodermatosclerosis ('inverted champagne bottle leg'; increased venous pressure causes inflammatory cells to fibrose subcutaneous tissue)
  3. Venous ulcers
- **Venous dilatation and tortuosity** (*varicose veins*)

PALPATION
Palpate with the patient supine.
- **Temperature:** feel for temperature differences between legs (minimum three places each side)
- **Tenderness:** palpate for calf tenderness with knee slightly flexed (squeeze near ankle and then up calves while watching face)
- **Pitting oedema:** if present, establish how far oedema extends (and also check JVP)
- **Calf diameters:** measure circumference 10 cm below tibial tuberosity (>3cm difference = significant)
- **Palpate pulses**

TO COMPLETE
- Thank patient and restore clothing
- 'To complete my examination, I would perform full cardiovascular and respiratory examinations. I would review the patient's observations, including oxygen saturations and respiratory rate. If these are abnormal, I would consider the possibility of a pulmonary embolism.'
- Summarise and suggest further investigations you would consider after a full history, for example:
  - FBC, U&Es (if anticoagulation is needed, choice depends on renal function), coagulation blood tests
  - D-dimer if *DVT Wells score* <2 (can rule out DVT)
  - If Wells score ≥2 or positive D-dimer: compression ultrasound (shows veins not collapsing under pressure)

NB: the DVT Wells score takes into account risk factors (cancer, patient immobility/recent surgery, leg immobility, previous DVT), symptoms (calf swelling >3cm, whole leg swelling, venous tenderness, unilateral oedema, presence of superficial veins), and likelihood of an alternative diagnosis (Wells et al. 2003).

VARICOSE VEINS FOCUSSED EXAMINATION

INTRODUCTION
- **W**ash hands; **I**ntroduce self; ask **P**atient's name, DOB and what they like to be called; **E**xplain examination and obtain consent
- Expose patient's legs and feet. Check for any pain in legs.

GENERAL INSPECTION
- **Patient:** well/unwell, breathless, pain/discomfort

LEG INSPECTION
- **Observe gait**
- **Inspection:** ask patient to stand and inspect carefully from all angles, then inspect again with patient lying supine
  - Skin: colour changes
  - Ankle/leg swelling (*DVT, heart failure*)
  - Venous insufficiency (describe)
    1. Venous eczema and haemosiderin deposits (damaged capillaries leak blood → red-brown patches)
    2. Lipodermatosclerosis (inflammation of subcutaneous fat → woody hard skin, pigmentation, swelling, redness, 'inverted champagne bottle leg')
    3. Venous ulcers/*atrophie blanche*
- **Venous dilatation and tortuosity** (*varicose veins*)
  - Distribution (long saphenous vein is all the way up the medial part of the leg; short saphenous vein is up the posterolateral part of the lower leg)
  - Colour
  - Prominence

PALPATION
- **Varicosities:** palpate all the way along varicosities for tenderness and hardness (*phlebitis*)
- **Saphenofemoral junction:** 2.5cm below and 2.5cm lateral to pubic tubercle
  - Feel for a saphena varix (large varicosity at saphenofemoral junction)
  - Ask patient to cough and feel for thrills/dilatations (*suggest saphena varix*)
- **Elevate limb** to 15° and note rate of venous emptying
- **Trendelenburg (/tourniquet) test:** if varicosities present, this can determine the location of venous regurgitation
  - Lift patient's leg as high as comfortable and milk leg to empty veins
  - While leg is elevated, apply tourniquet or press your thumb over saphenofemoral junction
  - Ask patient to stand while you maintain pressure over the saphenofemoral junction
  - Rapid filling of the varicosities with the tourniquet still on suggests incompetent perforator veins lie below the level of the saphenofemoral junction
  - Now repeat the test, moving the tourniquet down 3cm each time. When varicosities do not refill, the incompetent perforator is above the tourniquet but below where it was previously applied.
- **Calf tenderness** (*DVT*)

PERCUSSION AND AUSCULTATION
- **Percussion wave of varicosities:** tap distally and feel impulse proximally (*normal*); tap proximally and feel impulse distally (*incompetent valves*)
- **Auscultate** varicosities for a machinery–like rumbling sound if you suspect an *arteriovenous fistula*

FINALLY
- **Pitting oedema:** if present, establish how far oedema extends and also check JVP at 45°
- **Palpate arterial pulses**

TO COMPLETE
- Thank patient and restore clothing
- 'To complete my examination, I would perform full abdominal and pelvic examinations (*for masses causing venous obstruction*).'
- Summarise and suggest further investigations you would do after a full history (e.g. duplex USS)

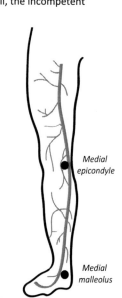

Medial epicondyle

Medial malleolus

Long saphenous vein

ABDOMINAL EXAMINATION

INTRODUCTION

- Wash hands; Introduce self; ask Patient's name, DOB and what they like to be called; Explain examination and obtain consent
- Expose and **lie patient flat**

GENERAL INSPECTION

- **Patient:** well/unwell, pain/discomfort, jaundice, pallor, muscle wasting/cachexia
- **Around bed:** vomit bowls, intravenous infusions, nutrition, catheter etc.

HANDS

- **Flapping tremor**: patient should hold their arms out straight, with their wrists 'cocked back' (*flap = hepatic encephalopathy*)
- **Nails:** clubbing (*cirrhosis, IBD, coeliac disease*), leukonychia (*hypoalbuminaemia in liver cirrhosis/enteropathy*), koilonychia (*iron deficiency*)
- **Palms:** palmar erythema (*hyperdynamic circulation due to ↑oestrogen levels in liver disease/pregnancy*), Dupuytren's contracture (*can be related to alcoholism/liver disease*), fingertip capillary glucose monitoring marks (*diabetes*)

FACE

- **Eyes:** sclera for jaundice (*liver disease*), conjunctival pallor (*anaemia, e.g. due to GI bleeding, malabsorption*), periorbital xanthelasma (*hyperlipidaemia in cholestasis*)
- **Mouth:** glossitis/stomatitis (*iron/B$_{12}$ deficiency*), aphthous ulcers (*IBD*), breath odour (*e.g. feculent in obstruction; fruity/ketotic in ketoacidosis; sweet/fetor hepaticus in portal hypertension; alcohol odour*)

NECK AND TORSO

Ask patient to sit forwards:
- **Neck:** examine for cervical lymphadenopathy from posteriorly – especially Virchow's node in left supraclavicular fossa (*classically gastric malignancy*)
- **Back inspection:** spider naevi (significant if >5), skin lesions (*immunosuppression*)

Ask patient to sit back:
- **Chest inspection:** spider naevi (significant if >5), gynaecomastia, loss of axillary hair (*all due to ↑oestrogen levels in liver disease/pregnancy*)

ABDOMEN

- **Inspection:** scars (*see p116*), distension (**5Fs:** *Fluid, Flatus, Fat, Fetus, Faeces*), striae (*pregnancy, Cushing's syndrome*), spider naevi, umbilical/incisional/spigelian hernias (ask patient to cough), movement with respiration (*absent in peritonitis*), obvious pulsations, distended abdominal wall veins/'caput medusae' (*portal hypertension*), stomas (*see p130*)
- **Palpation:** first ask if the patient has any pain and begin palpation away from painful areas

Superficial palpation	Crouch to patient's level and gently roll fingers of your right hand over each of the nine regions while watching the patient's face. Check for: tenderness, guarding (*peritonitis*), rebound tenderness (*peritonitis*).
Deep palpation	Palpate again but deeply using both hands – the upper hand to exert pressure, the lower hand to feel. (You can be standing for this.) Check for: masses, deep tenderness and, if relevant, Rovsing's sign (*appendicitis*) and Murphy's sign (*cholecystitis*).
Liver palpation	Ask the patient to breathe in and out deeply. Using the radial border of the right hand, palpate in increments from the RIF to the right costal margin – push in on each inspiration. (*Hepatomegaly may be caused by: metastasis/hepatocellular carcinoma, hepatitis, RVF, leukaemia/lymphoma, fatty liver, alcoholic liver disease.*)
Spleen palpation	Palpate the spleen in the same way as the liver, but diagonally from the RIF to the left costal margin. The spleen can be felt better if patient rolls onto their right side with tucked legs. (*Splenomegaly may be caused by: lymphoma/leukaemia, myelofibrosis, myeloproliferative disorders, portal hypertension, extravascular haemolysis, malaria/EBV.*) ***Spleen vs. kidney:*** *cannot get above spleen, spleen notched, spleen not ballotable, spleen moves down on inspiration*
Kidney palpation	One hand anterior and one posterior. Ask patient to expire as you press up into renal angle with your posterior hand and press down with your anterior hand. As patient breathes in, you may feel the kidney between your hands. Ballot the kidney by flexing the MCP joints of your posterior hand. Do *flick, flick, stop* and then repeat as necessary.
Aorta palpation	Press down with finger tips (one hand each side) in the horizontal plane midway between the umbilicus and xiphoid process, starting laterally and moving medially. The ulnar borders of your hands should be parallel with the costal margins. (*Pulsatile mass, i.e. upward movement, can be normal; expansile mass, i.e. outward movement, suggests AAA.*)

- **Percussion**
  - o **General percussion quality** (*tympanic = flatus; percussion tenderness = peritoneal irritation*)
  - o **Liver:** percuss upwards from the RIF to find the lower border of the liver (normally beneath right costal margin). The percussion note should become dull over the liver. Next, percuss the chest downwards in the right mid-clavicular line to find the upper border of the liver (normally beneath 5th costal cartilage). Ideally, percuss with the patient in expiration.
  - o **Spleen:** percuss diagonally from the RIF towards the spleen. The dull percussion note of the spleen is only heard when it is enlarged. Also percuss in Traube's space, which is just above the left costal margin in the mid-clavicular line (*if resonant, there is no splenomegaly*).
  - o **Flank:** percuss all the way across abdomen in each direction laterally from the midline. The flank should be resonant. If a dull percussion note is heard, go on to demonstrate **shifting dullness** (have patient roll to other side and percuss again – *it should become resonant if the cause is ascites*). You could also demonstrate **fluid thrill** (have patient press hand firmly on abdominal midline while you tap one side and feel the other; *fluid wave = ascites*).
- **Auscultation**
  - o Use diaphragm to listen for bowel sounds at ileocaecal valve in RLQ until heard, up to 1 minute (*tinkling = obstruction; absent = paralytic ileus/peritonitis*)
  - o Use bell to listen for aortic bruit (midline between xiphisternum and umbilicus; *may indicate AAA*); and renal bruits (5cm superior and lateral to umbilicus bilaterally; *renal artery stenosis*)

FINALLY

- Check for **pitting oedema** (*hypoalbuminaemia*)

TO COMPLETE

- Thank patient and restore clothing
- 'To complete my examination, I would examine the external hernial orifices, the external genitalia, and perform a digital rectal examination.'
- Summarise and suggest further investigations you would consider after a full history

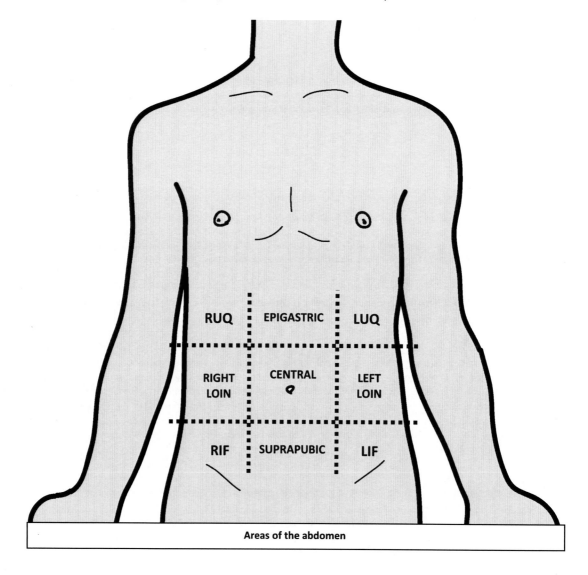

Areas of the abdomen

CHRONIC LIVER DISEASE

- Clubbing
- Leukonychia
- Palmar erythema
- Dupuytren's contracture
- Jaundice
- Spider naevi
- Gynaecomastia
- Loss of axillary hair
- Distended abdominal wall veins/'caput medusae' *(portal hypertension)*
- Hepatomegaly (but liver is often small in cirrhosis)
- Splenomegaly *(portal hypertension)*
- Ascites

Signs of aetiology: Afro-Caribbean (*sarcoid*), slate-grey pigmentation/capillary glucose monitoring marks (*haemochromatosis*), track marks/tattoos (*hepatitis C*), xanthelasma (*PBC*), goitre/middle-aged female (*autoimmune*), emphysema (*α1-antitrypsin deficiency*)
Signs of decompensation: flapping tremor/confusion *(encephalopathy)*, jaundice, ascites

TRANSPLANTED KIDNEY

- Old AV fistula
- Rutherford-Morrison scar (usually RIF)
- Smooth mass underlying scar (transplanted kidney)

Signs of aetiology: fingertip capillary glucose monitoring marks (*diabetes*), hearing aid (*Alport syndrome*), collapsed nasal bridge (*granulomatosis with polyangiitis*), butterfly rash (*SLE*), sternotomy (*renovascular disease*), flank masses (*PKD*)
Functionality: flap/excoriations (*uraemia*), active marks in AV fistula, pale conjunctiva (*anaemia*), fluid retention
Previous renal replacement therapy: AV fistula, central line and peritoneal dialysis scars
Complications of immunosuppression: tremor (*calcineurin inhibitor*), cushingoid/bruising (*steroids*), skin lesions/excisions (*immunosuppression*)

HEPATOSPLENOMEGALY

- Hepatomegaly/splenomegaly/both

Signs of hepatomegaly aetiology: signs of chronic liver disease, lymphadenopathy (*malignancy/lymphoma*), peripheral oedema/raised JVP (*right ventricular failure*)
Signs of splenomegaly aetiology: hand deformity (*RA/Felty's syndrome*), signs of chronic liver disease, pale conjunctiva (*leukaemia/myeloproliferative/haemolytic anaemia*), lymphadenopathy (*lymphoma*)

POLYCYSTIC KIDNEYS

- AV fistula (if undergone dialysis)
- Hypertension
- Pale conjunctiva (anaemia)
- Flank scar (if either kidney has been removed)
- Bilateral ballotable flank masses
- Hepatomegaly (hepatic cysts)

LIVER TRANSPLANT

- Signs of chronic liver disease (but most resolve)
- Mercedes Benz modification scar

Signs of aetiology: Afro-Caribbean (*sarcoid*), slate-grey pigmentation/capillary glucose monitoring marks (*haemochromatosis*), track marks/tattoos (*hepatitis C*), xanthelasma (*PBC*), goitre/middle-aged female (*autoimmune*), emphysema (*α1-antitrypsin deficiency*)
Complications of immunosuppression: tremor (*calcineurin inhibitor*), cushingoid/bruising (*steroids*), skin lesions/excisions (*immunosuppression*)

COMBINED KIDNEY-PANCREAS TRANSPLANT

- LIF scar (renal graft)
- RIF scar (pancreas graft)
- Smooth mass underlying LIF scar (transplanted kidney)

Signs of diabetic complications: visual aids (*retinopathy*), Charcot joints, toe ulcers/amputations, neuropathy
Renal graft functionality: flap/excoriations (*uraemia*), active marks in AV fistula, pale conjunctiva (*anaemia*), fluid retention
Pancreas graft functionality: fingertip capillary glucose monitoring marks, insulin injection marks
Previous renal replacement therapy: AV fistula, central line and peritoneal dialysis scars (but transplant may have been done pre-emptively)
Complications of immunosuppression: tremor (*calcineurin inhibitor*), cushingoid/bruising (*steroids*), skin lesions/excisions (*immunosuppression*)

POLYCYTHAEMIA RUBRA VERA

- Dusky cyanosis
- Hypertension
- Facial plethora
- Splenomegaly

HEREDITARY SPHEROCYTOSIS

- Pale conjunctiva
- Mild jaundice
- Splenomegaly

PRIMARY BILIARY CHOLANGITIS

- Middle-aged female
- Jaundice
- Skin hyperpigmentation
- Excoriations
- Xanthelasma
- Hepatomegaly

Signs of complications: signs of chronic liver disease

RENAL EXAMINATION

As you examine, look for evidence of renal disease aetiology, graft function (if transplant present), and complications of immunosuppression.

INTRODUCTION

- **W**ash hands; **I**ntroduce self; ask **P**atient's name, DOB and what they like to be called; **E**xplain examination and obtain consent
- Expose and **lie patient flat**

GENERAL INSPECTION

- **Patient:** well/unwell, pain/discomfort, muscle wasting/cachexia, cushingoid appearance, confusion, excoriations (*uraemic pruritus*), breathless (*fluid overload*)
- **Around bed:** dialysis machine, fluid charts

HANDS

- **Tremors:** postural tremor (*calcineurin inhibitor side effect*), flapping tremor (*uraemia*)
- **Nails:** leukonychia (*hypoalbuminaemia in nephrotic syndrome*), koilonychia (*iron deficiency anaemia in nephritic syndrome*)
- **Fingertips:** fingertip capillary glucose monitoring marks (*diabetes*)
- **Pulse:** rate and volume (*tachycardia and low volume may be due to blood loss*)
- **Arms:** arteriovenous fistula (look for active needle marks to see if it's being used), bruising (*Cushing's syndrome*), blood pressure (*may be high due to hypertension, in renal graft rejection, or due a to calcineurin inhibitor*), skin lesions (*immunosuppression*)

HEAD AND NECK

- **Face:** yellow tinge (*uraemia*), butterfly rash (*SLE*), hearing aid (*Alport syndrome*), collapsed nasal bridge (*granulomatosis with polyangiitis*)
- **Eyes:** periorbital oedema (*nephrotic syndrome*), conjunctival pallor (*erythropoietin deficiency*), corneal arcus/xanthelasma (*hyperlipidaemia in nephrotic syndrome*)
- **Mouth:** mucus membranes (hydration), gingival hypertrophy (*immunosuppressive drugs*)
- **Neck:** JVP (*fluid overload in nephrotic syndrome*), central line scar (*from previous dialysis*)

CHEST

- **Inspection:** sternotomy scar (*renovascular disease*)
- Capillary refill and skin turgor on sternum
- **Heart sounds** (*uraemic pericardial rub*)

Sit forwards:
- **Lung base auscultation** (*pulmonary oedema in nephrotic syndrome or fluid overload*)
- **Inspect back:** skin lesions/excisions (*immunosuppression*)

ABDOMEN

- **Inspection:** distension (**5Fs:** *Fluid, Flatus, Fat, Fetus, Faeces*), scars (*loin scar, may appear on back; Rutherford Morrison scar in L/RIF from transplanted kidney – see p116*), fat hypertrophy/lipodystrophy (*insulin injections*), peritoneal dialysis scars
- **Palpation:** check for pain and begin palpation away from painful areas
    - **Superficial palpation** (for tenderness): you crouch to their level and roll fingers over nine regions while watching the patient's face. Check for: tenderness, guarding or rebound tenderness (*peritonitis*).
    - **Deep palpation** (for masses): feel particularly for smooth renal graft in iliac fossae if scar present (*tenderness = rejection*)
    - **Kidney palpation:** one hand anterior, one posterior. Ask patient to expire as you press up into renal angle with your posterior hand and press down with your anterior hand. As patient breathes in, you may feel it between your hands. Ballot the kidney by flexing the metacarpophalangeal joints of your posterior hand. Do *flick, flick, stop* and repeat as necessary (*palpable = polycystic kidney disease*).
- **Percussion of flank:** should be resonant (tap all the way across abdomen horizontally). If dull, demonstrate shifting dullness (have patient roll to side and percuss all the way across again), or demonstrate fluid thrill (have patient press hand firmly on abdominal midline while you tap one side and feel the other; *ascites in co-existent liver disease*)
- **Auscultation** for renal bruits (5cm superior and lateral to umbilicus bilaterally; *renal artery stenosis*)

LEGS

- **Peripheral oedema** (*nephrotic syndrome or fluid overload*)

TO COMPLETE

- Thank patient and restore clothing
- Summarise and suggest further investigations you would consider after a full history

DIGITAL RECTAL EXAMINATION

INTRODUCTION

- **W**ash hands; **I**ntroduce self; ask **P**atient's name, DOB and what they like to be called; **E**xplain examination and obtain consent
- Get a **chaperone**
- Explain that procedure is intimate and why it is necessary
- Explain what you want the patient to do: 'Undress from the waist down, then lie on your left side, bringing your knees up to your chest.'
- Give them a sheet to cover up until you are ready
- Use the patient's name and take care to explain carefully what you are doing. Check they are OK throughout.

EQUIPMENT

- Lubricant
- Gauze
- Paper towels
- Put on gloves and apron

INSPECTION

- Part the buttocks and look for: any blood, rashes, fistulae, fissures, excoriations, warts, haemorrhoids, skin tags
- Ask the patient to bear down and look for rectal prolapse

EXAMINATION

- Lubricate gloved index finger and approach anus from posteriorly. Pause when the finger is over the anus and wait until the sphincter relaxes.
- Warn patient then advance finger into anus
  - Comment on consistency of any faeces
  - Ask the patient to bear down (brings high rectal lesions lower)
  - Ask the patient to squeeze your finger (tests anal tone)
- Do a 360° sweep feeling for any masses or wall thickenings
- In men, feel the two lobes of the anterior surface of the prostate and comment on any masses, symmetry, consistency and size
- Remove finger and wipe on gauze – inspect for mucus, blood and melaena
- Clean the anus

TO COMPLETE

- Thank patient and restore clothing
- Dispose of waste
- Wash hands
- Document findings and note presence and identity of chaperone
- Summarise and suggest further investigations you would do after a full history, for example:
  - Prostate surface antigen
  - Rectal ultrasound
  - FBC (anaemia)
  - Sigmoidoscopy
  - Colonoscopy

INGUINAL HERNIA EXAMINATION

INTRODUCTION
- **W**ash hands; **I**ntroduce self; ask **P**atient's name, DOB and what they like to be called; **E**xplain examination and obtain consent
- Get a <u>chaperone</u>
- Expose patient from waist down and ask them to **stand up**
- Put on gloves

INSPECTION
- **General**
  - **Patient**: well/unwell, pain/discomfort (*incarceration*), pallor, muscle wasting/cachexia, abdominal distension (*obstruction*)
  - **Around bed:** vomit bowls
- **Local**
  - **Lumps**: size, shape, position, scrotal extension
  - **Observe cough impulse**

PALPATION
- **Scrotal contents:** palpate from anteriorly. If a lump is present, determine if you can get above it.
- **Lump/inguinal area** (both sides): palpate from laterally, with one hand on the patient's back, using the other to feel the lump/inguinal ligament region
  *Describe lump (**SSSCCCTTT**): **S**ite, **S**ize, **S**hape, **C**onsistency, **C**ontours, **C**olour, **T**enderness, **T**emperature (**T**ransillumination not required here)*
- **Feel cough impulse** (on each side separately): compress lump/inguinal area firmly. Ask the patient to turn their head to the opposite direction and cough. If the swelling becomes tense and expands, there is a positive cough impulse.
- **Reducibility**:
  - Locate the deep inguinal ring (midway between ASIS and pubic tubercle)
  - Press firmly on the lump and, starting inferiorly, try to lift it up and compress it towards the deep inguinal ring
  - Once it is reduced, slide your fingers up and maintain pressure over the deep inguinal ring
  - Ask patient to <u>cough</u>
  - If the hernia reappears, it is a direct hernia; if not, it is an indirect hernia
  - Release and watch hernia reappear if it has not already done so (indirect will slide down obliquely; direct will project forwards)

  NB: If you cannot reduce the hernia, try again with patient lying supine.

PERCUSSION AND AUSCULTATION
- **Percuss and auscultate lump**: this may reveal if bowel is present in a hernia

TO COMPLETE
- Thank patient and restore clothing
- 'To complete my examination, I would perform a full abdominal examination.'
- Summarise and suggest further investigations you would consider after a full history

---

See diagram p135

Types of hernia

- **Direct inguinal hernia** (<u>superior</u> to the pubic tubercle – position of superficial inguinal ring)
  - Herniated abdominal contents come **direct**ly out of abdomen in a straight line
  - Hernia emerges through the <u>superficial</u> inguinal ring
  - If reduced, hernia cannot be contained by applying pressure over the deep inguinal ring
- **Indirect inguinal hernia** (anywhere between the deep inguinal ring and the scrotum)
  - Herniated abdominal contents run with**in** the inguinal canal
  - Hernia emerges through the <u>deep</u> inguinal ring
  - Hernia can extend all the way down the canal into the scrotum in men (inguinal-scrotal hernia)
  - If reduced, hernia can be contained by applying pressure over the deep inguinal ring
- **Femoral hernia** (always <u>inferior and lateral</u> to pubic tubercle)

TESTICULAR EXAMINATION

INTRODUCTION
- **W**ash hands; **I**ntroduce self; ask **P**atient's name, DOB and what they like to be called; **E**xplain examination and obtain consent
- Get a **chaperone**
- Patient should **stand up** and be exposed from waist down
- Put on gloves

GENERAL INSPECTION
- **Patient:** well/unwell, pain/discomfort, cachexia, gynaecomastia (*teratoma – produces βHCG*)

INSPECTION
Inspect from the front but also ensure you lift the scrotum to inspect posteriorly.
- **Skin:** erythema, rashes, excoriations, scars, ulcers
- **Testes:** level (left usually lower), swelling, oedema, obvious masses
- **Inspect penis and retract foreskin:** check for phimosis, adhesions and glans abnormalities. (Make sure you replace the foreskin.)

PALPATION
Support the testes with your non-dominant hand and palpate with the index finger and thumb of your dominant hand.
- **Testes:** feel inferior, middle and superior parts of testes. Note size, consistency, and any lumps or masses.
  *Describe lump (**SSSCCCTTT**): Site, Size, Shape, Consistency, Contours, Colour, Tenderness, Temperature, Transillumination*
- **Epididymis:** feel around the posterior aspect of each testis for the epididymis (*tenderness/swelling = epididymitis*)
- **Spermatic cord:** with thumb anteriorly and index finger posteriorly, feel neck of scrotum for spermatic cord (superior to testes, feels like string)
- **Palpate for inguinal lymphadenopathy** (*infection/inflammation*)
- **Reflexes**
  - Prehn's test: if testicular pain is relieved by elevating the testes, suspect epididymitis; if not, suspect testicular torsion
  - Cremasteric reflex: stroke inside of leg and watch scrotal skin tighten (*usually absent in torsion*)

FINALLY
- **Palpate for supraclavicular lymphadenopathy:** testicular cancer commonly metastasises here (rather than superficial inguinal nodes)

TO COMPLETE
- Thank patient and restore clothing
- 'To complete my examination, I would perform a full abdominal examination and examine herneal orifices.'
- Summarise and suggest further investigations you would consider after a full history (e.g. urinalysis, testicular ultrasound)

Specific conditions

- **Hydrocele:** fluid accumulation around testicle
- **Varicocele:** dilated pampiniform venous plexus in scrotum (feels like a bag of worms, usually occurs on left)
- **Epididymal cyst (spermatocele):** fluid-filled cyst in epididymis above testicle
- **Testicular tumour:** hard, irregular lump that is inseparable from testicle
- **Inguinal-scrotal hernia:** cannot get above it
- **Epididymitis:** pain, swelling and tenderness of epididymis behind testicle
- **Testicular torsion:** painful, high-riding testicle with horizontal lie
- **Orchitis:** inflammation of a testicle

THYROID EXAMINATION

INTRODUCTION
- **W**ash hands; **I**ntroduce self; ask **P**atient's name, DOB and what they like to be called; **E**xplain examination and obtain consent
- **Sit patient** in the middle of the room (so you can stand behind them)
- Expose patient's neck

GENERAL INSPECTION
- **Patient:** well/unwell, anxious/nervous, hot/cold, facial complexion (*myxoedematous, flushed*), obvious muscle wasting, BMI, obvious thyroid swellings, dry hair/waxy skin
- **Around bed:** excess clothes

HANDS
- **Fine tremor:** ask patient to stretch out arms and hands with fingers straight and separated. A tremor is more easily visualised with a sheet of paper resting on top of the patient's hands (*fine tremor = thyrotoxicosis*).
- **Nails:** thyroid acropachy (*Graves' disease*), onycholysis (*thyrotoxicosis*)
- **Palms:** cold and dry (*hypothyroidism*), moist and sweaty (*thyrotoxicosis*), palmar erythema (*thyrotoxicosis*)
- **Pulse** (*tachycardia and AF in thyrotoxicosis*)

FACE
- **Generally:** waxy pale skin, hair thinning (including lateral third of eyebrows), myxoedema* (*all signs of hypothyroidism*)
- **Eyes**
  - Lid retraction of upper eye-lid (*thyrotoxicosis*)
  - Exophthalmos (sclera visible above and below iris)
  - Proptosis (forward protrusion of eye; inspect from above and side)
  - Chemosis/conjunctival oedema   *Graves' eye disease*
- **Extra-ocular muscles:**
  - Perform H-test (*see p67*) and ask about diplopia to test for ophthalmoplegia
  - Test central vertical eye movement (*'lid lag' on downward vertical gaze = thyrotoxicosis*)

NECK
- **Inspection** (from anteriorly): swellings and scars; ask patient to swallow (*thyroid and thyroglossal cysts move on swallowing*), stick out tongue (*thyroglossal cysts move on tongue protrusion*), and place their hands above their head (*Pemberton's sign = retrosternal goitre compresses superior vena cava and results in venous congestion*)
- **Palpation** (from posteriorly)
  - Palpate thyroid gland (over 2nd, 3rd and 4th tracheal cartilages), including feel while patient swallows and sticks out tongue
  - Full cervical lymph node exam (*see notes on neck examination p105*)
  NB: if you feel a mass/swelling, note its characteristics (**SSSCCCTTT**): **S**ize, **S**hape, **S**urface, **C**onsistency, **C**ontours, **C**olour, **T**emperature, **T**enderness, (**T**ransillumination not required for thyroid).
- **Percussion over sternum:** for retrosternal goitre
- **Auscultation:** thyroid bruit over each lobe

FINALLY
- **Proximal myopathy:** test resisted shoulder abduction, then ask patient to stand up from chair with arms crossed (*hypothyroidism or hyperthyroidism*)
- **Reflexes** (*brisk in hyperthyroidism; slow-relaxing in hypothyroidism*)
- Look for **pretibial myxoedema*** (*Graves' disease*)

TO COMPLETE
- Thank patient
- Summarise and suggest further investigations you would consider after a full history (e.g. TFTs, thyroid USS)

NB: myxoedema = soft tissue swelling.

Specific conditions
- Diffuse goitre
- Multinodular goitre
- Solitary thyroid nodule
- Thyroid malignancies
- Hyperthyroidism/Graves' disease
- Hypothyroidism
- Thyroiditis

DIABETIC FOOT/FOOT ULCER EXAMINATION

INTRODUCTION
- **W**ash hands; **I**ntroduce self; ask **P**atient's name, DOB and what they like to be called; **E**xplain examination and obtain consent
- Expose feet

INSPECTION
- **General:** gait, shoes (flat heel, pattern of wear), amputations
- **Skin:** vascular insufficiency (hairlessness, pallor), rubor/corns/callus at pressure points, texture, fissures, skin breaks/lesions/ulcers, diabetic dermopathy, infection (swelling, erythema, gangrene, cellulitis), oedema, venous eczema/lipodermatosclerosis
- **Nails:** dystrophy, ingrown nails
- **Webspaces:** cracking, ulcers, maceration, infections
- **Deformity:** clawed toes, bony prominences, Charcot joints (joint swelling with collapse of medial longitudinal arch – due to loss of protective pain sensation)

NB: describe any ulcer – size, site, characteristics (shape, edge, colour), secondary features.

ARTERIOPATHY ASSESSMENT
- **Temperature:** use dorsum of each hand to feel up legs
- **Pulses:** femoral, popliteal, posterior tibial, dorsalis pedis
- **Capillary refill** (should be <2 seconds)

NEUROPATHY ASSESSMENT
- **Sensory:** show patient how each feels on sternum before and ask them to close their eyes
    - **10g monofilament:** fully extend the monofilament and press with enough force to make it bend. First let patient feel the sensation on their sternum, then ask them to close their eyes and tell you when they feel you touch their feet. Test sensation in multiple places, e.g. hallux and metatarsal heads.
    - **128Hz Tuning fork:** use your fingers to twang prongs and hold circular base on the patient's joint. First let patient feel the sensation on their sternum, then ask them to close their eyes and tell you when they feel a vibration on their feet and when they feel it stop (stop the vibration yourself by gripping the prongs). Start over first MTP joint and move to proximal joints if the patient cannot feel it.
    - **Proprioception:** hold the distal phalanx of the big toe with a finger on each side (while stabilising the proximal phalanx with your other hand). Flex and extend the joint with the patient watching these movements and then ask them to close their eyes. Wiggle the distal phalanx up and down a few times, then stop and ask the patient if their toe is up or down. If they cannot tell, test more proximal joints in succession until they can.
- **Motor:** muscle wasting, pes planus, pes cavus, Charcot joints
- **Reflexes:** ankle jerk
- **Autonomic:** sweaty, dry, cracked skin

TO COMPLETE
- Thank patient and restore clothing
- 'To complete my examination, I would perform a full neurovascular examination.'
- Summarise and suggest further investigations you would consider after a full history, for example:
    - ABPI
    - Doppler arterial pulses
    - Blood glucose
    - HbA1C

Ulcer properties by type			
	Venous	**Ischaemic**	**Neuropathic**
Site	Gaiter region	Soles/pressure areas	
Depth	Superficial	Deep	
Edges	Sloping	Punched out	
Base	Granulating	Sloughy and pale	Sloughy and bloody
Colour	Pink	Pale	Red
Pain	Moderate	Painful	Painless
Other characteristics	May be varicosities, venous eczema, haemosiderin deposits, lipodermatosclerosis	Loss of peripheral pulses	Sensory neuropathy

CUSHING'S SYNDROME FOCUSSED EXAMINATION

NB: the OSCE instructions may be non-specific, for example: 'Examine this patient's endocrine status.' This could be Cushing's syndrome, acromegaly or hypothyroidism. Approach this situation by asking a few generic questions (if allowed) and by doing a general inspection to determine which condition you think is present. Then proceed with the relevant focussed examination to elicit other signs.

INTRODUCTION

- **W**ash hands; **I**ntroduce self; ask **P**atient's name, DOB and what they like to be called; **E**xplain examination and obtain consent

GENERAL INSPECTION

- Central adiposity
- Intra-scapular fat pad
- Hirsutism
- Osteoporosis effects, e.g. kyphosis
- **Around bed:** inhalers, nebulisers, oxygen (*may be used in COPD or interstitial lung disease*)

HANDS AND ARMS

- Capillary glucose stick marks on finger pulps (*secondary diabetes*)
- Pigmentation (*Cushing's disease*)
- Deforming polyarthritis (*a reason for corticosteroid use*)
- Thin skin and bruising
- Poor wound healing

FACE

- **Inspection:** cushingoid-like facial features ('facial mooning'), facial plethora, hirsutism, acne, telangiectasia, butterfly rash (*SLE*)
- **Inside mouth:** oral thrush, buccal pigmentation (*Cushing's disease*)
- Listen for hoarse voice
- Visual fields (*bitemporal hemianopia in pituitary adenoma*)

NECK

- Intrascapular fat pad
- Supraclavicular fat pads

CHEST AND ABDOMEN

- Skin thinning
- Classical purple striae
- Lipodystrophy from insulin injections (*secondary diabetes*)
- Signs of any conditions requiring prolonged steroid use (e.g. organ transplant scars, hyperexpanded chest in COPD)

FINALLY

- Proximal myopathy (check resisted shoulder abduction, then ask patient to stand up with arms crossed)

TO COMPLETE

- Thank patient
- 'To complete my examination, I would measure blood pressure, dipstick test urine for glucose, and formally assess visual fields.'
- Summarise and suggest further investigations you would do after a full history, for example:
  - 24 hour urinary free cortisol
  - Overnight/low dose dexamethasone suppression test

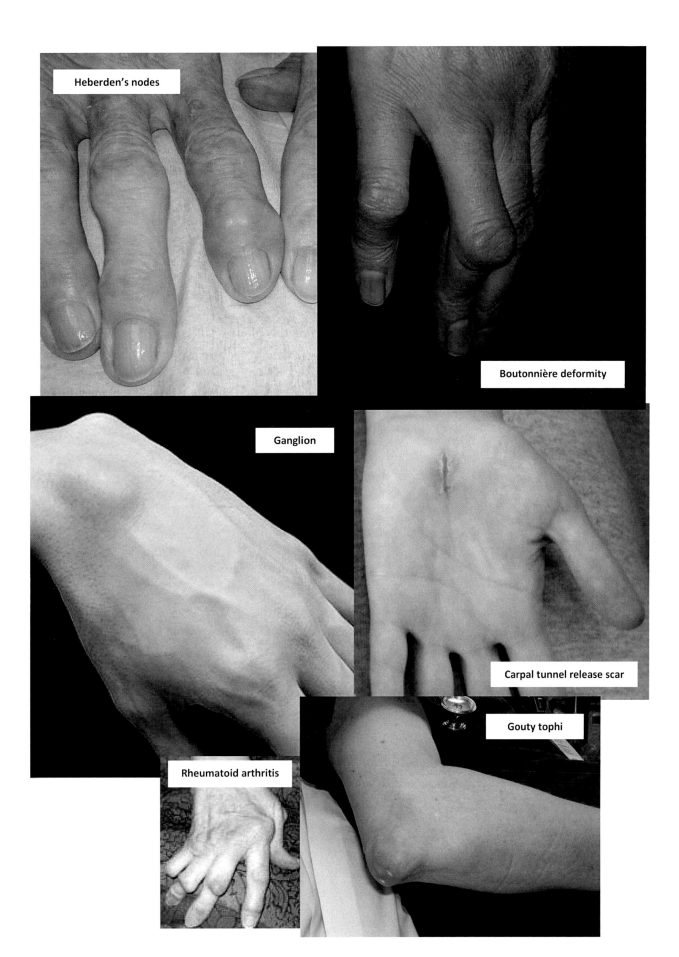

Heberden's nodes

Boutonnière deformity

Ganglion

Carpal tunnel release scar

Gouty tophi

Rheumatoid arthritis

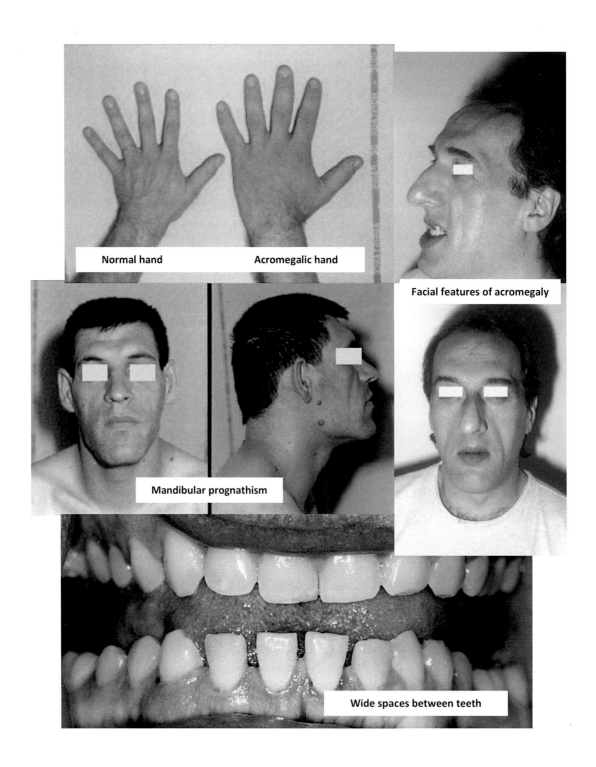

Normal hand   Acromegalic hand

Facial features of acromegaly

Mandibular prognathism

Wide spaces between teeth

ACROMEGALY FOCUSSED EXAMINATION

NB: the OSCE instructions may be non-specific, for example: 'Examine this patient's endocrine status.' This could be Cushing's syndrome, acromegaly or hypothyroidism. Approach this situation by asking a few generic questions (if allowed) and by doing a general inspection to determine which condition you think is present. Then proceed with the relevant focussed examination to elicit other signs.

Generic questions (acromegaly is usually obvious so ask questions to elicit symptoms you cannot examine for)

• What did you notice first when you developed this condition?
• Have you noticed a change in your appearance?

Determining if there is active acromegaly
• Do you notice excessive sweating?
• Do you have high blood pressure?

Other symptoms – work down body
• Headaches
• Visual problems
• Pins and needles
• Back ache
• Muscle weakness
• Change in shoe size

INTRODUCTION

- **W**ash hands; **I**ntroduce self; ask **P**atient's name, DOB and what they like to be called; **E**xplain examination and obtain consent

GENERAL INSPECTION

- Increased size of feet, hands, head
- Mildly hirsute
- Kyphosis

ARMS

- **Inspect and palpate** with patient's hands on pillow
    - Dorsum: large, spade-shaped, with signs of osteoarthritis
    - Palms: sweaty, doughy/boggy texture to palms, capillary glucose stick marks on finger pulps (*secondary diabetes*)
    - Signs of carpal tunnel syndrome (release scar or loss of thenar eminence and/or loss of sensation in median nerve distribution)
- **Blood pressure** (*hypertension*)

FACE

- **General:** coarse facial features, acne, enlarged nose and ears, macrognathia (large mandible), look for hypophysectomy scar under upper lip
- **Eyes:** visual fields (*bitemporal hemianopia in pituitary adenoma*), prominent supra-orbital ridges
- **Mouth:** prognathism (protrusion of mandible), splaying of teeth, macroglossia and ridges from teeth on sides of tongue

NECK

- Thyroid goitre (*increased thyroid vascularity*)
- JVP (*cardiomyopathy*)

CHEST

- Inspect: multiple skin tags
- Acanthosis nigricans in axillae
- Signs of cardiomyopathy (palpate apex, auscultate heart for murmurs/added sounds and lung bases for pulmonary oedema)

LIMBS

- Peripheral oedema (*cardiomyopathy*)
- Proximal myopathy (check resisted shoulder abduction, then ask patient to stand up with arms crossed)
- Gait: rolling gait with bowed legs

TO COMPLETE

- Thank patient
- 'To compete my examination, I would measure the blood pressure, perform thyroid and cardiovascular examinations and formally assess visual fields.'
- Summarise and suggest further investigations you would consider after a full history, for example:
    - Insulin-like growth factor-1
    - Growth hormone response to oral glucose tolerance test
    - MRI pituitary

NB: you may be asked to examine only the visual cranial nerves (CN 2, 3, 4 and 6) or the bulbar cranial nerves (CN 9, 10 and 12).

INTRODUCTION

- <u>W</u>ash hands; <u>I</u>ntroduce self; ask <u>P</u>atient's name, DOB and what they like to be called; <u>E</u>xplain examination and obtain consent

GENERAL INSPECTION

- **Patient**: posture, habitus, other signs of neurological conditions
- **Around bed**: mobility aids, NBM signs, fluid thickener, glasses, hearing aids etc.

1 OLFACTORY

- Test each nostril with smelling salts if available. If not, ask patient if they have noticed any change in smell.

2 OPTIC

AFRO (3 tests for each):

- **Inspection**: visual aids; pupil size and symmetry; screening test (ask if they can see your whole face clearly)
- **A**cuity: ask the patient to cover one eye with their palm and test each eye in turn
  - **Distant vision (visual acuity):** test with Snellen chart (the result is recorded as *distance/smallest font size read*, e.g. 6/9)
    - If the patient wears glasses, test with glasses on (corrected visual acuity)
    - A standard Snellen chart is read from 6 metres away but there are smaller versions which may be used at closer distances (e.g. 1 or 3 metres) – adjust the final acuity to '1/…' or '3/…' respectively
    - If the patient gets more than two letters wrong, the previous line should be recorded as their acuity. If they get two letters wrong, record acuity as the font size of this line but note '-2' in brackets, e.g. 6/9 (-2); and if they get one letter wrong, note '-1' e.g. 6/9 (-1).
  - **Near vision:** read a line of a letter/magazine
  - **Colour vision:** 'I would also like to test colour vision using Ishihara plates.'
- **F**ields: sit the patient 1 metre directly in front of you with both your eyes at the same level
  - **Visual inattention:** while the patient keeps both eyes open and focussed on you, hold out your hands in each of their outer visual fields. Ask them to point at the hand(s) which you are opening and closing. (*Inattention to one side, i.e. identification of only one moving hand when both are moving = contralateral parietal lesion.*)
  - **Visual fields:** ask the patient to cover one eye with their palm and close your eye on the same side (without using your palm if you can). Ask them to stay focussed on your open eye. Select a white visual fields pin and bring it in from the periphery, keeping it at mid-distance between you and the patient. Ask them to tell you when they can see it. Move in a diagonal direction into each of the four quadrants. Test both eyes individually, comparing their fields with yours.
    - *Mononuclear field loss = intra-ocular pathology or ipsilateral optic nerve lesion*
    - *Bitemporal hemianopia = optic chiasm compression*
    - *Left/right homonymous hemianopia = contralateral optic tract/radiation lesion, or occipital cortex if macular sparing is present*
  - **Blind spots** (offer to test): while the patient keeps both eyes open and focussed on you, hold a red pin mid-distance between you. Check they can see it as red in the middle (*central scotoma = optic nerve lesion*). Now move the pin horizontally towards the periphery in each direction and to tell you when it disappears. Map each of their blind spots against your own (*large blind spot = papilloedema*).
- **R**eflexes
  - **Accommodation:** ask the patient to focus on a distant object, then hold your finger close to their face and ask them to focus on it. Pupils should constrict and eyes should converge.
  - **Direct and consensual papillary reflexes:** in a dimmed room, ask the patient to hold an open hand between their eyes and focus on a distant point in the room. Shine the light at each pupil in turn from about 45°. Observe for direct and consensual papillary constriction.
    - *Afferent defect (i.e. pupils are symmetrical but when light is shone in the affected eye, neither pupil constricts) = CN2 (optic nerve) lesion*
    - *Efferent defect (affected pupil is persistently dilated, whilst other is reactive to light being shone in either eye) = CN3 lesion*
  - **Swinging light test:** swing the light between the two eyes – the pupil size should stay the same regardless of which eye the light is shone in. If pupils become more dilated when the light is shone in one eye, then that eye is less sensitive to light and, hence, there is a <u>relative</u> afferent pupillary defect in that eye (*partial optic nerve lesion on that side*).
- **O**ptic disc: 'I would also like to perform ophthalmoscopy to visualise the optic disc.' *See p102 if required.*

3,4,6 OCULOMOTOR, TROCHLEAR, ABDUCENS

Ask if the patient has any double vision and to tell you if they experience any during the test.

- **Inspect**: strabismus, ptosis (*partial = Horner's syndrome; complete = CN3 lesion*)
- **H-test**: ask patient to keep their head still (you may need to hold a finger on their forehead) and, with both eyes open, to follow your finger. Make an 'H' shape.
    - Pause when they are looking laterally (*nystagmus = cerebellar pathology*)
    - If there is complex ophthalmoplegia, ask them to look straight up while counting down from 20 (*fatigability suggests myasthenia gravis*)
- **Saccades test**: ask the patient to look back and forth between two widely spaced targets, e.g. your index finder on one hand and thumb on the other, while keeping their head still. Test horizontally and vertically. Check for conjugate eye movements and target accuracy. (*Delay, inaccuracy, or slow or disconjugate movements suggest a central nervous system pathology rather than a peripheral vestibular pathology.*)

NB: CN3 supplies all extra-ocular muscles except Superior Oblique (CN4) and Lateral Rectus (CN6) – SO4LR6

Hence, if the eye cannot move laterally, there is a CN6 lesion; if the eye cannot move inferiorly when facing medially, there is a CN4 lesion. If the majority of the eye's movements are impaired and the eye rests in a 'down and out' position, there is a CN3 lesion. If there are dramatically abnormal eye movements which do not fit with a single nerve lesion, there is complex ophthalmoplegia (Graves/ mitochondrial/myasthenia/brainstem lesion).

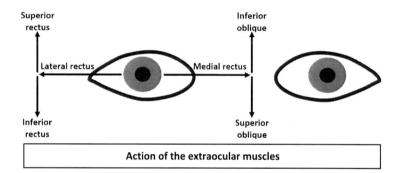

Action of the extraocular muscles

5 TRIGEMINAL

- **Inspect**: temporalis/masseter muscle wasting
- **Sensory:** ask the patient if they have any areas of pins and needles or numbness. With the patient's eyes closed, use a cotton wool ball ± a neurological pin to test sensation over the ophthalmic, maxillary and mandibular distributions of the trigeminal nerve. Ask the patient to tell you when they feel it and if it feels the same on each side.
- **Motor:** ask the patient to clench their jaw and feel the bulk of the temporalis and masseter muscles. Ask them to open the jaw against resistance.
- **Others**: 'I would also consider testing the **corneal reflex** (*afferent = CN 5; efferent = CN 7*) and **jaw jerk** (*afferent and efferent = CN 5*).'

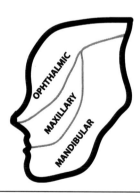

Cutaneous branches of trigeminal nerve

7 FACIAL

- **Inspect:** forehead wrinkles, nasolabial folds, angles of mouth for facial asymmetry
- **Motor**
    - Raise eyebrows
    - Scrunch up eyes (try to prise each open in turn with your thumbs)
    - Purse lips together (try to prise each open in turn with your thumbs)
    - Show teeth
    - Puff out cheeks (try to push air out)

NB: the forehead is spared in UMN lesions because the nucleus controlling the upper part of the face has bilateral UMN innervation. In a LMN lesion (e.g. Bell's palsy), the whole side of the face is affected.

8 VESTIBULOCOCHLEAR

- **Crude hearing test:** ask patient to occlude one ear and whisper a number into the other. Start at a distance and move towards the ear, asking them to tell you the number when they hear it. Repeat on the other side.
- **Weber's test:** use a 512Hz tuning fork. Twang the prongs and place the round base of the fork on the patient's forehead between their eyes. Ask them if one side is louder than the other.
  - *If one side is louder, either that side has a conductive deficit, or the contralateral side has a sensorineural deficit – Rinne's test can then confirm which*
- **Rinne's test:** use a 512Hz tuning fork. Twang the prongs and place the round base of the fork on the patient's mastoid process. Ask them to tell you when the sound stops. Then, place the prongs near the patient's ear and ask if they can hear it again. Air conduction should be louder than bone conduction.
  - *If they cannot hear it again, there is a conductive deficit in that ear*
- **Others**: 'I would also consider performing **vertigo tests** such as walking on the spot or vestibulo-ocular reflex testing.'

9,10 GLOSSOPHARYNGEAL, VAGUS

- **Inspect:** ask patient to open mouth and say 'ahhh' while you use a pen torch to inspect palate symmetry (CN 9) and uvula deviation (CN 10) – uvula deviates <u>away</u> from side of lesion
- **Motor:** assess speech, cough and swallow
- **Others**: 'I would also consider testing the **gag reflex** (*afferent = CN 9; efferent = CN 10*).'

11 ACCESSORY

- **Inspect:** sternocleidomastoid/trapezius muscle wasting
- **Motor:** ask the patient to turn their head to each side against resistance (tests contralateral sternocleidomastoid muscle), and shrug their shoulders against resistance (tests trapezius)

12 HYPOGLOSSAL

- **Inspect:** tongue while relaxed in mouth for muscle wasting and fasciculations (*LMN lesion, i.e. bulbar palsy*)
- **Motor:** stick out tongue (deviates <u>to</u> side of lesion), move from side to side and test power by resisting tongue pressed into cheek

TO COMPLETE

- Thank patient
- 'To complete my examination, I would perform full upper and lower limb neurological examinations.'
- Summarise and suggest further investigations you would consider after a full history

LOWER LIMB NEUROLOGICAL EXAMINATION

INTRODUCTION

- **W**ash hands; **I**ntroduce self; ask **P**atient's name, DOB and what they like to be called; **E**xplain examination and obtain consent
- Expose patient's legs (to underwear or shorts)

Diagnosing in neurology

Ask yourself throughout if the pathology is:

- **Unilateral/bilateral UMN** (pyramidal weakness)
- **Unilateral LMN** (weakness depends on lesion)
- **Bilateral LMN** (distal weakness)
- **Proximal weakness**

By the time you get to the sensory exam you should know what you are expecting to find and use it to confirm or narrow down differentials (*see notes on neurology differentials p73*).

INSPECTION

- **General inspection**
  - **Patient:** posture, habitus, other signs of neurological conditions (e.g. hypomimia, facial muscle wasting)
  - **Around bed:** mobility aids, orthoses
- **Gait** – first ask if they can walk and if they need assistance/aids
  - Normal walking (*hemiplegic = unilateral UMN; spastic = bilateral UMN; foot drop = LMN; ataxic = cerebellar; waddling = myopathic; festinating = parkinsonian*)
  - Heel-to-toe walking if stable (*ataxia = cerebellar pathology*)
  - Stand on heels and then toes (tests distal power)
  - Romberg's test if steady: close eyes while standing (*reduced stability = sensory ataxia due to proprioceptive deficit*)
- **Local inspection**
  - **Tremors**
  - **Muscles:** muscle wasting – in general and then look closely for plantar foot wasting and for dorsal foot guttering (*LMN lesion*); fasciculations (*LMN lesion*); associated bony deformity (e.g. pes cavus)
  - **Skin:** neurofibromas, *café au lait* spots, scars (including small muscle biopsy scars)

TONE

- **Tone:** patient should lie relaxed with legs flat. With one hand either side of the knee, roll each leg from side to side ($\uparrow$*tone, i.e. foot remains in line with knee = UMN lesion;* $\downarrow$ *tone = LMN lesion*).
- **Spasticity:** place hand under the patient's knee and briskly lift it up (*spasticity, i.e. foot kicks out involuntarily = UMN lesion*)
- **Clonus:** hold the sole of the patient's foot in one hand, and elevate it while holding their ipsilateral knee flexed in the other hand. Forcefully flex the ankle a few times quickly, and then hold it firmly in the flexed position. Feel for involuntary, rhythmic beats of gastrocnemius contraction (*>5 beats = UMN lesion*).

POWER

Test one joint at a time and compare sides. Always support the joint being tested with one hand (use it as a lever). Use all your strength!
MRC grades: 5 = full power; **4** = some resistance; **3 = GRAVITY; 2** = gravity eliminated; **1** = flicker of muscle contraction; **0** = nothing.

Hip flexion (L2/L3)	Patient should raise their leg off the bed with knee fully extended. Stabilise contralateral hip joint with one hand and push down on the quadriceps just above the knee of the raised leg. *'Don't let me push your leg down.'*
Hip extension (L4/L5)	With the same leg still raised to about 30°, stabilise the ipsilateral hip joint with one hand and hold the underside of the patient's knee with the other hand. *'Push my hand down into the bed.'*
Knee extension (L3/L4)	With the patient's knee flexed to about 90°, stabilise the joint with one hand and hold the anterior side of their ankle with your other hand and try to push it towards them. *'Try and kick your leg out. Don't let me push it towards you.'*
Knee flexion (L5/S1)	In the same position, but holding the posterior side of their ankle, try and pull it away. *'Try and pull your heel towards your bottom. Don't let me pull it away.'*
Ankle dorsiflexion (L4/L5)	With their leg straight on the bed and their ankle actively dorsiflexed, stabilise the ankle with one hand. Make a fist with your other and use the dorsal side of your fist to try and push the patient's foot downwards. *'Point your foot up towards your head. Don't let me push it down.'*
Ankle plantar-flexion (S1/S2)	With their leg straight on the bed and their ankle actively plantar-flexed, try to pull it up with your fingers around the ball of the patient's foot. *'Point your foot downwards towards the bottom of the bed. Don't let me pull it up.'*
Big toe extension (purely L5)	With their big toe actively flexed, isolate the toe's metatarsophalangeal joint with one hand and try to push it down with the index and middle fingers of your other hand. *'Point your big toe up towards your head. Don't let me push it down.'*

REFLEXES

Hold the tendon hammer by the <u>end</u> of the plastic rod to make a pendulum-like swing. Ensure the patient is fully relaxed. If you cannot elicit a reflex, ask them to close their eyes and grit their teeth when you strike the tendon.
Reflexes may be brisk, normal, reduced or absent.

- **Patellar (L3, 4 kick the door):** with the knee relaxed in passive flexion (hold it up with your left wrist under the patient's knee), locate the tibial tuberosity and inferior border of the patella, and strike the patellar tendon that lies between these.
- **Ankle (S1, 2 in the shoe):** externally rotate the patient's leg and flex their knee (so their lower leg rests over their contralateral shin). Hold their foot with your left hand and gently dorsiflex their ankle. Strike the Achilles tendon with the hammer in your right hand. *NB: to test their left ankle reflex, move to the base of the bed.*
- **Plantar (Babinski) reflex:** warn the patient and then, using an orange stick, gently scrape the plantar surface of their foot in a semi-circle from the heel, around the lateral edge and to the ball of the big toe (*big toe ↑ = UMN lesion; big toe ↓ = normal*).

CO-ORDINATION

- **Heel-to-shin test:** ask the patient to touch their heel to their contralateral knee. Then ask them to slide their heel down the tibia to their contralateral ankle. Now ask them to move it back up, through the air, to their contralateral knee again. Repeat this about three times for each side (*lower limb ataxia = cerebellar pathology*).

SENSATION

For pain and light touch, first show the patient how each should feel on their **sternum**, then start distally. If there is **distal sensory loss** *or if from the motor exam you suspect 'glove and stocking' sensory loss, or a sensory-level*, test from distal to proximal in 2-3 straight lines. If **distal sensation is intact**, *or if from the motor exam you suspect nerve/nerve root pathology*, test dermatomes ± peripheral nerves:

- **Pain (spinothalamic):** use neurological pin
- *'Close your eyes and say "yes" every time you feel the pin. Please also let me know if it feels blunt.'*
- **Light touch (dorsal column):** touch the skin with a cotton wool ball (don't stroke it)
  'Close your eyes and say "yes" every time you feel the cotton wool.'

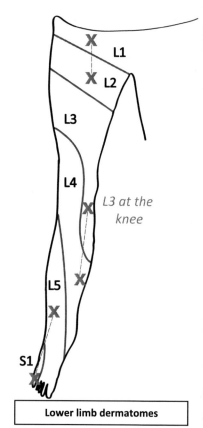

For the modalities below, start distally and only move proximally if the patient cannot feel you:

- **Proprioception (dorsal column):** hold the proximal phalanx of the patient's big toe with your index finger above and your thumb below. Move the distal phalanx up and down with the thumb and index finger of your other hand, holding it on each side. Show the patient the up and down positions. Now ask them to close their eyes and repeatedly wiggle the distal phalanx up and down. Stop in one position and ask them if it is up or down. Do this three times. If they get it wrong, move to the metatarsophalangeal joint, then the ankle, and so on until they can correctly state the position.
- **Vibration (dorsal column):** twang the prongs of a 128Hz (long) tuning fork. Place the round base on their sternum to demonstrate how it should feel. Now ask them to close their eyes and hold it over the interphalangeal joint of their big toe. Ask if they can feel it vibrate and when it stops vibrating. (Grip the prongs to stop the vibration yourself.) If they cannot sense the vibration, move to the metatarsophalangeal joint, then medial malleolus, then tibial tuberosity, and so on until they can.
- **Temperature (spinothalamic):** use the prongs of the tuning fork on the patient's sternum to test if they can identify them as cold. If so, touch a prong horizontally to the skin on the dorsum of the distal foot and ask if the patient can feel it as cold. If not, move proximally up the leg until they can.

Lower limb dermatomes

TO COMPLETE

- Thank patient and restore clothing
- 'To complete my examination, I would examine the cranial nerves and perform an upper limb neurological examination.'
- Summarise and suggest further investigations you would consider after a full history

| Clinical features of upper and lower motor neuron lesions ||
UMN Lesion	LMN lesion
Increased tone	Wasting and fasciculation
Spasticity	Hypotonia
Weakness	Weakness
Brisk reflexes, upgoing plantar reflex	Reduced reflexes

UPPER LIMB NEUROLOGICAL EXAMINATION

INTRODUCTION

- <u>W</u>ash hands; <u>I</u>ntroduce self; ask <u>P</u>atient's name, DOB and what they like to be called; <u>E</u>xplain examination and obtain consent
- Expose patient's upper body (leave bra on)

INSPECTION

- **General inspection**
  - ○ **Patient:** posture, habitus, other signs of neurological conditions (e.g. hypomimia, facial muscle wasting)
  - ○ **Around bed:** mobility aids, orthoses
- **Local inspection**
  - ○ **Tremors**
  - ○ **Muscles:** muscle wasting – look in general and then closely for thenar/hypothenar wasting and for dorsal hand guttering (*LMN lesion*); fasciculations (*LMN lesion*)
  - ○ **Skin:** neurofibromas, *café au lait* spots, scars (including small muscle biopsy scars)

TONE

- **Pronator drift:** ask patient to hold their arms out fully extended with palms facing upwards and their eyes closed (*pronator drift and distal flexion = pyramidal weakness; upward drift = cerebellar pathology*). Upward cerebellar drift can be accentuated by 'rebound' – pushing patient's wrists down briskly and then quickly letting go.
- **Tone** (↑ = *UMN lesion*; ↓ = *LMN lesion*; cogwheel rigidity = *Parkinsonian tremor superimposed on increased tone*)
  - ○ Elbow: hold the patient's hand as if you are shaking it. Support their elbow with your other hand and repeatedly flex and extend their elbow to full range.
  - ○ Forearm: in the same position, with their elbow at 90° flexion, repeatedly pronate and supinate their hand in alternating directions
  - ○ Wrist: hold their forearm just proximal to their wrist. Flex and extend, then rotate their hand on their wrist.

POWER

Test one joint at a time and compare sides. Always support the joint being tested with one hand (use it as a lever). Use all your strength!
MRC grades: 5 = full power; **4** = some resistance; **3** = GRAVITY; **2** = gravity eliminated; **1** = flicker of muscle contraction; **0** = nothing.

Shoulder abduction (C5)	Patient should abduct their shoulders to the horizontal plane with flexed elbows. Now push them down. *'Don't let me push your arms down.'*
Elbow flexion (C6)	Patient should bring arms into sagittal plane with elbows flexed. Hold the elbow with one hand and try to pull away at the wrist with the other. *'Hold your arms like this, as if you are boxing. I'm going to try and pull them away – don't let me.'*
Elbow extension (C7)	In the same position, try and push their wrist towards them. *'Now I want you to try to push me away while I hold your wrist.'*
Wrist extension (C7)	Patient should hold their arms out straight while making fists and extending their wrists. Stabilise their wrist with one hand and use the dorsum of your other fist to try to push theirs down. *'Hold your fists out like this. Now I'm going to try to push your fists downwards – don't let me.'*
Finger extension (C7)	Patient should hold their arms out straight with fingers extended. Stabilise their metacarpals with one hand and use the dorsal surface of your other hand's extended fingers to try and push theirs down. *'Hold your fingers straight out. Now I'm going to try and push your fingers downwards, don't let me.'*
Finger flexion (C8)	Interlock gripped fingers with the patient and try to open their hand. *'Grip my fingers and don't let me open your hand.'*
Finger abduction (T1)	Patient should spread their fingers. Try to push their little and index fingers inwards with your fingers, using the same digits as the ones you are touching. *'Spread your fingers. Don't let me push them inwards.'*
Thumb abduction (T1)	Patient should hold their palms facing up and point their thumbs up to the ceiling. Try to push their thumbs down into their palms. *'Don't let me push your thumbs down.'*

REFLEXES

Hold the tendon hammer by the <u>end</u> of the plastic rod to make a pendulum-type swing. Ensure the patient is fully relaxed. If you cannot elicit a reflex, ask them to close their eyes and grit their teeth when you strike the tendon.
Reflexes may be brisk (*UMN*), normal, reduced (*LMN*) or absent.

- **Biceps (C5/6):** ask patient to relax their arm across their lap with palm facing up. Place your index finger across their biceps tendon and then strike your finger.
- **Supinator (C4/6):** with the patient's arm still relaxed across their lap, place your index and middle fingers over the brachioradialis tendon (4 inches proximal to base of thumb on lateral border of forearm), and strike your fingers.
- **Triceps (C7):** hold up the patient's wrist against their torso with one hand to flex their elbow to 90°, while they let the arm go floppy. Strike their triceps tendon (just above the olecranon process) directly with the tendon hammer.

CO-ORDINATION

- **Finger-nose test:** ask the patient to hold their pointed index finger straight forwards. Now position your index finger tip touching theirs and ask them to alternate between touching the tip of their nose and your finger tip as fast as they can. Repeat on the other side (*intention tremor and past-pointing/dysmetria = cerebellar pathology*).
- **Dysdiadochokinesia:** ask the patient to hold one palm up and repeatedly hit the palmar surface of the extended fingers of their contralateral hand onto the palm. Then ask them to alternate hitting the palm with the palmar and dorsal surfaces of their extended fingers (*disorganisation of alternating movement, i.e. dysdiadochokinesia = cerebellar pathology*).

SENSATION

For pain and light touch, first show the patient how each should feel on their **sternum**. Then start distally. If there is **distal sensory loss** *or if from the motor exam you suspect 'glove and stocking' sensory loss*, test from distal to proximal in 2-3 straight lines. If **distal sensation is intact**, *or if from the motor exam you suspect nerve/nerve root pathology*, test dermatomes ± peripheral nerves:

- **Pain (spinothalamic):** use neurological pin
  'Close your eyes and say "yes" every time you feel the pin. Please also let me know if it feels blunt.'
- **Light touch (dorsal column):** touch the skin with a cotton wool ball (don't stroke it)
  'Close your eyes and say "yes" every time you feel the cotton wool.'

For the modalities below, start distally and only move proximally if the patient cannot feel you:

- **Proprioception (dorsal column):** hold the proximal phalanx of the patient's thumb with your index finger above and your thumb below. Move the distal phalanx up and down with the thumb and index finger of your other hand, holding it on each side. Show the patient the up and down positions. Now ask them to close their eyes and repeatedly wiggle the distal phalanx up and down. Stop in one position and ask them if it is up or down. Do this three times. If they get it wrong, move to the metacarpophalangeal joint, then the wrist, and so on until they can correctly state the position.

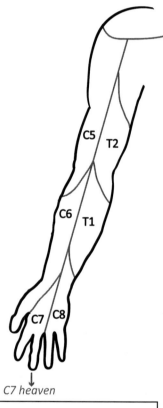

Upper limb dermatomes

- **Vibration (dorsal column):** twang the prongs of a 128Hz (long) tuning fork. Place the round base on their sternum to demonstrate how it should feel. Now ask them to close their eyes and hold it over the interphalangeal joint of their thumb. Ask if they can feel it vibrate and when it stops vibrating. (Grip the prongs to stop the vibration yourself.) If they cannot sense vibration, move to the metacarpophalangeal joint, radial styloid and so on until they can.
- **Temperature (spinothalamic):** use the prongs of the tuning fork on the patient's sternum to test if they can identify them as cold. If so, touch a prong horizontally to the skin on the dorsum of their hand and ask if the patient can feel it as cold. If not, move proximally up the arm until they can.

TO COMPLETE

- Thank patient and restore clothing
- 'To complete my examination, I would examine the cranial nerves and perform a lower limb neurological examination.'
- Summarise and suggest further investigations you would consider after a full history

| Clinical features of upper and lower motor neuron lesions ||
UMN Lesion	LMN lesion
Increased tone	Wasting and fasciculation
Spasticity	Hypotonia
Weakness	Weakness
Brisk reflexes, upgoing plantar reflex	Reduced reflexes

NEUROLOGICAL DIFFERENTIAL DIAGNOSIS

SENSORIMOTOR

*** = ACUTE ONSET**

UNILATERAL UMN (PYRAMIDAL WEAKNESS)

Work down (brain to cord):

- Intracranial - stroke*, SOL → *hemisensory loss*
- Brainstem - stroke*, SOL → *may be crossed signs*
- Spinal cord - MS, infarct/haemorrhage*, SOL, disc prolapse*, trauma*, syringomyelia, congenital → *sensory-level/segmental sensory loss*

NB: in the acute phase of stroke and transverse myelitis, there is initially hypotonia and hyporeflexia, so they may be confused with LMN lesions acutely.

BILATERAL UMN (PYRAMIDAL WEAKNESS)

3M's

- **M**S
- **M**otor neurone disease → *normal sensation*
- **M**yelopathy - cord compression (e.g. due to cervical myelopathy, SOL*, disc prolapse*, paraspinal infection*) trauma*, transverse myelitis*, syringomyelia, congenital → *sensory-level/segmental sensory loss*
- Others - brainstem stroke*, hereditary spastic paraplegia, cerebral palsy, HTLV-1, syphilis

UNILATERAL LMN (WEAKNESS DEPENDS ON SITE OF LESION)

Causes of unilateral LMN lesions – work down (nerve root to peripheral nerve)		
Lesion		**Causes**
Radiculopathy → *dermatomal sensory loss*		Disc herniation*/degenerative disc disease, spondylosis/OA with osteophytes
Plexopathy → *vast dermatomal sensory loss*	**Brachial**	Brachial neuritis*, trauma (e.g. dislocated shoulder)*, congenital (Erb's palsy, Klumpke's palsy), thoracic outlet syndrome, neoplastic infiltration/compression, radiotherapy
	Lumbosacral	Trauma*, congenital, neoplastic infiltration/compression, radiotherapy
Peripheral nerve palsy → *peripheral nerve sensory loss* ***NB: mononeuritis multiplex can cause any***	**Median**	Carpal tunnel syndrome (*associations = idiopathic, pregnancy, obesity, local pressure, hypothyroidism, acromegaly, diabetes*), distal radius fracture*, penetrating forearm injuries*, pronator teres syndrome
	Ulnar	Compression at elbow/cubital tunnel syndrome, fractures*, Guyon's canal/ulnar tunnel syndrome
	Radial	Trauma/compression at axilla (crutches*, sleeping over chair i.e. Saturday night palsy*, stabbing*), humeral shaft (fracture*), or elbow (fracture*, dislocation*, ganglion)
	Axillary	Shoulder dislocation*, surgical neck of humerus fracture*
	Common peroneal	Plaster cast compression*, trauma*

*NB: **polio*** sufferers may have asymmetrical limb paresis with LMN signs throughout the limb ± limb hypoplasia.*

BILATERAL LMN (DISTAL WEAKNESS)

Abnormal sensation distally i.e. sensorimotor polyneuropathy

ABCDE:

- **A**lcohol
- **B**$_{12}$/thiamine deficiency
- **C**harcot-Marie-Tooth, **C**arcinomas (paraneoplastic)
- **D**iabetes, **D**rugs (e.g. TB drugs, metronidazole/nitrofurantoin, vincristine/cisplatin, amiodarone)
- **E**very vasculitis (e.g. SLE, RA, polyarteritis nodosa) and some infections (e.g. herpes zoster, HIV, leprosy, syphilis)

PURE MOTOR

Normal sensation i.e. distal motor neuropathy

- Chronic inflammatory demyelinating polyneuropathy
- Myotonic dystrophy
- Inclusion body myositis (proximal in legs but distal in arms)
- Progressive muscular atrophy
- Lead poisoning
- Porphyria

Acute flaccid paralysis*

- Guillain-Barré syndrome
- Some rare infections (e.g. rabies, polio, West Nile)
- Cauda equina syndrome
- Acute transverse myelitis

NB: transverse myelitis is not a LMN lesion but initially presents with hypotonia and hyporeflexia. There is also usually a sensory level.

NB: cauda equina syndrome presents as LMN pathology but the weakness is usually asymmetrical and not usually distal, unlike other causes. There are also usually sensory deficits.

PROXIMAL WEAKNESS → *NORMAL SENSATION*

DENIM:

- **D**ystrophies - Becker's/Duchenne, limb girdle, facioscapulohumeral (shoulder, face and truncal weakness)
- **E**ndocrinological - Cushing's syndrome, hyper/hypothyroidism, diabetic amyotrophy (lower limbs)
- **N**euromuscular - myasthenia gravis (fatigable), Lambert–Eaton myasthenic syndrome
- **I**nflammatory - dermato-/polymyositis, inclusion body myositis (proximal in legs but distal in arms)
- **M**etabolic/congenital/mitochondrial myopathies

MONONEURITIS MULTIPLEX

- Vasculitis   -   granulomatosis with polyangiitis, eosinophilic granulomatosis with polyangiitis, polyarteritis nodosa, microscopic polyangiitis
- Autoimmune   -   RA, SLE, cryoglobulinaemia, Sjögren's syndrome, paraneoplastic
- Infectious   -   Lyme disease, HIV, leprosy
- Others   -   diabetes mellitus, amyloidosis, sarcoidosis

UMN + LMN

- Motor neurone disease (no sensory deficit)
- Dual pathology (e.g. cervical myelopathy + polyneuropathy)
- Myeloradiculopathy
- Subacute combined degeneration of the cord (symmetrical UMN signs with absent reflexes, impaired posterior column function, peripheral sensory neuropathy)

NB: spinal cord lesions can cause LMN signs at the site of the lesion and UMN signs below the lesion

CEREBELLAR DISEASE

MAVIS:
- **M**S
- **A**lcohol
- **V**ascular*   -   thromboembolic, haemorrhagic
- **I**nherited   -   Friedreich's ataxia, spinocerebellar ataxia, ataxia telangiectasia
- **S**OL

CRANIAL NERVE PALSIES

Commonest causes of cranial nerve lesions	
Lesion	**Causes**
Optic atrophy	Post-optic neuritis/MS, arteritic ischaemia (temporal arteritis)*, microvascular ischaemia*, compression (SOL, raised intracranial pressure), glaucoma*, toxins (methanol, ethambutol)
Third nerve palsy	**Medical (classically pupil-sparing), M's: M**icrovascular ischaemia (diabetes)*, **M**igraine*, **M**S/autoimmune disorders **Surgical (classically painful), C's:** posterior **C**ommunicating artery aneurysm (classic cause)*, **C**avernous sinus lesion, **C**ancer (SOL)
Sixth nerve palsy	Raised intracranial pressure*, microvascular ischaemia*, SOL, trauma*
Unilateral facial nerve palsy	Bell's palsy*, Ramsay Hunt syndrome*, SOL (e.g. acoustic neuroma, facial nerve tumour, meningioma), Lyme disease*, nerve infiltration (TB, sarcoidosis, lymphoma), parotid tumour/surgery*
Bilateral facial nerve palsy	Lyme disease*, sarcoidosis, Guillain-Barré syndrome*, amyloidosis *Other differentials for bilateral facial weakness: muscular dystrophies, myasthenia gravis*
Bulbar palsy (*LMN*)	Motor neurone disease, brainstem infarct/SOL, Guillain-Barré syndrome*, polio*, syringobulbia, neurosyphilis
Pseudobulbar palsy (*UMN*)	Motor neurone disease, high brainstem infarct/SOL, MS, bilateral internal capsule infarcts, traumatic brain injury*, progressive supranuclear palsy

MULTIPLE CRANIAL NERVE PALSIES

- Any = mononeuritis multiplex, SOLs, trauma*, sarcoidosis, Lyme disease*, Miller-Fisher syndrome*, neurosyphilis, vasculitis, botulism*
- CN 3-6 = cavernous sinus lesion*
- CN 5-8 + cerebellar = cerebellopontine angle lesion
- CN 9-10
  - + 11 = jugular foramen syndrome
  - + 12 = pseudobulbar/bulbar palsy
  - + Horner's syndrome + cerebellar + sensory disturbance (ipsilateral face, contralateral body) = lateral medullary (Wallenberg) syndrome*

COMPLEX OPHTHALMOPLEGIA

Work posteriorly (soft tissue to brainstem):
- Soft tissue   -   Graves' disease
- Muscle   -   mitochondrial myopathy
- Neuromuscular junction -   myasthenia gravis (test fatigability)
- Multiple CN's   -   cavernous sinus lesion*, mononeuritis multiplex, MS
- Brainstem   -   stroke*, SOL, trauma*

PTOSIS

- Unilateral
  - Third nerve palsy (pupil 'down and out', dilated) – complete ptosis
  - Horner's syndrome (pupil constricted) – partial ptosis
  - Idiopathic
- Bilateral
  - Myasthenia gravis
  - Myotonic dystrophy (frontal balding, facial muscle wasting)
  - Congenital
  - Neurosyphilis (Argyll Robertson pupils)

HORNER'S SYNDROME

- 1st order (central)   -   MS, spondylosis, SOL, syringomyelia, stroke/lateral medullary syndrome*
- 2nd order (pre-ganglionic)   -   Pancoast tumour, cervical rib, thyroid carcinoma/goitre
- 3rd order (post-ganglionic) -   carotid artery dissection*, radical neck dissection*

VISUAL FIELD DEFECTS

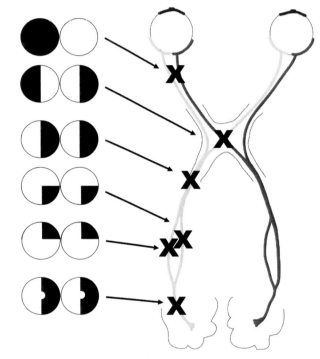

Monocular visual loss
Ipsilateral retinal or optic nerve lesion
Retinal, e.g. central retinal artery/vein occlusion, retinal detachment**
Optic nerve, e.g. optic neuritis, optic atrophy, glaucoma**

Bitemporal hemianopia
Optic chiasm lesion
e.g. pituitary tumour, craniopharyngioma

Homonymous hemianopia
Contralateral optic tract (or whole optic radiation) lesion
*e.g. middle cerebral artery occlusion (stem)**

PITS
Parietal
Inferior
Temporal
Superior

Homonymous inferior quadrantanopia
Contralateral parietal (upper) optic radiation lesion
*e.g. parietal tumour or middle cerebral
artery occlusion (superior branch)**

Homonymous superior quadrantanopia
Contralateral temporal (lower) optic radiation lesion
*e.g. temporal tumour or middle cerebral
artery occlusion (inferior branch)**

Homonymous hemianopia with macular sparring
Contralateral occipital visual cortex lesion
*e.g. posterior cerebral artery occlusion**

* = acute causes

CHOREOATHETOSIS

- Chorea   -   stroke*, Huntington's disease, Sydenham's chorea, drugs (e.g. anti-psychotics, levodopa)*, HIV
- Hemiballismus   -   subthalamic stroke (most)*, SOL, traumatic brain injury*, HIV
- Athetosis   -   asphyxia, neonatal jaundice, thalamic stroke*
- Dystonia   -   primary dystonia, brain trauma*, drugs*, Wilson's disease, PD, Huntington's disease, stroke*, SOL, encephalitis*, asphyxia*
- Myoclonus   -   epilepsy, essential myoclonus, metabolic*, psychological*, toxins/drugs*, SOL, MS, PD, Creutzfeldt-Jakob disease*

NB: Wilson's disease can cause any.

PARKINSONISM

- Parkinson's disease
- Vascular parkinsonism
- Parkinson-plus syndromes: multi-system atrophy, progressive supranuclear palsy, corticobulbar degeneration, Lewy body dementia
- Other causes: anti-dopaminergic drugs, Wilson's disease, communicating hydrocephalus, supratentorial tumours

NEUROLOGICAL HAND EXAMINATION

INTRODUCTION

- **W**ash hands; **I**ntroduce self; ask **P**atient's name, DOB and what they like to be called; **E**xplain examination and obtain consent
- Expose arms to above elbows; place pillow on their lap to rest hands on
- **General inspection:** mobility aids; posture; carpal tunnel syndrome risk factors (age, pregnancy, hypothyroidism, obesity, trauma, acromegaly)

HAND INSPECTION

- **Muscle wasting:** thenar (*median*) and hypothenar (*ulnar*) eminences; dorsal guttering (*ulnar*)
- **Scars** of previous surgery or trauma
- **Position:** claw hand (*ulnar*), wrist drop (*radial*)
- Tremors, fasciculations

> **Muscle innervation**
>
> Median nerve muscles (all thumb muscles except adductor pollicis)
> - **L**ateral two lumbricals
> - **O**pponens pollicis
> - **A**bductor pollicis brevis
> - **F**lexor pollicis brevis
>
> Ulnar nerve muscles (intrinsic hand muscles except most of thumb)
> - Adductor pollicis
> - Lumbricals (flex MCP joints and extend IP joints)
> - **P**almar interossei (**ad**duct fingers) **Pad Dab**
> - **D**orsal interossei (**ab**duct fingers)
>
> Radial nerve muscles (extensors)
> - Extensors

MOTOR POWER

- **Median** (*commonest causes: carpal tunnel syndrome, distal radial fracture, penetrating forearm injury, pronator teres syndrome*)
    - **Thumb abduction** (patient should lay hand flat on pillow with palm up and then point thumb towards ceiling – *'Don't let me push it down'*)
    - Pincer grip/thumb opposition (patient should touch tip of thumb to tip of little finger – *'Don't let me break it'*)
    - 'OK sign' (patient should touch tip of thumb to tip of index finger) – anterior interosseous nerve
- **Ulnar** (*commonest causes: compression at elbow/cubital tunnel syndrome, fractures, Guyon's canal/ulnar tunnel syndrome*)
    - **Finger abduction** (spread fingers against resistance)
    - <u>Grip card</u> between little and ring fingers with hands held vertically. Examiner tries to pull card away. (Tests adduction of little finger.)
    - <u>Grip card</u> between thumb and index fingers with hands held vertically. Examiner tries to pull card away. (If adductor pollicis is weak, patient will flex their thumb to grip the card – 'Froment's sign'.)
- **Radial** (*commonest causes: humeral shaft fracture, compression over spiral groove/Saturday night palsy*)
    - **Wrist <u>extension</u>**
    - Finger <u>extension</u> (all together at MCP joint) – posterior interosseous nerve
    - Thumb <u>extension</u> (with hand vertical, point thumb to ceiling – *'Don't let me push it down'*)

SENSORY (LIGHT TOUCH)

- **Palm facing up**
    - Over DIP joint of index finger (median nerve)
    - Over DIP joint of little finger (ulnar nerve)
- **Palm facing down**
    - Anatomical snuffbox (radial nerve)

SPECIAL TESTS FOR CARPAL TUNNEL SYNDROME

- **Phalen's test:** reverse prayer sign for 1 minute. Positive test = causes pain and paraesthesia in median nerve distribution.
- **Tinel's test:** tap median nerve at its course in wrist. Positive test = worsening paraesthesia.

FUNCTION

- **Function:** test pincer grip; prayer sign; carry out everyday tasks (e.g. undo buttons, write a sentence, hold cup, turn key)

TO COMPLETE

- Thank patient
- Summarise and suggest further investigations you would consider after a full history

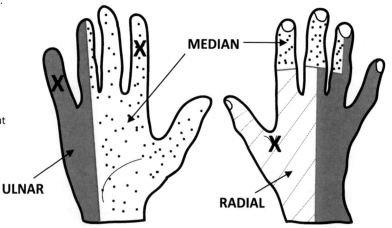

Cutaneous innervation of the ulnar, median and radial nerves

EXAMINATION OF SPEECH

INTRODUCTION

- **W**ash hands; **I**ntroduce self; ask **P**atient's name, DOB and what they like to be called; **E**xplain examination and obtain consent

GENERAL

- **Listen** to their speech
  - What's your name?
  - How old are you?
  - Describe how you got here today
  - Describe the room
- Determine if the pathology is dysarthria or dysphasia, then proceed to the appropriate examination
  - **Dysarthria** (difficulty with mechanics of speech)
    - Bulbar palsy = flaccid
    - Pseudobulbar palsy = spastic
    - Cerebellar = slurred, staccato (broken up into syllables, i.e. jerky), scanning (variability in pitch/volume)
    - Myasthenic = weak, quiet, fatigable
  - **Dysphasia** (difficulty with processing of speech)
    - Expressive (Broca's) = patient knows what they want to say but cannot say it
    - **R**eceptive (Wernicke's) = fluent, effortless speech but lacks meaning (talks **R**ubbish) + cannot understand language (written or spoken)

DYSARTHRIA

- **Repeat difficult phrases:** 'yellow lorry' (tests tongue), 'baby hippopotamus' (lips), 'we see three grey geese' (palate)
- **Repeat sounds:** 'pa' (facial and mouth), 'ta' (tongue), 'ka' (palate)
- **Count** to 30 (*fatigability in myasthenia gravis*)
- **Test cranial nerves 9, 10 and 12**
  - Look in mouth and say 'ahhh' to observe palatal movement
  - Look at uvula (deviates <u>away</u> from the side of lesion)
  - Look at tongue (*fasciculations = lower motor neuron, e.g. bulbar palsy*)
  - Assess cough and swallow
  - Stick tongue out (deviates <u>to</u> side of lesion)
  - Say you would also test gag reflex

DYSPHASIA

- **Commands** (receptive)
  - Single stage: 'open your mouth'
  - Two stage: 'with your right hand, touch your nose'
  - Three stage: 'with your right hand, touch your nose then your ear'
- **Word finding**
  - 'Say as many words as you can beginning with S' (<12 in 1 minute is abnormal)
- **Naming objects** (nominal)
  - Watch
  - Watch hands
  - Pen
  - Tie
  - Belt
- **Repetition** (receptive)
  - 'No ifs ands or buts'
- **Write** a sentence (expressive)
- **Read** a sentence (receptive)

TO COMPLETE EXAM

- Thank patient
- 'To complete my examination, I would perform a full neurological examination.'
- Summarise and suggest further investigations you would consider after a full history

PARKINSON'S DISEASE FOCUSSED EXAMINATION

NB: the OSCE instructions may be non-specific, for example: 'Examine this patient with a tremor', 'Examine this patient's gait and then proceed,' or 'Examine this patient neurologically'. Approach this situation by first asking a few generic questions (if allowed) or by inspecting for tremor/gait abnormalities. Then proceed with the relevant focussed examination to elicit other signs.

INTRODUCTION
- **W**ash hands; **I**ntroduce self; ask **P**atient's name, DOB and what they like to be called; **E**xplain examination and obtain consent

GENERAL OBSERVATIONS
- **General inspection:** patient, around bed (mobility aids etc.)
- **Tremor:** note any obvious tremor (if none, ask the patient to close their eyes and count down from 20 to distract them)
  - *Asymmetrical resting pill-rolling tremor (4-8 Hz)*
  - *Begins distally (fingers, hands, forearms), can involve chin and mouth*
  - *Reduced with finger to nose testing*
  - *Accentuated by distraction*
- **Gait:** ask patient to walk up and down the room
  - *Shuffling (reduced stride length)*
  - *Hesitant (difficulty initiating and turning (multiple steps))*
  - *Festinating (patient walks faster and faster so as to not fall over)*
  - *Lack of arm swing (early sign due to increased tone)*
  - *Unsteadiness (propulsion/retropulsion – tendency to fall forward or backward)*
- **Posture:** observe posture while walking *(stooped)*

Now work down the body:

FACE
- **Facial inspection** *(hypomimia, decreased blinking, drooling)*
- **Glabella tap test** (*Myerson's sign = blinking fails to cease with continued tapping*)
- **Speech:** ask the patient to say a sentence, e.g. describe the room they are in (*hypophonia, slow thinking, soft faint voice*)

FOCUSSED UPPER LIMBS
- **Tone:** increased tone can be accentuated with distraction by asking patient to move contralateral arm up and down (*lead pipe = increased tone; cogwheel rigidity = tremor superimposed on increased tone*)
- **Bradykinesia**
  - Open and close thumb and index finger like a 'snapper' as fast as possible (*lack or decay of amplitude; slow and asynchronous*)
  - Play imaginary piano *(slow)*
  - Open and close big imaginary doorknob (*difficulty pronating and supinating*)

FOCUSSED LOWER LIMBS
- **Bradykinesia:** heel tap (*lack or decay of amplitude; slow and asynchronous*)

EXTRAS
- **Function:** test undoing buttons, assess writing for *micrographia*
- **Exclude Parkinson-plus syndromes**
  - Vertical eye movements (*vertical limitation = progressive supranuclear palsy*)
  - Horizontal eye movements (*nystagmus = multisystem atrophy*)

TO COMPLETE
- Thank patient
- 'To complete my exam, I would look for cerebellar signs (*multisystem atrophy*), check postural blood pressure (*significant drop may be present in multisystem atrophy*) and undertake a mini-mental state exam (*Lewy body dementia*). I would also review any drug charts (*parkinsonism drugs*).'
- Summarise and suggest further investigations you would consider after a full history

---

Parkinsonism causes
- Parkinson's disease
- Vascular parkinsonism
- Parkinson-plus syndromes
- Other causes (e.g. anti-dopaminergic drugs, Wilson's disease)

Parkinson-plus syndromes
- Progressive supranuclear palsy: vertical limitation, axial rigidity
- Multi-system atrophy: cerebellar signs, autonomic problems
- Corticobulbar degeneration
- Dementia with Lewy bodies

Parkinson's disease tetrad
- Tremor
- Rigidity
- Bradykinesia
- Postural instability

CEREBELLAR DISEASE FOCUSSED EXAMINATION

NB: the instructions may be non-specific, for example: 'Examine this patient with a tremor', 'Examine this patient's gait and then proceed,' or 'Examine this patient neurologically'. Approach this situation by first asking a few generic questions (if allowed) or by inspecting for tremor/gait abnormalities. Then proceed with the relevant focussed examination to elicit other signs.

INTRODUCTION

- **W**ash hands; **I**ntroduce self; ask **P**atient's name, DOB and what they like to be called; **E**xplain examination and obtain consent

GENERAL OBSERVATIONS

- **General inspection**
  - Patient, e.g. posture
  - Around bed, e.g. mobility aids/wheelchair, neurological signs, posture, signs of neglect (*alcohol*)
- **Gait** (but first check that they can walk and accompany them in case they fall)
  - Stand from sitting with arms folded (*truncal ataxia*)
  - Walk away and, if stable, walk back heel-to-toe (*ataxic gait*)
- **Posture**
  - Stand with feet together
  - Romberg's test (only if steady): ask patient to close eyes and assess their stability (*sensory ataxia due to lack of proprioception*)

Now work down the body:

FACE

- **H-test** for extraocular muscle function (*see p67*) – look for *jerky pursuit movements* and pause at lateral gaze for *nystagmus*
- **Saccades test**: ask the patient to look back and forth between two widely spaced targets, e.g. your index finder on one hand and thumb on the other, while keeping their head still. Test horizontally and vertically. Check for conjugate eye movements and target accuracy. (*Hypometric saccades, i.e. slow movements, and saccadic dysmetria, i.e. difficulty fixing on target, are characteristic.*)
- **Repeat phrases**: 'West Register Street', 'baby hippopotamus' and 'British constitution' (*slurring; staccato (broken up into syllables, i.e. jerky); scanning (variability in pitch/volume)*)
- **Tongue:** move side to side

FOCUSSED UPPER LIMBS

- **Drift:** ask patient to hold arms out fully extended with palms facing upwards and their eyes closed (*pronator drift = weakness; upward drift = cerebellar pathology*)
- **Rebound test:** with the patient's arms still held up, push wrists down briskly and then quickly let go (*accentuates upward cerebellar drift*)
- **Tone** (*hypotonia*)
- **Co-ordination**
  - Finger-nose test (*intention tremor and dysmetria*)
  - Dysdiadochokinesia test (*inability to perform rapidly alternating movements*)

FOCUSSED LOWER LIMBS

- **Tone** (*hypotonia*)
- **Co-ordination:** heel-to-shin test (*ataxia*)
- **Knee jerks** over side of bed (*pendular reflex, i.e. multiple oscillations*)

TO COMPLETE

- Thank patient
- 'To complete my examination, I would examine the fundi for papilloedema (*space occupying lesion*) and perform a full neurological examination, including testing CN 5, 7 and 8 to exclude a cerebellopontine angle lesion.'
- Summarise and suggest further investigations you would consider after a full history

---

Generic questions

- What did you notice first when you developed this condition?
- How is it affecting you?
- When is your tremor worst?
- Do you have other problems, such as problems with balance or co-ordination?
- Do you have problems with buttons and shoe laces? Turning over in bed at night? Getting in and out of your car? (*All suggest Parkinsonism.*)

Examining for tremor

1. Resting tremor (rest hands on lap on ulnar border and close eyes and count down from 20)
2. Postural tremor (hold arms out)
3. Action tremor (finger-nose test)

Cerebellar signs

D	**D**ysdiadochikinesia and **D**ysmetria
A	**A**taxia
N	**N**ystagmus
I	**I**ntention tremor
S	**S**peech abnormality (slurring/scanning/staccato)
H	**H**ypotonia

Causes of cerebellar disease

M	**M**S
A	**A**lcohol
V	**V**ascular
I	**I**nherited ataxias
S	**S**pace occupying lesion

SHOULDER EXAMINATION

INTRODUCTION

- Wash hands; Introduce self; ask Patient's name, DOB and what they like to be called; Explain examination and obtain consent
- Expose upper body (but leave bra on in women)
- **General inspection**: patient, e.g. age, pain/discomfort, signs of trauma; around bed, e.g. mobility aids, sling

LOOK

You should inspect from the front, sides and behind.

- **Alignment and posture:** asymmetry of shoulders
- **Arm position** (*abducted and externally rotated = anterior dislocation; adducted and internally rotated = posterior dislocation*)
- **Bony prominences:** sternoclavicular joint, clavicle and acromioclavicular joint
- **Skin:** scars, bruising, sinuses, swelling
- **Muscles:** wasting (deltoid, supraspinatus, infraspinatus, pectorals)
- **Axilla:** obvious lymphadenopathy, large joint effusions, bruising

FEEL

Ask about any pain and then start by examining the normal side.

- **Skin:** palpate general area for temperature and soft tissue swelling/tenderness
- **Bony landmarks:** run hand from sternoclavicular joint along clavicle to acromioclavicular joint; then over the greater and lesser tuberosities and around the glenohumeral joint. Next feel the spine of the scapula, then around its inferior part back to the acromioclavicular joint. Watch the patient's face for tenderness.
- **Muscle bulk:** supraspinatus, infraspinatus, deltoid
- **Tendons:** look for biceps 'Popeye' sign/lump (*biceps tendon rupture*); flex elbow and feel long head of **biceps** tendon in bicipital groove while internally and externally rotating shoulder (*painful = tendinopathy*; check tendon is in groove and there is no subluxation); push arm posteriorly and feel the **supraspinatus** attachment at the greater tubercle just laterally

MOVE

Test active movements first, demonstrating them yourself beforehand.

- **Forward flexion (180°):** raise arms forward
- **Extension (65°):** swing arms backward
- **Abduction (180°):** raise each arm up sideways separately
  NB: if there is any pain, note at what angle it occurs (high arc pain = acromioclavicular joint pathology, e.g. arthritis; middle arc pain = rotator cuff pathology, e.g. supraspinatus tendonitis or partial rotator cuff tear). Passive movements will also help determine cause (no pain on passive movement = muscular; still painful on passive movement = mechanical/joint).
- **Adduction (50°):** move arms to midline and across body
- **External rotation (80°):** flex patient's elbows to 90° anteriorly, with their elbows fixed against their sides. Then ask them to turn their arms laterally (*external rotation lost early to <30° in adhesive capsulitis*).
- **Internal rotation:** ask patient to try to touch their scapula with their fingers behind their lower back (normal = can touch base of scapula, i.e. T6/7)
- **PASSIVE MOVEMENTS**: from behind, hold the patient's shoulder with one hand and their wrist with the other, then move their arm in all directions passively (feel for crepitus at acromioclavicular and glenohumeral joints)
- **SPECIAL TESTS:**

Muscle power	**Serratus anterior**	Patient should press hands on wall and lean forwards – look for scapula winging
	Deltoid (C5/6, axillary nerve)	Abduct shoulder against resistance at 90°
	Supraspinatus	Resisted 'empty can' test: patient should slightly forward flex their shoulder with their elbow extended, and pronate wrist ('empty a can of coke'); then ask them to push their wrist upwards against resistance
	Infraspinatus/teres minor	Resisted external rotation: arm in neutral position for infraspinatus; arm in 90° abduction for teres minor
	Subscapularis	Patient should place the dorsum of their hand over their lumbar spine; then move hand away posteriorly
	Neer's impingement test	From behind, stabilise the scapula with one hand, and use the other hand to internally rotate the patient's straight arm and passively forward flex it as high as possible. Pain is a positive test (*impingement syndrome*).
	Hawkins test	Patient should forward flex their shoulder to 90°, pronate hand ('empty a can of coke') and flex elbow medially to 90°. Now passively internally rotate shoulder (push their wrist downward while holding patient's elbow steady). Pain is a positive test (*impingement syndrome*).
	Apprehension test	Ask patient to hold hand out like a 'high five', then pull back elbow and push proximal humerus forward. Positive if patient shows fear of instability (*shoulder stabilisation problems, i.e. dislocation or subluxation*).
	Scarf acromioclavicular joint test	Position patient's hand over their opposite shoulder and push their elbow posteriorly (*pain = acromioclavicular joint pathology*)

FUNCTION

- **SCREENING**: test getting hands behind head and behind back

TO COMPLETE

- Thank patient and restore clothing
- 'To complete my examination, I would examine the cervical spine and elbows, and perform a distal neurovascular examination.'
- Summarise and suggest further investigations you would consider after a full history

---

Common shoulder pathology

- **Supraspinatus tendonitis (impingement syndrome)**
  - Supraspinatus tendon becomes inflamed due to impingement in the subacromial space
  - Signs: painful mid arc (60-120˚), positive impingement test
  - Treated with physiotherapy, analgesia, corticosteroid injection, arthroscopic acromioplasty
- **Rotator cuff tears**
  - Rotator cuff muscle tear, usually associated with impingement and tendonitis
  - Signs: supraspinatus wasting, weakness of abduction initiation
  - Incomplete tears managed conservatively, complete tears may require surgical repair
- **Adhesive capsulitis (frozen shoulder)**
  - Idiopathic
  - Severe pain initially, then persisting stiffness
  - Signs: loss of active and passive movement in all directions
  - NSAIDs/corticosteroid injection in painful phase; physiotherapy in stiff phase
- **Anterior shoulder instability (dislocation)**
  - Trauma or ligamentous laxity decreases stability and increases risk of dislocation or subluxation
  - Physiotherapy helps strengthen supporting muscles
  - MRI arthrogram and surgery may be required in persisting instability
- **Osteoarthritis**
  - Often secondary to chronic shoulder instability or chronic rotator cuff tear
  - Signs: painful movement restriction in all directions
  - Managed with analgesia, corticosteroid injection or surgery

---

Common elbow pathology

- **Olecranon bursitis**
  - Signs: localised swelling over olecranon tip, overlying erythema, preserved movements
- **Lateral epicondylitis (Tennis elbow)**
  - Inflammation at the common extensor origin on the lateral humeral epicondyle
  - Affects 30-50 year olds and is due to repetitive use
  - Lateral elbow pain worsens with use of extensor forearm muscles
  - Signs: tenderness over common extensor tendon origin (just distal to lateral epicondyle), pain on resisted wrist extension
  - Treated by avoiding painful activities, splints, NSAIDs, corticosteroid injections, physiotherapy, extracorporeal shock wave therapy, surgery
- **Medial epicondylitis (Golfer's elbow)**
  - Inflammation at the common flexor origin on the medial humeral epicondyle
  - Affects 30-50 year olds and is due to repetitive use
  - Medial elbow pain worsens with use of flexor forearm muscles
  - Signs: tenderness over common flexor tendon origin (just distal to medial epicondyle), pain on resisted wrist flexion
  - Treated by avoiding painful activities, splints, NSAIDs, corticosteroid injections, physiotherapy, surgery
- **Cubital tunnel syndrome**
  - Ulnar nerve entrapment just posterior to the medial humeral epicondyle (within the cubital tunnel)
  - Risk factors include cubitus valgus deformity, elbow osteoarthritis, and regular leaning on forearm with bent elbow

ELBOW EXAMINATION

Varus and valgus force application

• To apply a valgus force, press on the lateral side of the joint
• To apply a varus force, press on the medial side of the joint

INTRODUCTION

- **W**ash hands; **I**ntroduce self; ask **P**atient's name, DOB and what they like to be called; **E**xplain examination and obtain consent
- Expose arms
- **General inspection**: patient, e.g. age, pain/discomfort, signs of trauma; around bed, e.g. mobility aids, sling

LOOK

You should inspect from the front, sides and behind.
- **Carrying angle** (men 5-10°, women 10-15°): cubitus valgus = increased angle; cubitus varus ('gunstock' deformity) = reversed angle
- **Fixed flexion deformity**
- **Skin:** scars, bruising, sinuses, swelling, erythema
- **Rashes:** psoriatic plaques, rheumatoid nodules (feel up extensor surface)
- **Muscles:** wasting, look for biceps 'Popeye' sign/lump (*biceps tendon rupture*)

FEEL

Ask about any pain and then start by examining the normal side.
- **Skin:** palpate general area for temperature, effusions and soft tissue swelling/tenderness (*e.g. olecranon bursitis*)
- **Bony landmarks**
  - Palpate olecranon tip, medial epicondyle, lateral epicondyle (palpate in extension and in flexion)
  - Palpate radial head with thumb on rotation of forearm
- **Palpate tendons**
  - Common extensor origin – just distal to lateral epicondyle (*pain = Tennis elbow*)
  - Common flexor origin – just distal to medial epicondyle (*pain = Golfer's elbow*)
- **Palpate ulnar groove** between the olecranon process and the medial epicondyle (*paraesthesia in ulnar nerve distribution = cubital tunnel syndrome*)

MOVE

Test active <u>then</u> passive movements.
- **Flexion (145°)**
- **Extension (0°)**
- **Pronation (85°)** of wrist while elbow flexed to 90°
- **Supination (90°)** of wrist while elbow flexed to 90°
- **SPECIAL TESTS:**

Lateral collateral ligament	Flex elbow to 30° and apply varus force while forearm supinated
Medial collateral ligament	Flex elbow to 30° and apply valgus force while forearm pronated
Tennis elbow test	With elbow at 90°, forearm pronated, and wrist fully flexed, ask patient to extend wrist while applying resistance (pain at lateral epicondyle = positive test)
Golfer's elbow test	With elbow at 90°, forearm pronated, and wrist fully extended, ask patient to flex wrist while applying resistance (pain at medial epicondyle = positive test)

FUNCTION

- Move hand to mouth
- Place hands behind head

TO COMPLETE

- Thank patient and restore clothing
- 'To complete my examination, I would examine the shoulders and wrists, and perform a distal neurovascular examination.'
- Summarise and suggest further investigations you would consider after a full history

HAND AND WRIST EXAMINATION

INTRODUCTION

- **W**ash hands; **I**ntroduce self; ask **P**atient's name, DOB and what they like to be called; **E**xplain examination and obtain consent
- Expose arms to above elbows and place pillow on their lap to rest hands on
- **General inspection**: patient, e.g. age, pain/discomfort, signs of trauma; around bed, e.g. mobility aids, splint

LOOK

- **Dorsum**
  - o **General:** posture, obvious deformities, scars
  - o **Bone/joint swelling and deformity**
    - Osteoarthritis: Heberden's nodes (DIP joints), Bouchard's nodes (PIP joints)
    - RA: loss of knuckle guttering, 'swan neck' deformity (PIP joint hyperextension + DIP joint flexion), boutonnière deformity (PIP joint flexion + DIP joint hyperextension), Z-shaped thumb (IP joint hyperextension + MCP joint flexion), ulnar deviation at wrist, palmar subluxation of MCP joints
    - Seronegative spondyloarthropathy: dactylitis ('sausage digit' – inflammation of entire digit)
    NB: there is no DIP joint involvement in RA but there may be in OA or seronegative spondyloarthropathies.
  - o **Skin:** scars, thinning/bruising (*steroid use*), rashes, erythema
  - o **Muscles:** guttering (*ulnar nerve lesion, tendon ruptures, peripheral neuropathy*)
  - o **Nails:** psoriatic changes (e.g. pitting, onycholysis), nail fold vasculitis, clubbing
- **Palmar surface**
  - o **Look for:** posture abnormalities, muscle wasting of thenar eminence (*carpal tunnel syndrome*) and hypothenar eminence (*ulnar nerve lesion*), palmar erythema, carpal tunnel release scar, swellings (*e.g. ganglions – local small fluctuant swellings*)
- **Extensor surface of arm**
  - o **Feel up border:** psoriatic plaques, rheumatoid nodules, gouty tophi (whitish nodules of crystallised uric acid under skin around fingers/elbows)

FEEL

Ask about any pain before examining.

- **Palmar surface**
  - o **Bulk** of thenar/hypothenar eminences
  - o **Tendon thickening:** palpate palmar flexor tendons (*palmar tendon thickening with fixed flexion deformity = Dupuytren's contracture*); flex and extend fingers individually while palpating flexor tendons near MCP joints (*tendon thickening/bump near MCP joint with triggering = trigger finger*)
- **Dorsum**
  - o **Temperature** (forearm, wrist and MCP joints)
  - o **Squeeze joints** for tenderness and feel for bony swellings, effusions, synovitis, deformities
    - Distal radio-ulnar joint
    - Radial and ulnar styloids
    - Anatomical snuffbox (*tenderness = scaphoid fracture*)
    - Carpals (bimanual palpation)
    - MCP joints (squeeze along row then bimanual palpation if any pain elicited) and base of thumb (*squaring = osteoarthritis*)
    - IP joints (bimanual palpation of each joint; *Heberden's/Bouchard's nodes = osteoarthritis*)
  - o **Tendon tenderness**
    - Around radial styloid, i.e. 1st extensor compartment (*tenderness = de Quervain's tenosynovitis*)
    - Around ulnar styloid (*tenderness = extensor carpi ulnaris tendinopathy*)

MOVE

- **Wrist movements** actively <u>and</u> passively (feel for crepitus): extension 70° and flexion 80° ('prayer' sign and 'reverse prayer' sign respectively); pronation 70° and supination 80°; radial deviation 20° and ulnar deviation 40°
- **Finger movements**: straighten fingers fully against gravity (*difficulty = joint disease, extensor tendon rupture or neurological damage; triggering of a finger = trigger finger*); make fist (*cannot tuck fingers in = tendon/small joint involvement*); move each MCP and IP joint passively (assess for limited movement and crepitus)
- **Thumb movements**: extension (stretch thumb out laterally); resisted abduction (point thumb to ceiling with wrist supinated); opposition (touch thumb to little finger tip); flexion (thumb to palm); adduction (point thumb to floor with wrist supinated)
- **SPECIAL TESTS:**

Phalen's test	'Reverse prayer' sign for 1 minute (*pain/paraesthesia = carpal tunnel syndrome*)
Tinel's test	Tap over the carpal tunnel (*paraesthesia = carpal tunnel syndrome*)
Finkelstein's test	Ask patient to adduct their thumb to their palm and close fist around it; then tilt their wrist into ulnar deviation (*pain = de Quervain's tenosynovitis*)

FUNCTION

- **Function**: test pincer grip; carry out everyday tasks, e.g. undo buttons, write sentence, hold cup, turn key
- **Basic neurological hand exam:** quickly do the motor and sensory parts of the neurological hand exam

Basic neurological hand exam			
	Median	**Ulnar**	**Radial**
Motor	**Thumb abduction** (lie hand flat on pillow with palm up, then point thumb towards ceiling – *'Don't let me push it down'*)	**Finger abduction** (spread fingers against resistance)	**Wrist extension**
Sensory	Over DIP joint of **index finger** (palm facing up)	Over DIP joint of **little finger** (palm facing up)	Over **anatomical snuffbox** (palm facing down)

TO COMPLETE

- Thank patient
- 'To complete my examination, I would examine the elbows and perform a distal neurovascular examination.'
- Summarise and suggest further investigations you would consider after a full history

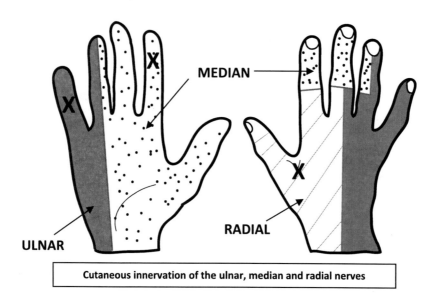

Cutaneous innervation of the ulnar, median and radial nerves

Common hand and wrist pathology

- **Rheumatoid arthritis**
  - Chronic autoimmune disorder resulting in symmetrical deforming polyarthropathy
  - Signs: synovitis, bony deformities (*described on previous page*), palmar erythema, small muscle wasting, reduced range of movement, tendon ruptures or subluxation
  - DIP joints sparred
  - Management: NSAIDs, steroids, DMARDs (e.g. methotrexate), surgery
- **Osteoarthritis**
  - Mechanical joint degradation with degeneration of articular cartilage, periarticular bone remodelling and inflammation
  - Signs: joint crepitus and limited range of movement, bony deformities (*described on previous page*)
  - Management: analgesia, corticosteroid injection, physiotherapy/splints, surgery
- **Carpal tunnel syndrome**
  - Median nerve entrapment neuropathy caused by compression of the median nerve in the carpal tunnel
  - Intermittent paraesthesia, pain/burning and numbness of thumb, first and middle fingers, and radial half of ring finger
  - Usually worse at night
  - Signs: loss of power and wasting of the thenar eminence, sensory loss in median nerve distribution
  - Management: splints, corticosteroid injection, carpal tunnel decompression
- **Trigger finger**
  - Thickening of the flexor tendon sheath causing entrapment at the A1 pulley (near MCP joint)
  - Discomfort and/or bump at base of digit and catching or clicking during extension
  - Management: splints, NSAIDs, corticosteroid injection, surgical release

SPINE EXAMINATION

INTRODUCTION

- **W**ash hands; **I**ntroduce self; ask **P**atient's name, DOB and what they like to be called; **E**xplain examination and obtain consent
- Expose upper body (but leave bra on in women)
- **General inspection**: patient, e.g. age, pain/discomfort, signs of trauma; around bed, e.g. mobility aids, spinal brace

LOOK

- **Gait:** walking aids, speed, phases of walking, stride length, arm swing
- **Inspect from behind**
  - Posture: asymmetry, scoliosis
  - Skin and muscles: muscle wasting, scars, redness
  - Soft tissue abnormalities: lipomas, hair growth (*spina bifida*), pigmentation, *café-au-lait* spots (*neurofibromatosis*)
- **Inspect from side** (stand against wall): check for normal cervical lordosis, thoracic kyphosis, and lumbar lordosis (*lost in spondylolisthesis and when in pain*)

FEEL

Ask about any pain before examining.

- **Spinous processes and over sacroiliac joints** for alignment and tenderness
- **Paraspinal muscles** for tenderness and increased tone
- Consider **spinal percussion** over thoracic/lumbar spinous processes, using the same technique as in a respiratory exam (*see p45*) or closed fist percussion (*percussion tenderness = serious pathology such as malignancy, osteomyelitis, or compression fracture*)

MOVE

Demonstrate movements first.

- **Lateral flexion:** *'Slide your hand down your leg'*
- **Lumbar flexion (10-20°) and extension:** flexion *'Touch your toes'*, extension *'Lean back as far as you can'*
- **Cervical spine movements:** flexion/extension (*'Touch your chin to your chest'*), rotation (*'Look over your shoulder'*), deviation (*'Touch you ear to you shoulder'*)
- **Thoracic rotation:** *'Rotate your chest while sitting with your arms crossed'*
- **SPECIAL TESTS:**

Schober's test	Mark midline 10cm above the dimples of Venus and 5cm below while standing, then re-measure distance in flexion (*<5cm difference implies lumbar flexion limitation that may be due to ankylosing spondylitis if there are other symptoms/signs*)
Chest circumference expansion	Measure chest circumference in expiration and inspiration. Around 7cm difference is normal (*<5cm suggests ankylosing spondylitis*).
Femoral nerve stretch test	With patient prone, passively flex knee and extend hip (*anterior thigh pain = femoral nerve irritation, usually due to L2-4 disc herniation*)
Straight leg raise (sciatic nerve stretch test)	With patient supine, lift a leg to full flexion or until significant leg pain, then depress it slightly and passively dorsiflex foot (*leg pain radiating down below knee = sciatic nerve irritation, usually due to L4-S1 disc herniation/facet joint impingement*)
Gaenslen's sacroiliac stress test	Ask patient to flex their hip and knee, then passively push that knee into the patient's chest and push the contralateral thigh into the bed (*pain = sacroiliac joint pathology*)

FUNCTION

- **(Gait:** already observed)
- **Brief lower limb neurological exam** (*see p69*)

TO COMPLETE

- Thank patient and restore clothing
- 'To complete my examination, I would examine the hips and perform a full lower limb neurological examination. I would also examine perianal sensation and anal tone if there was any concern about cauda equina syndrome.'
- Summarise and suggest further investigations you would consider after a full history

Common spine pathology

- **Osteoarthritis/facet joint degeneration:** stiffness (<30 minutes in morning), worse with movement; no neurology
- **Ankylosing spondylitis:** stiffness >30 minutes in morning; reduced range of movement in all directions
- **Sciatica:** nerve root impingement (commonly L4/5 or L5/S1); pain radiating down leg
- **Cauda equina syndrome:** compression of cauda equina nerves resulting in lower back pain, leg pain, urinary retention, perianal numbness and reduced anal tone – *requires emergency MRI and surgical decompression*

INTRODUCTION

- <u>W</u>ash hands; <u>I</u>ntroduce self; ask <u>P</u>atient's name, DOB and what they like to be called; <u>E</u>xplain examination and obtain consent
- Expose to underwear
- **General inspection**: patient, e.g. age, pain/discomfort, signs of trauma; around bed, e.g. mobility aids

LOOK

- **Gait:** speed, walking phases, stride length, arm swing, abnormal gaits (e.g. Trendelenburg's waddling gait (*abductor dysfunction*) or antalgic gait)
- **Standing inspection:** front (straight stance, pelvic tilt, any deformities of hip/knee/ankle/foot), side (stoop, lumbar lordosis), behind (scoliosis, gluteal atrophy)
    - **Trendelenburg test:** crouch down and hold the patient's ASIS's from the front, then ask them to stand on one leg by bending the contralateral knee. Then repeat on the other side. Normally their gluteal abducting muscles will tilt the pelvis so the contralateral (unsupported) side rises to balance. If the contralateral side dips, there is abductor muscle weakness on the side they are standing on.
- **Lying inspection:** observe legs and compare sides – look for symmetry and rotation (*one leg shortened and externally rotated = fractured neck of femur*), hip scars, sinuses, dressings or skin changes
- **Measure true/apparent leg lengths:** square hips then measure apparent leg length, i.e. xiphisternum/umbilicus to each medial malleolus (*unequal = spinal or pelvic deformity, e.g. scoliosis*). Next measure true leg length, i.e. ASIS to ipsilateral medial malleolus (*unequal = true limb shortening, e.g. in fracture or developmental problems*).

FEEL

Ask about any pain and then start by examining the normal side.

- **Bony landmark tenderness:** run hand up leg to greater trochanter (*tenderness may indicate trochanteric bursitis*), then to ASIS, then pubic rami
- **Skin:** palpate general area for temperature and soft tissue swelling/tenderness

MOVE

First test all active movements (except internal and external rotation), <u>then</u> test passive movements.

- Start by rolling each leg from side to side (assesses for hip fracture)
- **Flexion (120˚):** flex the patient's hip and knee and press their knee against their chest
- **Internal (30˚) and external (40˚) rotation:** with the knee and hip flexed to 90˚, turn shin inwards (external rotation) and outwards (internal rotation). *Internal rotation is lost early in osteoarthritis.*
- **Abduction (45˚) and adduction (30˚):** place your left hand on the patient's contralateral iliac crest to detect pelvic movement. Hold their calf in your right hand and abduct until pelvis tilts. Test adduction by crossing their leg over the other.
- **Extension (20˚):** ask patient to lie prone. Inspect for scars and muscle wasting. Extend hip actively then passively. Place your left hand on their pelvis/lumbar spine to detect movement while lifting each thigh.
- **SPECIAL TESTS:**

Thomas' test	Fully flex the patient's hip on one side (with their knee also in flexion) and place a hand under their lumbar spine. The lumbar lordosis should be reduced. If the contralateral thigh is forced off the couch, there is a fixed flexion deformity of that hip. Now repeat on the other side.
Trendelenburg's test	*Already performed*

FUNCTION

- **(Gait:** already observed)

TO COMPLETE

- Thank patient and restore clothing
- 'To complete my examination, I would examine the spine and the knees, and perform a distal neurovascular examination.'
- Summarise and suggest further investigations you would consider after a full history

Common hip pathology

- **Hip osteoarthritis:** pain and reduced range of movement (internal rotation often lost first),;Thomas and Trendelenburg tests positive in advanced osteoarthritis
- **Trochanteric bursitis:** pain and tenderness over the greater trochanter; cannot lie on affected side
- **Childhood problems**, e.g. dislocation, Perthes disease, slipped upper femoral epiphysis

KNEE EXAMINATION

Grading knee ligament injuries

- **Grade 1:** pain but knee stable
- **Grade 2:** pain and laxity
- **Grade 3:** very lax (no end point)

INTRODUCTION

- <u>W</u>ash hands; <u>I</u>ntroduce self; ask <u>P</u>atient's name, DOB and what they like to be called; <u>E</u>xplain examination and obtain consent
- Expose to underwear/shorts
- **General inspection**: patient, e.g. age, pain/discomfort, signs of trauma; around bed, e.g. mobility aids, splint

LOOK

- **Gait:** look for limp and movement restriction; assess knee movements during different phases of gait; check for normal heel-strike/toe-off
- **Standing inspection:** alignment (patella/legs), varus/valgus deformities, fixed flexion deformity, recurvatum (hyperextension), popliteal swelling (e.g. Baker's cyst, popliteal aneurysm)
- **Supine close inspection:** skin (scars/arthroscopic portals, bruising, erythema, psoriatic plaques), joints (swelling, effusions), alignment (patella, tibia), position (fixed flexion deformity), 'knobbly knees' (*osteoarthritis*)
- **Measure quadriceps muscle bulk:** measure quadriceps diameter 20 cm above tibial tuberosity; compare with contralateral side

FEEL

Ask about any pain and then start by examining the normal side with the patient supine.

- **Skin:** palpate general area for temperature and soft tissue swelling/tenderness
- **Joint:** flex patient's knee to 90° (and look for tibial lag), then feel along joint line (quadriceps tendon → patella → patella tendon → tibial tuberosity → tibial plateau → femoral epicondyles and over course of medial collateral ligament and lateral collateral ligament → popliteal fossa). Note any swelling, synovial thickening and tenderness.
- **Effusions** – test with knee extended
  - **Cross fluctuation test:** empty suprapatellar pouch by applying pressure with one hand. Hold your other hand just below the patella and alternate compressions each side. Positive test = impulses transmitted from side to side (*large effusion*).
  - **Patella tap test:** empty suprapatellar pouch, then sharply tap patella with index finger. Positive test = patella sinks, striking femur, then comes back up (*moderate effusion*).
  - **Bulge test:** empty suprapatellar pouch, then systematically stroke around the knee starting from the inferomedial position, up the medial side (drains medial compartment), then down the lateral side to end in the inferolateral position. Positive test = ripples on medial surface (*small effusion*).

MOVE

Test active <u>then</u> passive movements, keeping one hand on the knee to feel for crepitus.

- **Flexion (140°)**
- **Extension (0°)**
- Passively raise leg at ankle and look for knee hyperextension (up to 10° normal; *greater in collagen disorder/ hypermobility*)
- **SPECIAL TESTS:**

Collateral ligaments	Hold the patient's ankle/lower leg in one hand and their knee in the other. Apply varus and valgus knee forces to the knee. This stresses lateral and medial collateral ligaments respectively. Test at 0° and 30° of knee flexion. (You can hold their foot between your elbow and your side.) Look/feel for excessive movement (*collateral ligament laxity*).
Drawer test	First check for foot pain, then flex knee to 90°, sit on the side of their foot, and hold upper tibia with thumbs on tibial tuberosity and fingers in popliteal fossa. Pull anteriorly (*anterior lag = anterior cruciate ligament laxity*); then push posteriorly (*posterior lag = posterior cruciate ligament laxity*).
Lachman's test	With the patient's knee flexed to 30°, hold one hand on top of their thigh and the other on their posteromedial proximal tibia. Pull tibia anteriorly (*more sensitive for anterior cruciate ligament laxity*).
McMurray's test	Warn patient this test may cause pain. Flex knee as much as possible. Use one hand to externally rotate their foot and hold it over to the contralateral side of the patient. Then apply varus force to knee with the other hand, while extending the knee joint (stresses medial meniscus). Then test the opposite side (stresses lateral meniscus). Positive test = painful click felt or heard (*meniscal tear*).
Patellofemoral apprehension test	Flex knee while pressing patella laterally. If patella is unstable, patient will anticipate dislocation and stop you.
Apley's grind test	With patient prone and knee flexed to 90°, apply axial load to the knee and rotate foot (*pain = meniscal damage*)

FUNCTION

- **Squat test**

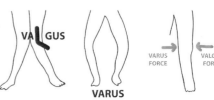

Valgus and varus

TO COMPLETE

- Thank patient and restore clothing
- 'To complete my examination, I would examine the hips and the ankles, and perform a distal neurovascular examination.'
- Summarise and suggest further investigations you would consider after a full history

---

Common knee pathology

- **Anterior cruciate ligament tear**
  - Usually torn in twisting injury
  - May feel pop; swelling usually develops immediately or within 1 hour (haemarthrosis)
  - Pain makes full examination difficult before 2 weeks
  - Signs: increased laxity on anterior draw test
  - Treated with physiotherapy and/or surgical reconstruction (if ongoing instability)
- **Posterior cruciate ligament tear**
  - Usually due to high energy trauma; associated with multiligament knee injury, hip dislocation and fracture
  - Signs: increased posterior laxity on posterior draw test
  - Treated with physiotherapy and/or surgical reconstruction (if multiligament, fracture, or ongoing instability)
- **Meniscal tears**
  - Usually torn in twisting injury
  - Swelling develops a number of hours later
  - Sharp localised medial or lateral pain exacerbated by hyperflexion/twisting
  - Knee may lock or give way (due to pain)
  - Signs: tender over medial/lateral joint line; good range of movement unless knee is locked; positive McMurray's/Apley's test
  - MRI or arthroscopy can confirm; meniscal tear is usually excised arthroscopically
- **Collateral ligament tears**
  - Signs: varus laxity (lateral collateral ligament) or valgus laxity (medial collateral ligament), effusion, tenderness over affected ligaments
  - Treated with rest, physiotherapy and hinged brace
- **Osteoarthritis**
  - Pain and stiffness
  - Signs: reduced range of movement, crepitus
- **Prepatellar bursitis ('Housemaid's knee')**
  - Localised swelling over patella
  - Precipitated by period of kneeling
  - Signs: tenderness over patella, normal range of movement
  - Treated with rest and NSAIDs
  - Aspiration and corticosteroid injections may also be used

---

Common foot and ankle pathology

- **Pes planus ('flat foot')**
  - Loss of medial arch
  - May be flexible (correctable on tip-toe standing) or rigid (non-correctable)
  - Flexible pes planus is normal in toddlers and is often asymptomatic in adults
  - Rigid pes planus may be due to tarsal coalition or sequelae of tibialis posterior tendon rupture
- **Hallux valgus**
  - Lateral angulation of big toe
  - Usually occurs in older women
  - Can result in pain at the medial aspect of MTP joint (from shoe pressure) and a bony bump ('bunion')
  - May be treated with alteration in footwear, osteotomy or fusion
- **Gout**
  - Monoarthropathy caused by deposition of monosodium urate crystals in hyperuricaemia
  - Signs: tender, erythematous, inflamed joint
  - MTP joint most commonly affected
  - Acutely managed with NSAIDs/colchicine
  - Prevented by allopurinol, avoiding purine rich foods/drinks, and stopping thiazide and loop diuretics
- **Achilles tendon rupture**
  - Patient feels like someone 'kicked them in the back of the leg' while pushing off with foot (e.g. while running)
  - Signs: unable to plantar-flex; Simmonds' test positive
  - May be treated by surgical repair, or conservatively in an equinus cast or boot (if minor tear/older/comorbidities/less athletic)
- **Charcot foot**
  - Pain-free joint destruction after minor trauma
  - Usually occurs in patients with peripheral neuropathy due to diabetes
  - In developing countries, tabes dorsalis and leprosy are common causes
  - Signs: erythema and swelling in the acute phase only; gross joint deformity; instability
  - Managed by educating patient, treating underlying cause, podiatry and joint immobilisation with a cast/boot in the acute phase
- **Morton's neuroma**
  - Benign neuroma of digital nerve in foot (between $2^{nd}/3^{rd}$ or $3^{rd}/4^{th}$ metatarsals)
  - Feeling of walking on a marble
  - May be treated with footwear changes, orthoses, steroid injections or surgical excision
- **Lateral ligament sprain**
  - Inversion injury causing anterior talofibular ligament injury
  - Usually managed with physiotherapy ± splints
- **Syndesmosis injury (high ankle sprain)**
  - Usually associated with external rotation injuries and other pathology (e.g. fractures)
  - Surgical fixation often required

FOOT AND ANKLE EXAMINATION

INTRODUCTION

- **W**ash hands; **I**ntroduce self; ask **P**atient's name, DOB and what they like to be called; **E**xplain examination and obtain consent
- Expose knees and below
- **General inspection**: patient, e.g. age, pain/discomfort, signs of trauma; around bed, e.g. mobility aids, splint

LOOK

- **Gait:** look for limp and movement restriction; assess knee, ankle and foot movements; check for normal heel-strike/toe-off
- **Standing inspection**
  - **Front:** hallux deformities (*lateral angulation of big toe = hallux valgus*), lesser toe deformities (*flexed PIP joints = hammer toes; flexed DIP joints = mallet toes; flexed PIP joints and DIP joints with pes cavus = claw toes*)
  - **Sides:** foot arches (*pes planus = flat foot; pes cavus = high arch, usually with clawed toes*)
  - **Behind:** alignment of hindfoot (5° valgus normal)
  - **Tip-toe standing inspection:** re-inspect foot arch if there was pes planus (*if it corrects on tip-toe standing, it is flexible pes planus; if it does not correct, it is rigid pes planus*); big toe flexion (*no flexion = hallux rigidus*); hindfoot varus/valgus angulation change (*normal hindfoot 5° valgus should correct into varus*)
- **Lying inspection:** skin (scars/arthroscopic portals, bruising, erythema), joints (swelling, effusions), muscles (wasting), heel (callosities), between toes (ulcers), nails (psoriatic changes), feel up extensor surface of lower leg (psoriasis plaques, rheumatoid nodules, gouty tophi)
- **Measure calf muscle bulk:** measure calf diameter 10 cm below tibial tuberosity and compare with contralateral side

FEEL

Ask about any pain and then start by examining the normal side.

- **Skin:** palpate general area for temperature and soft tissue swelling/tenderness
- **Ligaments:** deltoid ligament (anteroinferior to medial malleolus), anterior talofibular ligament (anterior to lateral malleolus), calcaneofibular ligament (inferior to lateral malleolus), and posterior talofibular ligament (posterior to lateral malleolus)
- **Bony landmarks** – assess joints for tenderness and feel for bony swellings, effusions, synovitis, deformities
  - Ankle: medial malleolus, lateral malleolus, anterior joint line
  - Hindfoot and midfoot: feel around joints in an 'n' pattern (distolateral → proximolateral → across dorsum → proximomedial → distomedial)
  - Forefoot: feel all joints in circle (tarsometatarsal joints, metatarsal heads, MTP joints and IP joints)
- **Plantar fascia:** feel for thickening, tenderness, fibromatosis

MOVE

Movements are best assessed with patient's legs hanging over bed.

- **Ankle movements** (actively, <u>and</u> passively while feeling for crepitus): dorsiflexion 20° and plantar-flexion 40°; inversion and eversion at subtalar joint (stabilise ankle with one hand and move heel with the other)
- **Midtarsal movements:** hold calcaneus with one hand and abduct (10°) and adduct (20°) forefoot with your other hand
- **Toe movements:** ask patient to: straighten toes fully (*difficulty = joint disease, extensor tendon rupture or neurological damage*); curl toes (*can't curl toes in = tendon/small joint involvement*); abduct (spread) toes and adduct toes (hold paper between); move MCP joints and IP joints passively (assess for limited movement and crepitus)
- **SPECIAL TESTS:**

Muscles		
Tibialis anterior	Foot inversion and dorsiflexion against resistance
Tibialis posterior	Foot inversion and plantar-flexion against resistance
Peroneus longus and brevis	Foot eversion against resistance
Anterior drawer test	Hold calcaneum still and push lower leg posteriorly (tests anterior talofibular ligament)
Tilt test	Invert foot at ankle and compare to other side (tests calcaneofibular ligament)
Syndesmosis test	Squeeze mid-lower leg to test syndesmosis (*pain at distal tibia/fibula joint = syndesmosis injury*
Simmonds' test	Ask patient to kneel on a chair with feet hanging over edge, then squeeze both calves. Feet should plantar-flex (*no plantar-flexion = Achilles tendon rupture*).
Mulder's sign	Squeeze metatarsal heads together in horizontal plane with one hand while applying pressure to the interdigital space with other hand (*pain ± Mulder's click in 2nd/3rd or 3rd/4th webspace = Morton's neuroma*)

FUNCTION

- **Balance** – stand on one leg (*often poor with peroneal weakness/ligament sprains*)

TO COMPLETE

- Thank patient and restore clothing
- 'To complete my examination, I would examine the knees and perform a distal neurovascular examination.'
- Summarise and suggest further investigations you would consider after a full history

PELVIC EXAMINATION

INTRODUCTION

- **W**ash hands; **I**ntroduce self; ask **P**atient's name, DOB and what they like to be called; **E**xplain examination, why it's necessary, and obtain consent
- Get a **chaperone**
- Explain procedure
  - o Be impersonal, e.g. 'It is an internal examination from down below. It will involve placing two fingers into the vagina, and also inserting a small plastic tube to look at the cervix.'
  - o 'It shouldn't be painful, but if at any point you are uncomfortable or want to stop, just say so. One of the nurses will also be present to ensure you are comfortable and act as a chaperone.'
  - o Patient should be lying flat in lithotomy position but remain covered initially: 'You will need to undress from the waist down, put your heels together and bring them as close to your bottom as possible, then flop your knees outwards.'
- Ask a few questions before starting: last menstrual period, intra-menstrual bleeding, discharge, contraception, last smear
- Ask if patient needs to use the toilet before the procedure

NB: keep talking to and reassuring the patient using their name throughout.

EXTERNAL EXAMINATION

- **Basic lower abdominal exam:** inspect for distension/scars; feel for masses/tenderness; feel groin for inguinal lymphadenopathy
- Put on gloves
- Part labia with forefinger and thumb of left hand
- **Inspect vulva:** tumours, lesions, warts/ulcerations, cysts (sebaceous/Bartholin's), erythema, atrophy, labial fusion, whitening, scarring, discharge, bleeding
- **Ask patient to <u>cough</u>** to assess for uterovaginal prolapse

SPECULUM EXAMINATION (± SWABS)

- Warm the speculum if necessary with warm water, lubricate the sides, and warn the patient prior to insertion
- Part the labia and insert the speculum with the screw sideways
- Rotate speculum as you advance it so that the screw is facing upwards. Open speculum and tighten screw when resistance is met.
- Direct light to visualise cervix and look for: discharge, erosions, ulcerations, growths, cervicitis, blood, polyps, ectropion
- Take swabs at this point if required (*see procedure notes on gynaecological swabs p230*)
- Close speculum blades (but not fully to avoid pinching vaginal wall)
- Remove speculum while rotating it back sideways

INTERNAL (BIMANUAL/PV) EXAMINATION

- Explain and reassure patient
- Lubricate fingers
- Part labia with non-dominant hand, and insert your dominant hand's index finger first, then introduce middle finger. Enter with palm facing sideways then rotate so it is facing up.
- With the two fingers facing upwards, move along posterior wall of vagina. Move up and over **cervix** (*cervical excitation = pelvic inflammatory disease or ectopic pregnancy*), and gently palpate it (smoothness, bleeding propensity, mobility, firmness).
- Now place one finger under cervix and push upwards, while simultaneously pushing down on the lower abdomen to depress the fundus with your other hand
  - o Assess **uterus** size (*enlargement = pregnancy, fibroids, malignancy, endometrial fluid collection*)
  - o Determine if anteverted or retroverted (fundus palpable in posterior fornix)
  - o Note tenderness, mobility, shape
- Now place fingers in each lateral fornix in turn, while simultaneously pushing down in the ipsilateral iliac fossa with the other hand to feel for **adnexal tenderness** (*salpingitis, ovarian torsion, ectopic pregnancy*) and masses
- Remove fingers slowly and inspect for blood or discharge
- Give patient gauze to wipe off lubricant

TO COMPLETE

- Thank patient and restore clothing
- Summarise and suggest further investigations you would consider after a full history

PREGNANT ABDOMEN EXAMINATION

INTRODUCTION

- **W**ash hands; **I**ntroduce self; ask **P**atient's name, DOB and what they like to be called; **E**xplain examination and obtain consent
- Position patient lying at 15° and expose their abdomen
- Reassure throughout (e.g. congratulate patient, ask how it's going so far, and if they have thought of a name)

GENERAL INSPECTION

- **General:** well/unwell, comfortable, breathlessness, pallor
- **Pulse rate**
- **Head and neck:** chloasma/jaundiced sclera (*obstetric cholestasis*), conjunctival pallor (*anaemia*), nasal congestion, facial oedema
- **Legs and feet:** swelling, oedema and varicose veins

ABDOMINAL INSPECTION

- **Distension**
- **Fetal movements**
- **Scars:** especially previous lower segment transverse/longitudinal scars (*C-section*) or laparoscopic scars (*may indicate ectopic*)
- **Skin changes**
    - **Linea nigra:** dark line from umbilicus or xiphisternum to suprapubic region
    - **Striae gravidarum:** purplish striae of no clinical significance
    - **Striae albicans:** old silvery-white striae (*parity*)
    - **Excoriations** (*obstetric cholestasis*)
    - **Distended superficial veins** (*increased inferior vena cava pressure due to gravid uterus*)
    - **Umbilicus eversion** (*occurs due to increased abdominal pressure*)
- **Cough for hernias**

ABDOMINAL PALPATION

Warm hands first, ask about pain, and always watch mother's face while examining.

- **Fundal height:** use the ulnar edge of your left hand to press down in a stepwise fashion from xiphisternum downwards to find the fundus (first bit of resistance); then measure from there to the pubic symphysis with measuring tape. To eliminate bias, measure with the inches side upwards, <u>then</u> turn over for centimetres reading. See box for normal fundal height.
    - *Bigger than expected = macrosomia, polyhydramnios, multiple pregnancy, wrong dates, fibroids*
    - *Smaller than expected = intrauterine growth restriction, oligohydramnios, small baby*
- **Lie:** face the mother's head and place your hands each side of the top pole of the uterus, applying gentle pressure. Walk hands down the sides of the abdomen using your palms and all four fingers (one side feels <u>firm</u> and is the back; on the other side you <u>may</u> be able to feel limbs). You can support each side in turn and push the fetus up against it with the other hand. You can also palpate around and on top for parts (the head should be ballotable).
    - *Longitudinal = baby vertical; oblique = baby diagonal; transverse = baby horizontal*
- **Presentation** (important over 37 weeks):
    - Feel for a presenting part by pressing on either side of the lower pole of the uterus simultaneously (one hand on each side), while facing mother's feet. If you are unable to feel a presenting part, press progressively more medially until you are able to (*cephalic = round presenting part, i.e. head; breech = broader soft presenting part, e.g. bottom*). Ballot head by pushing it gently from one side to the other. Be as gentle as possible and watch mother's face for pain throughout.
    - **Engagement:** note how many fifths of the head are palpable. See if your hands can come together below the head (unengaged), or if hands remain separate (engaged). Some people do a finger pinch of the head from below but it is not recommended because it is painful. (*'Engaged' = >50% of the presenting part is inside pelvis.*)
- **Liquor volume:** palpate around and ballot fluid to assess the approximate quantity (*oligohydramnios, polyhydramnios*)

FETAL HEART AUSCULTATION

- Find the back of the fetus and place the Pinard Horn or Doppler fetal monitor (Sonicaid) just behind the anterior shoulder, i.e. halfway between mother's umbilicus and ASIS on the side of the fetus' back. (Try both sides if unsure.) Feel the mother's pulse at the same time. Calculate the fetal heart rate (should be 120-160 bpm). Listen for 1 minute.

TO COMPLETE

- Thank patient and restore clothing
- 'To complete my examination, I would measure blood pressure and dipstick the urine.'
- Summarise and suggest further investigations you would consider after a full history

Normal fundal height
• Fundal height in centimetres should approximate the number of weeks' gestation from 20 weeks onwards (± 2cm until 36cm, and ±3cm from 36cm as may engage after)
• At **12 weeks**: uterus should be palpable
• At **20-22 weeks**: fundus should be near umbilicus
• At **36 weeks**: fundus should be near xiphisternum

INTRODUCTION

- <u>W</u>ash hands; <u>I</u>ntroduce self to parents; ask <u>B</u>aby's name and DOB; <u>E</u>xplain examination to parents and obtain consent
- Congratulate parents
- Undress baby completely

GENERAL INSPECTION

- **Cry:** feeble, pitch
- **Colour:** cyanosis, pallor, jaundice (*haemolysis*), rashes/petechiae
- **Birth trauma:** caput succedaneum, subconjunctival haemorrhages (*pressure*), cephalhaematoma (*ventouse*), forceps marks
- **Dysmorphic features:** dysmorphia, cleft lip, low set ears/epicanthic folds (*Down's syndrome*), small jaw (*Pierre Robin syndrome*)
- **Posture, tone and movements:** hypotonia (*Down's syndrome*), hypertonicity, hemiparesis, opisthotonos, myoclonus

> **Questions to ask mother**
>
> Labour
> - How long since delivery
> - Type of delivery
> - Problems in labour (including breech, premature rupture of membranes)
> - Medications in labour
>
> Mother
> - Any temperatures
> - Overall health in pregnancy
> - History of congenital hip dysplasia
>
> Baby
> - Pre-term/term/post-term
> - Weight
> - Breast-/bottle-feeding (latching OK?)
> - Urine (within 12 hours)
> - Meconium (sticky black stool within 48 hours)
> - Breathing

TOP TO TOE

- **Cranium:** look for cephalhaematoma, caput succedaneum, cranial moulding/deformities, micro-/macrocephaly, feel fontanelles (*bulging = raised intracranial pressure, e.g. hydrocephalus; sunken = dehydration*), feel sutures (check fused)
- **Face:** dysmorphic features, cleft lip, ears (*low set/preauricular skin tags/deformity = Down's syndrome*), feel with little finger inside roof of mouth (*cleft palate; high-arched palate = Marfan syndrome*) and determine presence of suck reflex
- **Eyes:** check red reflex using ophthalmoscope (*absent = congenital cataracts; white = retinoblastoma*), erythema/discharge (*conjunctivitis*), icteric sclera, subconjunctival haemorrhages (*trauma during delivery*)
- **Shoulders:** check aligned, feel clavicles
- **Upper limbs:** extend and check equal length; look for single palmar creases (*Down's syndrome*), extra digits (*polydactyly*), or fused digits (*syndactyly*)
- **Chest**
    - Respiratory rate
    - Capillary refill
    - Look for signs of respiratory distress (indrawing of intercostal muscles)
    - Feel for chest expansion
    - Auscultate lung and heart sounds (check for murmurs; normal heart rate is 120-150bpm)
- **Abdomen**
    - Inspect for distension (*bowel obstruction*), scaphoid abdomen (*diaphragmatic hernia*), and comment on umbilical stump (any erythema, bleeding, discharge)
    - Palpate for masses, hepatosplenomegaly and ballot kidneys (*Wilms tumour*)
- **Genitalia:** boys – feel testes (check both are descended and for a hydrocele); check foreskin and for hypo-/epispadias; girls – check for labial fusion and for cysts/tags; both – check anus is patent
- **Femoral pulses** (*absence suggests coarctation*)
- **Hip tests:** for both tests grasp their <u>flexed</u> knees in your palms, placing your thumbs over the medial aspects of their knees and your fingers over the lateral aspects. Hold both knees throughout but test one side at a time.

Barlow's test	Detects dislocatable hip. Flex adducted hip to 90°, then push posteriorly in the line of the femoral shaft. Dislocation is felt as a click.
Ortolani's test	Detects hips which are already dislocated ('<u>out</u>'). Flex hip to 90°, then abduct hip (turn it <u>out</u>). On full abduction, apply anteriorly directed force to the upper leg (pull upper thigh towards you with your fingers, keeping the knee steady in your palm). Relocation is felt as a click.

- **Lower limbs:** extend and check equal length; test range of movement at ankles; check feet for talipes ('club foot') and calcaneovalgus (abducted forefoot and dorsiflexed ankle); look for extra digits (*polydactyly*), or fused digits (*syndactyly*)
- **Back:** turn baby prone
    - Inspect for lipomas, tufts of hair (*spina bifida*), 'port wine' stains, and Mongolian blue spot
    - Palpate for spinal abnormalities (*spina bifida*) and natal cleft

FINALLY

- **Reflexes**
  - Grasp reflex: place finger in baby's palm. They should grasp it.
  - **Moro reflex:** warn parents first. Hold the baby in a sitting position a few inches above a soft surface, supporting their head in one of your hands and their bottom in the other. Allow the baby to rock backwards quickly but very slightly towards the bed (with your hands still supporting their head and bottom). Their arms should abduct, adduct, then the baby will usually cry.

TO COMPLETE

- Thank parents and redress baby
- 'To complete my examination, I would measure the head circumference, length and weight of the baby. I would also check preductal (*right hand*) and postductal (*left hand or either foot*) oxygen saturations to assess for critical congenital heart disease (*both should be ≥95%*).'
- 'I would fully document my findings in the notes and in the child's healthcare record book.'
- Summarise

KEY TIPS FOR COMMUNICATING WITH AND EXAMINING CHILDREN

MAJOR POINTS

- Keep using their **name**!
- Make it a **game** (e.g. in an abdominal exam, pretend you are trying to find out what they had for breakfast and keep naming cereals)
- Keep **interacting and asking questions** (e.g. 'So Billy, are you missing school today?', 'What lesson would you be in?', 'What's your favourite subject?', 'So is that what you want to do when you're older, Billy?')

OTHER TIPS

- If child is crying, let them calm down and see you talking to parents/siblings
- **Involve child** wherever possible
- Even babies like to hear a **reassuring voice**
- **Befriend child** before examining
- Position yourself at their **level**
- Distract with **toys**
- You can **pretend** to listen with stethoscope on parent's knee and then on child's arm to reassure them; or examine a teddy
- Use **parents** to distract them
- Use **simple words**, e.g. hurt, sore, funny, brave
- Undress in **stages**
- Sometimes you just need to persevere
- **Reward** and praise them
- If noisy, try using toys or bottles etc.
- Keep checking they're OK
- Warm your hands before touching them

GENERAL CHILD ASSESSMENT

A general assessment should be done for every unwell child along with an in-depth relevant system examination.

> **DON'T look in the throat if there's stridor!**

INTRO

- **W**ash hands; **I**ntroduce self; ask **P**atient's name, DOB and what they like to be called; **E**xplain examination and obtain consent

AIRWAY

- **Listen:** stridor (*croup, foreign body*), secretions, grunting (*bronchiolitis, pneumonia, asthma*)

BREATHING

- **Inspect**
  - Respiratory rate
  - Recession (subcostal, intercostal, sternal), nasal flaring, tracheal tug, accessory muscle use
- **Oxygen saturation** (*>97% normal, <94% significant illness, <90% alarming*)
- **Auscultation:** note any wheezing (*asthma, viral-induced wheeze*), crepitations (*secretions, bronchiolitis, infection*), or bronchial breathing (*pneumonia*). If the child is crying, try to listen during inspirations. Listen anteriorly and posteriorly.

CIRCULATION

- **Colour:** pallor, mottled arms/legs, blue (*poor perfusion*)
- **Radial pulse rate** (brachial if <6 months)
- **Hydration signs**
  - Wet nappies
  - Mucous membranes
  - Skin turgor
  - Capillary refill (central and peripheral; press for 5 seconds; normal refill time is <2 seconds) and
  - Temperature of hands and feet compared with trunk (*peripheries will be cooler in sepsis or dehydration due to peripheral vasoconstriction*)
- **Auscultate** heart sounds
- **Blood pressure** if very unwell (*maintained until late in shock*)
- Palpate for **hepatomegaly** (*sign of cardiac failure*)

DISABILITY (NEURO)

- **Alertness and activity**
  - Note how alert and reactive to surroundings (*may be drowsy after fit or fever*)
  - Look at behaviour (*true irritability, i.e. cannot be consoled = raised intracranial pressure or meningitis*)
  - AVPU score/GCS
  - Fontanelle (*bulging = raised intracranial pressure*)
- **Pupils:** check with torch if very unwell (*sluggish response = post-ictal or drug toxicity; changing sizes = seizure; asymmetrical = SOL, e.g. sub-/extradural; gaze may be abnormal after a seizure*)
- **Limb tone and movement** (also check for joint swelling)
- **Rash** (inspect everywhere) and check for **neck stiffness**
- **Capillary glucose:** measure if decreased alertness

Normal paediatric observations					
	<1 year	**1-2 years**	**2-5 years**	**5-12 years**	**>12 years**
Resp rate	30-40	25-35	25-30	20-25	15-20
Heart rate	110-160	100-150	95-140	80-120	60-100

EVERYTHING ELSE

<u>ENT</u>

Ensure you tell the parent what you need to do and give clear instructions.

- **Ears:** the child must be stable and held tight, sitting sideways on parent's lap. The parent should keep one hand on the child's head and the other encircling their arms and body. Use your free hand to hold the head in against the parent's chest. *NB: healthy eardrums often pink.*
- **Throat:** position the child facing you on parent's lap. They should use one arm to hold the child's forehead back and the other to encircle their arms. You may need to use a tongue depressor. *NB: children often have large red tonsils.*

<u>Temperature</u>

- **Measure temperature** (axilla recommended in babies)

<u>Abdomen</u>

- **Feel** – best if lying flat but child can be examined in parent's lap
  - Ask child to point to pain with finger (start away from painful areas)
  - Palpate gently first, then deeper
  - Check for organomegaly (liver, spleen, kidneys)
  - Check inguinal region and umbilicus for hernias
  - Auscultate for bowel sounds

	Warning features *Produced using NICE 'CG160 fever in under 5s: assessment and initial management' 2013*	
	Amber flags	**Red flags**
A		Stridor
B	Nasal flaring, tachypnoea, sats ≤95%, crackles	Respiratory distress (RR>60), grunting, moderate-severe chest in-drawing
C	Pallor, tachycardia, reduced capillary refill, reduced UO, dry mucus membranes, poor feeding	Pale/mottled/ashen/blue, reduced skin turgor
D	Reduced activity, not responding normally to social cues	No response to social cues/won't stay awake, non-blanching rash, neck stiffness, seizures/neurology, bulging fontanelle
E	Fever in 3-6month old (or for ≥5 days), rigors, limb or joint swelling/not using limb	Fever in <3 month old

PAEDIATRIC RESPIRATORY EXAMINATION

Do a full adult respiratory examination with the following additional components.

GENERAL

- Dysmorphic features
- Work of breathing
- Colour (pallor, cyanosis, mottling)
- Alertness and interest in surroundings
- Nutritional status

LISTEN TO BREATHING

- Wheezing (*bronchiolitis, asthma, viral-induced wheeze*)
- Stridor, harsh voice (*croup, foreign body*)
- Grunting (*bronchiolitis, pneumonia, asthma*)
- Secretions
- Cough (*barking = croup; dry = URTI; coughing fits with inspiratory whoop = whooping cough; fruity cough = bronchiectasis*)

NAILS

- Clubbing (*CF, bronchiectasis*)

RESPIRATORY RATE

- Count for 1 minute – usually best with chest exposed (*tachypnoea = respiratory distress; bradypnoea = final stages of respiratory failure*)
- Prolonged expiration (*bronchoconstriction in bronchiolitis or asthma*)

CHEST DEFORMITIES

- Barrel chest (*asthma*)
- Harrison's sulcus (*permanent groove in chest wall at insertion of diaphragm in chronic asthma*)
- Pectus carinatum
- Pectus excavatum

WORK OF BREATHING

- Nasal flaring
- Tracheal tug
- Recession
  - Supraclavicular
  - Intercostal (*in-drawing between ribs – an earlier feature in younger children because the chest wall is less firm*)
  - Subcostal
- Use of accessory muscles and head bobbing caused by sternocleidomastoid contractions (*quite severe respiratory distress*)

CHEST AUSCULTATION

- If child is crying, try to listen during inspirations
- Noises transmit all over chest as they are small
  - Crepitations crackles (*secretions, bronchiolitis, infection*)
  - Bronchial breathing (*pneumonia*)
  - Wheeze (*asthma, viral-induced wheeze*)

TO COMPLETE

- Observations
- Growth charts
- Ear, nose and throat exam

Normal paediatric observations					
	<1 year	1-2 years	2-5 years	5-12 years	>12 years
Resp rate	30-40	25-35	25-30	20-25	15-20
Heart rate	110-160	100-150	95-140	80-120	60-100

PAEDIATRIC CARDIAC EXAMINATION

Do a full adult cardiac examination with the following additional components.

GENERAL

- Dysmorphic features (*Down's, Williams and DiGeorge syndromes associated with congenital heart disease; Turner syndrome associated with AS; Noonan syndrome associated with PS*)
- Work of breathing
- Colour (pallor, cyanosis, mottling)
- Alertness and interest in surroundings
- Nutritional status

AUSCULTATION

- Also listen in the left interscapular area (*systolic murmur = coarctation of the aorta*), and in the left infraclavicular area (*systolic murmur = coarctation of the aorta; continuous machinery-like murmur = patent ductus arteriosus*)

TO COMPLETE

- Observations including blood pressure
- Preductal (*right hand*) and postductal (*left hand or either foot*) oxygen saturations to assess for critical congenital heart disease (*both should be ≥95%*)
- Growth charts

PAEDIATRIC ABDOMINAL EXAMINATION

Do a full adult abdominal examination with the following additional components.

GENERAL

- Dysmorphic features
- Colour (pallor, mottling)
- Alertness and interest in surroundings
- Nutritional status

> **Note**
>
> • Do **not** say you would do a digital rectal exam as you would with an adult
> • Examination of hernial orifices may be appropriate – incarcerated inguinal hernias may be a cause of obstruction
> • Examination of external genitalia may be appropriate, for example if there are concerns about congenital adrenal hyperplasia or safeguarding

HYDRATION STATUS

1. Capillary refill
2. Heart rate
3. Mucous membranes
4. Skin turgor
5. Wet nappies (depending on age)

POINTS

- Look for Grey-Turner's and Cullen's signs
- Liver can be up to 2cm below costal margin in children
- Faecal loading may be felt in umbilical region and LIF

TO COMPLETE

- Observations
- Growth charts

Normal paediatric observations					
	<1 year	**1-2 years**	**2-5 years**	**5-12 years**	**>12 years**
Resp rate	30-40	25-35	25-30	20-25	15-20
Heart rate	110-160	100-150	95-140	80-120	60-100

INTRODUCTION

- **W**ash hands; **I**ntroduce self; ask **P**atient's name and what they like to be called; **E**xplain examination and obtain consent from parents
- Ask parents if they have any developmental concerns
- **Observe** child for 30 seconds
- Tips
    - The modalities below can be assessed in any order, so if the child is comfortable on the parent's lap, for example, it may be better to assess the other modalities before gross motor
    - Ask the parents questions about anything you cannot get the child to demonstrate (e.g. if they are not rolling, ask if the parents have seen them roll)
    - You should know the ages for a few milestones in each category

GROSS MOTOR

- Check parent is happy for you to put the child on a play-mat on the floor
- Lie child on back – see if they can **roll**
- Put child in a sitting position – look for **head control** (*3 months*)
- See if they can **sit** aided/unaided (*6-9 months*)
    - Look at curvature of spine and sitting reflexes
- Pull to a **standing** position – see how much support is needed (*9-12 months*)
- Get them to **walk** if able (*15-18 months*) or run (*2 years*)
- Lastly, place prone – see if child **lifts head**/**chest** or **crawls** (*10 months*)

FINE MOTOR AND VISION

- Get child to take a toy and observe
    - **Transfers** (*6 months*)
    - Type of **grip** (*palmar grasp at 6 months; pincer grip at 9-10 months*)
- Offer bricks
    - 3-cube **tower** (*18 months*)
    - Builds **bridge** (*3 years*)
- Give paper and pen if old enough
    - **Scribbles** (*18 months*)
    - Circular scribbles and **lines** (*2 years*)
    - Copies **circle** (*3 years*)
    - Copies **cross** (*4 years*)
- Vision – wave toy
    - **Fixes** and follows (*3 months*)

HEARING AND LANGUAGE

- Click fingers or use rattles (see if they turn to sounds)
    - **Startles** to noise (*neonate*)
    - Turns to **sounds** (*6 months*)
    - Turns to **name** (*12 months*)
- Talk to child and ask parents what words/noises the child can say/make
    - **Babble** (*6 months*)
    - **'Mamma' and 'Dadda'** (*12 months*)
    - 2-word **phrases** (*2 years*)
    - Knows own name and colours (*3 years*)
- Commands
    - One-step command, e.g. 'take the brick' (*18 months*)
    - Two-step command, e.g. 'take the brick and place it in the cup' (*2 years*)

SOCIAL

- Observe interaction with people/environment
    - **Smiles** (*6 weeks*)
    - **Laughs** (*3 months*)
    - **Stranger anxiety** (*9 months*)
    - Plays **'peek-a-boo'** (*9 months*)

- o **Waves goodbye** (*12 months*)
- Ask parents about the child's diet
  - o **Solids** (*6 months*)
  - o **Fork and spoon** (*2 years*)

TO COMPLETE

- Thank child and parents
- 'To complete my examination, I would review growth charts and measure weight, height and head circumference.'
- 'I would also like to take a full history.'
- Summarise
  - o If age unknown: estimate developmental age
  - o If age known: comment if the development is appropriate for age, globally delayed, or asymmetrically delayed

Normal developmental milestones				
	Gross motor	**Fine motor and vision**	**Hearing and language**	**Social**
Neonate	Moves all limbs	Looks, startles	Startles to noise	Cries Smiles (6 weeks)
3 months	Head control	Reaches for objects Fixes and follows	Cries, laughs, vocalises (4 months)	Laughs
6 months	Rolls over Pushes up	Co-ordination Transfers	Localises sound Babbles	Alert and interested Starts solids
9 months	Sits alone Crawls	Pincer grip	Inappropriate sounds	Stranger anxiety
12 months	Stands alone		Babbles Understands simple commands Says 'Mamma'/ 'Dadda'	Socially responsive Wave bye
18 months	Walks alone	Uses spoon	Uses words	Stranger shyness Tantrums
2 years	Runs Stairs (2 feet per step)	Circular scribbles and lines	2-word phrases	Knows identity Parallel play
3-4 years	Stand on one foot Stairs (climbs with one foot per step at 3 years)	Builds bridge with bricks	Short sentences Knows colours	Interactive play
5 years	Skips/hops	Full drawings	Fluent speech	Dresses self

Common stations

- **Normal child** – you may be asked to estimate developmental age or the examiner may lie about the child's age
- **Global developmental delay**
  - o Prenatal causes: chromosome disorders (e.g. Down's syndrome), cerebral dysgenesis, hypothyroidism, alcohol/drugs in pregnancy, rubella/CMV/ toxoplasmosis
  - o Perinatal causes: intraventricular haemorrhage, hypoxic brain injury, hypoglycaemia
  - o Postnatal causes: meningitis/encephalitis, hypoxic/anoxic events, head injury, hypoglycaemia
- **Asymmetrically delayed**
  - o Motor (manifest in 1st year): cerebral palsy, congenital myopathy, spinal cord lesions, visual impairment, balance problems
  - o Language (manifest in 2nd year): hearing loss, anatomical deficits (e.g. cleft palate), normal variant/familial, environmental deprivation
  - o Social (manifest in 3rd year): autism, hyperactivity, attention deficit hyperactivity disorder

DERMATOLOGICAL SKIN EXAMINATION

INTRODUCTION
- **W**ash hands; **I**ntroduce self; ask **P**atient's name, DOB and what they like to be called; **E**xplain examination and obtain consent
- Get a **chaperone**
- Expose patient to underwear

GENERAL INSPECTION
- **Patient:** well/unwell, pain/discomfort
- **Describe the pattern of any rash:** site, number of lesions, distribution pattern

CLOSE INSPECTION
- **Nails:** psoriatic nail changes (pitting, onycholysis, subungual hyperkeratosis)
- **Hands**
- **Anterior arms**
- Ask patient to put hands behind head
    - **Posterior arms**
    - **Axilla**
- **Scalp:** look through hair and behind ears
- **Face**
- **Inside mouth**
- **Chest and abdomen**
- **Back**
- **'At this point, I would also like to look at the genital region.'**
- **Legs**
- **Feet and toe nails**

TO COMPLETE
- Thank patient and restore clothing
- 'To complete my examination, I would examine any suspicious moles with a dermatoscope and perform other relevant system examinations (e.g. vascular for an arterial ulcer).'
- Summarise and suggest further investigations you would consider after a full history

DESCRIBING LESIONS IN DERMATOLOGY

INSPECT LESIONS
- **Distribution and size**
    - e.g. acral (distal), central, flexor/extensor, localised/generalised, dermatomal, follicular, seborrhoeic
- **Characteristics (SEC)**
    - **Shape**, e.g. circular, linear, annular, irregular
    - **Edge and elevation**, e.g. well-demarcated, ill-defined, raised/flat
    - **Colour**, e.g. erythematous, depigmented/pigmented, purpuric
- **Secondary features**
    - e.g. crust, scale, pigmentation, keratosis, lichenification, erosion, excoriation, fissure, ulceration

PALPATE LESIONS
- **Temperature**
- **Texture**

Definitions in dermatology		
	<0.5cm	**>0.5cm**
Flat	Macule	Patch
		Plaque (palpable)
Raised	Papule	Nodule
	Vesicle (fluid-filled)	Bulla (fluid-filled)
	Pustule (pus-filled)	

VISUAL SYSTEM EXAMINATION

INTRODUCTION
- **W**ash hands; **I**ntroduce self; ask **P**atient's name, DOB and what they like to be called; **E**xplain examination and obtain consent

INSPECTION
- **Patient:** well/unwell, posture etc.
- **Around bed:** mobility aids, glasses
- **Eyes inspection:**
  - Pupil size and symmetry
    - Unilateral dilated pupil (*mydriatic eye drops, CN3 lesion, Holmes-Adie pupil, acute glaucoma, trauma*)
    - Unilateral constricted pupil (*miotic eye drops, Horner's syndrome*)
  - Strabismus (*CN3 lesion = pupil 'down and out'; CN6 lesion = cannot look laterally*)
  - Ptosis (*unilateral = CN3 lesion, Horner's syndrome; bilateral = myasthenia gravis, myotonic dystrophy*)
  - Proptosis (*thyrotoxicosis, retro-orbital tumour*)
  - Sclera (erythema, lesions)
  - Around eyes (scarring, lesions, pus, discharge, swelling)

ACUITY
Ask the patient to cover one eye with their palm to test <u>each eye in turn</u>.
- **Distant vision (visual acuity):** test with Snellen chart (the result is recorded as *distance/smallest font size read*, e.g. 6/9)
  - If the patient wears glasses, do this with glasses on (corrected visual acuity) and off (uncorrected visual acuity)
  - A standard Snellen chart is read from 6 metres away but there are smaller versions which may be used at closer distances (e.g. 1 or 3 metres) – adjust the final acuity to '1/...' or '3/...' respectively
  - If the patient gets more than two letters wrong, the previous line should be recorded as their acuity. If they get two letters wrong, record acuity as the font size of this line but note '-2' in brackets, e.g. 6/9 (-2); and if they get one letter wrong, note '-1' e.g. 6/9 (-1).
- **Near vision:** read a line of a letter/magazine
- **Colour vision:** 'I would also like to test colour vision using Ishihara plates.'

FIELDS
Sit the patient 1 metre directly in front of you with both your eyes at the same level.
- **Visual inattention:** while the patient keeps both eyes open and focussed on you, hold out your hands in each of their outer visual fields. Ask them to point at the hand(s) which you are opening/closing. (*Inattention to one side = contralateral parietal lesion.*)
- **Visual fields:** ask the patient to cover one eye with their palm and close your eye on the same side (without using your palm if you can). Ask them to stay focussed on your open eye. Select a white visual fields pin and bring it in from the periphery, keeping it at mid-distance between you and the patient. Ask them to tell you when they can see it. Move in a diagonal direction into each of the four quadrants. Test both eyes individually, comparing their fields with yours.
  - *Mononuclear field loss = intra-ocular pathology or ipsilateral optic nerve lesion*
  - *Bitemporal hemianopia = optic chiasm compression*
  - *Left/right homonymous hemianopia = contralateral optic tract/radiation lesion, or occipital cortex if macular sparing is present*
- **Blind spots** (offer to test): while the patient keeps both eyes open and focussed on you, hold a red pin mid-distance between you. Check they can see it as red in the middle (*central scotoma = optic nerve lesion*). Now move the pin horizontally towards the periphery in each direction and to tell you when it disappears. Map each of their blind spots against your own (*large blind spot = papilloedema*).

REFLEXES
- **Accommodation:** ask the patient to focus on a distant object, then hold your finger close to their face and ask them to focus on it. Pupils should constrict and eyes should converge.
- **Direct and consensual papillary reflexes:** in a dimmed room, ask the patient to hold an open hand between their eyes and focus on a distant point in the room. Shine the light at each pupil in turn from about 45°. Observe for direct and consensual papillary constriction
  - *Afferent defect (i.e. pupils are symmetrical but when light is shone in affected eye, neither pupil constricts) = CN2 (optic nerve) lesion*
  - *Efferent defect (affected pupil is persistently dilated, whilst other is reactive to light being shone in either eye) = CN3 lesion*
- **Swinging light test:** swing the light between the two eyes – the pupil size should stay the same regardless of which eye the light is shone in. If pupils become more dilated when the light is shone in one eye, then that eye is less sensitive to light and, hence, there is a <u>relative</u> afferent pupillary defect in that eye (*partial optic nerve lesion on that side*).

AFRO (three parts to each)

OPHTHALMOSCOPY

- Ask the patient to remove glasses if present; consider preparing pupils with mydriatic drops (e.g. tropicamide); and use a darkened room
- Ask the patient to focus on a point in the distance until you tell them otherwise
- **Red reflexes:** look through ophthalmoscope at patient's pupil from 1 metre away (*lost in: cataract, retinoblastoma, vitreous haemorrhage*)
- Hold the patient's right shoulder with your left hand and the ophthalmoscope in your right to examine the right eye (and vice versa for the left). First focus the ophthalmoscope to your vision by looking through it at a point in the distance and adjusting the focus wheel. Now look in the patient's eye and adjust the wheel to focus the ophthalmoscope on their retina. When their retina is in focus, look at:
    - **Optic disc:** visualised by aiming the ophthalmoscope slightly nasally. Check the **3Cs**:
        - **C**up – normal cup to disc ratio is 0.3 or less, i.e. the cup occupies 3/10 of the diameter of the entire disc (*enlarged = glaucoma*)
        - **C**olour (*grey/pale = optic atrophy*)
        - **C**ontours (*swelling = papilloedema*)
    - **Four quadrants:** follow the blood vessels out from the optic disc in each direction to visualise each of the four quadrants. Observe for:
        - Hypertensive retinopathy signs (silver wiring, AV nipping, cotton wool spots, papilloedema)
        - Diabetic retinopathy signs (dot and blot haemorrhages, cotton wool spots, neovascularisation, retinal fibrosis)
        - Other characteristic appearances, e.g. drusen (*macular degeneration*), peripheral pigmentation (*retinitis pigmentosa*)
    - **Macula:** visualise by asking the patient to focus on the light of the ophthalmoscope. Should be pink (*dark = macular degeneration*).

EXTRA-OCULAR MUSCLES

Ask if the patient has any double vision and to tell you if they experience any during the test.
- **H-test:** ask patient to keep their head still (you may need to hold a finger on their forehead) and, with both eyes open, to follow your finger. Make an 'H' shape.
    - Pause when they are looking laterally (*nystagmus = cerebellar pathology*)
    - If there is complex ophthalmoplegia, ask them to look straight up while counting down from 20 (*fatigability suggests myasthenia gravis*)

*NB: CN3 supplies all extra-ocular muscles except **S**uperior **O**blique (CN**4**) and **L**ateral **R**ectus (CN**6**) – **SO4LR6***

Hence, if the eye cannot move laterally, there is a CN6 lesion; if the eye cannot move inferiorly when facing medially, there is a CN4 lesion. If the majority of the eye's movements are impaired and the eye rests in a 'down and out' position, there is a CN3 lesion. If there are dramatically abnormal eye movements which do not fit with a single nerve lesion, there is complex ophthalmoplegia (Graves/ mitochondrial/myasthenia/brainstem lesion).

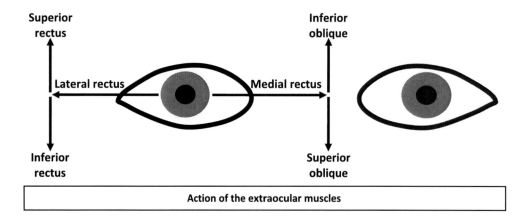

Action of the extraocular muscles

TO COMPLETE

- Thank patient
- Summarise and suggest further investigations you would consider after a full history

LYMPH NODE EXAMINATION

INTRODUCTION

- **W**ash hands; **I**ntroduce self; ask **P**atient's name, DOB and what they like to be called; **E**xplain examination and obtain consent
- Get a **chaperone**
- General inspection: well/unwell, pain/discomfort, cachexia
- For each lymph node group
    - Local inspection: obvious lymphadenopathy, surgical scars, overlying skin (erythema, rashes)
    - Palpation (technique discussed below): determine site, size (diameter <1cm is normal), shape, consistency (*hard = malignancy; rubbery = lymphoma*), tethering to other structures (*malignancy*)

Work down the body feeling each lymph node group:

CERVICAL LYMPH NODES

- Sit patient upright in a chair and stand behind them to palpate the following groups of nodes in order: submental, submandibular, jugulodigastric/tonsillar (commonly palpable), anterior cervical chain (shotty nodes common), posterior cervical chain, occipital, postauricular, preauricular
- These groups are palpated with finger pulps (do not 'play the piano', i.e. palpate using finger tips). Palpate as if you are giving a massage, and feel each group thoroughly – especially the anterior and posterior cervical chains, for which your whole hand should be placed around the patient's neck. Roll the lymph nodes over the deep muscles/bone to feel them (don't just press the superficial soft tissues).
- From in front of the patient, palpate the supraclavicular nodes with your fingertips in the supraclavicular fossae – Virchow's node is left supraclavicular (*classically gastric cancer metastasises here*)

AXILLARY LYMPH NODES

- To examine the right: ask the patient to hold your right biceps muscle while you support the weight of their right arm at the elbow with your right hand. Now place your left arm over your right and place your left hand into the patient's axilla. Palpate the apical, lateral, medial, anterior and posterior lymph node groups by firmly pressing the soft tissues and rolling them over the underlying harder tissues.
- Repeat on left
NB: to feel the medial lymph node group, you really have to push your hand high up into the axilla and press it firmly medially, rolling the nodes across the ribs with all your fingers. It helps if you bring the patient's elbow closer to their chest at this point.

EPITROCHLEAR LYMPH NODES

- To examine the right: hold the patient's right wrist with your left hand and their right elbow in your right palm. Use your right thumb to feel for lymph nodes.
- Repeat on left

INGUINAL LYMPH NODES

- Palpate horizontal chain (inferior and parallel to inguinal ligament) and vertical chain (alongside terminal great saphenous vein)
- Lymph nodes here are normal up to 1.5cm in diameter

POPLITEAL LYMPH NODES

- Flex knee and palpate in popliteal fossa

FINALLY

- Palpate for hepatosplenomegaly (*see notes on abdominal examination p53*)
- Examine any areas drained by palpable lymph nodes

TO COMPLETE

- Thank patient and restore clothing
- Summarise and suggest further investigations you would consider after a full history

Patient sitting upright

Patient lying flat

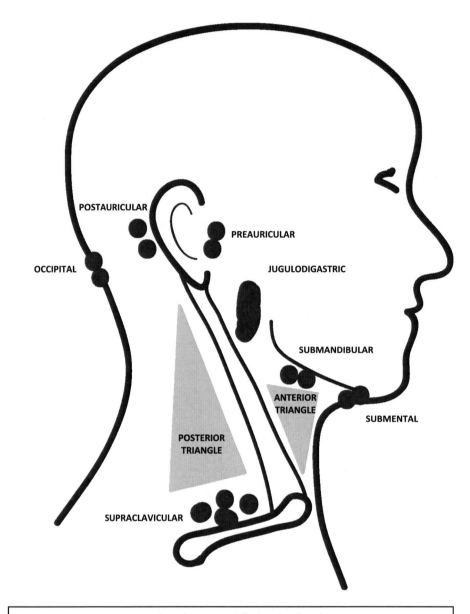

POSTAURICULAR

PREAURICULAR

OCCIPITAL

JUGULODIGASTRIC

SUBMANDIBULAR

ANTERIOR
TRIANGLE

POSTERIOR
TRIANGLE

SUBMENTAL

SUPRACLAVICULAR

Lymph node groups of the head and neck

NECK EXAMINATION

INTRODUCTION

- **W**ash hands; **I**ntroduce self; ask **P**atient's name, DOB and what they like to be called; **E**xplain examination and obtain consent
- Expose neck and sit patient in centre of room
- **General inspection**: well/unwell, cachexia, lethargic, sweaty, signs of hypo-/hyperthyroidism, abnormal voice etc.
- Check that the examiner does not want you also to examine thyroid status (*if so, see notes on thyroid exam p60*)

INSPECTION

- Obvious masses or lymphadenopathy
- Surgical scars
- Overlying skin (erythema, rashes)
- Goitre
- Ask patient to swallow and then stick tongue out while watching thyroid gland (*thyroid lumps and thyroglossal cysts rise on swallowing; thyroglossal cysts rise on tongue protrusion*)

PALPATION

- Check for any pain and explain you will be examining from behind initially

From posteriorly:
- Anterior lymph nodes, salivary glands and thyroid:
    - **Submental** lymph nodes
    - **Sublingual** gland
    - **Submandibular** lymph nodes and gland (*gland swelling may occur due to salivary duct calculi that may be palpable*)
    - **Jugulodigastric** (tonsillar) lymph nodes
    - **Parotid** gland
    - Down **anterior cervical chain** of lymph nodes
    - Stop at **thyroid gland** (over 2nd-4th tracheal rings): note size, consistency and any abnormal masses. Feel the two lobes and isthmus. With your fingers over the thyroid gland:
        - Ask patient to swallow (*thyroid masses and thyroglossal cysts will rise*)
        - Ask patient to stick out tongue (*thyroglossal cyst will rise*)
    - Complete the anterior cervical chain
- Posterior lymph nodes
    - Feel **posterior cervical chain** of lymph nodes from the bottom of the posterior triangle to the mastoid process
    - **Occipital** lymph nodes
    - **Postauricular** lymph nodes
    - **Preauricular** lymph nodes

From anteriorly:
- **Supraclavicular lymph nodes:** examine these from in front by placing fingertips in supraclavicular fossae (Virchow's node is left supraclavicular)
- Palpate each **carotid artery** in turn

*NB: palpate for lymphadenopathy with your finger pulps (do not 'play the piano', i.e. palpate using finger tips). Palpate as if you are giving a massage, and feel each group thoroughly – especially the anterior and posterior cervical chains, for which your whole hand should be placed around the patient's neck. Roll the lymph nodes over the muscles/bone to feel them (don't just press the superficial soft tissues). For any mass, note its characteristics (**SSSCCCTTT**): Size, Shape, Surface, Consistency, Contours, Colour, Temperature, Tenderness, Transillumination. It's important to determine if any palpable lymph nodes are hard (malignancy), rubbery (lymphoma), tethered (malignancy), or irregular (malignancy).*

PERCUSSION

- Percuss over sternum for retrosternal goitre

AUSCULTATION

- Thyroid and carotid bruits

TO COMPLETE

- Examine any areas drained by palpable lymph nodes; thank patient and restore clothing; summarise

---

Common pathology

Anywhere
- **Lymphadenopathy**
- **Lipoma:** painless smooth soft mass

Midline
- **Thyroid pathology:** moves with swallowing
- **Thyroglossal cyst:** fluctuant midline lump on thyroid migration path that moves up on tongue protrusion
- **Dermoid cyst:** cyst containing dermal structures at embryonic cutaneous junctions; patient usually <20 years

Anterior triangle
- **Branchial cyst:** cyst due to non-disappearance of cervical sinus, felt at upper anterior border of sternocleidomastoid; patient usually <20 years
- **Laryngocele:** painless air sac at larynx; mobile; worse with blowing
- **Carotid body tumour:** pulsatile mass at carotid bifurcation; very rare

Posterior triangle
- **Cystic hygroma (lymphangioma):** present since childhood; transilluminates brightly; felt at left base of neck
- **Pharyngeal pouch:** pouch from pharynx; may protrude on swallowing

BREAST EXAMINATION

INTRO

- **W**ash hands; **I**ntroduce self; ask **P**atient's name, DOB and what they like to be called; **E**xplain examination and obtain consent
- Get a **chaperone**
- Expose and position patient (**sitting** first, then lying at **30°**)

GENERAL INSPECTION

- **Patient**: age, well/unwell, cachexia

LOOK WITH PATIENT SITTING OVER EDGE OF BED

- Look for: asymmetry, local swelling, skin changes (erythema, dimpling, *peau d'orange*, scars), nipple changes (Paget's disease of the breast, inversion)
- Look in four positions:
  - **Arms relaxed**
  - **Hands rested on thighs**
  - **Hands actively pressed into hips** (tenses pectorals)
  - **Hands behind head** leaning slightly forwards (to expose whole breast and accentuate dimpling)
- Also lift the breast to look in the submammary fold

FEEL WITH PATIENT LYING

Position patient lying at 30°. When examining the right breast, the patient's right hand should be behind their head, and vice versa for the left. Ask if there is any pain first and start by examining the normal side.

- Examine using both hands, massaging the breast tissue using the whole of the palmar surface of your middle three fingers
- Move your hands in step-wise increments around breast in a systematic manner, e.g. a spiral motion from outside in
- Examine the axillary tail between your first two fingers and thumb
- Describe any lump (**SSSCCCTTT**): **S**ite, **S**ize, **S**hape, **C**onsistency, **C**ontours, **C**olour, **T**enderness, **T**emperature (**T**ransillumination not required here)
- Ask the patient to gently massage each nipple to attempt to express any discharge (*yellow/green = infection; bloody = malignancy*)

LYMPH NODES

Ask patient to sit over the side of the bed again to examine the axillary lymph nodes.

- **Axillary lymph nodes:** to examine the right, ask the patient to hold your right biceps while you support the weight of their right arm at the elbow with your right hand. Place your left arm over your right and place your left hand into their axilla. Now palpate the apical, lateral, medial, anterior and posterior lymph node groups by firmly pressing the soft tissues and rolling them over the underlying harder tissues. Repeat using opposite hands for the left side.
- **Supraclavicular lymph nodes:** feel with your fingertips pressed into the supraclavicular fossae from anteriorly

TO COMPLETE

- Thank patient and restore clothing
- Summarise and suggest further investigations you would consider after a full history
  - Two week wait referral for triple assessment (examination + imaging + tissue sampling)
  - Imaging depends on age: ultrasound if <35 years; mammogram if >35 years
  - Tissue sampling depends on mass: fine needle aspiration if cystic; core biopsy if solid

MENTAL STATE EXAMINATION

INTRODUCTION

- **W**ash hands; **I**ntroduce self; ask **P**atient's name, DOB and what they like to be called; **E**xplain examination and obtain consent

APPEARANCE AND BEHAVIOUR

You don't need to ask this!
- **Appearance:** dress, physical appearance, neglect
- **Behaviour:** suspicious, paranoid, irritable, aggressive, eye contact
- **Distractions:** preoccupied, distractible, withdrawn, quiet

SPEECH

You don't need to ask this!
- **Rate:** pressure of speech, slow
- **Volume/tone:** monotonous
- **Fluency and rhythm**

MOOD AND AFFECT

Ask about their mood (e.g. 'How are you feeling?', 'What is your mood like?', 'Have you felt low/anxious recently?')
- **Mood** (sustained emotion over prolonged period of time)
  - **Subjective:** low, high, anxious
  - **Objective:** depressed, elated, euthymic, labile
- **Affect** (immediately expressed emotion): facial expressions, overall demeanour

THOUGHTS

Ask about delusions (e.g. 'Have you noticed any strange thoughts, or thoughts that others find strange?', 'Can anyone interfere with or hear your thoughts?', 'Do you feel you are in control of your actions?', 'Do you ever get thoughts which keep going round and round in your head?', 'Are there any actions you feel you need to do repeatedly?')
Ask about risk to self and others (e.g. 'Some people in your situation feel like harming themselves or taking their own life, have you had such thoughts?')
- **Form:** coherence, muddled, flight of ideas, knight's move thinking, preoccupations
- **Content:** harm to self/others, suicidal ideas, delusions, over-valued ideas, thought insertion/withdrawal/broadcasting, control of thoughts

PERCEPTIONS

Ask about hallucinations (e.g. 'Have you ever heard or seen anything you can't explain?', 'Have you ever heard people commenting on what you do?', 'Do you ever feel events have a special meaning for you?', 'Have the voices ever told you to harm yourself or anyone else?')
- **Hallucination** (sensory perceptions without stimulus)
- **Illusion** (misinterpreted stimulus)
- **Pseudohallucination** (a hallucination that the patient is aware is not real)

COGNITION

Assess cognition
- **Concentration and attention**
- **Short-term memory**
- **Orientation** to time/person/place and **cognition test**, e.g. mini mental state examination

INSIGHT

Assess insight
- **Awareness** of illness
- **Understanding** of the need for medications and willingness to take them

Never forget to ask about risk to self/others
e.g. Have the voices ever told them to harm themself/others? Have they taken any measures to protect themself? Do they feel like taking their own life?

TO COMPLETE

- Other parts of psychiatric history; summarise

HYDRATION STATUS EXAMINATION

A hydration status examination is useful when assessing unwell patients and also when prescribing intravenous fluids (*see p281*).

INTRODUCTION
- **W**ash hands; **I**ntroduce self; ask **P**atient's name, DOB and what they like to be called; **E**xplain examination and obtain consent

GENERAL INSPECTION
- **Patient:** well/unwell, alert, breathless, fever, portals of infection/wounds/drains
- **Around bed** (if present, look at quantities of fluids going in/coming out)
  - In: IV fluids, NG feed, parenteral nutrition
  - Out: catheter, stoma, NG tube, vomit bowl
  - Charts: observations, fluid balance, drug chart (e.g. for diuretics, infusions etc.)

HANDS AND ARMS
- **Temperature** (*fever increases insensible losses*)
- **Pulse rate** (*tachycardia in dehydration*)
- **Blood pressure** and postural drop (*hypotension and postural drop in dehydration*)

HEAD AND NECK
- **Eyes** (*sunken in dehydration*)
- **Oral mucus membranes** (*dry in dehydration*)
- **JVP** (*raised in overload; reduced/not visible in dehydration*)
- **Carotid pulse** volume and character

CHEST
- **Sternum:** capillary refill (*>2 seconds in hypoperfusion*), skin turgor (*reduced in dehydration*)
- **Palpation:** apex beat (*may be displaced in LVF*)
- **Auscultation:** heart (*3rd heart sound in overload*), lung bases (*pulmonary oedema in overload*)

ABDOMEN
- **Ascites**

LEGS
- **Peripheral oedema** (*overload*)

TO COMPLETE
- Thank patient
- 'To complete my hydration status assessment, I would take a full history, look at U&Es, observations, and the fluid balance chart.'
- Summarise and suggest further investigations, for example:
  - Serial weights
  - Catheterise and monitor urine output
  - U&Es
  - ABG and serum lactate

NUTRITIONAL STATUS EXAMINATION

INTRODUCTION
- **W**ash hands; **I**ntroduce self; ask **P**atient's name, DOB and what they like to be called; **E**xplain examination and obtain consent

GENERAL INSPECTION
- **Patient**: well/unwell, approximate BMI, alert, breathless, fever, portals of infection/wounds/drains, long lines (may be used for parenteral nutrition)
- **Around bed** (if present look at quantity of fluids going in/coming out)
  - In: NG feed/parenteral nutrition, IV fluids, nutritional supplements, food/drink/NBM notes
  - Out: catheter, stoma, NG tube, vomit bowl
  - Charts: observations, fluid balance, drug chart

HANDS AND ARMS
- **Nails:** clubbing (*cirrhosis, IBD, coeliac disease*), leukonychia (*hypoalbuminaemia*), koilonychia (*iron deficiency anaemia*)
- **Palms:** temperature, xanthomata (*hypercholesterolaemia*)
- **Pulse rate** (*tachycardia in dehydration*)
- **Arms:** bruising (*coagulopathy in vitamin K deficiency*), extensor rash (*dermatitis herpetiformis in coeliac disease*)
- **Blood pressure** and postural drop (*hypotension and postural drop in dehydration*)

HEAD AND NECK
- **Eyes:** sunken (*dehydration*), corneal arcus/xanthelasma (*hypercholesterolaemia*), xerophthalmia (*vitamin A deficiency*), conjunctival pallor (*anaemia, e.g. due to bleeding or malabsorption*)
- **Mouth/tongue:** glossitis/stomatitis (*iron/B12 deficiency anaemia*), aphthous ulcers (*Crohn's disease*), breath odour (*e.g. feculent in obstruction; ketotic in ketoacidosis; alcohol*), dry mucous membranes (*dehydration*), gingivitis (*scurvy*)
- **JVP** (*heart failure in wet beriberi*) and carotid pulse (volume and character)
- **Goitre** (*iodine deficiency*)

CHEST
- **Sternum:** capillary refill, skin turgor (*reduced in dehydration*)

ABDOMEN
- **Ascites** (*hypoalbuminaemia, liver disease*)
- **Adiposity**
- **Loose skin/striae** (*rapid weight loss*)

LEGS
- **Peripheral oedema** (*hypoalbuminaemia*)
- **Bowed legs** (*rickets/osteomalacia*)
- **Peripheral neuropathy** (*B12 deficiency, dry beriberi*)

TO COMPLETE
- Thank patient
- 'To complete my nutritional status assessment, I would take a full history, calculate BMI, check observations, look at the food and fluid balance charts, and take refeeding bloods (*U&Es, Ca^{2+}, Mg^{2+}, PO_4^{3-}*).'
- Summarise and suggest further investigations (e.g. OGD/colonoscopy for iron deficiency anaemia, anti-TTG for coeliac disease, parietal cell and intrinsic factor antibodies for B12 deficiency, dual energy X-ray absorptiometry (DEXA) scan)

Vitamin deficiencies	
Vitamin	**Deficiency**
A	Xerophthalmia (dry conjunctiva); night blindness
D	Rickets/osteomalacia
E	Haemolysis; neurological defects; retinopathy
K	Coagulopathy (vitamin K required for factors II, VII, IX, X and protein C/S)
B1 (thiamine)	Dry beriberi (peripheral neuropathy); wet beriberi (heart failure)
	Wernicke's encephalopathy (ophthalmoplegia + ataxia + confusion)
	Korsakoff syndrome (amnesia, confabulation, apathy)
B3 (niacin)	Pellagra (4Ds: Diarrhoea, Dermatitis, Dementia, Death)
B6 (pyridoxine)	Dermatitis, glossitis, neuropathy, conjunctivitis
B12	Macrocytic anaemia; polyneuropathy; subacute combined degeneration of the cord; glossitis; pancytopenia
C	Scurvy (listlessness, gingivitis, bleeding gums/hair follicles, rough dry scaly skin, anorexia, bruising)

NB: vitamins ADEK are fat soluble so may be low in fat malabsorption.

EAR EXAMINATION

INTRODUCTION

- **W**ash hands; **I**ntroduce self; ask **P**atient's name, DOB and what they like to be called; **E**xplain examination and obtain consent
- Explain procedure, asking them to stay completely still when you use the otoscope
- Position patient – seat at same level as you with both ears accessible
- Note and remove any hearing aids
- Prepare otoscope, speculum, 512Hz tuning fork

INSPECTION

- **General inspection:** symmetry, position (*low set = genetic syndromes*), shape
- **Close ear inspection**
    - Skin in front of and behind ear: skin tags, erythema, scars, preauricular sinuses/pits
    - Pinna: any skin changes (*e.g. neoplasia*), deformities (*e.g. accessory auricle*), scars, erythema (*erysipelas, chondritis*), perichondrial haematoma (*trauma*)
    - External auditory meatus: erythema, pus/discharge (*otitis externa*)
    - Mastoid: erythema/swelling (*mastoiditis*)

External ear anatomy

PALPATION

- **Pinna:** tug gently (*tenderness may suggest mastoiditis*)
- **Mastoid:** palpate mastoid (*tenderness may suggest mastoiditis*)
- **Lymph nodes:** feel for pre/postauricular lymphadenopathy (*infection*)

OTOSCOPY

- Apply new speculum to otoscope and turn on light
- Hold the otoscope like a pencil (in your right hand for the right ear and vice versa) with the handle pointing anteriorly
- Start with non-affected ear
- Pull the pinna up and backwards (down and backwards in children) with your other hand to straighten the external auditory canal
- Insert the speculum tip into the external auditory meatus
- Rest the ulnar border of your hand on their cheek to stabilise it
- Gently advance the speculum while looking through the otoscope
- Look at:
    - **Auditory canal:** wax, foreign bodies, skin quality (*thick white growth = cholesteatoma*), erythema/discharge (*otitis externa*)
    - **Tympanic membrane**
        - Colour: should be pinkish-grey (*erythematous = otitis media; scarred = tympanosclerosis*)
        - Structure: look for perforation, tympanostomy ('grommet'), bulging (*otitis media*), or retraction (*Eustachian tube dysfunction*)
        - Fluid (*effusion, haemotympanum*)
    - **Behind tympanic membrane** for any visible features (pars tensa, pars flaccida, handle/lateral process of malleolus, cone of light)
- Slowly withdraw the otoscope
- Dispose of speculum in clinical waste bin

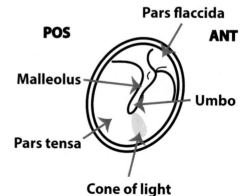

Otoscopic view of right tympanic membrane

HEARING TESTS

Crude hearing test	Ask patient to occlude one ear. Whisper a number, starting peripherally and then moving closer towards their ear. Ask them to tell you the number when they hear it. Repeat on other side.
Weber's test	Use a 512Hz tuning fork. Twang the prongs and place the round base of the fork on the patient's forehead between their eyes. Ask them if one side is louder than the other (*if one side is louder, either that side has a conductive deficit, or the contralateral side has a sensorineural deficit – Rinne's test can then determine which*).
Rinne's test	Use a 512Hz tuning fork. Twang the prongs and place the round base of the fork on the patient's mastoid process. Ask them to tell you when the sound stops. Then, place the prongs near the patient's ear. Ask them if they can then hear it again – air conduction should be louder than bone conduction (*if they cannot hear it, there is a conductive deficit in that ear*).

LASTLY

- Test **facial nerve function** if serious pathology observed

TO COMPLETE

- Thank patient
- Summarise and suggest further investigations you would consider after a full history (e.g. audiometry, tympanometry)

Common ear pathology

- **Otitis externa ('swimmer's ear'):** inflamed swollen narrow canal with discharge/flaking skin. Treated with antibiotic/steroid eardrops (if acute) or anti-fungal/steroid eardrops (if chronic).
- **Acute otitis media:** swollen red tympanic membrane. May be effusion or perforation. Treated with oral antibiotics, e.g. amoxicillin.
- **Otitis media with effusion ('glue ear') :** fluid level behind tympanic membrane due to Eustachian tube dysfunction. Observe for at least 3 months as many resolve, but may require tympanostomy.
- **Cholesteatoma:** slowly expanding growth of squamous epithelium that can invade surrounding tissues. Treated by excision
- **Perforation:** hole in eardrum. Most heal spontaneously.
- **Wax**

PRESENTING IN OSCE EXAMINATIONS

FOR EVERY EXAM

BEFORE

W Wash hands
I Introduce self (including full name and grade)
P Patient's name, DOB and what they like to be called
E Explain examination (± chaperone if intimate exam) – *also tell the patient you will be talking to the examiner throughout*

DURING

- Tell them the exam should not be painful but, if there's any discomfort, to let you know
- For general inspection, always <u>stand back</u> at the foot of the patient's bed with your arms behind your back and then present. Comment on the general appearance first, e.g. 'On general inspection, this patient looks well.' Then go on to present other relevant patient details (e.g. 'There is no evidence of jaundice, cachexia or pallor.') and comment on the presence/absence of things around the bed.
- Ask if they have pain anywhere before touching them and use the patient's name and talk to the patient during the exam
- Examine from the patient's right-hand side – a medical tradition
- Most medical schools like you to talk through your findings as you go. If this is the case, turn to the examiner in between each part of your examination (e.g. the hands), and confidently present your findings, for example: 'On examination of the hands, there was stage three clubbing, but no evidence of leukonychia, koilonychia or palmar erythema.' Then do the same for the next section (e.g. eyes, then mouth etc.). DON'T SAY, 'I am looking for koilonychia.' Say instead, 'There is no evidence of koilonychia.'

AFTER

Thank the patient and restore clothing. Then take your stethoscope off and hold it in your hand. Stand straight with your arms behind your back, look the examiner in the eyes and say with confidence:

1. **'I would complete my examination by** ...' (state other examinations, NOT investigations)
2. **'In summary**, this is Mr X and I have examined his respiratory system.'
   a. Major finding(s): 'The major finding was...' (state the most striking finding(s) first to capture their attention)
   b. Additional findings to back up your case: 'In addition...' (state other important positive and relevant negative findings)
      - Don't list irrelevant negative findings
      - Avoid presenting a long list of findings without thinking about their clinical significance
      - If you know the diagnosis, think about the cause and consequences of the condition
   c. Diagnosis/differential: 'These findings would be consistent with...' or 'My differential diagnosis would include...'
3. 'After taking a full history, **further investigations** might include...' – make these relevant to the presenting complaint

BE SYSTEMATIC WHEN ANSWERING QUESTIONS

e.g. 'What is the treatment for Dupuytren's contracture?'
'The management for Dupuytren's contracture can be divided into conservative, medical or surgical.' 'Medical management can include...'

Causes	If many, use a surgical sieve, e.g. **VITAMIN**: **V**ascular, **I**nfective/inflammatory, **T**raumatic, **A**utoimmune, **M**etabolic, **I**atrogenic/idiopathic, **N**eoplastic
Investigations	Bedside tests, bloods, radiological tests, specialised tests
Treatment	Conservative, medical, surgical
Complications	Immediate, early, late

TOP TIPS

- OSCEs are about **acting**. Even if you don't feel confident or haven't seen something before, act as if you have done it 100 times!
- How you say things matters as much as what you say. Be **confident** but not arrogant.
- **Flaunt your knowledge!** If you have good background knowledge, show it to the examiner whenever you can.
- Try to use **buzzwords**, e.g. 'There is a symmetrical deforming polyarthropathy, with no active synovitis.'
- **Read the question** carefully – there will always be one station where you will lose marks for not reading the question correctly
- Some **examiners act grumpy** and uninterested even though they may actually be very nice and generous. Go in expecting every examiner to act like this and you won't be thrown when they are.
- **Pauses to think are absolutely fine**. Don't mumble, say 'errrr', or speak before you know what you want to say.
- Never forget to **wash your hands**. It should be the first thing you do when you go in.
- For orthopaedics, don't forget to say you would like to examine joints above and below, and assess neurovascular status
- In all psychiatry stations, don't forget about risk to self and others
- If you don't know what to do, just go back to basics: inspection/palpation/percussion/auscultation for most exams; or look/feel/move/special tests/function for orthopaedics
- Lastly, and most importantly, try to enjoy yourself. Take satisfaction in demonstrating your knowledge and spotting rare signs. Examiners are all very generous in finals and the stations are usually basic: the medical school and examiners do not want you to see you fail.

CHAPTER 3: VIVAS AND SPOTTERS

This page is intentionally left blank

THORACIC SCARS

MINI-THORACOTOMY/MINI-STERNOTOMY

- Aortic valve accessed via right anterior mini-thoracotomy (2nd intercostal space) or mini-sternotomy
- Mitral valve accessed via right lateral mini-thoracotomy (below nipple or in breast crease)
- INDICATIONS: minimally invasive valve replacement/repair

MEDIAN STERNOTOMY

- Mainly for **open heart surgery**
- Sternum is cracked open and chest opened
- INDICATIONS: valve surgery, congenital cardiac defect corrections, CABG (if seen, ask to look for vein harvesting scar on legs)

PACEMAKER SCAR

- Usually on left but can be on right
- INDICATIONS: pacemaker/ICD/ loop recorder insertion

AXILLARY THORACOTOMY

- Muscle-sparing approach
- INDICATIONS: pneumothorax, pleurectomy, pulmonary resections (pneumonectomy/ lobectomy/wedge)

ANTEROLATERAL THORACOTOMY

- Under breast
- Left anterolateral thoracotomy is used for **open chest massage**

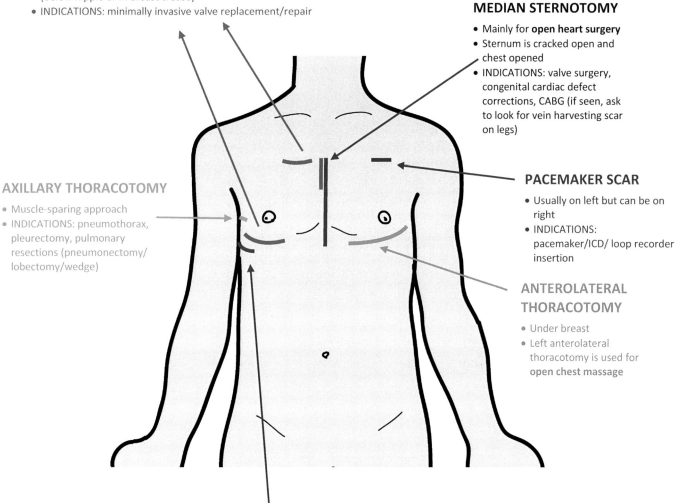

POSTEROLATERAL THORACOTOMY

- Most common thoracotomy
- Performed with patient in lateral decubitus position
- Cut through intercostal space beginning inferomedially to tip of scapula
- INDICATIONS: **pulmonary resections** (pneumonectomy/ lobectomy/wedge), oesophageal surgery

SMALL INCISIONS/PORTS may be used for thoracoscopy (e.g. for diagnosis, biopsies, pleurodesis) or video-assisted thoracic surgery (e.g. for pleural operations, lobectomies, lung resections)

ABDOMINAL SCARS

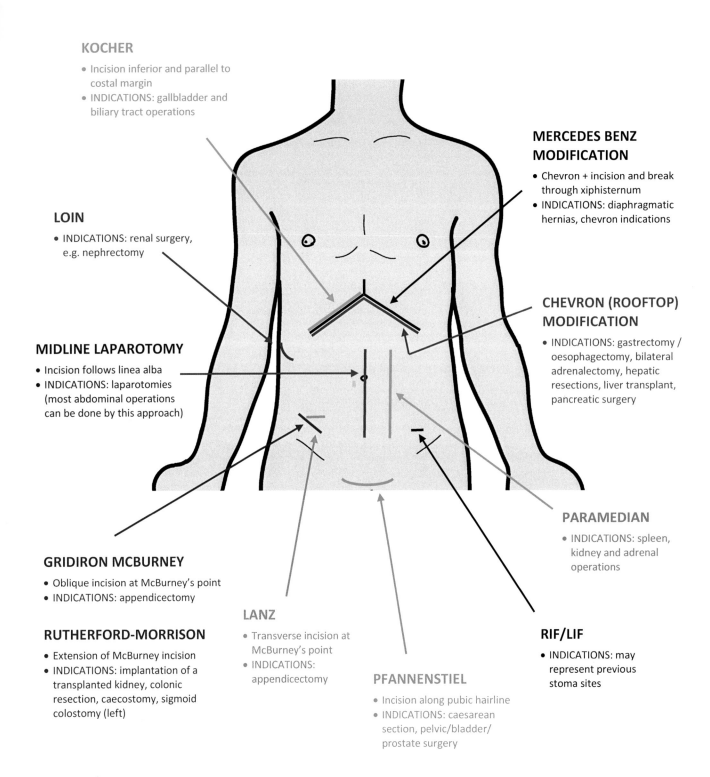

KOCHER
- Incision inferior and parallel to costal margin
- INDICATIONS: gallbladder and biliary tract operations

MERCEDES BENZ MODIFICATION
- Chevron + incision and break through xiphisternum
- INDICATIONS: diaphragmatic hernias, chevron indications

LOIN
- INDICATIONS: renal surgery, e.g. nephrectomy

CHEVRON (ROOFTOP) MODIFICATION
- INDICATIONS: gastrectomy / oesophagectomy, bilateral adrenalectomy, hepatic resections, liver transplant, pancreatic surgery

MIDLINE LAPAROTOMY
- Incision follows linea alba
- INDICATIONS: laparotomies (most abdominal operations can be done by this approach)

PARAMEDIAN
- INDICATIONS: spleen, kidney and adrenal operations

GRIDIRON MCBURNEY
- Oblique incision at McBurney's point
- INDICATIONS: appendicectomy

LANZ
- Transverse incision at McBurney's point
- INDICATIONS: appendicectomy

RIF/LIF
- INDICATIONS: may represent previous stoma sites

RUTHERFORD-MORRISON
- Extension of McBurney incision
- INDICATIONS: implantation of a transplanted kidney, colonic resection, caecostomy, sigmoid colostomy (left)

PFANNENSTIEL
- Incision along pubic hairline
- INDICATIONS: caesarean section, pelvic/bladder/prostate surgery

LAPRASCOPIC INCISIONS may be used for many abdominal operations

VALVE REPLACEMENTS

CLINICAL EXAMINATION

- **Metallic valves**
    - Metallic mitral valve: S1 sounds metallic
    - Metallic aortic valve: S2 sounds metallic
    - There is often a click audible without a stethoscope
- **Tissue valves**
    - Relevant heart sounds may be normal, loud or quiet
- Systolic **flow murmurs** are normal for aortic valve replacements
- Assess for **valve function** (signs of regurgitation of replaced valve), **cardiac decompensation** (signs of heart failure), and signs of **infective endocarditis**
- Also look for signs of **over-anticoagulation** (bruising) and **anaemia** (haemolysis)

INDICATIONS FOR SURGERY

- **Left-sided valve dysfunction**
    - Any valve: associated LVF, symptomatic
    - If regurgitation, also: acute onset, associated LV dilation
    - If mitral, also: presence of pulmonary hypertension

    NB: for MR, valve repair is preferred when possible; for MS, balloon valvuloplasty is preferred unless contraindicated (i.e. coexistent MR, thrombus or calcified valve).
- **Infective endocarditis**
    - Associated heart failure
    - Uncontrolled infection (fistula, enlarging vegetation, false aneurysm, aortic root abscess, persistently positive blood cultures, fungal/multidrug-resistant organism)
    - High embolic risk (persistent large vegetation)

    NB: If prosthetic valve, surgery also indicated if: <2 months post-op, valve dysfunction or Staphylococcus aureus infection.

TYPES

- **Tissue valve**
    - Usually porcine xenograft
    - Needs replacing after 10-15 years; sooner if patient is active
    - No need for warfarin
    - Recommended for older people, people with low life expectancy and females of child-bearing age
- **Mechanical valve**
    - Longer lasting (older valves 20-30 years, newer valves >30 years)
    - Lifelong warfarin
    - Makes a quiet clicking noise
    - Recommended for younger people (<60 years) so they don't need repeat surgeries (unless female and of child-bearing age because warfarin is teratogenic)

PROCEDURE

- Pre-operative: transthoracic ± transoesophageal echo, coronary angiography
- May be performed by:
    - **Open surgery:** via midline sternotomy
    - **Minimally invasive surgery**
        - **Aortic valve:** via right anterior mini-thoracotomy (2nd intercostal space) or mini-sternotomy
        - **Mitral valve:** via right lateral mini-thoracotomy (below nipple or in breast crease)
- Patient is put on cardiopulmonary bypass while valve is replaced

NB: if there is also coronary artery disease, CABG is usually performed concurrently – check the legs for a vein grafting scar.

> **Complications of valve replacements**
>
> - **Perioperative risks:** arrhythmias, stroke/TIA, infections (wound/lung/endocarditis), bleeding/haemothorax, thromboembolism, pulmonary oedema/acute respiratory distress syndrome, acute kidney injury
> - **Valve complications:** leakage, dehiscence, obstruction, thromboembolism, haemolytic anaemia, infective endocarditis
> - **Warfarin side effects:** bleeding

PACEMAKERS

Pacemakers are used to treat bradyarrhythmias. They are usually inserted subcutaneously below the left clavicle. A wire connects the pacemaker to the myocardium of the right atrium and/or right ventricle. This supplies electrical stimulation which initiates myocardial depolarisation and subsequent contraction. It can be programmed externally. The battery lasts 5-10 years.

COMMON INDICATIONS

For permanent pacing
- Mobitz type 2 second degree heart block
- Complete heart block
- Symptomatic bradycardias (e.g. sick sinus syndrome)
- Symptomatic pauses (>3 seconds)
- Trifascicular block with syncope/pre-syncope

For temporary pacing
- Haemodynamically unstable bradycardia unresponsive to atropine
- Haemodynamically unstable heart block post-myocardial infarction (rare)

NB: temporary pacing may also be used to supress drug-resistant tachyarrhythmias (e.g. VT storm) by pacing at a higher rate than the native heart rate ('overdrive pacing').

BASIC TYPES

- **Dual-chamber** pacemaker (two leads, one in right atrium and one in right ventricle): paces both chambers; used for most patients requiring a pacemaker unless they meet the criteria below for a single chamber pacemaker
- **Single-chamber** pacemaker
  - One lead in right ventricle: used in patients with permanent AF because there is no point pacing a fibrillating atrium
  - One lead in right atrium: sometimes used for sick sinus syndrome <u>with</u> normal AV conduction because the pacemaker only needs to replace the SA node when the rest of the heart functions normally – *although generally a dual-chamber pacemaker would still be used in this situation because there is an increased risk of AV problems in the future*

NB: implantable cardioverter defibrillators look like pacemakers but have a different function – they are used for automatic defibrillation in patients who are at risk of VF or VT and sudden cardiac death (e.g. patients with previous episodes of ventricular arrhythmias and haemodynamic compromise or poor ejection fraction; repaired congenital heart disease; or familial cardiac conditions). Some implantable cardioverter defibrillators may also function as pacemakers.

CODING

3 letter codes
The pacemaker can pace the right ventricle, the right atrium or both. The pacemaker can also sense spontaneous heart depolarisations through the same lead(s), and pacing can either be triggered by that spontaneous heart depolarisation or inhibited by it (most).
- **Letter 1:** indicates which chamber is paced (<u>A</u>tria, <u>V</u>entricles, <u>D</u>ual chamber)
- **Letter 2:** indicates which chamber is sensed (<u>A</u>tria, <u>V</u>entricles, <u>D</u>ual chamber)
- **Letter 3:** indicates pacemaker response (<u>T</u>riggered, <u>I</u>nhibited, <u>D</u>ual)

Further letters which may be used
- **Letter 4:** if rate responsive features present (<u>R</u>ate responsive), e.g. rate can increase during exercise
- **Letter 5:** anti-tachycardia features
  - <u>P</u>: in tachycardia, it will pace
  - <u>S</u>: in tachycardia, it will shock
  - <u>D</u>: dual ability to pace and shock

NB: <u>O</u> can mean none for any letter.

Examples
- **VVI:** ventricles are paced, but pacing is inhibited when spontaneous ventricular depolarisations are sensed
- **AAI:** as above but for atria – *rarely used for reasons above*
- **DDD:** both chambers are paced, but atrial pacing is inhibited when spontaneous atrial depolarisation is sensed (within a predetermined maximum RP interval), and ventricular pacing is inhibited when spontaneous ventricular depolarisation is sensed (within a predetermined maximum PR interval).

ECG OF PACED RHYTHM

- The ECG of a paced rhythm has vertical pacing spikes when it is pacing (but they may be difficult to see) – *you cannot interpret a paced ECG for other abnormalities*
  - If the atrium is paced, a pacing spike is seen immediately before a P wave
  - If the ventricle is paced, a pacing spike is seen immediately before a broad QRS complex
  - In dual chamber pacing, both of these pacing spikes are seen

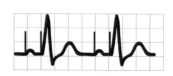

Atrial and ventricular pacing spikes on ECG

HEART FAILURE

Heart failure is a clinical syndrome characterised by the symptoms and signs that occur due to a reduced cardiac output and/or increased filling pressures.

TYPES

- **Heart failure with reduced ejection fraction – *'systolic heart failure'***
    - Reduction in contractility of ventricles
    - *Causes below*
- **Heart failure with preserved ejection fraction – *'diastolic heart failure'***
    - Reduction in compliance of ventricles (i.e. stiff ventricles)
    - Usually related to old age/chronic hypertension

CAUSES

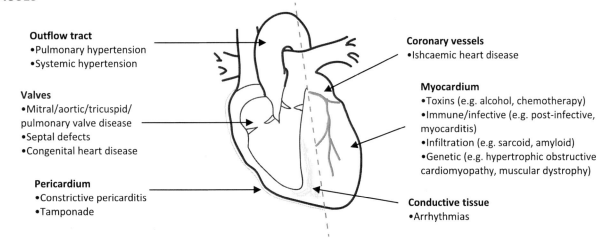

Outflow tract
- Pulmonary hypertension
- Systemic hypertension

Valves
- Mitral/aortic/tricuspid/ pulmonary valve disease
- Septal defects
- Congenital heart disease

Pericardium
- Constrictive pericarditis
- Tamponade

Coronary vessels
- Ishcaemic heart disease

Myocardium
- Toxins (e.g. alcohol, chemotherapy)
- Immune/infective (e.g. post-infective, myocarditis)
- Infiltration (e.g. sarcoid, amyloid)
- Genetic (e.g. hypertrophic obstructive cardiomyopathy, muscular dystrophy)

Conductive tissue
- Arrhythmias

CLINICAL FEATURES

Clinical features of heart failure			
	Reduced perfusion	**Pulmonary congestion (LVF)**	**Systemic congestion (RVF)**
Symptoms	•Fatigue •Exercise intolerance	•SOB on exertion, orthopnoea •Paroxysmal nocturnal dyspnoea •White/pink frothy sputum •Cardiac wheeze	•Peripheral oedema •Weight gain •Bloating and reduced appetite
Signs	•Cyanosis •Tachypnoea/ tachycardia •Cool extremities •Oliguria	•Pulmonary oedema (fine basal creps) •Pleural effusions •S3/ventricular gallop	•Raised JVP •Peripheral oedema (pedal, sacral, scrotal) •Hepatomegaly •Ascites

INVESTIGATIONS

To confirm diagnosis
- Serum natriuretic peptide
- Chest X-ray (**ABCDE**): **A**lveolar shadowing (bat's wings sign), **B**-lines (interstitial oedema), **C**ardiomegaly, **D**iversion of blood to upper lobes, **E**ffusion
- Echocardiography: diagnostic test and may help determine cause

To determine cause
- Bloods: FBC, U&Es, TFTs, LFTs, ferritin, lipid profile, HbA1C
- ECG: look for ischaemia, arrhythmias, small complexes (*amyloid/pericardial effusion*)
- Angiogram or functional imaging: if suspect ischaemic heart disease
- Cardiac MRI: if poor echo windows, suspected infiltrative cause or unclear cause

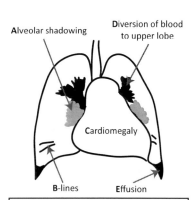

Alveolar shadowing

Diversion of blood to upper lobe

Cardiomegaly

B-lines

Effusion

CXR changes in heart failure

MANAGEMENT

- Treat cause where possible
- Pharmacological treatments
  - Core medications
    - ACE inhibitor (<u>or</u> angiotensin receptor blocker <u>or</u> angiotensin receptor-neprilysin inhibitor)
    - β-blocker
    - Diuretic, e.g. furosemide/bumetanide, *if peripheral or pulmonary oedema* (weight monitoring can be useful for titration – weight changes with fluid retention)
  - Other medications: add aldosterone antagonist (e.g. spironolactone, eplerenone) *if uncontrolled with core treatments*; add ivabradine *if in sinus rhythm ≥70 bpm despite maximum β-blocker dose*
- Non-pharmacological treatments
  - Cardiac resynchronisation therapy device: considered if QRS significantly prolonged
  - Implantable cardioverter defibrillator: considered if risk of ventricular arrhythmias

NB: this is the long-term management of heart failure; the management of acute pulmonary oedema is described on p186.

VARICOSE VEINS

Varicose veins are tortuous, dilated veins of the superficial venous system.

PATHOPHYSIOLOGY

- Incompetent valves in perforating veins cause retrograde blood flow from the deep to superficial veins of the leg
- This results in increased pressure and dilation of the superficial veins
- **Risks:** age, female > male, previous DVT, obesity, pregnancy

CLINICAL FEATURES

<u>Symptoms</u>
- Most are asymptomatic except for aesthetic problems but patient may have pain, cramps, heaviness, tingling and restless legs

<u>Signs</u>
- Oedema
- Varicose eczema
- Venous ulcers
- Haemosiderin deposits
- Phlebitis
- Lipodermatosclerosis (subcutaneous fibrosis due to chronic inflammation and fat necrosis)
- *Atrophie blanche* (white scarring around healing ulcer)
- **Saphena varix:** dilation of the saphenous vein at its confluence with the femoral vein (transmits a cough impulse)

INVESTIGATIONS

- Colour flow duplex ultrasound

MANAGEMENT

- Refer if: bleeding, pain, ulceration, thrombophlebitis, severe impact on quality of life
- Management options
  - **Conservative:** avoid prolonged standing, graduated compression stockings (if no peripheral arterial disease), regular walking, weight loss
  - **Injection sclerotherapy:** sclerosant injected at multiple sites in varicosities
  - **Phlebectomy:** stab avulsion or mechanical avulsion
  - **Endovenous laser ablation**
  - **Radiofrequency ablation**
  - **Surgical stripping**

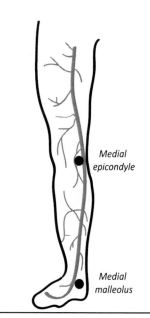

Medial epicondyle

Medial malleolus

Long saphenous vein distribution

PERIPHERAL ARTERIAL DISEASE

CLINICAL FEATURES

Acute limb ischaemia – *due to thrombus (acute on chronic) or emboli*
- **6 P's:** **P**ale, **P**ulseless, **P**araesthesia, **P**aralysis, **Pa**in, **P**erishingly cold

Intermittent claudication
- Calf pain on exertion which is relieved by rest (check *claudication distance*)

Critical ischaemia
- Chronic rest pain (often at night, relieved by hanging legs over bed)
- Tissue loss (e.g. arterial ulcers, gangrene)

INVESTIGATIONS

- **Ankle-brachial pressure index**

> **<0.9** = intermittent claudication
> **<0.6** = rest pain
> **<0.3** = critical ischaemia

NB: ABPI may be falsely elevated in patients with calcified arteries.

- **Imaging**
  - Duplex ultrasound (first line imaging)
  - MR or CT angiography (second line imaging, MR preferred but CT more widely available)
  - Catheter angiography (third line)
- **Bloods:** lipid levels, fasting glucose, FBC (rule out anaemia), U&Es (to check renal function prior to contrast), coagulation screen
- **ECG:** to look for AF as a cause of emboli

MANAGEMENT

- **Risk factor control**
  - Anti-platelet therapy (aspirin or clopidogrel)
  - Lipid lowering therapy (statin)
  - Smoking cessation
  - Diet, weight management and exercise
  - BP and diabetes control
- **Supervised exercise** regimen (for intermittent claudication)
- **Naftidrofuryl oxalate** (for intermittent claudication) – *rarely successful*
- **Revascularisation for acute ischaemia**
  - Percutaneous catheter-directed thrombolytic therapy
  - Percutaneous transluminal angioplasty (stent)
  - Surgical embolectomy
- **Revascularisation for chronic ischaemia**
  1. Percutaneous transluminal angioplasty (stent) – *if possible (i.e. short segment, not at knee joint, good run-off)*
  2. Vascular bypass grafting
- **Debridement/amputation** for gangrene or non-viable limbs

Vascular bypass procedures			
Procedure	Details	Indication	Signs on examination
Aortobifemoral	Aorta to both femoral arteries *(open operation)*	Aortoiliac occlusive disease	•Midline laparotomy scar •Bilateral groin scars
Axillofemoral/ axillobifemoral	Axillary artery to one/both femoral arteries *(graft tunnelled subcutaneously)*	*Axillofemoral used for patients who are unable to tolerate aortobifemoral*	•Axillary scar •Unilateral/bilateral groin scars •Graft may be palpable
Femorofemoral	Femoral artery to femoral artery *(graft tunnelled subcutaneously or in pre-peritoneal space)*	Unilateral iliac disease	•Bilateral groin scars •Graft may be palpable
Iliofemoral	Iliac artery to femoral artery *(iliac artery on ipsilateral or contralateral side may be used)*		•2 groin scars (may be on the same or opposite sides depending on operation)
Femoropopliteal Femorotibial Femorodistal	Femoral artery to popliteal artery, a tibial artery or distally *(graft may be tunnelled subcutaneously or anatomically)*	Femoropopliteal disease	•Groin scar •Medial lower leg scar •Graft may be palpable

PULMONARY FIBROSIS

A restrictive lung disease characterised by accumulation of excess fibrous connective tissue in the lung parenchyma, causing reduced lung compliance and oxygen diffusion capacity. This leads to progressive hypoxia and shortness of breath.

CAUSES

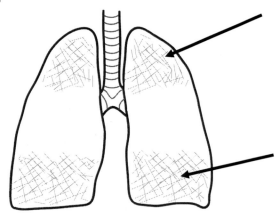

Upper zone fibrosis = CARTEx

Coal

Ankylosing spondylitis

Radiation

TB

Extrinsic allergic alveolitis

Lower zone fibrosis = CAID (*more common*)

Connective tissue disorders (scleroderma, rheumatoid)

Asbestos

Idiopathic pulmonary fibrosis

Drugs (nitrofurantoin, amiodarone, methotrexate, cyclophosphamide, gold, sulfasalazine)

CLINICAL FEATURES

Symptoms
- Chronic progressive shortness of breath
- Dry cough

Signs of pulmonary fibrosis
- Dyspnoea
- Reduced expansion
- Fine end-inspiratory crepitations

Signs of cause
- Clubbing (*idiopathic pulmonary fibrosis*)
- Hand deformity (*RA*)
- Telangiectasia, sclerodactyly and microstomia (*systemic sclerosis*)
- Butterfly rash (*SLE*)
- Lupus pernio (*sarcoidosis*)
- Radiation burns
- Kyphosis (*ankylosing spondylitis*)

INVESTIGATIONS

- Chest X-ray: reticulonodular shadowing
- High-resolution CT chest: honeycombing cysts, reticular septal thickening, ground glass changes (indicates inflammatory process which is often steroid responsive)
- Spirometry: restrictive defect with reduced diffusion capacity (*see interpretation notes on spirometry p251*)
- Blood tests: for likely causes, e.g. antinuclear antibody, rheumatoid factor, anti-centromere antibody
- Lung biopsy

MANAGEMENT

NB: fibrosis is permanent and there is no cure.
- Corticosteroids may help in acute exacerbations
- Anti-fibrotics (pirfenidone/nintedanib) may be used in idiopathic pulmonary fibrosis
- Treat/withdraw cause if possible (may include corticosteroids and immunosuppressants)
- Supplementary measures
  - Smoking cessation
  - Pulmonary rehabilitation
  - Long-term oxygen therapy – usually considered if PaO2<7.3kPa (or <8kPa in presence of pulmonary hypertension or secondary polycythaemia)
- Lung transplant (option for some patients)

PNEUMONECTOMY/LOBECTOMY

A pneumonectomy is the removal of an entire lung, and a lobectomy is the removal of a lobe of the lung.

PNEUMONECTOMY SIGNS
- Left/right thoracotomy scar
- On affected side:
    - Tracheal displacement to side of removal
    - Reduced expansion
    - Dull percussion note
    - Absent breath sounds (although there may be bronchial breathing in the upper zone due to tracheal deviation)

LOBECTOMY SIGNS
- Left/right thoracotomy scar
- May be no other signs due to compensatory hyperexpansion of the remaining lobes
- May be some reduced expansion, dullness to percussion and reduced air entry

CHEST X-RAY
- Fluid fills cavity of removed lung (radio-opaque)
- Organs shift into cavity of removed lung (i.e. heart and trachea displaced)

INDICATIONS
- Lung malignancy
- Localised bronchiectasis
- Aspergilloma
- Large bullectomy
- TB (historically – practice discontinued)

LUNG LESION WORKUP
- CT chest/abdomen/pelvis + PET
    - Confirm no metastasis
- Attain histology
    - CT-guided biopsy/bronchoscopy/mediastinoscopy
- Pulmonary function tests: to determine whether surgical resection is appropriate
    - $FEV_1 > 2L$ for pneumonectomy or >1.5L for lobectomy = suitable for resection
    - If not, ventilation-perfusion scanning may be considered to determine split lung function (lung with tumour may not be contributing to total FEV_1)

CHRONIC OBSTRUCTIVE PULMONARY DISEASE

CLINICAL FEATURES

- Symptoms: exertional dyspnoea, chronic productive cough, wheeze
- Signs: accessory muscle use, tar-stained fingers, bounding pulse, CO_2 retention flap, lip pursing, central cyanosis, tracheal tug, hyperexpanded chest, quiet breath sounds/wheeze/prolonged expiratory phase

INVESTIGATIONS

- **Spirometry**
  - Obstructive pattern: $\downarrow FEV_1$ (<80%), normal FVC (>80%), $\downarrow FEV_1/FVC$ ratio (<0.7)
  - FEV_1 grades severity
- **Chest X-ray**
  - Hyperinflation (>8 anterior ribs visible)
  - Flat hemi-diaphragms
  - Decreased lung markings
  - Black lesions (bullae)
  - Prominent hila

SEVERITY GRADING

Mild	FEV_1 >80%
Moderate	FEV_1 50-80%
Severe	FEV_1 30-50%
Very severe	FEV_1 <30%

MANAGEMENT

Pharmacological

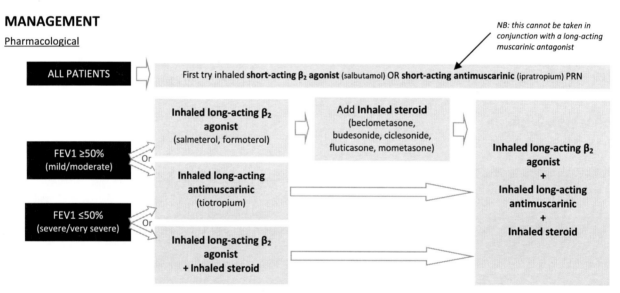

Produced using NICE 'CG101 chronic obstructive pulmonary disease in over 16s: diagnosis and management' 2010

- Common combination inhalers
  - **Seretide** = salmeterol + fluticasone
  - **Symbicort** = formoterol + budesonide
  - **Fostair** = formoterol + beclomethasone
- Tablets
  - Mucolytics, e.g. carbocisteine
  - Theophylline

- Abbreviations
  - **LABA** = long-acting β_2 agonist
  - **LAMA** = long-acting muscarinic antagonist
  - **ICS** = inhaled corticosteroid

Non-pharmacological

- Smoking cessation
- Exercise and pulmonary rehabilitation
- Long-term oxygen therapy – considered if PaO2<7.3kPa (or <8kPa in presence of pulmonary hypertension or secondary polycythaemia)
- Lung transplant
- Pneumococcal/influenza vaccines
  - *NB: this is the long-term management of COPD; the management of COPD exacerbation is described on p183.*

BRONCHIECTASIS

Abnormal dilation of distal airways, associated with chronic cough and excessive sputum production.

CAUSES

Genetic	CF, Young's syndrome, Kartagener's syndrome, yellow nail syndrome, α1-antitrypsin deficiency
Mechanical	Malignancy, foreign body
Childhood infection	Pertussis, measles, TB, pneumonia
Immunological	Allergic bronchopulmonary aspergillosis, hypogammaglobulinaemia, HIV, leukaemia, autoimmune

CLINICAL FEATURES

Symptoms
- Chronic productive cough
- Haemoptysis
- Recurrent chest infections

Signs of bronchiectasis
- Clubbing
- Inspiratory clicks
- Coarse inspiratory crepitations
- Large airway rhonchi

Signs of cause
- Curved yellow nails and lymphoedema (*yellow nail syndrome*)
- Dextrocardia (*Kartagener's syndrome*)
- Young and thin (*CF*)

INVESTIGATIONS

- **Diagnosis**
  - Chest X-ray: tramlines and ring shadows
  - High-resolution CT chest: 'signet ring sign' (bronchi larger than the adjacent vasculature) and bronchial wall thickening – *diagnostic test*
  - Spirometry: variable but often obstructive pattern
- **To ascertain cause**
  - Immunoglobulins and electrophoresis
  - Aspergillus precipitins and serum IgE
  - CF sweat test/genetic mutation analysis
  - HIV
  - Rheumatoid factor
  - α1-antitrypsin
- Sputum culture (to determine any colonising bacteria and sensitivities)

MANAGEMENT

- Exercise and improved nutrition
- Chest physiotherapy
- Prompt treatment of infections (choose antibiotics based on culture sensitivities)
- Rotating antibiotics may be used for prophylaxis if recurrent infections
- Trial of bronchodilator and nebulised hypertonic saline
- Pneumococcal/influenza vaccines
- Lung resection may be considered in localised disease with a poor response to medical management

DIALYSIS

Dialysis is a method of removing plasma waste products and excess fluid and maintaining normal electrolyte concentrations. It is used when the kidneys are unable to perform this function. It may be used temporarily in acute kidney injury or long-term in chronic kidney disease.

INDICATIONS

Acute kidney injury
Refractory:

A	**A**cidosis
E	**E**lectrolyte abnormalities (hyperkalaemia, hyponatraemia, hypercalcaemia)
I	**I**ntoxicants (methanol, lithium, salicylates)
O	**O**verload
U	**U**raemia

Chronic kidney disease
In chronic kidney disease, dialysis is required when the GFR is <15ml/minute.

TYPES OF DIALYSIS

Types of dialysis			
Type	**Use**	**Access routes**	**Details**

Haemodialysis	•Acute kidney injury
	•Chronic kidney disease
		•Arteriovenous fistula
		•Tunnelled central venous catheter ('dual lumen tunnelled cuffed catheter'; tunnelled under skin to reduce infection; lasts weeks/months)
		•Non-tunnelled central venous catheter (lasts 10 days)
			•Blood is removed from a vein and pumped along a semi-permeable membrane by a haemodialysis machine. Dialysate fluid is pumped in the opposite direction on the other side. The dialysate is a purified fluid with similar constituents to plasma but without the toxins. Toxins are removed from the blood due to the concentration-gradient.
			•With training, haemodialysis can also be performed at home. There are three types:
			  - **Conventional:** for 4 hours, 3 times a week (like in hospital)
			  - **Short daily:** for 2 hours, 5-7 times a week
			  - **Nocturnal:** for 6-8 hours overnight, 6 times a week or every other night
			•Several lifestyle modifications are needed while undergoing haemodialysis: fluid restriction, salt restriction, potassium restriction, phosphate restriction

Peritoneal dialysis	•Chronic kidney disease	•Tenckhoff catheter	•Types:
			  - **Continuous ambulatory peritoneal dialysis:** patient replaces peritoneal dialysate manually with fluid bags 3-5 times daily (each exchange takes 30-40 minutes)
			  - **Automated peritoneal dialysis:** machine automatically replaces peritoneal dialysate overnight (over 8-10 hours)
			•Peritoneal dialysis is an alternative to haemodialysis for patients with chronic kidney disease and can be performed at home. The peritoneum is used as a semi-permeable membrane.

Continuous venovenous haemofiltration	•Acute kidney injury (in intensive care)	•Central venous catheter	•Haemofiltration involves filtering blood through a high-pressure column with a semi-permeable membrane. Small molecules and water pass across the membrane and are removed. Fluid is replaced with a fluid of optimal biochemical composition. •Haemofiltration causes less haemodynamic instability than haemodialysis so is used for critically ill patients

COMPLICATIONS OF DIALYSIS PROCESS

- Common non-severe side effects: headache, itching, muscle cramps
- Disequilibrium syndrome: osmotic changes lead to cerebral oedema
- Hypotension
- Haemolysis (may cause hyperkalaemia)
- Sepsis
- Problems with fluid balance

ARTERIOVENOUS FISTULA

An arteriovenous fistula is a surgically created anastomosis between an artery and a vein. Its main use is to dilate a vein for easier access in patients requiring regular haemodialysis.

EXAMINING AN AV FISTULA

Look
- **General inspection**
  - Patient well/unwell
  - In pain
- **Fistula**
  - Type of fistula
    - Radiocephalic (most) = at wrist
    - Brachiocephalic = at antecubital fossa
    - Upper arm basilic vein transposition
  - Scars
  - Signs of inflammation: rash, erythema, swelling
  - Arm elevation test (for outflow obstruction): fistula should collapse on arm elevation
- **Veins**
  - Presence of collateral veins (*suggest venous stenosis*)
- **Hands** – *compare to other side*
  - Oedema
  - Signs of ischaemia (*Steal syndrome = vascular insufficiency secondary to AV fistula*)

Feel
- **Thrill:** a thrill is normal but it shouldn't be pulsatile
- **Consistency:** should be soft and easily compressible
- **Augmentation test** (for anastomotic stenosis): occlude vein 1-2 cm above anastomosis. If arterial pressure is adequately conducted (i.e. there is no anastomotic stenosis), a pulsation in the vein will be seen. *NB: if vein is pulsatile anyway, there is venous outflow stenosis.*

Listen
- **Bruit:** should be a soft machinery–like rumbling sound (*high-pitched = stenosis*)

NOTES ON AV FISTULAS

Why is it needed?
The blood volume that needs to be removed and returned during haemodialysis is too great for a normal vein. If a vein and an artery are joined, the pressure of arterial blood entering the vein dilates it and increases the flow rate. After the vein is sufficiently dilated, it can be used for haemodialysis.

How long before an AV fistula becomes patent?
It takes 4-6 weeks to sufficiently dilate the vein.

How is it used?
Once the vein is dilated, two needles are inserted into the vein:
- Afferent needle: takes blood from the vein to the haemodialysis machine (placed distally)
- Efferent needle: returns blood from the haemodialysis machine to the vein (place proximally)

What are the complications of an AV fistula?
Common complications include: thrombosis, venous stenosis, aneurysm, infection, Steal syndrome (distal ischaemia)

Special instructions for the patient
- Do not let anyone take blood from or cannulate the arm on the side of the AV fistula
- Do not let anyone measure blood pressure on the arm on the side of the AV fistula
- Keep the arm clean
- Check the fistula daily for pulse/thrill

What are the advantages of an AV fistula over a central venous catheter?
- Lower re-circulation rate: afferent and efferent needles can be placed quite far apart up the vein, so only a tiny proportion of the blood returned to the patient (via the efferent needle) it taken back up again (by the afferent needle). Central venous catheter haemodialysis has a higher re-circulation rate because the afferent and efferent tubes are very close to one another.
- Lower infection rate
- Higher blood flow rate (allowing more efficient dialysis)
- Lower incidence of thrombosis

TENCKHOFF CATHETER

A Tenckhoff catheter is a catheter placed through the abdominal wall that provides access to the peritoneum. It is used to perform peritoneal dialysis.

EXAMINING A TENCKHOFF CATHETER

Look
- **General inspection**
    - Patient well/unwell
    - In pain
- **Abdomen**
    - Signs of acute abdomen/peritonitis
    - Scars
- **Tenckhoff catheter**
    - Patency
    - Signs of inflammation

Feel
- **Abdomen**
    - Brief abdominal exam to determine if any signs of peritonitis or areas of tenderness
- **Skin around catheter**
    - Temperature
    - Swelling

NOTES ON TENCKHOFF CATHETERS AND PERITONEAL DIALYSIS

What are the different types of peritoneal dialysis?
- **Continuous ambulatory peritoneal dialysis:** patient replaces peritoneal dialysate manually with fluid bags 3-5 times daily (each exchange takes 30-40 minutes)
- **Automated peritoneal dialysis:** machine automatically replaces peritoneal dialysate overnight (over 8-10 hours)

What are the contraindications to peritoneal dialysis?
- Peritoneal adhesions
- Stoma
- Hernias
- Inflammatory bowel disease

What are the complications of peritoneal dialysis?
1. Peritonitis
2. Infection around catheter site
3. Constipation
4. Pleural effusions
5. Hernias and weight gain

What are the advantages of peritoneal dialysis?
- Can be done at home
- Easier to travel/go on holiday

RENAL TRANSPLANT

RENAL TRANSPLANT EXAMINATION

- Perform **renal exam** (*see examination notes on renal exam p56*)
- Look for:
  1. **Aetiology:** fingertip capillary glucose monitoring marks (*diabetes*), flank masses (*PKD*), butterfly rash (*SLE*), hearing aid (*Alport syndrome*), collapsed nasal bridge (*granulomatosis with polyangiitis*), sternotomy (*renovascular disease*)
  2. **Previous renal replacement therapy:** AV fistula, central line and peritoneal dialysis scars
  3. **Graft functionality:** active marks in AV fistula, fluid retention, anaemia, uraemia
  4. **Immunosuppression side effects:** tremor (*calcineurin inhibitor*), cushingoid/bruising (*steroids*), skin lesions/excisions (*immunosuppression*)

INDICATIONS

- End stage chronic kidney disease (GFR <15ml/minute)
- Commonest causes: diabetes mellitus, polycystic kidney disease, hypertension, autoimmune glomerulonephritis

CONTRAINDICATIONS

- Cardiac/pulmonary insufficiency
- Hepatic disease
- Cancer
- Active infection

PROCEDURE

- **Pre-operative donor and recipient screening:** HLA, cross-match, infection screen (HIV, hepatitis B/C, CMV/EBV, human T-lymphotropic virus, Varicella zoster virus, syphilis, Toxoplasma)
- **Additional donor screening:** renal ultrasound, blood tests (U&Es, FBC, LFTs, fasting glucose, coagulation screen), urine tests (dipstick, MC&S, protein-creatinine ratio)
- Remove donor kidney (loin scar)
- Anastomose in recipient's iliac fossa (Rutherford-Morrison scar)
  - Renal vein to **external** iliac vein
  - Renal artery to **external** iliac artery

POST-OPERATIVE IMMUNOSUPPRESSION (FOR LIFE)

- **Triple immunosuppression** is usually required:
  - Prednisolone
  - Calcineurin inhibitor (e.g. ciclosporin, tacrolimus)
  - Antimetabolite (e.g. azathioprine, mycophenolate mofetil)

COMPLICATIONS

- **Rejection**
  - Hyper-acute rejection (immediate): thrombosis and occlusion of graft vessels during surgery
  - Acute rejection (weeks to months): deterioration in renal function ± flu-like symptoms and graft tenderness
  - Chronic rejection (months to years): gradual deterioration in renal function
- **Immunosuppression complications**
  - Opportunistic infections and sepsis
  - EBV-mediated post-transplant lymphoproliferative disorder
- **Other**
  - UTIs
  - Renal graft thrombosis

PROGNOSIS

- Graft usually lasts 12-15 years
- Affected by: 'cold time' (time out of donor/recipient body); type of donor (live/cadaveric); donor age

STOMAS

STOMA EXAM

- **Patient:** well/unwell, signs of malnutrition/hydration
- **Abdomen:** signs of acute abdomen/obstruction, scar from operation
- **Stoma**
  - Site
  - Surrounding skin
  - Opening
    - Spout (*ileostomy*) or flush with skin (*colostomy*)
    - Loop (2 openings) or end (1 opening)
  - Contents: liquid faeces (*ileostomy*), solid faeces (*colostomy*) or urine (*urostomy*)
  - Patient cough: look for signs of parastomal herniation
- **Palpate around stoma:** also get patient to cough while feeling over stoma (*parastomal herniation*)

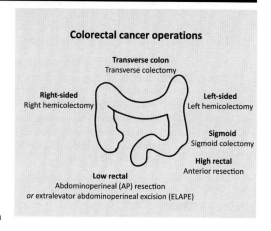

Colorectal cancer operations

TYPES OF STOMA

Summary of stoma types			
	Colostomy	**Ileostomy**	**Urostomy**
Site	Left iliac fossa	Right iliac fossa	Right iliac fossa
Content	Solid faeces	Liquid faeces	Urine
Opening	Flush with skin	Spouted (to protect skin from enzymes)	Spouted

Colostomy

- **End colostomy** (sigmoid/descending colon): proximal bowel opening brought to surface and distal bowel removed or stapled off/oversewn. Uses include:
  - Abdominoperineal (AP) resection for low rectal tumours (all distal bowel removed so permanent colostomy required)
  - Hartmann's procedure for emergency resection of rectosigmoid lesions where primary anastomosis is unfavourable due to obstruction/inflammation/contamination (proximal bowel made into end colostomy and distal bowel stapled off/oversewn – may be reversed after inflammation settled)
- **Loop colostomy** (transverse/descending colon): two openings made in a <u>loop of intact bowel</u> that is brought to the surface through one incision to form a stoma. The proximal opening drains faeces and the distal opening can drain mucus. It may be initially supported by a plastic rod. It is most commonly performed to divert the faecal stream away from distal bowel because of:
  - Impending or actually obstructed large bowel
  - Colonic lesions where the patient may not survive extensive surgery but still maintains a certain quality of life (such as contained tumour perforations or fistulae)
  - A distal bowel resection with primary anastomosis (to protect the anastomosis while sutures heal; reversed after around 6 weeks) – *however, loop ileostomies are now more commonly used for this indication*
- **Double barrel colostomy** (transverse/descending colon): a segment of bowel removed and both ends brought to the surface <u>separately</u> to form a stoma. The proximal end drains faeces and the distal end (called a 'mucous fistula') can drain mucus from the non-functioning bowel. Used *infrequently* after a segment of colon removed and primary anastomosis is unfavourable.

Ileostomy

- **End ileostomy** (terminal ileum): previously, a permanent ileostomy was required when the whole colon and anus were removed in a *panproctocolectomy* (e.g. for ulcerative colitis, familial adenomatous polyposis, Hirschsprung's disease). However, newer sphincter-saving procedures allow ileoanal anastomosis so this is now less commonly performed. End ileostomies may still be created with subtotal colectomies (e.g. for toxic megacolon, ischaemic bowel or synchronous tumours) and may be reversible.
- **Loop ileostomy** (distal ileum): as *loop colostomy*. Commonly used to protect ileoanal or low colorectal anastomoses, or to prevent stool passing through anorectum (e.g. in perianal Crohn's disease, anorectal trauma or malignancy).

Urostomy

- **Ileal conduit**: short segment of ileum removed to act as bladder. One end sutured to skin, other end sutured to ureters. Replaces bladder after cystectomy (for bladder carcinoma).

COMPLICATIONS OF STOMAS

- **Early**: high output stoma >1L/day (→ dehydration, hypokalaemia), retraction, bowel obstruction/ileus, ischaemia of stoma
- **Late**: parastomal hernia, prolapse, fistulae, stenosis, psychological complications, skin dermatitis, malnutrition

Stoma care

- **Stoma nurse** is a good source of support
- Most bags have an **emptying tap**. These are emptied when ²/₃ full, irrigated with water daily, and changed every 2-4 days.
- Some bags are single use and are changed when full
- Bags can be left on in the **shower**
- **Initial diet:** take lots of fluids, small amounts of fibre for first 2 months
- **Foods that may cause blockage:** nuts, sweetcorn, mushrooms, orange pith, celery, dried fruits, fruit skins
- **Foods that may cause diarrhoea:** fruit juice, fruits, vegetables, salad, bran cereals, caffeine, alcohol
- **Foods that may cause odour/flatulence:** brassica vegetables, beans, fizzy drinks

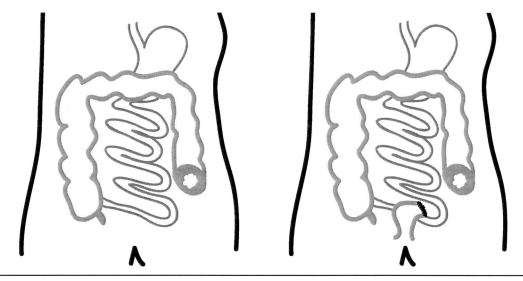

End colostomy after abdominoperineal resection (left) and Hartmann's procedure (right)

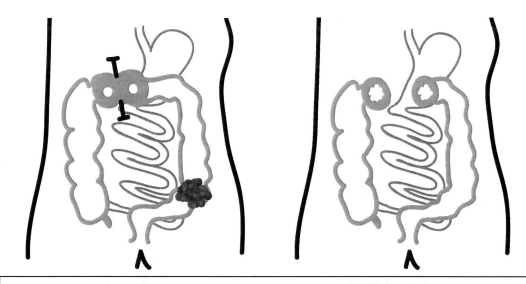

Loop colostomy   Double barrel colostomy

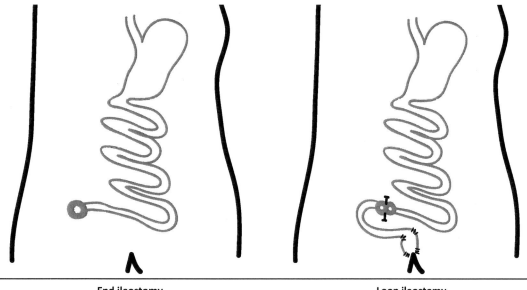

End ileostomy   Loop ileostomy

CAUSES OF HEPATOSPLENOMEGALY

HEPATOMEGALY

- **Malignancy**
    - o Primary or secondary
- **Hepatic congestion**
    - o Right heart failure
    - o Hepatic vein thrombosis (Budd-Chiari syndrome)
- **Haematological**
    - o Lymphoma/leukaemia/myeloproliferative
- **Infection**
    - o Infectious mononucleosis
    - o Viral hepatitis
- **Anatomical**
    - o Riedel's lobe
- **Other**
    - o Non-alcoholic fatty liver disease
    - o Alcoholic liver disease
    - o Sarcoidosis
    - o Amyloidosis
    - o Infective endocarditis

NB: the liver is often not palpable in cirrhosis because it shrinks. Splenomegaly due to portal hypertension is a more common finding.

SPLENOMEGALY

- **Infiltration**
    - o Leukaemia
    - o Lymphoma
    - o Myeloproliferative disorders
- **Increased function**
    - o ↑Extravascular haemolysis (haemoglobinopathy, thalassaemia, spherocytosis)
    - o ↑Extramedullary haematopoiesis (myelofibrosis, malignant bone marrow infiltration)
    - o ↑Response to infection (HIV/AIDS, glandular fever, infective endocarditis, malaria, autoimmune disorders)
- **Vascular congestion**
    - o Cirrhosis (causing portal hypertension)
    - o Splenic vein obstruction
    - o Budd-Chiari syndrome

*NB: Massive splenomegaly is usually due to: chronic **M**yeloid leukaemia, **M**yelofibrosis, **M**alaria (or less commonly splenic lymphoma or visceral leishmaniasis).*

HEPATOSPLENOMEGALY

- **Chronic liver disease with portal hypertension**
    - o Any cause of chronic liver disease
- **Haematological**
    - o Leukaemia
    - o Lymphoma
    - o Myeloproliferative disorders
- **Infections**
    - o Acute viral hepatitis
    - o CMV/EBV
    - o Malaria
    - o Visceral leishmaniasis
- **Infiltration**
    - o Amyloidosis
    - o Sarcoidosis

CHRONIC LIVER DISEASE

The signs of chronic liver disease are described on p55.

MOST COMMON CAUSES IN THE UK

1. Alcohol
2. Non-alcoholic fatty liver disease
3. Viral hepatitides
4. Autoimmune (e.g. autoimmune hepatitis, primary biliary cholangitis)
5. Metabolic (e.g. haemochromatosis)

INVESTIGATING CAUSE

- Hepatitis B surface antigen, hepatitis C IgG
- Autoimmune liver screen: anti-smooth muscle (*autoimmune hepatitis type 1*), anti-mitochondrial (*primary biliary cholangitis*), anti-liver-kidney microsomal (*autoimmune hepatitis type 2, hepatitis C/D, drug-induced hepatitis*), anti-nuclear (*autoimmune hepatitis type 1, SLE*)
- α-fetoprotein (*hepatocellular carcinoma*)
- Metabolic/infiltrative: ferritin and transferrin saturation (*haemochromatosis*), serum copper and caeruloplasmin ± 24-hour urinary copper (*Wilson's disease*), fasting glucose and lipids (*fatty liver disease*), α_1-antitrypsin (*α_1-antitrypsin deficiency*)
- Immunoglobulins and protein electrophoresis (*IgM raised in primary biliary cholangitis, IgA raised in alcoholic liver disease, IgG raised in autoimmune hepatitis*)
- Tissue transglutaminase antibody (*Coeliac disease*)
- Abdominal ultrasound/CT
- Liver biopsy if cause unclear

LONG-TERM MANAGEMENT

- **Treat cause**
- **General:** optimise nutrition, alcohol abstinence
- **Monitoring**
  - Bloods, including FBC, LFTs, albumin, coagulation screen, and α- fetoprotein *every 6 months* (for liver function and hepatocellular carcinoma)
  - USS *every 6 months* (for hepatocellular carcinoma, hepatic vein thrombus, reversed portal flow)
  - Upper GI endoscopy *every 3 years* (for varices)
- **Treat/prevent complications**
  - Varices: banding, propranolol, transjugular intrahepatic portosystemic shunt (for refractory ascites/varices/hepatic pleural effusion)
  - Ascites: spironolactone, low salt diet, fluid restriction
  - Encephalopathy: lactulose, rifaximin
  - Coagulopathy: vitamin K

NB: elastography may be used to non-invasively grade liver cirrhosis.

ACUTE COMPLICATIONS

<u>Investigations</u>
- Bloods: FBC, U&Es, LFTs, CRP, coagulation screen, glucose, blood cultures (if any signs of infection)
- Chest X-ray
- Urine dip and MSU
- Abdominal USS
- Ascitic tap (if ascites present)

<u>Types</u>
1. **Decompensation**
   - Signs: jaundice, ascites, encephalopathy
   - Causes: spontaneous bacterial peritonitis/sepsis, dehydration/AKI, upper GI bleed/constipation, others (portal vein thrombosis, drugs, liver ischaemia, hepatocellular carcinoma)
   - Management: treat cause, lactulose/enemas, avoid sedatives, nurse in intensive care if required
2. **Hepatorenal failure**
   - Worsening renal function in advanced chronic liver disease with no other cause (and no response to fluids)
   - Management: fluid balance monitoring and daily weights, suspend diuretics and nephrotoxic drugs, human albumin solution (to increase effective intravascular blood volume), arterial vasoconstrictors (e.g. terlipressin)
3. **Spontaneous bacterial peritonitis**
   - Sepsis/signs of infection in patient with ascites
   - Management: diagnostic ascitic tap, IV antibiotics, human albumin solution (to prevent renal dysfunction)

NB: if there is a history of alcohol excess, prescribe Pabrinex and chlordiazepoxide for withdrawal.

INGUINAL HERNIAS

An inguinal hernia is the protrusion of abdominal contents through the inguinal canal.

ANATOMY

- **Inguinal ligament** = ASIS to pubic tubercle
- **Inguinal canal** = deep inguinal ring to superficial inguinal ring
    - Inguinal ring positions
        - Deep inguinal ring (start of inguinal canal) = midpoint of the inguinal ligament
        - Superficial inguinal ring (end of inguinal canal) = superior to the pubic tubercle
    - Borders of the inguinal canal **MALT**
        - **M**uscle (internal oblique)   - *ROOF*
        - **A**poneurosis (external oblique)   - *ANTERIOR*
        - **L**igament (inguinal ligament)   - *FLOOR*
        - **T**endon (transversalis fascia)   - *POSTERIOR*
    - Contents
        - Males: spermatic cord and ilioinguinal nerve
          Spermatic cord contains:
            - 3 arteries: testicular artery, artery to vas deferens, cremasteric artery
            - 3 nerves: genitofemoral nerve, autonomic nerves, ilioinguinal nerve (outside cord)
            - 3 other structures: vas deferens, pampiniform plexus of veins, lymphatic vessels
        - Females: round ligament of the uterus and ilioinguinal nerve
- **Points to remember**
    - Midpoint of the inguinal ligament (midpoint between the ASIS and pubic tubercle) = deep inguinal ring position
    - Mid-inguinal point (midpoint between the ASIS and pubic symphysis) = femoral artery position

DIRECT VS. INDIRECT INGUINAL HERNIA

- **Direct** inguinal hernia (40%)
    - Herniated abdominal contents come **directly** out of abdomen in a straight line
    - Penetrate through the superficial inguinal ring
    - If reduced, cannot be controlled by applying pressure over the deep inguinal ring
- **In**direct inguinal hernia (60%)
    - Herniated abdominal contents run **in** the inguinal canal
    - Penetrate through the deep inguinal ring
    - Can go right the way down the canal into the scrotum in men (inguinal-scrotal hernia)
    - May occur due to failure of the closure of the processus vaginalis
    - If reduced, can be controlled by applying pressure over the deep inguinal ring

INGUINAL HERNIA VS. FEMORAL HERNIA

- **Femoral hernia** is inferior and lateral to the pubic tubercle (through femoral canal) – *more common in females*
- **Direct inguinal hernia** is superior to the pubic tubercle (position of superficial inguinal ring) – *more common in males*
- **Indirect inguinal hernia** can occur anywhere between the deep inguinal ring and the scrotum

HERNIA TERMINOLOGY

Reducible	Can be pushed back into the abdomen by applying pressure
Irreducible	Cannot be pushed back into the abdomen by applying pressure
Obstructed	Lumen if herniated part of bowel is compressed so contents cannot pass, causing obstructive symptoms
Strangulated	Vasculature to herniated bowel is compressed, causing ischaemia

MANAGEMENT

- Watch and wait: for small, asymptomatic hernias
- Open repair: for irreducible, obstructed or strangulated hernias
- Open/laparoscopic mesh repair: for large or symptomatic hernias

Differential diagnosis for a groin lump

- Psoas abscess (lateral to femoral artery)
- Femoral neurofibroma (hard swelling lateral to femoral artery; painful if pressed)
- Inguinal lymph nodes (medial to femoral vein)
- Saphena varix (dilation of the saphenous vein at junction with the femoral vein)
- Femoral aneurysm (pulsatile)
- Ectopic testes (rare congenital anomaly)
- Hydrocele of spermatic cord (loculated fluid collection along the spermatic cord)
- Inguinal canal lipoma (extraperitoneal fat in inguinal canal)

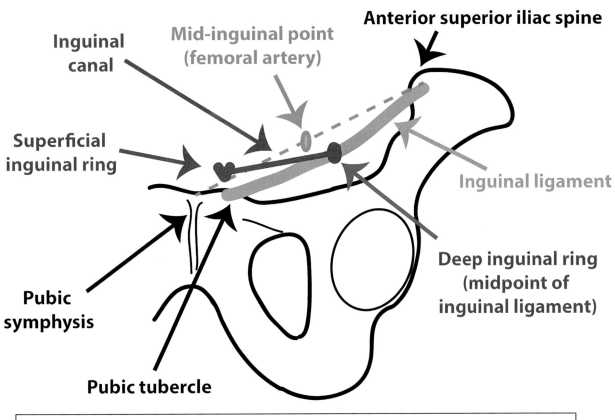

Anatomy of the inguinal canal and inguinal ligament

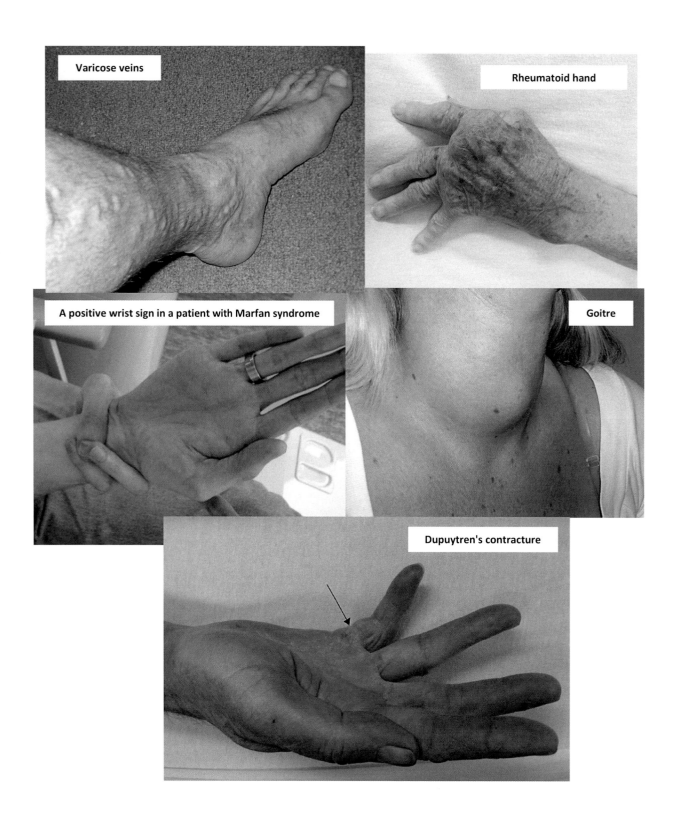

Varicose veins

Rheumatoid hand

A positive wrist sign in a patient with Marfan syndrome

Goitre

Dupuytren's contracture

GOITRES

A goitre is the term used for an enlarged thyroid gland.

MOST COMMON CAUSES IN THE UK

1. Graves' disease
2. Multinodular goitre (*NB: a multinodular is an ultrasound diagnosis because they usually feel smooth or only slightly irregular*)
3. Physiological goitre (pregnancy/puberty)

CLASSIFICATION OF POSSIBLE CAUSES

- **Diffuse**
  - Simple = euthyroid gland enlargement without inflammation or cancer (e.g. physiological, iodine deficiency)
  - Autoimmune (e.g. Graves' disease, Hashimoto's thyroiditis)
  - Infective (e.g. acute viral/De Quervain's thyroiditis) – *painful*
  - Iatrogenic (e.g. lithium, amiodarone)
- **Nodular**
  - Multinodular goitre (euthyroid)
  - Toxic multinodular goitre (hyperthyroid)
  - Solitary nodule (e.g. cancer, adenoma, cysts)

INVESTIGATIONS

- Thyroid function tests
- Thyroid autoantibodies: TSH-receptor antibodies, thyroid peroxidase antibodies, thyroglobulin antibodies
- Imaging
  - Ultrasound
  - Radioiodine uptake scan
  - CT (if retrosternal)
- Ultrasound-guided fine needle aspiration

MANAGEMENT

- **Conservative:** if patient is euthyroid, reassure
- **Medical:** make patient euthyroid
  - Hyperthyroid: β-blocker (symptomatic), carbimazole (thyroid peroxidase inhibitor), radioiodine-131 therapy
  - Hypothyroid: thyroxine
- **Surgical** thyroidectomy/resection if:
  - Malignant
  - Compression of surrounding structures
  - Cosmetic
  - Alternative option for treating hyperthyroidism

COMPLICATIONS

- Hyper/hypothyroidism
- Compression of surrounding structures
  - Trachea compression → breathlessness
  - Recurrent laryngeal nerve damage → dysphonia
  - Oesophageal compression → dysphagia
  - Superior vena cava obstruction → facial swelling, dizziness, headache, blurred vision, syncope
  - Pre-ganglionic Horner's syndrome → ptosis, meiosis, anhidrosis
- Cosmetic issues

CUSHING'S SYNDROME

Cushing's syndrome is a clinical syndrome characterised by the symptoms and signs that occur due to chronic glucocorticoid excess.

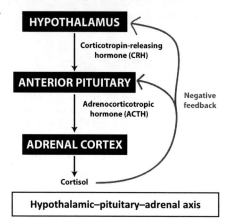

HYPOTHALAMUS
Corticotropin-releasing hormone (CRH)

ANTERIOR PITUITARY
Adrenocorticotropic hormone (ACTH)

Negative feedback

ADRENAL CORTEX
Cortisol

Hypothalamic–pituitary–adrenal axis

TERMINOLOGY

- **Cushing's syndrome** = symptoms/signs resulting from chronic glucocorticoid excess
- **Cushing's disease** = ACTH-producing pituitary tumour causing Cushing's syndrome
- **Nelson's syndrome** = symptoms resulting from rapid enlargement of a pre-existing pituitary tumour after bilateral adrenalectomy

CAUSES

- **ACTH-dependent**
    - Cushing's disease (i.e. ACTH-secreting pituitary tumour)
    - Ectopic ACTH secretion (small cell lung cancer most common cause)
- **ACTH-independent**
    - Iatrogenic (steroid treatment) – most common
    - Adrenal adenoma/carcinoma
    - Adrenal hyperplasia

CLINICAL FEATURES

- **Fat redistribution:** weight increase, central obesity, cushingoid facial features (facial mooning), interscapular and supraclavicular fat pads
- **Skin:** bruising, skin thinning, purple abdominal striae
- Hyperpigmentation (ACTH-dependent causes)
- Mood changes
- Proximal myopathy

INVESTIGATIONS

Confirming Cushing's syndrome
- First-line tests – use one of:
    - Overnight dexamethasone suppression test (*normally cortisol is suppressed by exogenous steroids, but not in Cushing's syndrome*)
    - 24-hour urinary cortisol
- Second-line tests (if needed)
    - 48-hour dexamethasone suppression test
    - Midnight cortisol

Localising causative lesion
1. Plasma ACTH
2. **If ACTH is low:** CT adrenals (*look for adrenal tumour/hyperplasia*)
   If ACTH is high: high-dose dexamethasone suppression test (*ACTH from a pituitary tumour is still suppressible at high exogenous steroid doses, whereas ectopic ACTH is not*)
       ↘ if cortisol is not suppressed, CT thorax (*look for ectopic ACTH source*)
       ↘ if cortisol is suppressed, MRI pituitary – if tumour not seen, it may be too small to visualise and bilateral petrosal sinus sampling may be required to make diagnosis

MANAGEMENT

- Metyrapone/ketoconazole to control symptoms if needed
- Treat cause
    - Resect tumour (e.g. transsphenoidal adenomectomy in Cushing's disease)
    - Bilateral adrenalectomy (if source cannot be localised/recurrent post-surgery/bilateral adrenal hyperplasia)
    NB: Nelson's syndrome is a complication if Cushing's disease was the cause.

COMPLICATIONS

- Impaired glucose tolerance and diabetes mellitus
- Hypertension
- Osteoporosis

ACROMEGALY

Acromegaly is a disorder caused by excess growth hormone. Over 99% of cases are due to a growth hormone-secreting pituitary macroadenoma.

CLINICAL FEATURES
- **Pituitary enlargement symptoms**
  - Hypopituitarism
  - Bitemporal hemianopia
  - Headache
- **Excessive soft tissue growth**
  - Increased hand and feet size
  - Coarsening of facial features
  - Prognathism, macrognathia, wide spaces between teeth, macroglossia
  - Hoarse voice
  - Osteoarthritis and arthralgia
  - Carpal tunnel syndrome
- **Active acromegaly signs**
  - Excessive sweating
  - Hypertension

INVESTIGATIONS
- Confirm acromegaly
  - Insulin-like growth factor 1 – *initial screening test*
  - Failure to suppress growth hormone during glucose tolerance test – *diagnostic test*
- Pituitary function tests and serum prolactin: to rule out coexistent hypopituitarism
- MRI pituitary: to visualise tumour

MANAGEMENT
- Transsphenoidal resection
- Second line options: somatostatin analogues (e.g. octreotide), growth hormone receptor antagonist (e.g. pegvisomant), radiotherapy

COMPLICATIONS
- Impaired glucose tolerance (40%) and diabetes mellitus
- Cardiomyopathy
- Colon cancer (colonoscopy surveillance)

DUPUYTREN'S CONTRACTURE

Progressive palmar fascia thickening that results in tethering, fixed finger flexion and skin puckering.

ASSOCIATIONS
- Family history
- Liver disease/alcohol
- Anti-epileptics
- Diabetes mellitus
- As a feature of other collagen tissue disorders: Peyronie's disease (curvature of the penis), Ledderhose disease (callus under foot ± toe curling), Garrod's disease (dorsal knuckle pads)

CLINICAL FEATURES
- Fixed flexion of fingers (especially little and ring fingers)
- Thickened palmar fascia
- Positive table top test (functional test)

MANAGEMENT

- *Non-surgical*
    - o Conservative management if not limiting function
    - o Splinting and physiotherapy
    - o Corticosteroid injections
    - o Collagenase injections (collagenase enzymes break down collagen)
- *Minimally invasive*
    - o Needle aponeurotomy (parts of contracted cord weakened by needle manipulation)
    - o Percutaneous fasciotomy (parts of contracted cord weakened by multiple incisions)
    - o Segmental aponeurotomy (segments of contracted cord removed by small incisions)
- *Surgical (open)*
    - o Partial fasciectomy (diseased fascia removed)
    - o Dermofasciectomy (skin also removed and replaced with skin graft) – lowest recurrence rate ↘

COMPLICATIONS

- Recurrence **(50%)**
- Bleeding
- Scarring
- Infection
- Neurovascular complications

CARPAL TUNNEL SYNDROME

Carpal tunnel syndrome is a median nerve entrapment neuropathy caused by compression of the median nerve in the carpal tunnel.

CAUSES

- Idiopathic
- Pregnancy
- Obesity
- Rheumatoid arthritis
- Local extrinsic pressure, e.g. ganglion, lipoma, fracture, haematoma
- Endocrinological
    - o Diabetes
    - o Hypothyroidism
    - o Acromegaly

CLINICAL FEATURES

- Intermittent paraesthesia, pain/burning and numbness of thumb, first, middle and radial half of ring finger
- Loss of strength and wasting of the thenar eminence
- Symptoms often worse at night
- Phalen's test +ve
- Tinel's test +ve

DIFFERENTIAL DIAGNOSIS

- Thoracic outlet syndrome
- Pronator teres syndrome (compression of median nerve at elbow)

MANAGEMENT

- **Conservative**
    - o Watch and wait (spontaneous resolution occurs in 25% over 1 year)
    - o Wrist splint (especially at night)
    - o Corticosteroid injection
    - o NSAIDs may help
- **Surgical carpal tunnel release:** transverse carpal ligament over volar aspect of wrist incised under local anaesthesia) – *recurrence rare*

OSTEOARTHRITIS

Osteoarthritis is the mechanical degradation of a joint with degeneration of the articular cartilage, periarticular bone remodelling and inflammation.

RISK FACTORS

- **Primary osteoarthritis** risk factors
  - Increasing age
  - Obesity
  - Family history
  - Female gender
  - Sports activities
- **Secondary osteoarthritis** causes
  - Pre-existing joint damage: trauma, RA, gout, spondyloarthropathy, septic arthritis, Paget's disease, avascular necrosis
  - Metabolic disease: chondrocalcinosis, haemochromatosis, acromegaly
  - Systemic disease: haemophilia (haemarthrosis), neuropathy, haemoglobinopathy

CLINICAL FEATURES

Symptoms
- **Joint pain:** worse on exercise and relieved by rest, morning pain <30 minutes
- **Commonly affected joints:** knees, hips, interphalangeal joints of fingers, carpometacarpal joint of thumb

Signs
- **Joint examination**
  - Crepitus
  - Pain on movement
  - Reduced range of movement
  - May be bony swellings (osteophytes), joint instability, joint effusions
- **Characteristic hand deformities:** Heberden's nodes, Bouchard's nodes, squaring of carpometacarpal joint of thumb

INVESTIGATIONS

- **X-Rays**
- **Bloods:** FBC, CRP/ESR
  - Only useful for **ruling out** inflammatory and infectious causes (inflammatory markers **not** raised in osteoarthritis)

MANAGEMENT

- **Conservative:** exercise, physiotherapy, weight loss, mobility aids, supportive footwear
- **Analgesia**
  1. Topical analgesia (e.g. capsaicin, NSAIDs)
  2. Add paracetamol
  3. Add NSAID
  4. Add opioid
- **Intra-articular corticosteroid injections**
- **Joint replacement** aims to reduce pain and improve mobility

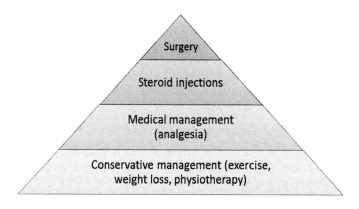

GOUT

Gout is a monoarthropathy caused by deposition of monosodium urate crystals in hyperuricaemia.

HYPERURICAEMIA RISK FACTORS

- Male gender
- Chronic kidney disease
- Diuretics
- Purine rich diet: alcohol, meat, seafood
- Obesity

CLINICAL FEATURES

- Tender, inflamed joint
    - Usually a monoarthritis
    - Commonly affects first metatarsophalangeal joint
    - Other joints include ankles, knees, wrists, finger joints
    - Arthralgia worse at night
- Acute episodes last around 2 weeks
- Other features of hyperuricaemia
    - Gouty tophi
    - Renal nephrolithiasis

INVESTIGATIONS

- Bloods: uric acid level (hyperuricaemia seen in gout, but uric acid level may be falsely low or normal during attack)
- Needle aspiration of synovial fluid – _gold standard_
    - Send for polarising microscopy
        - Gout = negatively-birefringent needle shaped crystals (Negative Needles)
        - Pseudogout = positively-birefringent rhomboid shaped crystals
    - Send for microbiology: to rule out septic arthritis
- X-Ray

MANAGEMENT

- **Treat cause**
    - Lifestyle: keep hydrated, avoid purine rich food/drink, avoid fasting, lose weight
    - Medication review: thiazides and loop diuretics can trigger gout
- **Acute management:** NSAIDs, colchicine or corticosteroids
- **Prevention:** allopurinol (_NB: starting allopurinol can trigger an acute episode of gout so wait 2 weeks for symptoms to subside and offer NSAID/colchicine cover for first 1-3 months_); febuxostat may be used if there is a contraindication to allopurinol

RHEUMATOID ARTHRITIS

Rheumatoid arthritis is a chronic autoimmune disorder resulting in a symmetrical deforming polyarthropathy and various extra-articular features.

RISK FACTORS

- Female gender
- Age 30-50
- Genetics: HLA-DR4 and HLA-DR1
- Smoking

CLINICAL FEATURES

- **Polyarthritis**
  - Morning stiffness
  - Tender, erythematous inflamed joints
  - Usually symmetrical
  - Any synovial joint can be affected
    - Mostly small joints (hands, feet, cervical spine)
    - MCP joints most commonly affected; DIP joints rarely affected
    - Cervical spine – odontoid peg erosion can result in fracture and atlanto-axial subluxation
- **Joint deformities**
  - Loss of knuckle guttering
  - Swan neck deformity (PIP joint hyperextension + DIP joint flexion)
  - Boutonnière deformity (PIP joint flexion + DIP joint hyperextension)
  - Z-shaped thumb (IP joint hyperextension + MCP joint flexion)
  - Ulnar deviation
  - Palmar subluxation of MCP joints
- **Others**, e.g. palmar erythema, small muscle wasting, reduced range of movement, carpal tunnel syndrome signs
- **Extra-articular features:**

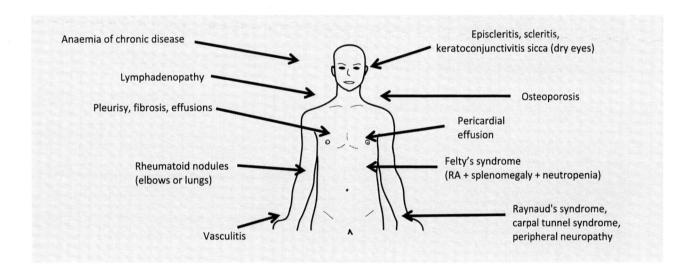

INVESTIGATIONS

- **Bloods**
  - Raised inflammatory markers (ESR, CRP)
  - Rheumatoid factor (autoantibody to Fc portion of IgG)
  - Anti-cyclic citrullinated peptide (CCP) – *more specific*
- **X-Rays**

*The **DAS28 score** is used to assess severity and guide treatment (includes assessment of the number of swollen joints, the number of tender joints, the ESR and a patient self-assessment)*

MANAGEMENT

- **NSAIDs:** for symptomatic relief
- **Steroids:** short course prednisolone at diagnosis to induce remission
- **Disease Modifying Anti-Rheumatic Drug (DMARD) therapy** (e.g. methotrexate, sulfasalazine, hydroxychloroquine): dual agents commenced early to prevent long-term progression
- **TNF-α blockers** (e.g. etanercept, infliximab): can halt or even reverse disease process; offered to patients with severe disease who have not responded to combination DMARDs
- **Other therapies**
  - Surgery: can improve mobility and reduce pain in patients with deformities
  - Physiotherapy
  - Occupational therapy

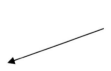

Prednisolone- Induces remission	2 DMARDs – Maintain remission	NSAIDs – Symptomatic relief

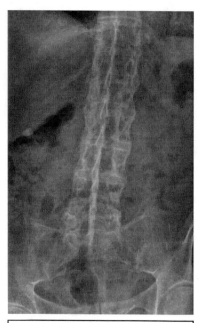

'Bamboo spine': vertebral body fusion by marginal syndesmophytes

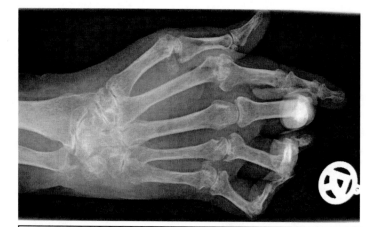

Classic features of rheumatoid arthritis on X-Ray:

- Loss of joint space
- Soft tissue swelling
- Periarticular osteopenia
- Marginal erosions

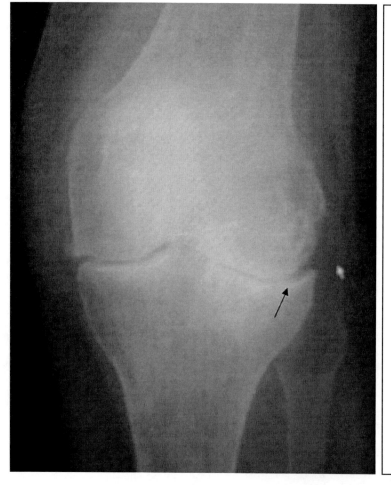

Classic features of osteoarthritis on X-Ray (LOSS):

- **L**oss of joint space
- **O**steophytes
- **S**ubchondral sclerosis
- **S**ubchondral bone cysts

ANKYLOSING SPONDYLITIS

Ankylosing spondylitis is a chronic seronegative spondyloarthropathy which primarily involves the axial skeleton.

RISK FACTORS

- HLA-B27 (positive in 90-95%)
- Age: peak onset 15-25 years
- Male gender
- Family history

CLINICAL FEATURES

Symptoms
- **Low back pain**
    - Progressive
    - Relieved by exercise
    - Night pain
    - Radiates to sacroiliac joints and hips
- **Morning stiffness**
- **Systemic features:** fever, weight loss, fatigue

Signs
- Question mark posture (loss of lumbar lordosis and thoracic kyphosis)
- Sacroiliac joint tenderness (*sacroiliitis*)
- Schober's test: mark midline 10cm above the dimples of Venus and 5cm below while standing, then re-measure distance in flexion (*<5cm difference implies lumbar flexion limitation that may be due to ankylosing spondylitis*)
- <5cm chest circumference expansion on inspiration

Extra-articular features
- **Extra-articular features:**

A	**A**nterior uveitis
A	**A**ortitis
A	**A**ortic regurgitation
A	**A**V node block
A	**A**pical pulmonary fibrosis
A	**A**myloidosis → glomerulonephritis
A	**A**chilles tendon (and other tendon) enthesitis

INVESTIGATIONS

- Clinical diagnosis
- **X-Rays:** pelvis and spine ('bamboo spine' is a characteristic sign caused by vertebral body fusion by marginal syndesmophytes)
- **MRI:** more sensitive than X-Ray
- **Bloods:** FBC (anaemia), ESR (raised), CRP (raised), HLA B27 (+ve)

MANAGEMENT

- **Exercise and physiotherapy:** essential
- **NSAIDs** (e.g. ibuprofen, naproxen, diclofenac): may need to try two or more
- **TNF-α inhibitors** (e.g. etanercept) may be used when two or more NSAIDs have failed
- **Interleukin-17A inhibitors** (e.g. secukinumab): may be used in place of TNF-α inhibitors
- **Other therapies:** corticosteroid joint injections, short courses of corticosteroids, intravenous bisphosphonates

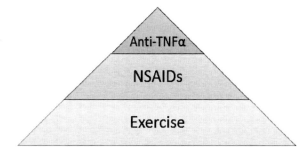

SYSTEMIC SCLEROSIS (SCLERODERMA)

Systemic sclerosis is a systemic autoimmune condition resulting in excessive collagen deposition by fibroblasts.

TYPES

- **Limited cutaneous systemic sclerosis:** cutaneous sclerosis limited to below elbows
- **Diffuse cutaneous systemic sclerosis:** cutaneous sclerosis extends above elbows – *more likely to get organ involvement*

CLINICAL FEATURES

Symptoms
- **Skin**
  - Thick, tight, itchy skin
  - Usually affects the face, hands and feet but can progress to affect the whole body
- **CREST** features

C	Calcinosis
R	Raynaud's (*hands change colour in cold: White→Blue→Red –* White Before Red)
E	Esophageal dysfunction (*heartburn*)
S	Sclerodactyly (*thickening and tightness of skin of fingers/toes*)
T	Telangiectasia

Signs
- **Hands**
  - Look: sclerodactyly, tight waxy skin, ulceration, blanching, finger-pulp atrophy
  - Feel: subcutaneous calcinosis, cool hands
  - Move: prayer sign lost (*fixed flexion deformity of fingers*)
- **Face**
  - Mask-like face
  - Skin tethering
  - Telangiectasia
  - Microstomia
  - Beaked nose

Fibrotic organ involvement

Lungs	Fibrosis, pulmonary hypertension
Heart	Myocardial fibrosis → arrhythmias
Kidneys	Acute or chronic kidney injury, hypertension, acute renal hypertensive crises
Gut	Reflux, dysphagia, faecal incontinence

INVESTIGATIONS

- Auto-antibodies
  - Anti-nuclear (commonly positive but non-specific)
  - Limited: anti-**C**entromere (**C**REST)
  - Diffuse: anti-topoisomerase (anti-Scl-70)
- Assess extent of organ involvement (e.g. CXR/high-resolution CT, echocardiogram, ECG, U&Es, urinalysis, barium swallow)
- Hand X-rays (calcinosis)

MANAGEMENT

- No cure
- **Symptomatic treatment**
  - Raynaud's: hand warmers, Ca^{2+} antagonists, IV prostacyclins, phosphodiesterase-5 inhibitors
  - GI: proton pump inhibitor
- **Prevention of complications**
  - Lung fibrosis: immunosuppressants (e.g. cyclophosphamide, mycophenolate)
  - Pulmonary hypertension: prostaglandins, endothelin antagonists, phosphodiesterase-5 inhibitors, supplemental oxygen
  - Renal crises: low dose ACE inhibitor

PAGET'S DISEASE

Paget's disease is caused by increased bone remodelling by osteoclasts and osteoblasts. This results in in bone enlargement, pain, deformity and weakness. The cause is unknown.

EPIDEMIOLOGY

- 1-2% of white >55 year olds
- High incidence in UK; low incidence in Asia

INVESTIGATIONS

- **Imaging:** plain X-rays (bone enlargement and 'cotton wool' lytic/sclerotic pattern), bone scan (scintigraphy/technetium scan)
- **Blood tests:** ALP (increased), calcium/phosphate/vitamin D (all normal)
- **Other tests:** urine/serum hydroxyproline, urine pyridinoline, serum procollagen I N-terminal peptide (PINP)

CLINICAL FEATURES

Symptoms
- Bony pain
- Pathological fractures

Signs
- **General inspection**
  - Kyphosis
  - Paraplegia (spinal disease)
  - Bone pain
- **Hands inspection**
  - Osteoarthritis
- **Face**
  - Frontal bossing of skull
  - Nerve deafness and tinnitus (due to bony compression of CN8)
  - Enlarged maxilla
- **Neck**
  - Raised JVP (heart failure due to hyperdynamic circulation)
- **Legs**
  - Bowed femur
  - Sabre (bowed) tibia
  - Feel warm
  - Pathological fractures
  - Osteoarthritis

MANAGEMENT

- Analgesia (e.g. NSAIDs)
- Bisphosphonates (e.g. alendronic acid)
- Ensure adequate vitamin D and calcium intake
- Physiotherapy

COMPLICATIONS

- Secondary osteosarcoma
- Nerve compression

MARFAN SYNDROME

Marfan syndrome is a genetic disorder of connective tissue primarily affecting the skeletal system, eyes and cardiovascular system.

CAUSE
- Autosomal dominant FBN-1 gene mutation which transcribes Fibrillin-1, a major constituent of elastin in connective tissues.

CLINICAL FEATURES
- **General**
  - Tall and thin
  - Scoliosis
- **Upper limbs**
  - Arachnodactyly (ask them to wrap their fingers around their wrist)
  - Wide arm span
  - Hyperextensible joints
- **Face**
  - Long thin face
  - Myopia/lens dislocation
  - High-arched palate
- **Chest and abdomen**
  - Pectus carinatum/excavatum
  - Stretch marks
  - Auscultate heart for murmurs (especially aortic regurgitation)
- **Lower limbs**
  - Long legs
  - Flat feet

DIAGNOSIS
- Genetic tests – *diagnostic*

MANAGEMENT
- No cure
- Symptomatic treatment
- Prevention of and surveillance for complications
  - Multidisciplinary team regular check ups
  - Annual echocardiogram (to assess aortic root and heart valves)
  - 5-yearly MR/CT aorta (to asses whole aorta)
  - β-blockers (to prevent aortic dilatation)
  - Composite valve conduit/aortic root graft replacement (for aortic dilatation)
  - Regular eye examinations
- Screening of family members

COMPLICATIONS
- Eyes: lens dislocation (50%), myopia
- Weak thoracic aorta: aneurysms, dissection
- Valves: aortic regurgitation, mitral prolapse/regurgitation

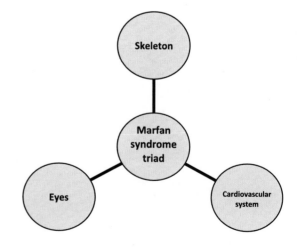

STROKE

TYPES OF STROKE

- **Ischaemic stroke** (risk factors: age, AF, diabetes, hypertension, obesity, hypercholesterolaemia, smoking, obesity, family history)
  - Total anterior circulation stoke (TACS)   3/3 ⎤
  - Partial anterior circulation stroke (PACS) 2/3 ⎬ of -**H**igher function (speech/apraxia/neglect)
  - Lacunar stroke (LACS)   1/3 ⎦   -**H**emianopia
  - Posterior circulation stroke (POCS) – vertebrobasilar arterial system occlusions -**H**emi-loss (motor/sensory)
    - Occipital → isolated contralateral homonymous visual field defect
    - Cerebellar → ipsilateral cerebellar signs
    - Brainstem → ipsilateral cranial nerve palsies, bilateral sensory/motor deficit, disorder of eye movements
- **Intracerebral haemorrhage** (risk factors: age, anticoagulation, alcohol, hypertension, stress, smoking)

POSSIBLE CLINICAL FEATURES BY VASCULAR TERRITORY

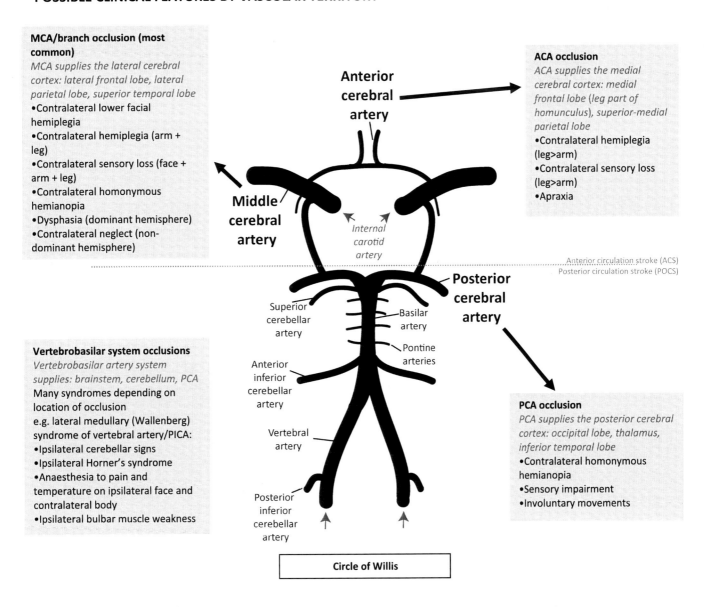

MCA/branch occlusion (most common)
MCA supplies the lateral cerebral cortex: lateral frontal lobe, lateral parietal lobe, superior temporal lobe
- Contralateral lower facial hemiplegia
- Contralateral hemiplegia (arm + leg)
- Contralateral sensory loss (face + arm + leg)
- Contralateral homonymous hemianopia
- Dysphasia (dominant hemisphere)
- Contralateral neglect (non-dominant hemisphere)

ACA occlusion
ACA supplies the medial cerebral cortex: medial frontal lobe (leg part of homunculus), superior-medial parietal lobe
- Contralateral hemiplegia (leg>arm)
- Contralateral sensory loss (leg>arm)
- Apraxia

Anterior circulation stroke (ACS)
Posterior circulation stroke (POCS)

Vertebrobasilar system occlusions
Vertebrobasilar artery system supplies: brainstem, cerebellum, PCA
Many syndromes depending on location of occlusion
e.g. lateral medullary (Wallenberg) syndrome of vertebral artery/PICA:
- Ipsilateral cerebellar signs
- Ipsilateral Horner's syndrome
- Anaesthesia to pain and temperature on ipsilateral face and contralateral body
- Ipsilateral bulbar muscle weakness

PCA occlusion
PCA supplies the posterior cerebral cortex: occipital lobe, thalamus, inferior temporal lobe
- Contralateral homonymous hemianopia
- Sensory impairment
- Involuntary movements

Anterior cerebral artery

Middle cerebral artery

Internal carotid artery

Posterior cerebral artery

Superior cerebellar artery

Basilar artery

Pontine arteries

Anterior inferior cerebellar artery

Vertebral artery

Posterior inferior cerebellar artery

Circle of Willis

NB: carotid artery dissection is a cause of anterior circulation stroke and vertebral artery dissection is a cause of posterior circulation stroke. Think about dissection if there is neck pain, the patient is young or there is associated trauma.

INVESTIGATIONS AND MANAGEMENT

- *See acute management notes on stroke p195*

PARKINSON'S DISEASE

Parkinson's disease is caused by degeneration of the dopaminergic neurons in the substantia nigra (part of the basal ganglia). This results in rigidity, tremor, bradykinesia and postural instability.

CLINICAL FEATURES – TETRAD

Rigidity	Lead pipe rigidity, cogwheel rigidity, festinant gait
Tremor	4-6Hz, resting, pill-rolling
Bradykinesia	Slow shuffling gait, flexed trunk, slow monotonous speech, expressionless face, reduced blink rate, micrographia
Postural instability	Falls

DIFFERENTIAL DIAGNOSIS OF PARKINSONISM

- **Parkinson's disease**
- **Vascular parkinsonism**
- **Parkinson-plus syndromes**
    - Multi-system atrophy (cerebellar signs, autonomic problems)
    - Progressive supranuclear palsy (vertical gaze palsy, axial rigidity)
    - Corticobulbar degeneration (apraxia, dementia, aphasia)
    - Lewy body dementia (dementia with some parkinsonian features)
- **Other causes**
    - Iatrogenic, e.g. secondary to anti-dopaminergic drugs
    - Wilson's disease
    - Communicating hydrocephalus
    - Supratentorial tumours

INVESTIGATION

Parkinson's disease is a clinical diagnosis – however, investigations may be required if the diagnosis is unclear:
- Structural MRI: may be used to exclude some other causes of parkinsonism
- Single-photon emission CT: may be used to differentiate Parkinson's disease from other causes of tremor
- Serum caeruloplasmin or 24-hour urinary copper excretion: to exclude Wilson's disease

MANAGEMENT

Pharmacological
Low potency:
- **Monoamine oxidase B inhibitors** (e.g. rasagiline, selegiline)
    - For mild symptoms (no functional disability)

Moderate potency:
- **Dopamine agonists** (e.g. ropinirole, pramipexole)
    - For moderate symptoms (most at diagnosis)
    - Take several weeks to work
    - Notable side effects: sleep attacks, impulse control disorders

High potency:
- **Levodopa** (e.g. Madopar, Sinemet)
    - For severe symptoms/elderly
    - Given with peripheral decarboxylase inhibitor (e.g. carbidopa) to prevent peripheral conversion to dopamine
    - Notable side effects: 'on-off'/'wearing off' phenomenon (increased immobility before the next dose is due after prolonged levodopa use); dyskinesias

Adjuncts to levodopa:
- Dopamine agonists   -   reduce motor complications and levodopa dosage needs
- Monoamine oxidase B inhibitors   -   reduce 'off time'
- COMT inhibitors (e.g. entacapone)   -   reduce 'off time'
- Apomorphine (subcutaneous)   -   for rescue therapy during 'off time'
- Amantadine (glutamate antagonist)   -   for levodopa-induced dyskinesias

Non-pharmacological
- Multidisciplinary approach: input from neurologist, physiotherapist, occupational therapist, specialist nurse, GP, speech and language therapist
- Supervised exercise
- Home modifications
- Consider associated conditions: dementia, depression, psychosis, sleep disturbance

MULTIPLE SCLEROSIS

Multiple sclerosis is a chronic inflammatory disorder characterised by plaques of demyelination in central nervous system that cause neurological symptoms and disability.

TYPES OF MS

- **Relapsing-remitting (85%):**   intermittent relapses with subsequent total or partial recovery
- **Primary progressive (15%):**   sustained, progressive disability from the start
- **Secondary progressive:**   65% of people with relapsing-remitting MS will develop secondary progressive MS with sustained, progressive disability

CLINICAL FEATURES

Any part of central nervous system can be affected but common deficits include:

- **Optic nerve:**   reduced visual acuity, central scotoma
- **Medial longitudinal fasciculus:**   internuclear ophthalmoplegia (disorder of lateral conjugate gaze)
- **Cerebellum:**   **DANISH**: **D**ysdiadochokinesia, **A**taxia, **N**ystagmus, **I**ntention tremor, **S**peech abnormality (slurring/scanning/staccato), **H**ypotonia
- **Spinal cord:**   spastic paraparesis, lower limb sensory loss, urinary symptoms

INVESTIGATIONS

Diagnosis requires demonstration of demyelinating lesions 'disseminated in time and space'

- MRI brain/spinal cord: shows demyelination
- Evoked potentials: may reveal delayed visual/auditory/sensory potentials due to demyelination
- Cerebrospinal fluid analysis: oligoclonal bands

MANAGEMENT

Management requires a multi-disciplinary approach (including neurologist, specialist nurse, physiotherapist, occupational therapist, GP, speech and language therapist)

Acute relapses

- Methylprednisolone (IV or oral)

Preventing relapses (disease-modifying agents)

Suitable for some patients with relapsing-remitting or secondary progressive MS:

- **Highly effective:**   alemtuzumab, natalizumab
- **Good:**   dimethyl fumarate, fingolimod
- **Moderate:**   glatiramer, β-interferon, teriflunomide

Symptomatic management

- **Neuropathic pain:**   tricyclic antidepressants, gabapentin
- **Incontinence:**   intermittent self-catheterisation for overflow, anticholinergics for urge
- **Spasticity:**   physiotherapy, baclofen, gabapentin
- **Oscillopsia:**   gabapentin
- **Fatigue:**   exercise, diet, amantadine

NEUROFIBROMATOSIS

Neurofibromatosis is an autosomal dominant condition resulting in the growth of nerve tumours.

SUGGESTED APPROACH TO NEUROFIBROMATOSIS TYPE 1 OSCE STATION

Describing lesions
- **Neurofibromas**
  - 'There are multiple, well-demarcated brown circular nodules and papules present across the back in a generalized distribution.'
  - 'There are no secondary features (such as crusting, scaling or erosion).'
  - 'On palpation, these lesions are soft and non-tender, with some exhibiting the button-hole sign.'
  - 'These lesions are consistent with neurofibromas.'
- *Café au lait* spots
  - 'There are also irregularly shaped, evenly pigmented, flat brown patches.'
  - 'These are characteristic of *café au lait* spots.'
- **Other areas**
  - 'I would like to look for axillary and inguinal freckling, and abdominal scars (e.g. for phaeochromocytoma surgery).'
- **Conclusion**
  - 'Given there are 2 or more neurofibromas and 6 or more *café au lait* spots, the likely diagnosis is neurofibromatosis type 1.'
  - 'In addition to examining the rest of the skin and taking a full history, I would like to measure blood pressure, do a full neurological exam for signs of spinal cord neurofibromas, examine the eyes for signs of optic nerve gliomas, and use a slit lamp to look for Lisch nodules on the iris.'

If you are allowed to ask the patient questions
- Family history
- Eyes, ears, blood pressure
- Any nerve lesions

Differential diagnosis
- Neurofibromatosis type 2
- Tuberous sclerosis (multi-system hamartoma formation)

TYPES OF NEUROFIBROMATOSIS

Type 1 (peripheral) – *most common*
- NF-1 gene defect (chromosome 17) resulting in **peripheral neurofibromas** (i.e. in skin or subcutaneous tissue)
- Skin
  - Neurofibromas (2 or more): well-demarcated nodules which are erythematous and varied in size and shape
  - *Café au lait* spots (6 or more): flat patch of asymmetrical darkened skin (brown/black)
  - Axillary freckling
- Other features
  - Optic nerve glioma → non-correctable visual loss
  - Lisch nodules (iris hamartomas, i.e. brown spots on iris seen with slit lamp)
  - Dorsal root spinal cord tumours
  - Plexiform neurofibromas (diffuse and invasive → bony erosion)

Type 2 (central)
- Merlin protein gene defect (chromosome 22) resulting in **central schwannomas**
- Most common presenting condition is bilateral acoustic neuromas (CN8) causing hearing loss, typically at 20-30 years of age
- Other conditions include: meningiomas, gliomas, juvenile cataracts
- Other symptoms include: headache, balance loss, vertigo, facial weakness, deafness, tinnitus
- Skin symptoms uncommon

INVESTIGATIONS

- Diagnosed on clinical features and MRI

MANAGEMENT

- Lifelong annual monitoring: vision, heart and blood pressure, hearing
- Treat complications
- Education

> **Complications of neurofibromatosis type 1**
>
> - Malignant nerve sheath tumours
> - Hypertension
> - Phaeochromocytoma
> - Renal artery stenosis
> - GI neurofibromas → bloating, pain, dyspepsia, haemorrhage, constipation

PSORIASIS

Psoriasis is a chronic, inflammatory skin disease characterised by keratinocyte hyperproliferation. The most common type is plaque psoriasis, which causes erythematous raised plaques on extensor surfaces.

SUGGESTED APPROACH TO PSORIASIS OSCE STATION

Examine
- **Dermatological skin exam**
  - Skin
  - Scalp
  - Ears
- **Nails**
- **Hand joints**

Describing lesions
- **Plaques**
  - 'There are multiple well-demarcated, raised erythematous plaques over the extensor surfaces.'
  - 'These range in size from 1-6cm.'
  - 'There is scaling across the surface of these lesions, but no other secondary features.'
  - 'These lesions are consistent with chronic plaque type psoriasis.'
- **Nails**
  - 'There is also evidence of pitting, subungual hyperkeratosis, onycholysis and Beau lines on the finger nails.'
  - 'These are characteristic psoriatic nail changes.'
- **Joints**
  - 'I can also see a symmetrical polyarthropathy of the distal inter-phalangeal joints with active synovitis.'
  - 'This could be evidence of psoriatic arthritis.'

Differential diagnosis
- Other types of psoriasis
- Eczema

TYPES OF PSORIASIS

Chronic plaque	Most common and described here
Guttate	Raindrop lesions
Seborrhoeic	Lesions around nose and ears
Flexural	Flexural surfaces affected
Pustular	Pustular lesions on palms/soles
Erythrodermic	>90% of skin affected

ASSOCIATIONS

- Multiple HLA subtypes
- Post-streptococcal guttate psoriasis
- Medications (β-blockers, antimalarials, lithium)
- Alcohol
- Stress
- Trauma (Koebner phenomenon)
- HIV

MANAGEMENT

- Avoid precipitants
- Emollients
- Topical treatments
  - Vitamin D analogues, e.g. calcipotriol
  - Topical corticosteroids
  - Coal tar
  - Dithranol
  - Topical retinoids
- Phototherapy
- Systemic rheumatological drugs (methotrexate, ciclosporin, infliximab)

Combination (e.g. Dovobet ointment or Enstilar foam) often used first line

Complications of psoriasis

- Nail changes: pitting, subungual hyperkeratosis, onycholysis, Beau lines
- Psoriatic arthropathy
- Erythroderma

ATOPIC ECZEMA

Atopic eczema is the most common type of eczema (dermatitis) that results in a pruritic erythematous rash and usually affects flexor surfaces.

SUGGESTED APPROACH TO ATOPIC ECZEMA OSCE STATION

Examine
- **Dermatological skin exam**

Describing lesions
- **Lesions**
  - 'There are multiple papules and vesicles with an erythematous base distributed over the flexor surfaces.'
  - 'These range in size from 1-6mm.'
  - 'There is some evidence of lichenification and scaling but no evidence of secondary infection or eczema herpeticum.'
  - 'These lesions are consistent with atopic eczema.'

Differential diagnosis
- Other types of eczema

If allowed to ask patient questions
- Personal/family history of asthma, hay fever, eczema

TYPES OF ECZEMA

- **Exogenous:** irritant contact, allergic contact, photocontact/photosensitive, photo-allergic
- **Endogenous**

Atopic	Most common and described here
Seborrhoeic	Greasy/scaly erythematous rash around nose, ears and scalp
Asteatotic	Cracked skin, often on lower limbs
Discoid	Coin-like lesions
Pityriasis alba	Pink scaly patches that later leave hypopigmentated areas of skin
Pompholyx	Itchy blisters on hands and feet
Varicose	Associated with chronic venous insufficiency; affects lower limbs

ASSOCIATIONS

- Atopic individuals/families (i.e. asthma, hay fever, eczema)
- Exacerbations may be associated with:
  - Allergens (e.g. chemicals, food, dust, pet fur)
  - Infection
  - Heat/sweating
  - Stress

MANAGEMENT

- **Topical treatments**
  1. Emollients and bath/shower substitutes
  2. Corticosteroids (e.g. hydrocortisone, mometasone)
  3. Calcineurin inhibitors (e.g. pimecrolimus, tacrolimus)
- **Others**
  - Identify and avoid allergens
  - Antihistamines for persistent pruritus/sleep disturbance
  - Phototherapy if other treatments fail
  - Antibiotics if secondary infection

Fingertip units

Fingertip unit = amount of cream/ointment expressed to reach from the **index finger's distal skin crease to the tip**

1 fingertip unit will treat an area **twice the size of an adult's flat hand** (with fingers together)

COMPLICATIONS

- Secondary infection
- Eczema herpeticum

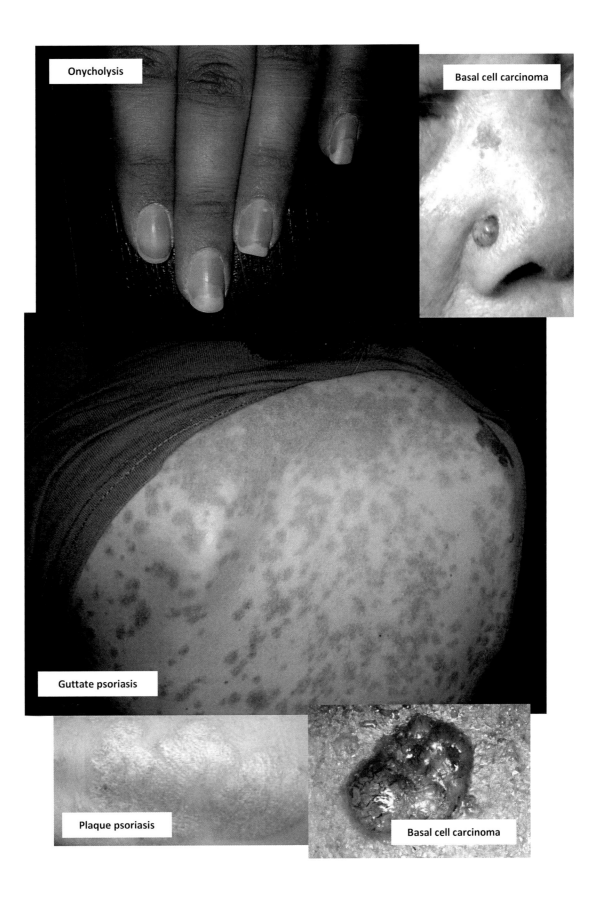

Onycholysis

Basal cell carcinoma

Guttate psoriasis

Plaque psoriasis

Basal cell carcinoma

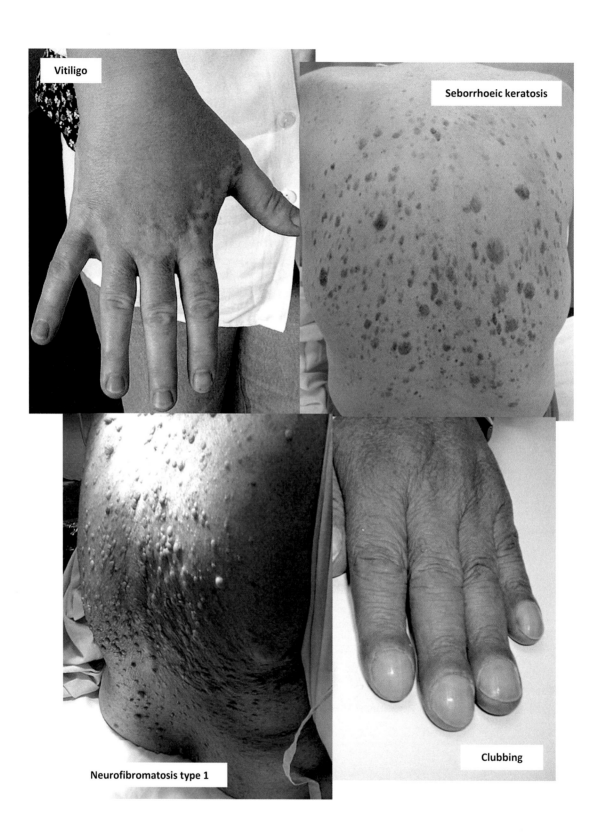

Vitiligo

Seborrhoeic keratosis

Neurofibromatosis type 1

Clubbing

BASAL CELL CARCINOMA

Basal cell carcinoma is the most common skin malignancy. It is a slow-growing tumour that is invasive but rarely metastasises. It usually occurs on sun-exposed skin, especially of the head and neck.

SUGGESTED APPROACH TO BASAL CELL CARCINOMA OSCE STATION

Describing lesions
- **Lesion**
  - 'There is a skin-coloured papule/nodule present on the left cheek. It has a pearly rolled edge and there is surface telangiectasia.'
  - 'It is approximately 13mm in diameter.'
  - 'There is no ulceration, necrosis or secondary features (such as crusting, scaling or erosion).'
  - 'On palpation, it is firm and not hot or tender.'
  - 'This lesion is characteristic of a basal cell carcinoma.'

Differential diagnosis
- Squamous cell carcinoma
- Seborrhoeic keratosis
- Malignant melanoma

MANAGEMENT

- **First line**
  - Conventional surgery
  - Mohs surgery (cancerous skin removed in layers and examined microscopically until only non-cancerous skin remains)
- **Other treatment options**
  - Curettage and electrodessication
  - Cryotherapy
  - Topical therapies (e.g. imiquimod, fluorouracil)
  - Radiotherapy

Complications of basal cell carcinoma

- Local tissue invasion
- Ulceration
- Metastasis (very rare)

SEBORRHOEIC KERATOSIS (SEBORRHOEIC WART)

Seborrhoeic keratosis is a benign skin growth originating from keratinocytes.

SUGGESTED APPROACH TO SEBORRHOEIC KERATOSIS OSCE STATION

Describing lesions
- **Lesion**
  - 'There is a well-demarcated dark brown papule on the upper left part of the patient's back.'
  - 'This is 4mm in diameter and has a regular border, with a *stuck-on* appearance.'
  - 'The lesion is raised, with a rough surface, but there are no secondary features.'
  - 'This lesion is characteristic of a seborrhoeic keratosis.'

Differential diagnosis
- Melanoma
- Melanocytic naevus
- Dermatofibroma
- Pigmented basal cell carcinoma
- Acanthosis nigricans

MANAGEMENT

- Reassurance
- Remove surgically *if diagnostic uncertainty*
- Remove using cryotherapy or curettage and cautery *if cosmetic concerns*
- Topical corticosteroids *for itchy/irritated lesions*

Complications of seborrheic warts

- Irritation or chafing from clothes
- Cosmetic dislike

VITILIGO

Vitiligo is a chronic patchy depigmenting skin condition due to T-cell-mediated melanocyte destruction.

SUGGESTED APPROACH TO VITILIGO OSCE STATION

Describing lesions

- **Areas of depigmentation**
  - o 'There are multiple well-demarcated patches of depigmentation in a generalised distribution.'
  - o 'They range in size from 1-4cm and have irregular borders.'
  - o 'These lesions are flat and there are no secondary features.'
  - o 'These lesions are consistent with vitiligo.'

Differential diagnosis

- Tinea versicolor
- Post-inflammatory hypopigmentation
- Pityriasis alba
- Scarring
- Tuberculoid leprosy

ASSOCIATIONS

- Other autoimmune conditions (e.g. thyroid disease, pernicious anaemia, diabetes, Addison's disease)
- 20% of cases are familial
- Lesions may be triggered by stress, skin trauma or exposure to chemicals

MANAGEMENT

- General: avoid sun and use strong sun cream (sun-exposed areas will not tan but will burn), avoid skin trauma
- Screen for other autoimmune diseases
  - o Thyroid disease
  - o Pernicious anaemia
  - o Diabetes
  - o Addison's disease
- Cosmetic camouflage creams
- Topical corticosteroids (e.g. clobetasol, mometasone)
- Topical calcineurin inhibitors (e.g. tacrolimus)
- Phototherapy

FOOT ULCERS

A foot ulcer is a break in skin continuity on or around the feet that may be of arterial, venous or neuropathic aetiology.

SUGGESTED APPROACH TO FOOT ULCER OSCE STATION

Describing lesions
- **Arterial ulcer**
  - 'There is a well-demarcated ulcer on the tip of the right great toe.'
  - 'It has a diameter of 1cm and a punched-out appearance.'
  - 'The ulcer has a necrotic base.'
  - 'The surrounding skin is cool and pale, and the dorsalis pedis and posterior tibial pulses are very weak.'
  - 'This lesion is characteristic of an arterial ulcer.'
- **Venous ulcer**
  - 'There is a large superficial ulcer on the medial gaiter region of the right leg.'
  - 'This has a diameter of approximately 14cm and has an irregular border.'
  - 'The ulcer has an exudative, granulating base.'
  - 'There is associated venous eczema and lipodermatosclerosis.'
  - 'This lesion is characteristic of a venous ulcer.'
- **Neuropathic ulcer**
  - 'There is a well-demarcated ulcer on the dorsal aspect of the first metatarsophalangeal joint.'
  - 'It has a diameter of 1cm and a punched-out appearance.'
  - 'The ulcer has a granulating base.'
  - 'The surrounding skin is hyperkeratotic and there is reduced sensation peripherally.'
  - 'This lesion is characteristic of a neuropathic ulcer.'

Other aspects of examination
- Surrounding skin (including temperature)
- Peripheral pulses and capillary refill
- Peripheral sensation

If you are required to ask the patient questions
- Associated pain and when this is worse
- Loss of sensation
- History of diabetes, vascular disease, varicose veins, DVT

TYPES

Types of foot ulcers				
Type of ulcer	Commonest sites	History	Exam findings	Management
Arterial	•Areas of poor blood supply (e.g. tips of toes, pre-tibial area)	•Nocturnal pain •Worse with leg elevation	•Small deep ulcer •Well-demarcated •Punched out •Necrotic base •**Associated:** weak pulses, cool pale skin, loss of hair, nail dystrophy	•Vascular reconstruction •Avoid pressure to areas affected
Venous	•Gaiter region	•Mild pain •Worse on standing •Associated varicose veins	•Large superficial ulcer •Irregular border •Exudative, granulating based •Sloping edges •**Associated:** varicosities, oedema, venous eczema, lipodermatosclerosis, haemosiderin deposition, *atrophie blanche*	•Compression bandaging (after arterial insufficiency excluded by ABPI)
Neuropathic	•Pressure points (e.g. metatarsal heads, soles, heels, toes) •Often under calluses	•Painless •Associated reduction in peripheral sensation	•Small deep ulcer •Well-demarcated •Punched out •Granulating base •**Associated:** overlying hyperkeratosis, 'glove and stocking' sensory loss	•Debridement •Appropriate footwear •Regular repositioning •Foot checking advice •Don't walk bare foot

POSSIBLE INVESTIGATIONS TO DETERMINE CAUSE

- Fasting glucose: to exclude diabetes
- Ankle brachial pressure index: <0.9 = peripheral vascular disease
- Duplex ultrasound: to look for peripheral vascular disease or venous incompetence
- X-ray: to exclude osteomyelitis
- Swabs for MC&S: if signs of infection

ABNORMAL FUNDOSCOPIC APPEARANCES

Condition	Symptoms	Fundoscopic appearance	Management
Retina			
Diabetic retinopathy	•Often none unless severe or complications (e.g. vitreous haemorrhage)	Non-proliferative – *graded mild-severe* •Microaneurysms (dots) – *only change in mild* •Haemorrhages (blots) •Venous beading •Intraretinal microvascular anomalies •Hard exudates – lipid deposits (well-demarcated) •Cotton wool spots – infarcts (not well-demarcated) Proliferative • Any neovascularisation	•Panretinal photocoagulation (for severe non-proliferative or proliferative retinopathy) •Focal or grid laser photocoagulation (for maculopathy) •Intravitreal anti-vascular endothelial growth factor injections (for clinically significant macular oedema) •Optimise diabetic control
Retinal laser photocoagulation scars	N/A	Panretinal laser photocoagulation scars •Hundreds of dots of laser burns across wide area of retina (avoiding major vessels and macula) Focal or grid laser photocoagulation scars •Smaller areas of laser burns in dots or grids near macula	N/A
Hypertensive retinopathy	•Most patients have no symptoms	Grade 1 •Arteriolar narrowing Grade 2 • + AV nicking • + Silver wiring Grade 3 • + Retinopathy (flame haemorrhages, hard exudates, cotton wool spots) Grade 4 • + Papilloedema	•Treat hypertension
Retinal artery occlusion	•Sudden painless loss of all (central occlusion) or part (branch occlusion) of vision	•Swollen, pale (oedematous) retina •Cherry red spot (in macula)	•Reduction of intraocular pressure (within 6 hours)
Retinal vein occlusion		•Tortuous dilated vessels •Widespread retinal flame haemorrhages ('stormy sunset') •Optic disc oedema	•No specific treatment •Photocoagulation for neovascularisation
Retinal detachment	•**4 F's:** Floaters, Flashes, Fall in acuity, Field loss •'Curtain falling over vision'	•Grey opalescent retina, ballooning forwards	•Surgical vitrectomy (most) or scleral buckle surgery •+ cryopexy/laser retinopexy to secure break
Retinitis pigmentosa	•Deteriorating night vision •Tunnel vision	•Bone spicule-shaped peripheral pigmentation •Arteriolar narrowing •Waxy disc pallor	•No cure •Genetic counselling •Symptomatic management
Macula			
Dry macular degeneration	•Progressive central visual deterioration	•Drusen in macula area (tiny yellow/white deposits)	•No treatment •Stop smoking •Antioxidant supplements
Wet macular degeneration		•Subretinal haemorrhages in/around macula •Localised retinal elevation and retinal oedema	• Intravitreal anti-vascular endothelial growth factor injections •Photodynamic therapy •Laser photocoagulation
Disc			
Optic neuritis	•Reduced visual acuity •Loss of red colour vision •Central scotoma •Afferent pupillary defect	•Unilateral swollen optic disc (blurred margin)	•Methylprednisolone for MS-associated optic neuritis (most)
Optic atrophy		•Pale, featureless optic disc (like setting sun)	•No specific treatment •Treat cause to preserve remaining function
Papilloedema	•Signs of raised intracranial pressure •Vision usually normal	•Bilateral swollen optic discs (blurred margins)	•Treat cause of raised intracranial pressure
Chronic open angle glaucoma	•Asymptomatic until vision severely impaired	•Optic disc cupping (optic cup > $\frac{1}{3}$ of disc) •Optic disc atrophy	•β-blocker eye drops •Prostaglandin eye drops •α-agonist eye drops •Carbonic anhydrase inhibitor eye drops •Laser trabeculoplasty (2nd line)
Acute closed angle glaucoma	•Eye pain/headache •Halos and visual blurring •Red eye	•Ciliary flush + mid-dilated irregular pupil •Optic disc cupping may be present	•IV/PO acetazolamide •α-agonist/β-blocker drops •Laser peripheral iridectomy
Vitreous			
Vitreous haemorrhage	•Sudden painful visual loss or haze	•No red reflex •Difficult/impossible to visualise retina	•Treat cause, e.g. diabetic retinopathy, retinal detachment/tear

VISUAL FIELD DEFECTS

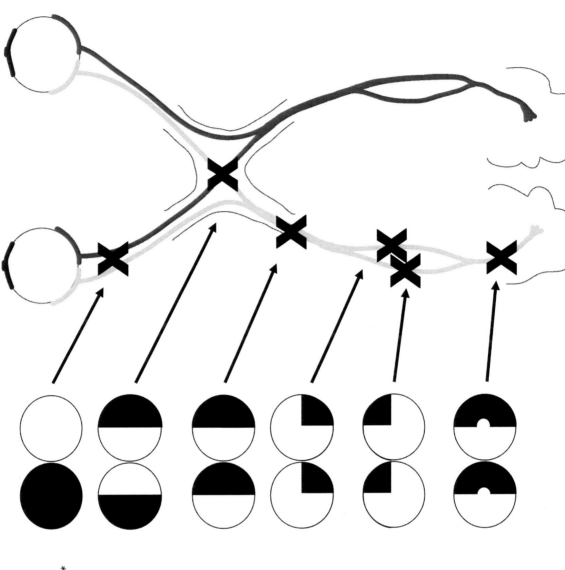

Monocular visual loss

Ipsilateral retinal or optic nerve lesion

Retinal, e.g. central retinal artery/vein occlusion*, retinal detachment*
Optic nerve, e.g. optic neuritis*, optic atrophy, glaucoma*

Bitemporal hemianopia

Optic chiasm lesion

e.g. pituitary tumour, craniopharyngioma

Homonymous hemianopia

Contralateral optic tract (or whole optic radiation) lesion

e.g. middle cerebral artery occlusion (stem)*

Homonymous inferior quadrantanopia

Contralateral parietal (upper) optic radiation lesion

e.g. parietal tumour or middle cerebral
artery occlusion (superior branch)*

Homonymous superior quadrantanopia

Contralateral temporal (lower) optic radiation lesion

e.g. temporal tumour or middle cerebral
artery occlusion (inferior branch)*

Homonymous hemianopia with macular sparring

Contralateral occipital visual cortex lesion

e.g. posterior cerebral artery occlusion*

PITS
Parietal
Inferior
Temporal
Superior

* = acute causes

DIGITAL CLUBBING

Digital clubbing is the term used to describe the bulbous soft-tissue swelling that affects the finger's distal phalanges in certain systemic conditions.

STAGES OF CLUBBING

1 **Fluctuant** nail bed

2 Loss of nail **angle** (Schamroth's window is obliterated)

3 Increased **curvature** of nail

4 **Broadening** of distal phalanx

CAUSES OF CLUBBING

Respiratory	**Cardiovascular**	**Abdominal**	**Others**
Idiopathic pulmonary fibrosis	Cyanotic congenital heart disease	IBD	Pregnancy
Lung cancer	Infective endocarditis	Liver cirrhosis	Acromegaly
Suppurative lung disease (bronchiectasis, cystic fibrosis)			Thyroid acropachy
Sarcoidosis/TB			Familial clubbing

SCHAMROTH'S WINDOW

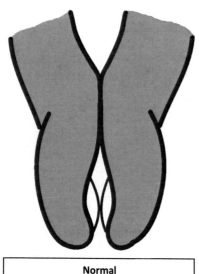

Normal

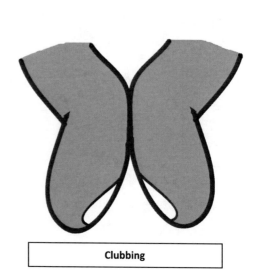

Clubbing

MECHANISMS OF LABOUR

Labour = expulsion of products of conception after 24 weeks' gestation.

1ST STAGE

1ST STAGE OF LABOUR (CERVIAL DILATION)

- **Timing:** 12-15 hours if primiparous (1cm/2 hours), 7.5 hours if multiparous (1cm/hour). It is usually divided into the latent phase (cervical dilation 0-3cm) and active phase (cervical dilation 3-10cm).
- **Signs:**
  - Regular painful contractions (3-4 in 10 minutes)
  - 'Show' (passage of blood stained mucus)
  - Rupture of membranes
- **Mechanism:** fetal head descends into pelvis
- **Complications: 3 Ps**
  - **Passenger:** cephalopelvic disproportion, fetal malpresentation (e.g. persistent occipito-posterior position)
  - **Passage:** fibroids, cervical stenosis, narrow mid-pelvis
  - **Power:** primary uterine inertia
- **Interventions may include:** C-section (e.g. for cephalopelvic disproportion), oxytocin (for contractions)
- **Other points:** induction of labour may be required and is usually initiated with prostaglandin gel/pessary or artificial rupture of membranes

2ND STAGE

2ND STAGE OF LABOUR (EXPULSION OF FETUS)

- **Timing:** 45-120 minutes if primiparous, 15-45 minutes if multiparous
- **Signs:** first sign is desire to bear down
- **Mechanism:**
  1. Flexed fetus descends: head very flexed on spine. Descends and engages.
  2. Internal rotation: whole fetus internally rotates (until facing towards maternal back, head at level of ischial spines)
  3. Extension of head: head extends around pubic symphysis until delivery
  4. Restitution (external rotation): after head delivered, fetus rotates back to its original position, i.e. shoulders AP, and comes out sideways
  5. Delivery of shoulders: anterior shoulder comes out first, then rest in pelvic axis (i.e. anteriorly)
- **Complications:** *as 1st stage*
- **Intervene when:** maternal/fetal distress, incomplete internal rotation causing failure to progress
- **Interventions may include:** instrumental delivery/C-section (for fetal distress or failure to progress), oxytocin (for contractions), McRoberts manoeuvre (for shoulder dystocia)

3RD STAGE

3RD STAGE OF LABOUR (EXPULSION OF PLACENTA)

- **Timing:** Around 5-10 minutes with syntometrine (30 minutes - 1 hour without) – *IM syntometrine is usually given when the head is born to reduce time and post-partum haemorrhage risk*
- **Signs:**
  - Gush of blood (50-100ml)
  - Lengthening of cord
- **Management:** controlled cord traction
- **Complications:**
  - Post-partum haemorrhage (*>500ml blood loss*)
    - Primary (within 24 hours) = **4 Ts:** **T**one (uterine atony), **T**issue (retained placenta/clots), **T**rauma (to perineum), **T**hrombin (coagulopathy)
    - Secondary (24 hours–6 weeks) = retained placenta/clots
  - Retained placenta
  - Inversion of uterus

OTHER POINTS

- **Pelvic anatomy**
    - Pelvic inlet (brim) formed by: sacral prominence, arcuate and pectineal lines, upper margin of pubic symphysis
    - Pelvic outlet formed by: coccyx tip, sacrotuberous ligament, ischial tuberosities, pubic arch
    - False (greater) pelvis = part of pelvis above pelvic brim
    - True (lesser) pelvis = part of pelvis below pelvic brim
- **Female pelvic features (compared to male)**
    - Wider and shallower
    - Round/oval pelvic inlet (male is heart shaped)
    - Larger pelvic outlet
    - Pubic arch >100° (male is <90°)
    - Wider greater sciatic notch
    - Curved sacrum
- **Common fetal orientations**
    - Lie:
        - Longitudinal (baby vertical)
        - Transverse (baby horizontal)
        - Oblique (baby diagonal)
    - Presentation:
        - Cephalic (head is presenting part)
        - Breech (bottom is presenting part)
    - Position (of occiput relative to pelvic rim):
        - Left/right occiput-anterior (LOA/ROA)
        - Left/right occiput-transverse (LOT/ROT)
        - Left/right occiput-posterior (LOP/ROP)

    NB: left occiput-anterior is most common position.

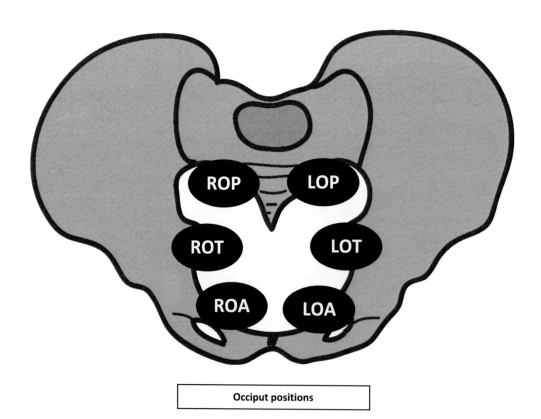

Occiput positions

CHAPTER 4: MANAGEMENT OF ACUTELY UNWELL PATIENTS

Produced using UK Resuscitation Council 'Adult basic life support' 2015

ASSESSMENT

DR's ABCD:

- **Danger:** check around patient and environment for danger
- **Response:** question (e.g. 'Hello, can you hear me?'), shake and command (e.g. 'Open your eyes')
- **Shout:** 'help, help, help' if unresponsive
- **Airway:** open airway with head-tilt/chin-lift or jaw-thrust and look for/remove obstructions
- **Breathing:** assess breathing for up to 10 seconds by listening and feeling with your ear, while watching for chest movements and palpating carotid pulse

  NB: you should do this while maintaining the head-tilt/chin-lift or jaw-thrust (e.g. place your forearm on the patient's forehead, apply positive pressure to tilt the head back, and reach around their face to pull up the angle of the jaw with the index and middle fingers, whilst palpating the carotid pulse with the other hand).
- **CPR and Call ambulance:** if patient is not breathing, start CPR (*described in detail below*) and ask a helper to call 999 and explain there is a cardiac arrest and the location. If there are no helpers, you must call yourself (even if you have to leave the scene to do so). Also ask the helper to get an automated external defibrillator if one is available (but do not leave the scene yourself to get this).
- **Defibrillation:** if an automated external defibrillator arrives, attach the pads to the patient's bare chest (one below right clavicle and one over cardiac apex). If there is more than one rescuer, continue CPR while attaching electrodes. Follow the defibrillation spoken/visual prompts on the machine.

CARDIOPULMONARY RESUSCITATION

Perform **30:2** chest compressions to rescue breaths. If there is another trained helper, take turns; if not, continue until you tire and can no longer physically continue.

- **30 chest compressions:** perform at a rate of **100-120/minute** and a **depth of 5-6cm**. You must fully extend your elbows, wrists and fingers. Have both hands palm downwards with fingers interlocked. Place the carpal area of the hand over the lower sternum and apply all of the pressure over this point.
- **2 rescue breaths:** at the patient's side, place part of your palm and your little finger firmly on the patient's forehead and occlude the nostrils using the index finger and thumb of the same hand. Perform a head-tilt, and lift the chin with the other hand. Now, with a good seal around the patient's lips, breathe a normal expiration for 1 second, watching the patient's chest to check it expands.

  NB: if you have a pocket mask, position yourself at the head of the patient and firmly press the mask around the patient's face with the index finger and thumb of each hand on either side. Place your little fingers either side around the angle of the patient's mandible to pull it up into the mask and then perform the 2 breaths while watching the chest.

SPECIAL CASES

Algorithm differences in children
- Pulse check
  - Infant (<1 year): feel brachial pulse
  - Children (>1 year): feel carotid pulse
- Compression:ventilation ratio
  - At birth: 3:1 ratio
  - Infants/children: start with 5 rescue breaths, then 15:2 ratio
- Compressions
  - Compress to at least one-third the AP chest diameter
  - Infant:
    - Lone rescuer: compress the sternum with the tips of two fingers
    - Two or more rescuers: encircling technique – performed by placing both thumbs flat on the lower sternum pointing towards the infant's head and the fingers around the rib cage
  - Children: as for an adult but only use one hand
- If you are on your own, perform CPR for 1 minute before leaving to get help

Drowning
- Give 5 initial ventilations first, then continue at normal 30:2 ratio
- If you are on your own, perform CPR for 1 minute before leaving to get help
- Dry the patient's chest prior to defibrillation

Pregnancy
- Manually displace the uterus to the left (prevents caval compression during CPR)
- Prepare for emergency C-section if >20 weeks gestation – should be performed within 5 minutes of cardiac arrest

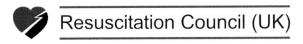

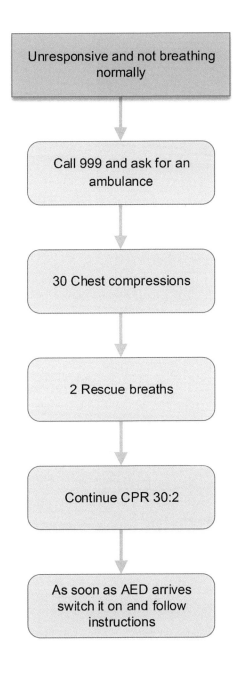

Unresponsive and not breathing normally

Call 999 and ask for an ambulance

30 Chest compressions

2 Rescue breaths

Continue CPR 30:2

As soon as AED arrives switch it on and follow instructions

Resuscitation Council (UK)

GUIDELINES 2015

Adult Advanced Life Support

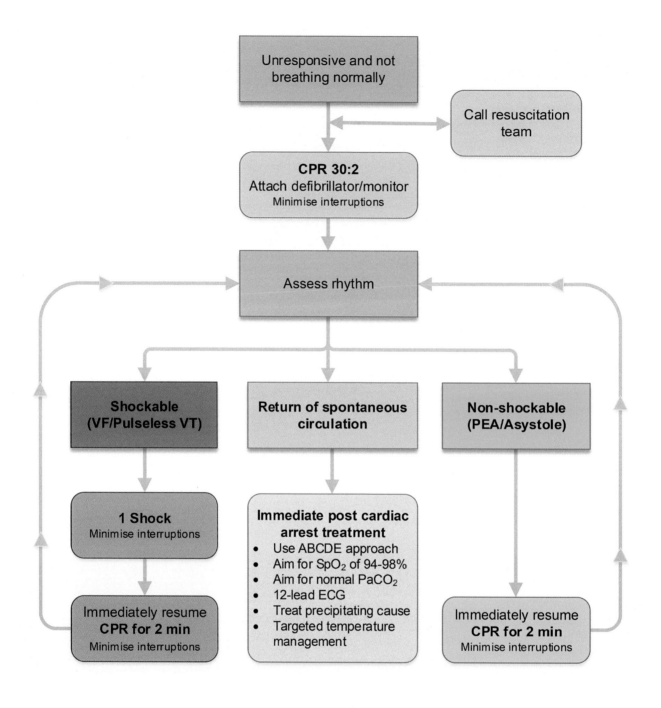

Unresponsive and not breathing normally

Call resuscitation team

CPR 30:2
Attach defibrillator/monitor
Minimise interruptions

Assess rhythm

Shockable (VF/Pulseless VT)

Return of spontaneous circulation

Non-shockable (PEA/Asystole)

1 Shock
Minimise interruptions

Immediate post cardiac arrest treatment
- Use ABCDE approach
- Aim for SpO$_2$ of 94-98%
- Aim for normal PaCO$_2$
- 12-lead ECG
- Treat precipitating cause
- Targeted temperature management

Immediately resume CPR for 2 min
Minimise interruptions

Immediately resume CPR for 2 min
Minimise interruptions

During CPR
- Ensure high quality chest compressions
- Minimise interruptions to compressions
- Give oxygen
- Use waveform capnography
- Continuous compressions when advanced airway in place
- Vascular access (intravenous or intraosseous)
- Give adrenaline every 3-5 min
- Give amiodarone after 3 shocks

Treat Reversible Causes
- Hypoxia
- Hypovolaemia
- Hypo-/hyperkalaemia/metabolic
- Hypothermia

- Thrombosis - coronary or pulmonary
- Tension pneumothorax
- Tamponade – cardiac
- Toxins

Consider
- Ultrasound imaging
- Mechanical chest compressions to facilitate transfer/treatment
- Coronary angiography and percutaneous coronary intervention
- Extracorporeal CPR

ADULT ADVANCED LIFE SUPPORT

Produced using UK Resuscitation Council 'Adult advanced life support' 2015

Start by assessing the patient as below (basic life support until defibrillator trolley arrives):

DR's ABCD:

- **Danger:** check around patient and environment for danger
- **Response:** question (e.g. 'Hello, can you hear me?'), shake and command (e.g. 'Open your eyes')
- **Shout:** 'Can I get some help over here please?' and make the bed flat
- **Airway:** open airway with head-tilt/chin-lift or jaw-thrust and look for obstructions
- **Breathing:** assess breathing for up to 10 seconds by listening and feeling with your ear, while watching for chest movements and palpating carotid pulse
  NB: you should do this while maintaining the head-tilt/chin-lift or jaw-thrust (e.g. place your forearm on the patient's forehead, apply positive pressure to tilt the head back, and reach around their face to pull up the angle of the jaw with the index and middle fingers, whilst palpating the carotid pulse with the other hand).
- **CPR and Call cardiac arrest team:** if patient is not breathing, start CPR (*described in detail below*) and ask a helper to call 2222 and explain there is an adult/paediatric/neonatal/trauma cardiac arrest and the location. Ask the helper to bring the resuscitation trolley back with them.
- **Defibrillation:** *as described below*

Tasks needing to be performed simultaneously are shown below in order of priority:

Roles of the team leader

- Delegate tasks (leader should be hands-off)
  - **Timer and scribe** (keep this person close to you and ask them to clearly tell you when each cycle ends, the cycle number and remind you when drugs are due if competent to)
  - **Compressions** (2-3 people rotating)
  - **Airway and ventilation** (anaesthetist if present)
  - **Defibrillation** (if shockable)
  - **IV access, bloods/gases and drugs** (x 2 people)
- Co-ordinate above tasks
- Go through reversible causes

CHEST COMPRESSIONS

Perform **30:2** chest compressions to ventilations (until airway is secure).

- Perform at a rate of **100-120/minute** (i.e. 2/second) and a depth of **5-6cm**. Fully extend your elbows, wrists and fingers. Have both hands palm downwards with fingers interlocked. Place the carpal area of the hand over the lower sternum and apply all pressure over this point.
- ONLY stop CPR for 5 second rhythm checks, electrical shocks, and the 2 rescue breaths (before the airway is secure). Ask the person doing compressions to tell the airway person each time 30 compressions are complete.
- Chest compressions should be continuous once the airway is secured with either a supraglottic airway or endotracheal tube
- Switch CPR provider during the rhythm check every 2 minutes (or earlier if they tire)

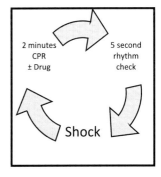

2 minutes CPR ± Drug → 5 second rhythm check → Shock

DEFIBRILLATION

<u>Setup</u>

- Working around the person performing compressions, place the two defibrillation pads in the correct positions on the chest (below right clavicle and over cardiac apex). You may need to shave or dry the chest. Leave jewellery on, but move it out the way. *NB: if a pacemaker is present, ensure pads are >8cm away from it (you can put the pads on AP if needed).*
- Connect pads to defibrillator and set monitoring trace to 'pads'
- Delegate someone to manage timing and say when 2 minute cycles are up and remember the cycle number. Cycle 1 starts when the defibrillator is connected.

<u>Rhythm check</u>

- Perform a rhythm check ± shock every 2 minutes
- When pads are in place and defibrillator is on, immediately ask for CPR to be stopped for a 5 second rhythm check. Determine if the rhythm is **shockable** ('wavy lines' – VF, VT) or **non-shockable** (asystole, PEA).
  - If a rhythm that could be compatible with a pulse is seen (i.e. sinus or VT) during the rhythm check, also feel for a central pulse and stop compressions if present
- Then immediately continue CPR

<u>Shock</u>

- If shockable rhythm, follow these extra steps
  - Select correct energy level for device, **usually 150J biphasic**. If unsure, give the highest energy level shock.
  - Ask for oxygen to be removed and everybody except the person doing compressions to move away. Tell the person doing compressions to continue and that you will alert them to move away before the shock.
  - Charge defibrillator by pressing 'charge' (button 2) and then move hand away from machine
  - Once charged, ask the compressions to now be stopped and shout 'Everybody stand clear!'
  - Check the area is clear (i.e. check no one is in contact with the patient/bed and that the oxygen is away)
  - Deliver shock by pressing 'shock' (button 3)
  - Immediately ask for CPR to be restarted
NB: while operating defibrillator, always look outwards around the bed (not at the machine) and never float your hand near the buttons.

AIRWAY MANAGEMENT

- Airway options (*see procedure notes on airways p235*)
  - Face mask with bag (30 compressions to 2 ventilations): if able to ventilate whilst maintaining seal and jaw-thrust, one person can do this alone. If not, one person should hold the rigid part of the mask while pulling the jaw up into the mask, while another person squeezes the bag.
    Consider also placing an oropharyngeal (Guedel) or nasopharyngeal airway under the mask if struggling.
  - Supraglottic airway (laryngeal mask airway, i-gel): once placed, **ventilate every 6 seconds** with continuous compressions, providing the seal is good and there is no significant air leak
  - Intubation with endotracheal tube(gold standard): once placed, **ventilate every 6 seconds** with continuous compressions
- Attach 15L/minute oxygen
- Attach end-tidal CO_2 monitoring if supraglottic mask or endotracheal tube inserted
- Avoid hyperventilation

DRUGS

- Obtain IV access and have drugs ready
  - If you cannot get IV access after 2 attempts, get intraosseous access via head of humerus or tibial tuberosity
  - Take blood from the cannula (**VBG** + send FBC, U&Es, Mg^{2+}, G&S) and give IV fluids
- **Adrenaline 1mg IV** (10ml of 1:10,000):
  - **Shockable rhythm:** give after 3rd shock (during CPR). Flush with 20ml saline.
  - **Non-shockable rhythm:** give as soon as IV access is established. Flush with 20ml saline.
  NB: this is given to cause peripheral vasoconstriction and so maximise cardiac blood flow.
  <u>Repeat adrenaline dose during every other CPR cycle thereafter</u> (i.e. repeat every 3-5 minutes once given, regardless of any rhythm changes)
- **Amiodarone 300mg IV:** if shockable rhythm only. Give once after 3 shocks have been administered (during CPR).
  NB: amiodarone is given to stabilise the myocardium in VF and VT.
  This is usually a single dose but a further 150mg bolus may be given, followed by an infusion if necessary.

CONSIDER REVERSIBLE CAUSES

The team leader should assess the reversible causes by assessing the patient, speaking to nurses/relatives and reviewing their drug chart and notes. Each of the following reversible causes should be eliminated/treated (**4 H's, 4 T's**):

Reversible causes of cardiac arrest		
Reversible cause	Assessing it	Treating it
<u>H</u>ypoxia	Ventilation adequacy, oxygen flow rate, ABG	15L/minute oxygen and good ventilation
<u>H</u>ypovolaemia	History, drains, haemorrhage, fluid collections (expose patient)	Fluid resuscitation
<u>H</u>ypo/hyperkalaemia	ABG and latest blood results	↑K$^+$: 10ml 10% calcium chloride and 10 units Actrapid insulin in 50ml 50% dextrose ↓ K$^+$: 20mmol KCl over 10 minutes
<u>H</u>ypothermia	Patient's temperature on recent observations, warmth	Warm patient
<u>T</u>hrombosis (coronary or pulmonary) *Commonest cause*	History, risk factors, legs (DVT signs), post-surgery?	Thrombolysis if PE, call cardiology if MI
<u>T</u>ension pneumothorax	Tracheal deviation, hyper-resonance, decreased breath sounds	Insert cannula into second intercostal space, mid-clavicular line
<u>T</u>amponade, cardiac	Recent chest trauma/surgery, focussed ultrasound	Pericardiocentesis
<u>T</u>oxins	History, drug chart, gather info, capillary glucose	Treat toxaemia, e.g. naloxone for opioids

WHAT NEXT?

<u>Return of circulation</u>
- Full ABCDE assessment
- Controlled oxygenation (aim 94-98%)
- Consider therapeutic hypothermia 32-36° for 24 hours (avoid hyperthermia)
- Post-arrest investigations (<u>CXR</u>, <u>12 lead ECG</u>, <u>full set of bloods</u>, echo, ABG, capillary glucose and cardiac monitoring)
- Treat cause
- Consider transfer to intensive care if still requiring ventilation or high-dependency care if not

<u>No return of circulation</u>
- In general, CPR should be continued as long as there is a shockable rhythm
- Only stop if a registrar or above makes the decision with the team

<u>Afterwards</u>
- Retrospectively document everything that happened

SPECIAL CASES

Pregnancy
- Manually displace the uterus to the left (prevents caval compression during CPR)
- Prepare for emergency C-section if >20 weeks gestation – should be performed within 5 minutes of cardiac arrest

Algorithm differences in children
- Pulse check
  - o Infant (<1 year): feel brachial pulse
  - o Children (>1 year): feel carotid pulse
- Compression:ventilation ratio
  - o At birth: 3:1 ratio
  - o Infants/children: start with 5 rescue breaths, then 15:2 ratio
- Compressions
  - o Compress to at least one-third the AP chest diameter
  - o Infant (<1 year):
    - ▪ Lone rescuer: compress the sternum with the tips of two fingers
    - ▪ Two or more rescuers: encircling technique – performed by placing both thumbs flat on the lower sternum pointing towards the infant's head with the fingers around the rib cage
  - o Children (>1 year): as in an adult but can use one or two hands (as needed to achieve depth)
- Defibrillation
  - o Energy:
    - ▪ Manual defibrillator: **4J/kg**
    - ▪ If using automated defibrillator for child <8 years: use paediatric-attenuated adult shock energy
    - ▪ If using automated defibrillator for child >8 years: use adult shock energy
  - o Infants: 4.5cm pads
  - o Children: 8-12cm pads
  - o If paediatric electrodes are unavailable, it is acceptable to use the adult defibrillator and settings – ensure the pads are not touching each other
- Drug doses
  - o Adrenaline 10mcg/kg (0.1ml/kg of 1:10,000 solution)
  - o Amiodarone 5mg/kg – repeat same dose after 5th shock if still in shockable rhythm

Asthma
- Intubate the trachea early
- Treat asthma exacerbation
- Consider tension pneumothorax
- Consider higher shock energies if initial attempts fail as chest may be hyperexpanded

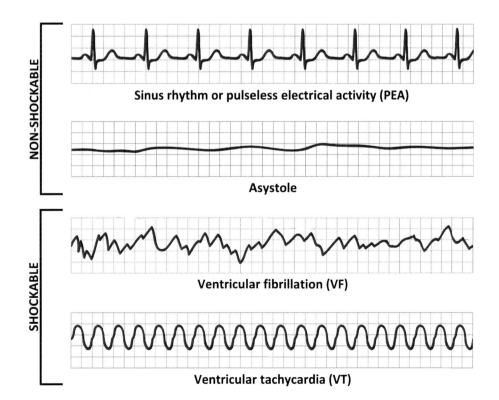

NON-SHOCKABLE

Sinus rhythm or pulseless electrical activity (PEA)

Asystole

SHOCKABLE

Ventricular fibrillation (VF)

Ventricular tachycardia (VT)

This protocol should be used for critically ill patients (i.e. with very unstable observations or reduced GCS).

	Assessment	Management
A AIRWAY	•It's patent if the patient can talk •It's not if there are secretions, the patient has aspirated, or is snoring/GCS<8 •Look inside the mouth – are there any obstructions?	•Consider: suction, airway opening manoeuvres (e.g. jaw-thrust or head-tilt/chin lift), oropharyngeal/nasopharyngeal airways, intubation (if GCS <8) •Cricothyroidotomy may be required in upper airway obstruction where intubation is not possible •*See procedure notes on airways p235* **Treat cause** •Treat any evident causes (e.g. anaphylaxis, foreign body)
B BREATHING	•**Pulse oximetry** •**RR** •**Chest exam**: cyanosis, tracheal deviation, chest inspection (accessory muscles, deformities), expansion, percussion, auscultation •**Calves** *Tests* •**ABG** (*if low saturations or low GCS*) •**CXR** (*if lung pathology suspected*)	•15L/minute O_2 via non-rebreather mask (*see prescribing notes on oxygen p280*) ***WARNING***: *take care if COPD* (*unless they are in respiratory distress/critically unwell and need high-flow oxygen, start at 24-28% i.e. 2-4L venturi and aim for sats 88-92%. Titrate to ABG results.*) •Consider non-invasive or invasive ventilation if hypoxic or hypercapnic despite maximal therapy •If respiratory effort is inadequate, it must be supported (e.g. ventilate with bag-mask) **Treat cause** •Treat any evident causes (e.g. pneumothorax, asthma/COPD exacerbation, opiate overdose, PE)
C CIRCULATION	•**Capillary refill** (central) •**Pulse** rate, rhythm and volume •**Blood pressure** (look at trend) •**Temperature** •**Auscultate** heart, check JVP and look for signs of fluid overload •Assess **fluid balance** and organ perfusion (IN e.g. fluids, intake; OUT e.g. catheter/urine, drains, vomit) *Tests* •*Place **wide-bore IV Cannula** and take bloods (also do VBG for fast results if ABG not required)* •*Apply 3-lead **cardiac monitoring*** •***ECG** (if any concern)* •***Catheter** and fluid balance monitoring (if hypotensive/unwell)*	**Hypotension** •Lay supine and elevate legs •Fluid challenge = 500ml 0.9% saline/Hartmann's solution STAT and monitor response by HR, BP and UO (*see prescribing notes on fluids p281*) ***WARNING***: *take care if significant heart failure history* (*use 250ml challenge*) **Shock** •2 large bore IV cannulas •Fluid challenge = 1L 0.9% saline/Hartmann's solution STAT •Replace blood with blood (can give O negative or typing takes 15 minutes). In massive blood loss, call 2222/lab and activate the *massive blood loss protocol* to get packed red cells + FFP ± platelets **Further management** •Respond fully: give maintenance fluids •Responds but BP falls again: more fluids (adequate resuscitation depends on patient and degree of deficit but is usually 20-30ml/kg given quickly) •No response: patient is either fluid overloaded (don't give any more fluids) or very depleted (give lots of fluids) **Escalation** •If patient is hypotensive <u>and</u> overloaded, they need inotropes •If patient is still hypotensive despite adequate fluid resuscitation (30ml/kg), they need vasopressors **Treat cause** e.g. arrhythmia (*further management in arrhythmia notes*), sepsis, bleeding etc.
D DISABILITY	•**DEFG** – Don't Ever Forget Glucose •**GCS**/AVPU score •**Pupils** reactivity and symmetry •**Pain** assessment *Tests* •*CT brain* (*if intracerebral pathology needs to be excluded*)	•Correct glucose •Give analgesia if pain (e.g. morphine 10mg in 10ml slow IV injection titrated to pain) **Look for and treat cause** •Look for and treat causes of low GCS, e.g. morphine/sedative use, focal neurology to suggest intracranial pathology, hypercapnia, post-ictal
E EVERYTHING ELSE	•**Exposure** (look for bleeds, rashes, injuries, drain/catheter output, lines) •Examine **abdomen** •**Focussed exam** of relevant systems	•Manage any other abnormal findings as appropriate

NB: only move to the next letter when the one before has been treated, and keep re-assessing ABCDE from the start as necessary.

INVESTIGATIONS TO FIND CAUSE

- Review patient's notes
- **BOXES**

Bloods (mark as urgent)	ABG (if low saturations/low GCS), venous bloods (group and save, FBC, U&Es, CRP, LFTs ± amylase, clotting, troponin, VBG etc.), capillary glucose, blood cultures (if pyrexial)
Orifice tests	Urine dip, urine/sputum/faeces culture, urine βHCG
X-rays/imaging	Portable CXR, CT brain (if neurology or low GCS in the absence of other causes)
ECG	± 3-lead cardiac monitoring
Special tests	Depending on likely cause

CONDITION SPECIFIC TREATMENT

- *See acute management notes on specific conditions p185* e.g. MONAC for MI, furosemide for heart failure, anticoagulation/thrombolysis for PE, sepsis six, fluids and insulin for DKA, terlipressin and OGD for bleeding varices

REQUEST HELP AS REQUIRED

- Inform senior
- Refer to other specialty if indicated
  - Medical registrar: medical problems
  - Endoscopist on call: upper GI bleeding
  - Surgical registrar: surgical problems and bleeding
  - Cardiology registrar: MI/arrhythmia
  - Gynaecological registrar: ruptured ectopic
  - Intensive/high-dependency care registrar: if likely to be required

DOCUMENT IN PATIENT'S NOTES

- Document with a brief case summary, ABCDE headings with findings and management
- Review patient and results as necessary

ACUTE PRESENTATION ASSESSMENT

INTRODUCTION

- **W**ash hands; **I**ntroduce self; ask **P**atient's name and DOB; **E**xplain you want to ask them some questions and examine them
- If they are critically ill, use an ABCDE approach
- Give oxygen, fluids, analgesia **as soon as** you realise the patient needs them ('ask a nurse' to do it while you continue assessing)

FOCUSSED HISTORY

- **Presenting complaint**
- **History of presenting complaint**
  - Explore symptoms, e.g. SOCRATES for pain (*see history notes on exploring symptoms p3*)
  - Important parts of relevant systems reviews to include or exclude differential diagnoses (*see history notes on systems review p7*)
- **PMHx** (focus on PMHx relevant to problem)
- **DHx + allergies**
- **FHx:** if relevant to PC (e.g. family cardiovascular history if patient presents with chest pain)
- **SHx:** smoking and alcohol

CHECK OBSERVATIONS

Determine the patient's **observations**:
- HR and BP
- Respiratory rate and O_2 saturations
- Temperature

FOCUSSED EXAMINATION

- Quick **general exam**
  - Surroundings: drips, medications, catheters, monitoring
  - General inspection: well/unwell, breathing pattern, in pain, pale, sweaty/clammy
  - Hands: shut down, tremor, capillary refill
  - Pulse: rate, rhythm, volume (central and peripheral)
  - Eyes: pallor, jaundice
  - Mouth: dry mucus membranes, cyanosis
- Perform the **appropriate focussed system examination** – *examples in table on next page*

INVESTIGATIONS

- **BOXES** – *choose relevant ones to include or exclude differentials*
  - **B**loods + cannulate (mark as urgent): e.g. VBG and venous bloods (FBC, CRP, U&Es, LFTs ± amylase, G&S, INR), blood culture, ABG, capillary glucose
  - **O**rifice tests: e.g. urine dip, urine βHCG, sputum culture, stool culture
  - **X**-rays/imaging: e.g. CXR, abdominal X-ray
  - **E**CG
  - **S**pecial tests: depending on likely cause (*see notes on relevant condition's acute management p185*)

MANAGEMENT

Acute management tetrad:
- **Oxygen** - if low sats (e.g. 15L via non-rebreather mask *if no COPD*)
- **Fluids** - if hypotensive or dehydrated (e.g. bolus 500ml 0.9% saline/Hartmann's solution *if no heart failure*)
- **Analgesia** - e.g. 10mg morphine IV titrated slowly to pain if severe ± anti-emetic ± anti-pyretic
- **Disease-specific treatments** - depends on cause (*see notes on relative condition's acute management p185*)

NB: use ABCDE approach if critically unwell.

FINALLY

- Check for patient concerns and explain what's going on
- Document in notes
- Chase investigation results (and change plan as necessary)
- Discuss with seniors if required and refer to relevant team if necessary

Suggested approaches to common acute presentations				
Presenting complaint	Key differentials	Focussed history	Focussed examination	Investigations
Shortness of breath	**Life-threatening** 1. PE 2. Pneumothorax 3. Asthma/COPD 4. Pneumonia 5. Acute LVF 6. ACS	**Exploring** •When did it start? How did it come on? •Getting worse? •Exercise tolerance (current vs. normal) •Orthopnoea, paroxysmal nocturnal dyspnoea **Systems reviews (important parts)** •General: how patient feels, fever •Cardiorespiratory: chest pain, wheeze, cough, sputum, leg swelling **PMHx** •Happened before? Other medical conditions •If asthma/COPD: baseline and severity (including home nebs/oxygen), exacerbation history (spectrum: home → GP → ward → non-invasive ventilation → ICU/intubated), normal peak flow •Recent surgery **DHx + allergies** •Remember inhaler compliance **SHx** •Smoking, alcohol, long-haul travel	**Cardiorespiratory** •Tracheal deviation and JVP •Inspect chest •Expansion, apex, heaves •Percuss •Auscultate heart and lungs •Legs (swelling/tenderness/ oedema) •Peak flow if asthmatic	**Bloods** •FBC, CRP, U&Es •D-dimer (to exclude PE if Wells score low) •BNP (if suspect heart failure) •Blood cultures if pyrexial •ABG **Orifice tests** •Sputum culture **X-rays/imaging** •CXR •CTPA (if PE suspected) **ECG**
Chest pain	**Life-threatening** 1. ACS 2. PE 3. Aortic dissection 4. Pneumothorax 5. Pneumonia	**Exploring** •SOCRATES **Systems reviews (important parts)** •General: how patient feels, fever, clammy •Cardiorespiratory: SOB, wheeze, cough, sputum, leg swelling **PMHx** •Happened before? Other medical conditions •Cardiovascular risk factors **DHx + allergies** •Including cardiovascular medications **FHx** •Cardiovascular events in close family **SHx** •Smoking, alcohol, long-haul travel	**Cardiorespiratory** •Tracheal deviation and JVP •Inspect chest •Expansion, apex, heaves •Percuss •Auscultate heart and lungs •Legs (swelling/tenderness/ oedema)	**Bloods** • FBC, CRP, U&Es •Troponin (STAT and at 12 hours) **X-rays/imaging** •CXR •CTPA (if PE suspected) •CT angio (if aortic dissection needs to be excluded) **ECG**
Abdominal pain	**Life-threatening** 1. Peritonitis 2. AAA 3. Ischaemic bowel 4. Medical causes (DKA, pneumonia, MI, Addisonian crisis) **Upper abdomen** Hepatitis, cholecystitis, peptic ulcer, pancreatitis **Lower abdomen** GI (appendicitis, IBD, diverticulitis), urinary (UTI/pyelonephritis, renal calculi), gynaecological (ectopic, ovarian torsion, PID)	**Exploring** •SOCRATES **Systems reviews (important parts)** •General: how patient feels, fever •Gastro: nausea and vomiting, bowel habit, blood/melaena, weight loss •Urological: dysuria, urinary frequency •Gynaecological: last menstrual period, PV discharge, contraception, chance of pregnancy **PMHx** •Happened before? Other medical conditions **DHx + allergies** •Including relevant medications **SHx** •Smoking, alcohol	**Abdominal** •Inspect (movement with respiration, Grey Turner's/ Cullen's signs, scars) •Guarding and rebound tenderness •Murphy's sign, Rovsing's sign •Quickly palpate liver, spleen, kidneys and for AAA •Palpate for hernias •Percussion tenderness •Bowel sounds •Also examine external genitalia and perform a digital rectal exam if indicated	**Bloods** •FBC, CRP, U&Es •LFTs, amylase •INR, G&S •Capillary glucose •VBG (lactic acidosis in ischaemic bowel) **Orifice tests** •Urine dip •Urine βHCG **X-rays/imaging** •Erect CXR •AXR (if suspect bowel obstruction) •FAST scan (for AAA) •USS/CT abdomen **ECG**
Headache	**Life-threatening** 1. Subarachnoid haemorrhage 2.Meningitis/ encephalitis 3. SOL 4. Temporal arteritis 5. Pre-eclampsia **Common** Migraine, tension headache, cluster headache, sinusitis **Rarer but still important** Venous sinus thrombosis, dissection, hypertensive encephalopathy, CO_2 poisoning, acute glaucoma	**Exploring** •SOCRATES •Meningism symptoms: rash, fever, neck stiffness, photophobia •Temporal arteritis symptoms: visual problems, jaw claudication, scalp tenderness •Glaucoma symptoms: visual problems, red eyes, halos around lights **Systems reviews (important parts)** •General: how patient feels, fever, rash •Neurological: fits/falls/LOC, limb weakness, altered sensations, vision **PMHx** •Happened before? Other medical conditions **DHx + allergies** •Including anticoagulants, steroids, analgesia **FHx** •e.g. for berry aneurysms **SHx** •Smoking, alcohol, travel	•GCS, signs of photophobia, rash •Eyes: pupils, redness, vision •Feel sinuses and temporal arteries for tenderness •Neck stiffness: passively turn head side to side and touch ears to shoulder •Brudzinski's sign (passive flexion of neck causes involuntary flexion of knee and hip) •Kernig's sign (pain on passive knee extension with hip fully flexed) •Motor neuro exam: tone, power, reflexes •Cranial nerves exam •Fundoscopy to look for papilloedema (↑intracranial pressure) or haemorrhages (subarachnoid haemorrhage)	**Bloods** •FBC, CRP, U&Es •ESR •Blood cultures if pyrexial •Meningococcal PCR **X-rays/imaging** •CT head **Special tests** •Lumbar puncture

DIFFERENTIAL DIAGNOSIS OF ACUTE SHORTNESS OF BREATH

Cause grouping	Differentials	Classical history	Classic examination findings	Investigation findings (*initial test, **diagnostic test)	Definitive management (remember ABCDE first)
Respiratory	Pulmonary embolism	•Pleuritic chest pain •Haemoptysis and SOB •Risk factors (long haul flight, recent surgery, immobility)	•Cardiovascular: tachycardia, raised JVP, RV heave, loud P2, split S2 •Respiratory: tachypnoea, clear chest/pleural rub •Calves: look for DVT •SBP<90/pulselessness/persistent bradycardia = 'massive PE'	•D-Dimer* (consider if Wells score low): raised •CT pulmonary angiogram** •ECG: tachycardia, RV strain (T wave inversion in right chest and inferior leads), RBBB, right axis deviation, S1Q3T3 pattern rare •ABG: hypoxaemia, hypocapnia •CXR: may show wedge opacity, regional oligaemia, enlarged pulmonary artery, effusion	•Treatment-dose anticoagulation •Thrombolysis if massive PE
	Pneumonia	•Fever •SOB •Productive cough •Pleuritic chest pain •Confusion	•Tachypnoea, cyanosis •Coarse crepitations and bronchial breathing •Dullness to percussion •Increased vocal resonance/tactile vocal fremitus	•CXR**: consolidation, air bronchogram •Inflammatory markers: raised Identify cause •Sputum culture •Urinary pneumococcal and *Legionella* antigens •Blood cultures ± *Mycoplasma* serology	•Antibiotics
	Pneumothorax	•Sudden onset pleuritic chest pain •May have SOB if large enough •Risk factors, e.g. Marfan syndrome, COPD/asthma	•Reduced chest expansion •Absent breath sounds •Hyperresonance Tension pneumothorax •Raised JVP, hypotension, respiratory distress •Tracheal deviation (away from affected side)	•CXR**: air in pleural space	Primary •<2cm → CXR monitoring •>2cm or Sx → aspirate Secondary •<1cm → observe for 24 hours + high flow oxygen •1-2cm → aspirate •>2cm or Sx → chest drain
	Asthma exacerbation	•Dyspnoea •Wheeze •Known asthmatic	•Tachypnoea •Use of accessory muscles •Polyphonic wheeze •Reduced air entry •Reduced peak flow	*Clinical diagnosis* •CXR: exclude infection and pneumothorax •ABG: usually normal P_aO_2 and low P_aCO_2 (hyperventilation), if ↓P_aO_2 or ↑P_aCO_2, patient is tiring •Blood and sputum cultures if evidence of infection	•Salbutamol nebs •Ipratropium nebs •Steroids •Magnesium IV •Antibiotics if evidence of infection
	COPD exacerbation	•Dyspnoea •Wheeze •Change in sputum •Known COPD or lifelong smoker	•Tachypnoea •Use of accessory muscles •Polyphonic wheeze •Reduced air entry	*Clinical diagnosis* •CXR: exclude infection and pneumothorax •ABG: hypoxaemia, hypercapnia	•Salbutamol nebs •Ipratropium nebs •Steroids •Antibiotics •BiPAP if required
	Other respiratory differentials	Extrinsic allergic alveolitis, laryngitis, bronchitis, pneumonitis, bronchiectasis, LRTI, pleural effusion			
Cardiac	ACS	•Crushing central chest pain •Radiates to neck/left arm •Associated nausea/SOB/sweatiness •Cardiovascular risk factors	•May be normal •General: sweaty, SOB, in pain •Cardiovascular: signs of heart failure, brady/tachycardic	•ECG*: ST-elevation (or new LBBB), inverted T waves, Q waves •Troponin*: increased (but normal in unstable angina) •CXR: normal or signs of heart failure •Coronary angiography**	•**MONAC** (Morphine, Oxygen, Nitrate, Aspirin, Clopidogrel) •Percutaneous coronary intervention
	Acute LVF	•SOB, orthopnoea, paroxysmal nocturnal dyspnoea •Pink frothy sputum •Peripheral oedema •Cardiac history	•Tachycardia, tachypnoea •Raised JVP •Fine bi-basal crepitations •S3 gallop rhythm •Peripheral oedema	•CXR*: **ABCDE** (Alveolar shadowing, B-lines, Cardiomegaly, Diversion of blood to upper lobes, Effusion) •Echocardiogram** •BNP •ECG: look for MI	•**POD MAN** (Position siting up, Oxygen, Diuretics, Morphine, Anti-emetic, Nitrate infusion) •CPAP if required •Treat cause (if any)
	Other cardiac differentials	Cardiomyopathy, myocarditis, acute valvular disease, pericardial effusion, pulmonary hypertension			
Other	Hyperventilation in anxiety	•Tight chest pain, SOB, sweating, dizziness, palpitations, feeling of impending doom •Anxious personality/other symptoms of generalised anxiety disorder •Recurrent episodes triggered by a stimulus (e.g. crowds)	•Usually normal •Hyperventilation	*Diagnosis of exclusion* •ECG: exclude MI •Troponin: exclude MI •D-dimer: exclude PE •CXR: exclude infection •ABG: respiratory alkalosis	•Reassurance •Cognitive behavioural therapy •SSRI
	Other differentials	DKA, overdoses, metabolic acidosis, sepsis/systemic inflammatory response syndrome, foreign body, anaphylaxis, anaemia			

DIFFERENTIAL DIAGNOSIS OF ACUTE CHEST PAIN

Cause grouping	Differentials	Classical history	Classic examination findings	Investigation findings (*initial test, **diagnostic test)	Definitive management (remember ABCDE first)
Cardiac	ACS	•Crushing central chest pain •Radiates to neck/left arm •Associated nausea/SOB/ sweatiness •Cardiovascular risk factors	•May be normal •General: sweaty, SOB, in pain •Cardiovascular: signs of heart failure, brady/tachycardic	•ECG*: ST-elevation (or new LBBB), inverted T waves, Q waves •Troponin*: increased (but normal in unstable angina) •CXR: normal or signs of heart failure •Coronary angiography**	•MONAC (Morphine, Oxygen, Nitrate, Aspirin, Clopidogrel) •Percutaneous coronary intervention
	Aortic dissection	•Tearing chest pain of <u>very</u> sudden onset •Radiates to back •Pain in other sites, e.g. arms, legs, neck, head	•Unequal arm pulses or BPs •May develop acute aortic regurgitation •May be new neurological symptoms due to involvement of carotid/vertebral arteries	•CXR*: widened mediastinum •CT angiogram** •ECG: may show signs of MI (usually inferior)	•Type A → surgical repair •Type B → BP control
	Pericarditis	•Retrosternal/precordial pleuritic chest pain •Relieved by sitting forward •May radiate to trapezius ridge/neck/shoulder •Viral prodrome common	•Pericardial rub (stepping in snow) •Tachycardia •JVP distension and pulsus paradoxus may indicate tamponade	*Clinical diagnosis* •ECG: PR depression, saddle-shaped ST-elevation •CXR: may show globular heart if pericardial effusion present •Echo: if pericardial effusion suspected	•NSAIDs •Treat cause (if known)
	Myocarditis	•Chest pain •Palpitations •Fever •Fatigue •Dyspnoea	•Signs of heart failure •S3/summation gallop •Fever •Tachypnoea/tachycardia	•ECG: diffuse T wave inversions, ST-elevation/depression •Inflammatory markers: raised •Troponin: raised •Serology: identify cause •Myocardial biopsy** (if required)	•Treat cause •Treat complications, e.g. heart failure •Bed rest
	Other cardiac differentials	Stable angina, tamponade, mitral valve prolapse, pulmonary hypertension, aortic stenosis, arrhythmias				

Cause grouping	Differentials	Classical history	Classic examination findings	Investigation findings (*initial test, **diagnostic test)	Definitive management (remember ABCDE first)
Respiratory	Pulmonary embolism	•Pleuritic chest pain •Dyspnoea •Haemoptysis •Risk factors (long haul flight, recent surgery, immobility)	•Cardiovascular: tachycardia, raised JVP, RV heave, loud P2, split S2 •Respiratory: tachypnoea, clear chest/pleural rub •Calves: look for DVT •SBP<90/pulselessness/persistent bradycardia = 'massive PE'	•D-Dimer* (consider if Wells score low): raised •CT pulmonary angiogram** •ECG: tachycardia, RV strain (T wave inversion in right chest and inferior leads), RBBB, right axis deviation, S1Q3T3 pattern rare •ABG: hypoxaemia, hypocapnia •CXR: may show wedge opacity, regional oligaemia, enlarged pulmonary artery, effusion	•Treatment-dose anticoagulation •Thrombolysis if massive PE
	Pneumonia	•Fever •SOB •Productive cough •Pleuritic chest pain •Confusion	•Tachypnoea, cyanosis •Coarse crepitations and bronchial breathing •Dullness to percussion •Increased vocal resonance/tactile vocal fremitus	•CXR**: consolidation, air bronchogram •Inflammatory markers: raised <u>Identify cause</u> •Sputum culture •Urinary pneumococcal and *Legionella* antigens •Blood cultures ± *Mycoplasma* serology	•Antibiotics
	Pneumothorax	•Sudden onset pleuritic chest pain •May have SOB if large enough •Risk factors, e.g. Marfan appearance, COPD/asthma	•Reduced chest expansion •Absent breath sounds •Hyperresonance <u>Tension pneumothorax</u> •Raised JVP, hypotension, respiratory distress •Tracheal deviation (away from affected side)	•CXR**: air in pleural space	<u>Primary</u> •<2cm → CXR monitoring •>2cm or Sx → aspirate <u>Secondary</u> •<1cm → observe for 24 hours + high flow oxygen •1-2cm → aspirate •>2cm or Sx → chest drain
	Pleurisy	•Pleuritic chest pain •May have: dry cough, fever, dyspnoea	•Pleural rub	*Clinical diagnosis* •CXR: exclude pneumothorax, effusion and pneumonia	•NSAIDS •Treat cause (if known) •Treat complications (effusion, pneumothorax)

Cause grouping	Differentials	Classical history	Classic examination findings	Investigation findings (*initial test, **diagnostic test)	Definitive management (remember ABCDE first)
Other	Musculoskeletal	•Sharp chest pain •Exacerbated by movement and inspiration •Clearly localised •Exacerbated by palpation	•Tenderness over area of pain •Exam otherwise normal	*Diagnosis of exclusion* •D-dimer: exclude PE •CXR: exclude pneumothorax and infection •Inflammatory markers: normal	•Analgesia •Deep breathing exercises to prevent infection
	Costochondritis	•Costosternal joint pain •Worse with coughing, twisting and physical activity	•Tenderness at sternal edges •Normal exam otherwise	*Diagnosis of exclusion* •ECG: exclude MI •Troponin: exclude MI •CXR: normal	•NSAIDs •Physical therapy
	Gastro-oesophageal reflux disease	•Retrosternal burning chest pain •Related to meals, lying, straining •Water brash	•Usually normal •May be epigastric tenderness if associated gastritis	*Clinical diagnosis* •ECG: exclude MI •OGD** (if red flags) •Oesophageal pH monitoring** (if diagnostic uncertainty)	•Lifestyle advice •Proton pump inhibitor
	Anxiety/panic attack	•Tight chest pain, SOB, sweating, dizziness, palpitations, feeling of impending doom •Anxious personality/other symptoms of generalised anxiety disorder •Recurrent episodes triggered by a stimulus (e.g. crowds)	•Usually normal •May be hyperventilation	*Diagnosis of exclusion* •ECG: exclude MI •Troponin: exclude MI •CXR: exclude infection	•Reassurance •Cognitive behavioural therapy •SSRI
	Oesophageal spasm	•Intermittent crushing sub-sternal pain •Relieved by GTN •Associated dysphagia	•Normal	•Barium swallow: corkscrew oesophagus •Oesophageal manometry**	•Avoid precipitating foods •Try: PPI, nitrates, Ca^{2+} blockers, phosphodiesterase inhibitors, antidepressants
	Other differentials	Gastritis, peptic ulcer disease, acute cholecystitis, gastritis, pancreatitis, fibromyalgia, Tietze syndrome			

178

DIFFERENTIAL DIAGNOSIS OF ACUTE ABDOMINAL PAIN

Cause grouping	Differentials	Classical history	Classic examination findings	Investigation findings (*initial, **diagnostic test)	Definitive management (remember ABCDE first)
Surgical	Peritonitis/ perforation (e.g. peptic ulcer, colonic tumour, diverticulum, gallbladder, appendix, spleen, AAA, ectopic)	•Severe generalised abdominal pain	•Shock •No abdominal movement with respiration •Guarding •Firm, peritonitic abdomen •Rebound tenderness •Severe pain to light palpation •Percussion tenderness	•Erect CXR*: air under diaphragm •CT abdomen/pelvis**: help determine site of perforation	•Urgent surgical repair •Consider patient comorbidities and chance of survival
	Ruptured AAA	•Elderly •Severe generalised abdominal pain •Back pain •Reduced GCS/collapse	•Shock •Peritonitis •Expansile mass	•Bedside USS abdomen if freely available •CT angiography	•Aim for permissive hypotension (SBP 100) •Activate 'massive haemorrhage protocol' e.g. 10 units •Urgent open repair (or endovascular aneurysm repair if stable)
	Appendicitis	•Young patient •Periumbilical pain initially •Moves to RIF •Anorexia/nausea •Fever	•Tender RIF •Worse at McBurney's point •Guarding/local peritonitis •Rovsing's +ve	*Clinical diagnosis* •USS abdomen/pelvis if gynaecological differentials •Inflammatory markers: raised •βHCG: rule out ectopic	•Appendicectomy
	Gallstones	Biliary colic •Severe intermittent RUQ/epigastric pain •Exacerbated by fatty food Cholecystitis •Continuous RUQ/epigastric pain •Murphy's +ve •Tenderness and guarding RUQ Common bile duct stones •Jaundice •RUQ pain Cholangitis •Jaundice •Fever/rigors •RUQ pain		•LFTs: obstructive picture if common bile duct stones/cholangitis •Inflammatory markers: raised in cholecystitis/cholangitis •Abdominal USS** •CT if percutaneous biliary drainage or cholecystostomy required	Biliary colic •Analgesia •Fat-free diet •Outpatient cholecystectomy Cholecystitis •Antibiotics (e.g. ciprofloxacin, cephalosporin or co-amoxiclav) •Cholecystectomy ('hot' if mild, after 6 weeks if not) CBD stone •Continuous IV fluids (prevent renal injury) •ERCP Cholangitis •IV antibiotics (e.g. ciprofloxacin or Tazocin) •Treat cause
	Acute pancreatitis	•Severe epigastric/central pain •Radiating to back •Relieved by sitting forwards •Vomiting •History of possible cause, e.g. gallstones, alcohol, hypertriglyceridemia, trauma, surgery, medications etc.	•Epigastric tenderness •Tachycardia •Fever •Shock •Jaundice •Grey-Turner's and Cullen's signs (rare)	*Clinical diagnosis* •Amylase or lipase*: raised •LFTs: deranged •CT abdomen if diagnostic uncertainty •Apache II/Glasgow score (requires calcium and ABG) •Confirm cause ↘USS abdomen (exclude gallstones in all patients) ↘Triglycerides ↘Immunoglobulins	•Supportive management •Aggressive fluid resuscitation with Hartmann's solution, e.g. 1L every 4 hours (third space sequestration) – *titrate to UO* •NBM until nausea/pain improve (enteric feeding if prolonged) •No antibiotics unless proven infection, gas on CT or raised procalcitonin •Treat/withdraw cause •ICU may be required
	Diverticulitis	•Elderly •LIF pain •Pyrexia •Diarrhoea common	•Tender LIF •Guarding/local peritonism •PR (check for malignancy/abscess)	•Inflammatory markers: raised •CT abdomen/pelvis** (if needed)	•Clear fluids only initially, then build up over 2-3 days •Antibiotics (e.g. cefuroxime + metronidazole or co-amoxiclav)
	Renal colic	•Spasms of loin to groin pain (excruciating) •Nausea and vomiting •Cannot lie still	•Soft abdomen •May be renal angle tenderness	•Urine dip: microscopic haematuria •KUB X-ray* •CT KUB**	•Analgesia (e.g. diclofenac) •IV fluids •Antibiotics if infection •Removal ↘<1cm – smooth muscle relaxants (e.g. tamsulosin) ↘>1cm – ureteroscopy/ESWL ↘>2cm in renal pelvis – percutaneous nephrolithotomy •Ureteric stent/nephrostomy if obstruction
	Bowel obstruction	•Vomiting (may be feculent) •Colicky abdominal pain •No bowel motions or flatus	•Distended, tender abdomen •Tinkling bowel sounds	•AXR*: distended bowel loops •CT abdomen/pelvis**: confirm and look for cause •Gastrografin study in SBO	•NBM + IV fluids •Wide-bore NG tube (free drainage) •Laparoscopy/laparotomy (if complete or non-resolving partial obstruction)
	Acute mesenteric ischaemia	•Age >50 years •Severe abdominal pain •Diarrhoea •Risk factors: AF, cardiovascular risk factors	•Hypovolaemia/shock •Soft abdomen (pain out of proportion to exam)	•VBG: ↑lactate •CT abdomen/pelvis*: ischaemic bowel •Mesenteric angiography**: if required	•Aggressive IV fluids + NBM + NG decompression •Antibiotics (e.g. cefuroxime + metronidazole) •If infarction: bowel resection + post-operative heparinisation •No infarction: revascularisation
	Other surgical differentials	Testicular torsion, ischaemic colitis, volvulus, strangulated hernia, Meckel's diverticulum, mesenteric adenitis, adhesions, hepatic abscess, psoas abscess			

179

Cause grouping	Differentials	Classical history	Classic examination findings	Investigation findings (*initial, **diagnostic test)	Definitive management (remember ABCDE first)
Medical	Gastritis/peptic ulcer	•Epigastric pain •Related to meals (peptic ulcer = during meals; duodenal ulcer = before meals/at night) •Risk factors, e.g. NSAIDs, alcohol, spicy food	•Tender epigastrium •Soft abdomen	•FBC: may show microcytic anaemia •Erect CXR: exclude perforation •OGD**: if severe/ recurrent •*H. pylori* investigations	•Proton pump inhibitor (IV/PO) •*H. pylori* eradication (if +ve)
	Pyelonephritis	•Fever, rigors •Loin pain •Urinary frequency and dysuria	•Loin tenderness •Renal angle tenderness	•Urine dip + culture*: positive leukocytes and nitrites •Inflammatory markers: raised •USS to look for any structural abnormalities or nephronia/renal abscess	•Antibiotics (e.g. ciprofloxacin or cephalosporin)
	Other medical differentials	Gastroenteritis, constipation, Crohn's disease, ulcerative colitis, MI, pneumonia, sickle cell crisis, DKA, pyelonephritis, IBS, Budd-Chiari syndrome, addisonian crisis, hypercalcaemia, acute intermittent porphyria, hepatitis			
Gynae	Ectopic pregnancy	•Severe unilateral pelvic pain •~6-8 weeks pregnant/not using contraception/missed period •Shoulder tip pain •May have spotting	•Tenderness RIF/LIF •Guarding •Adnexal tenderness ± mass •Cervical excitation	•Urinary βHCG*: +ve •Serum βHCG + trend •Transvaginal USS**	Options include: •Methotrexate if uncomplicated •Laparoscopic salpingostomy/ salpingectomy •Laparotomy + Anti-D prophylaxis (if required)
	Ovarian cyst rupture/ torsion/ haemorrhage	•Sudden unilateral pelvic pain (very severe if torsion) •May have light vaginal bleeding •May have fever/vomiting	•Tenderness RIF/LIF •Guarding •Adnexal tenderness ± mass	•Transvaginal/abdominal USS** •βHCG: exclude ectopic	•Laparoscopy/laparotomy if torsion •Others mostly managed conservatively
	Pelvic inflammatory disease	•Bilateral pelvic pain (gradual onset) •Vaginal discharge •Dyspareunia and dysmenorrhoea •May have post-coital or intermenstrual bleeding	•Suprapubic tenderness •Vaginal discharge, cervicitis •Bilateral adnexal tenderness •Cervical excitation •May have fever	•Inflammatory markers: raised •Triple vaginal swabs**	•Broad spectrum antibiotics (e.g. metronidazole + doxycycline + quinolone)
	Other gynaecological differentials	Salpingitis, pregnancy, fibroid degeneration, Fitz-Hugh–Curtis syndrome, endometriosis			

DIFFERENTIAL DIAGNOSIS OF ACUTE HEADACHE

Cause grouping	Differentials	Classical history	Classic examination findings	Investigation findings (*initial, **diagnostic test)	Definitive management (remember ABCDE first)
Primary	Tension headache	•Bilateral tight band sensation •Recurrent •Occurs late in day •Association with stress	•Tension and tenderness in neck and scalp muscles	*Clinical diagnosis*	•Simple analgesia •Avoid triggers
	Cluster headache	•Short painful attacks around one eye •Lasts between 30 mins – 3 hours •Occurs 1-8x a day for 1-3 months •May have lacrimation and flushing	•Conjunctival injection •Lacrimation •Swollen eye-lid •Horner's syndrome during attack	*Clinical diagnosis*	•100% oxygen •Triptan •Verapamil may be used for prevention
	Migraine	•Unilateral pulsating •Occurs in trigeminal nerve distribution •Lasts hours – days •May have aura (usually visual) •Photophobia	•May be focal neurology with aura •Otherwise normal	*Clinical diagnosis*	•Abortive: 1. NSAID/aspirin 2. Triptan •Preventative: 1. β-blocker (propranolol) 2. TCA (amitriptyline) 3. Anticonvulsants
	Trigeminal neuralgia	•2 second paroxysms of stabbing pain in unilateral trigeminal nerve distribution •Face screws up with pain •Triggers (e.g. shaving) •Symptoms of underlying cause (e.g. aneurysm, tumour, MS)	•Normal	*Clinical diagnosis* •MRI to find cause	•Anticonvulsants •Treat cause, e.g. nerve compression

indications for imaging:
1. focal neurologic signs or symptoms
2. onset of HA c̄ exertion, cough or sexual activity
3. onset of HA p̄ age 40
4. alarming Δ in pattern frequency or severity
5. orbital bruits, carotid bruits
6. progressive worsening despite appropriate therapy

Cause grouping	Differentials	Classical history	Classic examination findings	Investigation findings (*initial test, **diagnostic test)	Definitive management (remember ABCDE first)
Secondary-intracranial	Meningitis	•Photophobia •Neck stiffness •Systemic symptoms, e.g. fever, non-blanching rash	•Photophobia •Neck stiffness •Kernig's and Brudzinski's +ve •Non-blanching rash (meningococcal) •Focal neurology (20%)	•Blood culture* and meningococcal PCR •Lumbar puncture** •Throat swab •CXR: pneumonia may be cause	•IV 3rd generation cephalosporin without delay (+ amoxicillin if >65 years/ immunocompromised) •IM benzylpenicillin if in community •Dexamethasone •Ciprofloxacin prophylaxis for close contacts
	Temporal arteritis	•Unilateral throbbing pain •Scalp tenderness and jaw claudication •>55 years •May have visual problems	•Ipsilateral blindness •Temporal tenderness •Optic nerve oedema	•ESR*: raised •Temporal artery biopsy** •Doppler temporal artery: ↓flow	•High dose corticosteroids
	Subarachnoid haemorrhage	•Very sudden onset •Very severe •'Like someone hit me over the head' •Meningism	•Meningism •GCS may be reduced	1. CT head*: blood within area of circle of Willis 2. Lumbar puncture** (if CT normal): xanthochromia	•Calcium antagonists (to reduce vasospasm) •Coiling/clipping of aneurysm
	Raised intracranial pressure (e.g. tumour, benign intracranial hypertension, acute hydrocephalus)	•Worse in morning and with coughing and bending •Vomiting and reduced GCS •Visual disturbance •May have neurological symptoms and/or seizures if due to tumour	•↓GCS •Papilloedema •CN6 (abducens) palsy •Ipsilateral mydriasis •Cushing response (↓pulse, ↑BP) •Cheyne-Stokes respiration	•CT head**: to confirm and determine cause •Intracranial pressure monitoring	•Mannitol + hyperventilation if severe •Treat cause
	Venous sinus thrombosis	•May build up over a few days or be of sudden onset •Nausea and vomiting •Seizures •History of hypercoagulable state, e.g. pregnancy	•Papilloedema •Visual field defects •Cranial nerve palsies •Focal neurology	•CT head* •MR venography**	•Treatment dose LMWH •Cavernous sinus thrombosis: also antibiotics (high risk of infection) and hypopituitarism treatment if required
	Intracerebral haemorrhage	•Symptoms of stroke + headache	•Neurological defects, e.g. hemiplegia, homonymous hemianopia, dysphasia	•CT head** •Catheter angiography: to look for arteriovenous malformations and arteriopathy if young/suspected •Further CT at 6 weeks and MRI at 3 months to look for underlying tumour	•BP control •Correct any coagulopathy •Treat cause, e.g. arteriovenous malformation if found •If large/raised intracranial pressure/midline shift/ superficial: consider craniotomy and clot evacuation, stereotactic aspiration or endoscopic evacuation
	Other differentials	Encephalitis, cerebral abscess, tumour, pituitary apoplexy, subdural haematoma, extradural haematoma			

Cause grouping	Differentials	Classical history	Classic examination findings	Investigation findings (*initial test, **diagnostic test)	Definitive management (remember ABCDE first)
Secondary-extracranial	Acute closed-angle glaucoma	•Pain around one eye •Swollen red eye •Visual blurring and halos	•Reduced acuity •Conjunctival injection •Cloudy cornea •Pupil mid-dilated and irregular	•Tonometry** >24mmHg (>21mmHg suspicious)	•IV/PO acetazolamide •α-agonist/β-blocker drops •Laser peripheral iridectomy
	Sinusitis	•Facial pain exacerbated by leaning head forward, coughing etc. •Rhinorrhoea/nasal congestion	•Sinus tenderness •Pain on percussion of frontal/temporal sinuses	*Clinical diagnosis*	•Antibiotics if bacterial •Warm face packs •Saline nasal drops •Analgesia
	Hypertensive encephalopathy	•Headache •Visual blurring •Vomiting	•Severe hypertension •Bilateral retinal haemorrhages •Papilloedema	*Clinical diagnosis* •Urine dip: microscopic haematuria •Look for cause •CT brain: may be required to exclude cerebral haemorrhage	•Controlled BP reduction with IV labetalol or nicardipine
	Pre-eclampsia	•3rd trimester or peripartum •Headache •Visual disturbance •Epigastric pain •Vomiting	•Hypertensive •Brisk reflexes •Oedema	•Urine dip: proteinuria •Bloods: HELLP syndrome (Haemolysis, Elevated Liver enzymes, Low Platelets) •Cardiotocography and fetal USS	•Delivery is only cure (aim to wait >34w) •BP control (labetalol, methyldopa) •Magnesium sulphate (prevent fits) •Aspirin may be used for prevention
	Carotid/vertebral artery dissection	•Most common cause of stroke in young adult •Dull pressure occipital headache •Neck and facial pain •Stroke symptoms (may be transient) •Risk factors, e.g. trauma, neck manipulation, connective tissue disease	•Signs of stroke	•CT or MR angiography** •Duplex carotid ultrasonography	•Treat stroke as usual (thrombolysis or antiplatelet) •Antiplatelets or anticoagulation for 6 months •Endovascular stent may be considered for recurrent ischaemia
	Other differentials	Drugs (e.g. nitrates, PPI, Ca2+ antagonists, caffeine, analgesia overuse, hormones), drug withdrawal, carbon monoxide poisoning, post-traumatic, Paget's disease, hypoxia, cervical spondylosis, otitis media, dental causes			

DIFFERENTIAL DIAGNOSIS OF COLLAPSE/FALL

Cause grouping	Differentials	Classical history	Classic examination findings	Investigation findings (*initial test, **diagnostic test)	Definitive management (remember ABCDE first)
Neurological	Generalised seizure	•Tonic-clonic (grand mal): sudden LOC, limbs stiffen then jerk, incontinence, tongue-biting, myalgia and confusion afterwards •Absence (petit mal): unresponsive, staring into space for a few seconds (typically in childhood) •Atonic: all muscles relax, patient drops to floor •Tonic: all muscles become rigid •Myoclonic: involuntary flexion	•May be post-ictal •Focal neurology may indicate cause	•Electroencephalogram (EEG)** if required Find cause •CT head: rule out intracranial cause •Electrolytes •Capillary glucose •Drug levels	•Treat cause •Anti-epileptics if ≥2 episodes •IV lorazepam or PR diazepam to terminate acute seizure •Driving restriction
	Parkinson's disease	•TETRAD = rigidity + tremor + bradykinesia + postural instability	•Resting tremor •Shuffling, festinant gait with lack of arm swing •Cogwheel rigidity •Bradykinesia	Clinical diagnosis •Functional neuroimaging/dopamine transporter imaging (e.g. DaTscan) may be useful if diagnostic uncertainty	•Levodopa •Dopamine agonists •Monoamine oxidase inhibitors •Physiotherapy + home modifications
	TIA/stroke	•Sudden onset neurological symptoms, e.g. limb/face weakness, slurred speech, hemianopia •Risk factors, e.g. age, hypertension, smoking, DM, vascular disease, AF	•Neurological defects, e.g. hemiplegia, homonymous hemianopia, dysphasia, sensory loss	•CT head** •ECG: check for AF •Coagulation screen •Carotid dopplers	•Acute: antiplatelet or thrombolysis if ischaemic stroke (± endovascular clot retrieval where available) •Long-term: clopidogrel + statin + BP control •Carotid endarterectomy (if stenosis >50% NASCET criteria/>70% ECST criteria)
	Vasovagal	•Occurs in response to stimuli, e.g. emotion, pain or prolonged standing •Preceding nausea, pallor, sweat, closing visual fields •Then transient LOC	•Normal	Clinical diagnosis •Tilt-table test** if syncope diagnosis unclear •Consider investigation to exclude other causes •ECG: normal	•Reassurance •Avoid triggers
	Situational syncope (e.g. cough syncope, micturition syncope)	•Transient syncope in certain circumstance, e.g. while coughing or during micturition/defecation	•Normal	Clinical diagnosis •Tilt-table test** if syncope diagnosis unclear •Consider investigation to exclude other causes •ECG: normal	•Reassurance
	Other neuro differentials	Neuropathy (e.g. MS), intracranial haemorrhages (extradural, subarachnoid, subdural), raised intracranial pressure			

Cause grouping	Differentials	Classical history	Classic examination findings	Investigation findings (*initial test, **diagnostic test)	Definitive management (remember ABCDE first)
Cardio-vascular	Postural hypotension	•Dizziness ± LOC on standing from lying/sitting •Recently started/changed anti-hypertensive	•Postural BP drop** of >20mmHg systolic and/or >10mmHg diastolic within 3 minutes of standing	Find cause •U&Es (dehydration) •Inflammatory markers (infection) •FBC (anaemia) •Synacthen test (Addison's) •Fasting glucose (diabetic autonomic dysfunction)	•Treat cause, e.g. rehydrate, change medications •Stand up in stages •Elastic stockings •Fludrocortisone may be tried if refractory
	Aortic stenosis	•Collapse on exertion •SOB on exertion	•Ejection systolic murmur •Slow-rising pulse •Narrow pulse pressure •Heaving apex beat •May be signs of LVF	•Echocardiogram**	•Surgical valve replacement (if symptomatic or LVF) •TAVI if not fit for surgery •Echo follow-up
	Cardiac syncope (arrhythmia)	•Fall after transient arrhythmia •Sudden LOC •May have palpitations or feel strange before collapse •Cardiac history or family history of sudden death •May have occurred during exercise or when supine	•May be normal	•ECG*: usually normal between attacks but may reveal underlying cause, e.g. Wolff-Parkinson-White syndrome, Brugada syndrome, long QT •24 hour tape* •Implantable loop recorder**: if episodes less frequent •Echocardiogram: look for structural heart disease	•Depends on arrhythmia •β-blockers or antiarrhythmics or ablation where appropriate •ICD (if risk of VT/VF) •Pacemaker (if: persistent symptomatic bradycardia, trifascicular block, Mobitz II, complete heart block or pauses >3 seconds)
	Other cardiac differentials	-Structural (e.g. hypertrophic obstructive cardiomyopathy, arrhythmogenic right ventricular dysplasia) -Carotid sinus hypersensitivity (precipitated by head turning/shaving – diagnosed by carotid sinus massage** → ≥3 second pauses) -Vertebrobasilar insufficiency (vertigo precipitated by head extension in elderly patients with cervical osteoarthritis) -Subclavian steal syndrome (proximal subclavian artery stenosis causes retrograde flow in one of the vertebral arteries as they become involved in a collateral circuit to bypass the obstruction)			

Cause grouping	Differentials	Classical history	Classic examination findings	Investigation findings (*initial test, **diagnostic test)	Definitive management (remember ABCDE first)
Other	Drug overdose/ toxicity	•History of drug use or taking drug with narrow therapeutic range •Drug use prior to collapse	•Depends on drug	•Therapeutic drug levels •Overdose drug levels (e.g. paracetamol, salicylate)	•Depends on drug
	Alcohol intoxication	•History of alcohol use	•Odour of alcohol	•Ethanol level (if required)	•Observation
	Mechanical fall	•Clear account of tripping •No syncope/LOC/symptoms	•Normal •Check for injuries	•Consider investigation to exclude other causes	•Reassurance •Treat any injuries
	Other differentials	Postural instability, polypharmacy, ectopic pregnancy, ruptured AAA, delirium, vertigo, anaemia, hypoglycaemia, hypercapnic acidosis, sepsis, eyesight problems, arthritis, leg weakness, anxiety, factitious blackouts, choking, heat syncope, multifactorial			

ACUTE ASTHMA AND COPD EXACERBATION MANAGEMENT

Type I IgE mediated hypersensitivity reaction causing smooth muscle contraction in airways.

CLASSIFYING ASTHMA SEVERITY

- Life-threatening (PEFR < 33%): **33, 92 CHEST**
  - o **33**: PEFR <33% predicted
  - o **92**: Sats <92%
  - o **C**yanosis
  - o **H**ypotension
  - o **E**xhaustion
  - o **S**ilent chest
  - o **T**achycardia
- Severe (PEFR < 50%): cannot complete sentences, respiratory rate > 25, heart rate >110
- Moderate (PEFR <75%)
- Mild (PEFR >75%)

TREATING ASTHMA EXACERBATION
O SHIT ME!

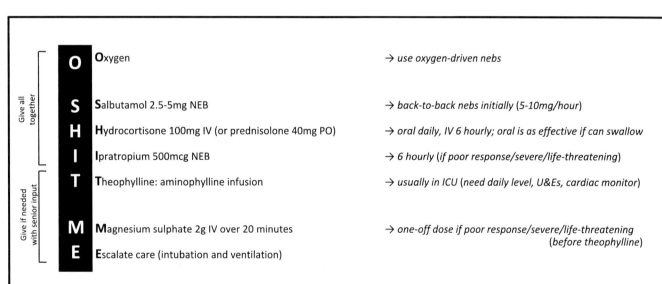

Give all together	**O**	**O**xygen	→ use oxygen-driven nebs
	S	**S**albutamol 2.5-5mg NEB	→ back-to-back nebs initially (5-10mg/hour)
	H	**H**ydrocortisone 100mg IV (or prednisolone 40mg PO)	→ oral daily, IV 6 hourly; oral is as effective if can swallow
	I	**I**pratropium 500mcg NEB	→ 6 hourly (if poor response/severe/life-threatening)
Give if needed with senior input	**T**	**T**heophylline: aminophylline infusion	→ usually in ICU (need daily level, U&Es, cardiac monitor)
	M	**M**agnesium sulphate 2g IV over 20 minutes	→ one-off dose if poor response/severe/life-threatening (before theophylline)
	E	**E**scalate care (intubation and ventilation)	

If hypoxaemia/hypercapnia is worsening despite maximal therapy, involve senior/anaesthetist with a view to intubation and ventilation.

TREATING COPD EXACERBATION

- **O SHIT** as in asthma but give controlled oxygen, i.e. 24-28% (venturi mask), and do regular ABGs to determine further oxygen therapy (*see prescribing notes on oxygen therapy p280*)
- **Antibiotics:** prescribe if any signs of infection as per local guidelines, e.g. doxycycline
- **Chest physiotherapy**
- **Consider BiPAP** if you cannot deliver enough oxygen to maintain sats of 88-92%, without depressing their respiratory drive and causing a hypercapnic acidosis

If hypoxaemia/hypercapnia is worsening despite maximal therapy, involve senior/anaesthetist with a view to intubation and ventilation.

INTENSIVE CARE INDICATIONS

- Requiring ventilator support
- Worsening hypoxaemia/hypercapnia/acidosis
- Exhaustion
- Drowsiness/confusion

PULMONARY EMBOLISM MANAGEMENT

ABCDE APPROACH
Follow usual ABCDE approach if critically ill.

INVESTIGATIONS
- **Confirm/exclude diagnosis**
  - D-Dimer if low *PE Wells score*
  - CTPA (or V/Q scan if contraindicated)
- **Investigate severity**
  - ECG may show: tachycardia; RV strain, i.e. T-wave inversion in right precordial and inferior leads; RBBB; right axis deviation; $S_1Q_3T_3$; RA enlargement, i.e. P pulmonale; RV dilation, i.e. dominant R in V1
  - CXR may show: wedge infarcts; regional oligaemia; enlarged pulmonary artery; effusion)
  - Echocardiogram: look for right heart strain/overload
- **Consider looking for cause if unknown**
  - Hereditary thrombophilia testing: if family history
  - Anti-phospholipid antibodies: consider if relevant
  - Investigate for occult malignancy with mammogram (if female and >40 years) and/or CT abdomen/pelvis (if >40 years)

MANAGEMENT ALGORITHM

Calculate the *PE Wells score* to predict the likelihood of PE. This score takes into account risk factors (recent surgery/immobility, previous VTE, cancer), symptoms of VTE (DVT symptoms, HR, haemoptysis), and the likelihood of alternative diagnosis (Wells et al. 2001).

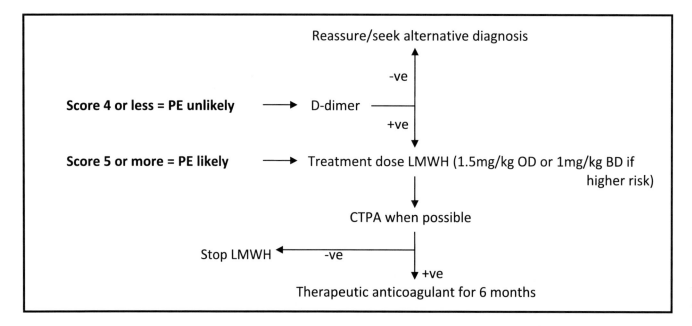

Reassure/seek alternative diagnosis

-ve

Score 4 or less = PE unlikely → D-dimer

+ve

Score 5 or more = PE likely → Treatment dose LMWH (1.5mg/kg OD or 1mg/kg BD if higher risk)

CTPA when possible

Stop LMWH ← -ve

+ve

Therapeutic anticoagulant for 6 months

THERAPEUTIC ANTICOAGULANT OPTIONS
- **DOACs:** most commonly used for anticoagulation. Rivaroxaban and apixaban have loading doses; edoxaban and dabigatran do not and so require 5 days of dual therapy with LMWH initially.
- **Warfarin:** usually used where DOACs are contraindicated (e.g. renal impairment) or if reversibility is required. If using warfarin, continue LMWH until had ≥5 days dual therapy and is INR 2-3.
- **LMWH:** less preferable because patient will have to give daily self-injections. Currently the only licenced treatment in cancer patients.

THROMBOLYSIS INDICATIONS
- In <u>massive PE</u> (SBP <90mmHg for >15 minutes, pulselessness or persistent bradycardia) → immediate thrombolysis with alteplase
- In <u>sub-massive PE</u> (RV dysfunction, myocardial necrosis or large clot burden, e.g. saddle PE) → give unfractionated heparin infusion (usually for 72 hours) so thrombolysis can be considered

ACUTE CORONARY SYNDROME MANAGEMENT

ABCDE APPROACH

Follow usual ABCDE approach if critically ill.

SHORT-TERM MANAGEMENT OF ACS

<u>Initial management</u>

M	**M**orphine: 10mg in 10ml slow IV – titrate to pain (+ 10mg metoclopramide IV)
O	**O**xygen: only if saturations below target range of 94-98%
N	**N**itrates: sublingual GTN if not hypotensive (then PRN) – *IV infusion can also be used*
A	**A**spirin: 300mg PO loading dose (then 75mg OD)
C	**C**lopidogrel: 300-600mg PO loading dose (then 75mg OD)

<u>Other medications to start</u>
In STEMI patients who should have immediate PCI, cardiologist will decide when to start these.
- Statin
- β-blocker
- ACE inhibitor (start 6-24 hours after admission)
- ACS-dose anticoagulation (fondaparinux or LMWH or heparin) for 5 days – *NSTEMI only*
- Glycoprotein IIb/IIIa inhibitor – *very select patients only*

<u>Reperfusion therapy</u>
- STEMI → within 2 hours
- NSTEMI or unstable angina
  - Haemodynamically unstable, arrhythmias or high ischaemic risk (e.g. ongoing/recurrent pain, ongoing ECG changes) → as soon as possible
  - Intermediate or high risk GRACE score → within 3 days
  - Low risk GRACE score → may be treated conservatively or investigated further as outpatient

*NB: **GRACE score** is a measure of 6-month mortality: above 6% is high risk, 3-6% is intermediate risk, below 3% is low risk. It takes into account age, heart rate, SBP, creatinine, and the presence of ST deviation, troponin, cardiac arrest or LVF (Eagle et al. 2004).*

Reperfusion therapy indications and contraindications		
	Indications	**Contraindications**
Percutaneous coronary intervention (PCI) *Gold standard*	Any ACS: • STEMI (inc. any amount of ST-elevation/new LBBB) • NSTEMI • Unstable angina	• Significant comorbidities (relative contraindication)

Thrombolysis
 	
Rarely used now – only if PCI unavailable within 2 hours
	STEMI with:
	• ST-elevation in two contiguous ECG leads
	  ○ >1mm in limb leads
	  ○ >2mm in chest leads
	• Or, new LBBB
	• Many contraindications
		• Many contraindications related to bleeding risk
		
		Examples include: active internal bleeding, bleeding disorder, aortic dissection, stroke (haemorrhagic at any time or ischaemic <6 months), surgery/trauma <2 weeks, history of CNS bleed/aneurysm/neoplasm, GI bleed <1 month

<u>Other points</u>
- All patients should have an echo to assess LV function
- Check electrolytes regularly and ensure patients are on cardiac monitoring while in hospital
- STEMI patients with complete revascularisation may be discharged after 2-3 days; low risk NSTEMI patients with complete revascularisation may be discharged within 24 hours

LONG-TERM MANAGEMENT OF ACS

- β-blocker (reduces myocardial demand – continue for 12 months, or lifelong if LV systolic dysfunction)
- ACE inhibitor (prevents adverse cardiac remodelling)
- GTN spray PRN if required
- Aldosterone antagonist (eplerenone) if LV function ≤40%
- Cardiovascular risk reduction
  - Aspirin (lifelong) + clopidogrel/ticagrelor (12 months)
  - Statin
  - BP control
  - Lifestyle modifications/cardiac rehabilitation and smoking cessation

---

Include in assessment

- **12 lead ECG** (then continuous cardiac monitoring)
- **Bloods**: usual bloods (FBC, U&Es, LFTs, CRP, glucose) plus cardiac enzymes (STAT and again at 10-12 hours post-pain onset), magnesium, phosphate, lipid profile
- **Chest X-ray** (LVF signs, alternative cause of chest pain)

Types of ACS

- **STEMI**: ST-elevation or new LBBB
- **NSTEMI**: ACS without ST-elevation/new LBBB but with raised troponin at 12 hours
- **Unstable angina**: ACS without ST-elevation/new LBBB or raised troponin at 12 hours

ACUTE PULMONARY OEDEMA MANAGEMENT

ABCDE APPROACH

Follow usual ABCDE approach if critically ill.

INITIAL TREATMENT

P	**P**osition (sit up)
O	**O**xygen (high-flow)
D	**D**iuretic (furosemide IV)
M	**M**orphine (may be used to cause venodilation and reduce preload)
A	**A**nti-emetic (metoclopramide 10mg IV)
N	**N**itrates in severe pulmonary oedema (GTN infusion if SBP >110, or 2 puffs GTN spray if SBP >90)

FURTHER INTERVENTIONS IF REQUIRED

- Look for and treat any cause, e.g. surgery for acute aortic/mitral regurgitation, PCI for ACS, arrhythmia management, BP management if hypertensive crisis, pericardiocentesis if tamponade
- CPAP *if hypoxic despite above interventions*
- Inotropes ± intra-aortic balloon pump in ICU *if in cardiogenic shock* (*hypotension + overload*)

LONG-TERM HEART FAILURE TREATMENTS

- Treat cause where possible
- Pharmacological treatments
  - Core medications
    - ACE inhibitor (<u>or</u> angiotensin receptor blocker <u>or</u> angiotensin receptor-neprilysin inhibitor)
    - β-blocker
    - Diuretic (e.g. furosemide, bumetanide) *if peripheral/pulmonary oedema*
  - Other medications: add aldosterone antagonist (e.g. spironolactone, eplerenone) *if uncontrolled with core treatments*; add ivabradine *if in sinus rhythm ≥70 bpm despite maximum β-blocker dose*
- Non-pharmacological treatments
  - Cardiac resynchronisation therapy device: considered if QRS significantly prolonged
  - Implantable cardioverter defibrillator: considered if risk of ventricular arrhythmias

ARRHYTHMIA MANAGEMENT

Produced partly using UK Resuscitation Council 'Peri-arrest Arrhythmias' 2015

INITIAL APPROACH

- Follow usual **ABCDE approach** if critically ill

- **No pulse** – follow cardiac arrest ALS algorithm
- **Adverse signs**
  - Tachyarrhythmia → synchronised DC cardioversion
  - Bradycardia → atropine ± pacing
- **No adverse signs** – *see specific sections below*

> **Adverse signs**
>
> 1. Shock (SBP<90)
> 2. Syncope
> 3. Myocardial ischaemia (chest pain or on ECG)
> 4. Heart failure

- All arrhythmias
  - Apply 3-lead cardiac monitoring
  - Treat any reversible causes, e.g. electrolyte abnormalities
- Review ECG – determine type of arrhythmia
  - Tachycardia (HR > 100 bpm)
    - Narrow complex tachycardia (QRS < 120 ms/3 small squares)
    - Broad complex tachycardia (QRS > 120 ms/3 small squares)
  - Bradycardia (HR < 60 bpm)

NARROW COMPLEX TACHYCARDIAS

Caused by *supraventricular tachyarrhythmias.*

> **Unmasking rhythm**
>
> If the cause of a regular narrow complex tachycardia is unclear, you can unmask the rhythm by transiently increasing AV node block with vagal manoeuvres or adenosine while an recording a 3-lead cardiac tracing.

<u>Sinus</u>
- **Sinus tachycardia** (ECG: regular with P waves before each QRS complex) → *managed by treating cause*

<u>'Paroxysmal' SVT</u>
- **Atrial tachycardia** due to abnormal depolarising focus in atrium (ECG: regular with abnormal P waves)
- **AV <u>nodal</u> re-entry tachycardia/'AVNRT'** due to an entire re-entry conduction circuit in AV node (ECG regular, often without discernible P waves because they may be buried in the QRS)
- **AV re-entry tachycardia/'AVRT'** due to an accessory conduction pathway allowing conduction *re-entry* between atrium and ventricle, e.g. Wolff-Parkinson-White syndrome (ECG: regular, often without discernible P waves because they may be buried in the QRS or retrograde). *NB: this refers to orthodromic AVRT. Antidromic AVRT looks like and is treated like VT.*
→ *managed by: vagal manoeuvres (1ˢᵗ), adenosine (2ⁿᵈ; <u>not in asthma</u> – use Ca²⁺ channel blocker, e.g. verapamil), β-blocker (3ʳᵈ)*

<u>Atrial fibrillation /flutter</u>
- **Atrial fibrillation** due to fibrillating atria (ECG: irregular with no P waves)
- **Atrial flutter** due to fluttering atria (ECG: regular with saw-tooth baseline)
→ *managed by rate or rhythm control <u>and</u> treating cause <u>and</u> therapeutic anticoagulation (depending on CHADS2VASC score).*

Rate vs. rhythm control

Rate control if patient is >65 years <u>and</u> has IHD/no Sx/is not suitable for cardioversion: use β-blocker, rate-limiting Ca²⁺ channel blocker (e.g. diltiazem), or digoxin if sedentary lifestyle/heart failure/hypotension.

Rhythm control if the above does not apply: acutely if clear onset <48 hours ago or after 4 weeks therapeutic anticoagulation (and rate control) if not. Options include electrical cardioversion or pharmacological cardioversion (using flecainide, or amiodarone if structural heart disease).

BROAD COMPLEX TACHYCARDIAS

May be caused by *ventricular tachyarrhythmias* or *supraventricular tachyarrhythmias* with abnormal conduction.

> **Broad complex tachycardias of supraventricular origin**
>
> - Mimic VT
> - The broad complex is caused by a pre-existing condition such as BBB
> - The tachycardia is of supraventricular origin
> - More likely supraventricular if: previous ECG with bundle branch block, delta waves (Wolff-Parkinson-White syndrome), same shape QRS or irregular QRS
> - Not supraventricular if: QRS >160ms, left axis deviation, AV dissociation

<u>Ventricular tachyarrhythmias</u>
- **Monomorphic VT** due to an abnormal depolarising focus in ventricles or a re-entry circuit within the ventricles (ECG: regular broad complex tachycardia) → *managed with amiodarone*
- **Polymorphic VT/'***Torsades de pointes***'** due to prolonged ventricular repolarisation, which is predisposed to by ↑QT (ECG: VT with varying amplitude) → *managed with magnesium sulphate*

<u>Broad complex tachycardias of supraventricular origin (treat as VT if unsure)</u>
- **Supraventricular tachyarrhythmia with aberrant conduction**, e.g. SVT or AF with L/RBBB (ECG: looks like VT but *see box* for how to distinguish; irregular if due to AF) → *treat as supraventricular*
- **Atrial fibrillation/flutter with pre-excitation**, e.g. in Wolff-Parkinson-White syndrome (ECG: irregular broad complex tachycardia and with different size complexes due to different AV conduction pathways) → *managed with flecainide or synchronised DC cardioversion (<u>don't</u> use AV nodal blocking medications – they will increase accessory path conduction and may cause VF)*

BRADYCARDIAS

Bradycardias at risk of asystole
1. Recent asystole
2. Mobitz II AV block
3. Complete heart block with broad QRS
4. Ventricular pauses >3 seconds

Differentials

- **Sinus bradycardia** may be caused by: drugs (e.g. β-blockers, digitalis), neutrally mediated syndromes (e.g. carotid sinus hypersensitivity, vasovagal syncope), hypothermia, hypothyroidism, SA node dysfunction
- **SA node dysfunction ('sick sinus syndrome')** may result in: sinus bradycardia, sinus pauses, or sinoatrial arrest with an 'escape rhythm'. Escape rhythms may be initiated by the AV node (ECG: 'junctional rhythm' – no p waves but normal QRS at 40-60bpm) or ventricles (ECG: 'ventricular escape rhythm' – no p waves and abnormal broad QRS at 20-40bpm)
- **AV node dysfunction ('heart block'):** 2nd degree or complete heart block (*see interpretation notes on ECGs p246*)

Management

- Treat cause
- If adverse signs present:
    1. Atropine
    2. If ongoing haemodynamic compromise or bradycardia is at risk of asystole (*see box*), transvenous pacing is required. In the interim, further atropine, transcutaneous pacing or infusion of isoprenaline/adrenaline may be required.
- If neither adverse signs nor risk of asystole: observe and treat cause if possible
    - Indications for permanent pacing: Mobitz type II second degree heart block, complete heart block, symptomatic bradycardias (e.g. sick sinus syndrome), symptomatic pauses (>3 secs), trifascicular block with syncope/pre-syncope

Practical aspects

Drug doses to memorise

- **Adenosine** 6mg IV (can be followed by 12mg then another 12mg if unsuccessful) *flushed quickly wide-bore cannula in the antecubital fossa*
- **Amiodarone** 300mg IV over 20-60 minutes followed by 900mg over 24 hours through a large vein (ideally central venous catheter)
- **Atropine** 500mcg IV (repeat every 3-5 minutes to maximum of 3mg if needed)
- **Magnesium sulphate** 2g IV over 10-15 minutes

Placement of 3-lead cardiac monitoring and anterior-posterior (AP) defibrillator pads

- 3-lead cardiac monitoring (clockwise from right arm: **Ride Your Green Bicycle**)
    - **Red**: anterior aspect of right shoulder
    - **Yellow**: anterior aspect of left shoulder
    - **Green**: left anterior superior iliac spine
    - **Black**: not present on defibrillation machine (would go on right anterior superior iliac spine)
- AP defibrillation pads
    - 'Right' pad: place longitudinally on left sternal edge
    - 'Left' pad: place longitudinally on left paraspinal muscles (in line with anterior pad)

Synchronised DC Cardioversion

- Anaesthetist/sedation-trained doctor should be present to sedate patient
- Apply 3-lead cardiac monitoring and connect lead to external monitor or defibrillator machine
- Apply defibrillator pads (AP position if atrial dysrhythmia; in anterolateral position if ventricular) after shaving chest if required
- Connect pads lead to defibrillator machine
- Set defibrillator machine monitoring trace to 'pads'
- Set defibrillator to synchronised mode (synchronises shock with R wave to avoid inducing VF)
- Set energy level (increase as shown if unsuccessful) – *energy protocols vary depending on defibrillator and hospital policy*
    - Broad-complex tachycardia or AF: **150J → 200J → 200J** (biphasic)
    - Narrow complex tachycardia or atrial flutter: **70J → 100J → 150J** (biphasic)
- Ask anaesthetist to sedate patient and wait until they are happy to proceed
- Ask for oxygen to be removed and everybody to move away from the patient
- Press 'charge', then move hand away from button
- Re-check everybody (and oxygen) is away from the patient, announce you are about to shock and, while looking at the patient, hold down the 'shock' button until the shock is delivered – it will wait for the R wave
- Re-assess the rhythm and pulse (even if patient reverts to sinus rhythm, ensure you feel pulse to check it is not PEA)
    - If unsuccessful, repeat at next energy
    - If successful, reassess patient (ABCDE) and perform another ECG to check rhythm and for any signs of ischaemia
- If cardioversion fails and the patient is unstable, give amiodarone 300 mg IV over 10–20 min and re-attempt electrical cardioversion
- Give all patients who are not anticoagulated therapeutic LMWH or heparin infusion, and continue anticoagulation for at least 4 weeks
- *NB: the above is for patients with a pulse. If pulseless, follow cardiac arrest ALS algorithm.*

Transcutaneous pacing

- A conscious patient will require some sedation (ask anaesthetist/sedation-trained doctor)
- Apply the defibrillator machine's 3-lead cardiac monitoring and defibrillator pads (in standard position) after shaving chest if required
- Ask sedating doctor to sedate patient and wait until they are happy to proceed
- Set defibrillator to pacing (NB: synchronous/demand mode means pacing will only occur if no complex is sensed within given time period; asynchronous/fixed rate mode means pacing will occur at programmed rate regardless of complexes – *demand mode usually used*)
- Set onscreen pacing rate (default usually 70bpm) and energy (default starting energy usually 30mA)
- Press button to start pacing
- Observe the monitor to see if QRS complexes follow every pacing spike. If not, gradually increase the energy until they do – *electrical capture* (usually occurs at 50-100mA).
- Next check the patient's pulse corresponds to the induced QRS complexes – *mechanical capture*. Now increase the energy by 10mA further.
- Now seek definitive management   *NB: you can touch the patient during pacing*

amazon.co.uk

SD3y9qhYHm

D3y9qhYHm/-1 of 1-/pri-eu-ag-world/0 A3

Packing slip for

Your order of 02 November 2020

Order ID 026-7147368-5095528

Packing slip number D3y9qhYHm

Shipping date 02 November 2020

Qty.	Item	Bin
	The OSCE Revision Guide for Medical Students Paperback, Mansbridge, Christopher, X00107GEPF : CQ-EFSB- ZA20: 9781999719807	

This shipment completes your order.

You can always check the status of your orders or change your account details from the "Your Account" link at the top of each page on our site.

Thinking of returning an item? PLEASE USE OUR ON-LINE RETURNS SUPPORT CENTRE.

Our Returns Support Centre (www.amazon.co.uk/returns-support) will guide you through our Returns Policy and provide you with a printable personalised return label. Please have your order number ready (you can find it next to your order summary, above). Our Returns Policy does not affect your statutory rights.

0/D3y9qhYHm/-1 of 1-//LH-LCY8/pri-eu-ag-world/0/1103-03:45/1102-23:05 Pack Type : A3

Adult Bradycardia Algorithm

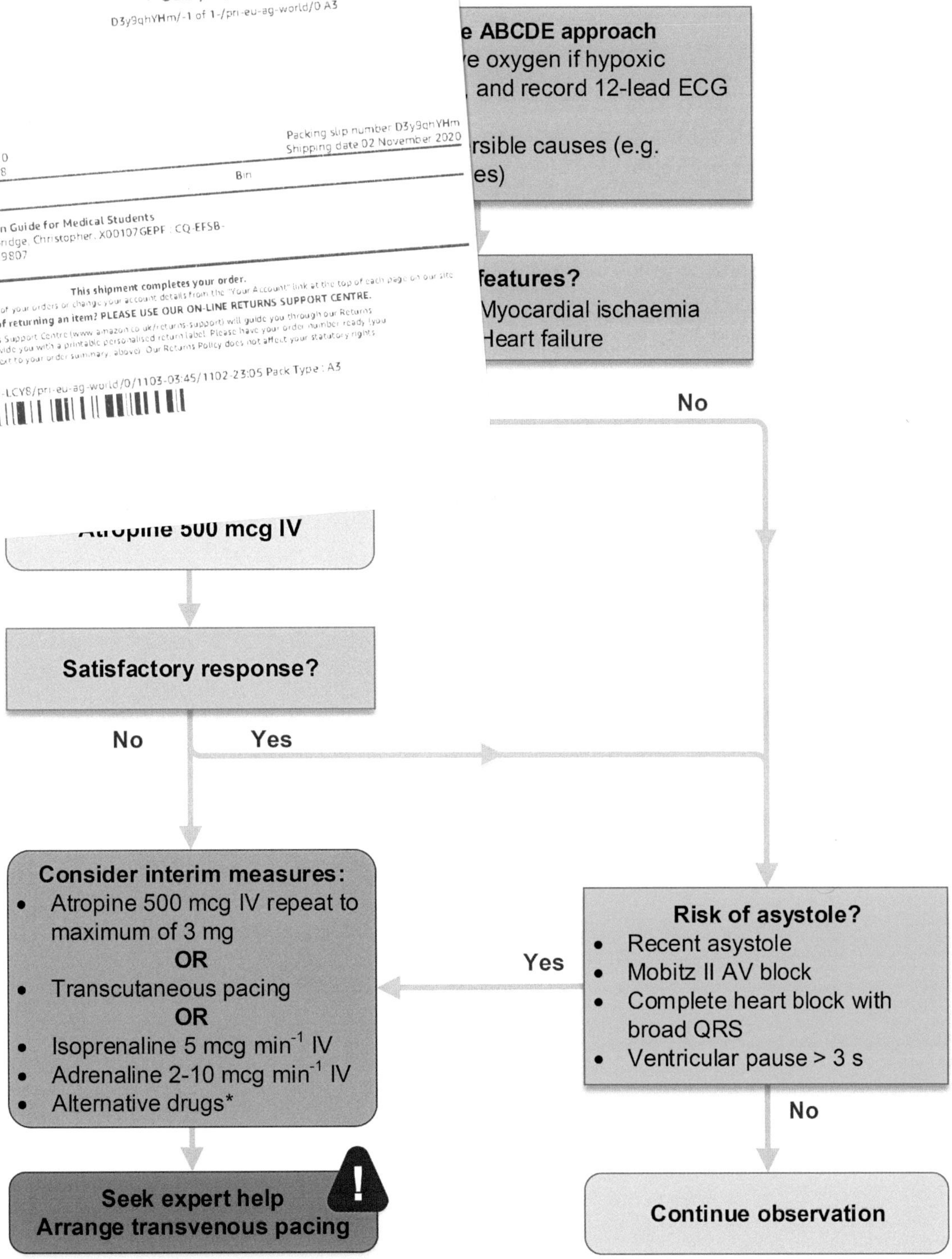

e ABCDE approach
e oxygen if hypoxic
, and record 12-lead ECG
rsible causes (e.g.
es)
features?
Myocardial ischaemia
Heart failure
No
Atropine 500 mcg IV
Satisfactory response?
No
Yes
Consider interim measures:
Atropine 500 mcg IV repeat to maximum of 3 mg
OR
Transcutaneous pacing
OR
Isoprenaline 5 mcg min-1 IV
Adrenaline 2-10 mcg min-1 IV
Alternative drugs*
Seek expert help
Arrange transvenous pacing
Yes
Risk of asystole?
Recent asystole
Mobitz II AV block
Complete heart block with broad QRS
Ventricular pause > 3 s
No
Continue observation

*** Alternatives include:**

- Aminophylline
- Dopamine
- Glucagon (if bradycardia is caused by beta-blocker or calcium channel blocker)
- Glycopyrrolate (may be used instead of atropine)

Resuscitation Council (UK)

GUIDELINES 2015

Adult Tachycardia (with pulse) Algorithm

Assess using the ABCDE approach
- Monitor SpO$_2$ and give oxygen if hypoxic
- Monitor ECG and BP, and record 12-lead ECG
- Obtain IV access
- Identify and treat reversible causes (e.g. electrolyte abnormalities)

Adverse features?
- Shock
- Syncope
- Myocardial ischaemia
- Heart failure

Yes - Unstable

Synchronised DC Shock*
Up to 3 attempts

Seek expert help

- Amiodarone 300 mg IV over 10-20 min
- Repeat shock
- Then give amiodarone 900 mg over 24 h

No - Stable

Is QRS narrow (< 0.12 s)?

Broad

Broad QRS
Is QRS regular?

Irregular

Seek expert help

Possibilities include:
AF with bundle branch block
- treat as for narrow complex
- Pre-excited AF
- consider amiodarone

Regular

- **If VT (or uncertain rhythm):**
  Amiodarone 300 mg IV over 20-60 min then 900 mg over 24 h
- **If known to be SVT with bundle branch block:**
  Treat as for regular narrow-complex tachycardia

Narrow

Narrow QRS
Is rhythm regular?

Irregular

Seek expert help

Probable AF:
- Control rate with beta-blocker or diltiazem
- If in heart failure consider digoxin or amiodarone
- Assess thromboembolic risk and consider anticoagulation

Possible atrial flutter:
- Control rate (e.g. with beta-blocker)

Regular

- Vagal manoeuvres
- Adenosine 6 mg rapid IV bolus
  if no effect give 12 mg
  if no effect give further 12 mg
- Monitor/record ECG continuously

Sinus rhythm achieved?

Yes

Probable re-entry paroxysmal SVT:
- Record 12-lead ECG in sinus rhythm
- If SVT recurs treat again and consider anti-arrhythmic prophylaxis

No

Seek expert help

*Conscious patients require sedation or general anaesthesia for cardioversion

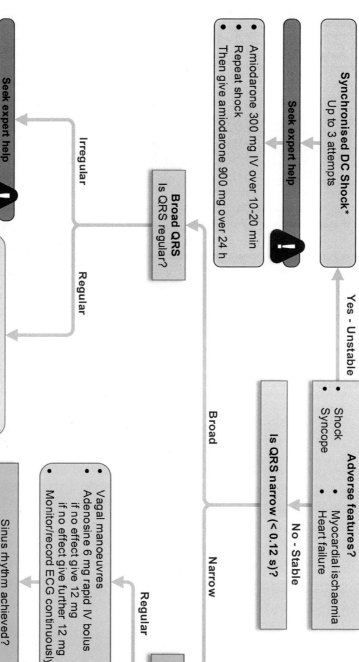

ASSESSMENT AND MANAGEMENT OF THE ACUTE ABDOMEN

	Peritonitis/perforation	Ruptured AAA	Renal colic	Appendicitis	Gallstones	Acute pancreatitis	Gastritis/peptic ulcer	Diverticulitis	Bowel obstruction	Ectopic pregnancy
Common differentials	• Perforated viscus (e.g. peptic ulcer, colonic tumour, diverticulum, gallbladder, appendix, spleen, AAA, ectopic)	• Other peritonitis causes	• Pyelonephritis • Biliary colic	• Meckel's diverticulum • Crohn's disease • Mesenteric adenitis • Ovarian cyst rupture/torsion/haemorrhage • Ectopic pregnancy		• Gastritis • Cholecystitis	• Pancreatitis • Cholecystitis	• Diverticular cyst • Diverticulosis • Mesenteric ischaemia • IBS • Ovarian cyst rupture/torsion/haemorrhage	• Gastroenteritis	• Appendicitis • Pelvic inflammatory disease • Meckel's diverticulum • Crohn's disease • Mesenteric adenitis • Ovarian cyst rupture/torsion/haemorrhage
Classical history	• Severe generalised abdominal pain	• Elderly • Severe generalised abdominal pain • Back pain • Reduced GCS/collapse	• Spasms of loin to groin pain (excruciating) • Nausea and vomiting • Cannot lie still	• Young patient • Periumbilical pain • Moves to RIF • Anorexia/nausea • Fever	<u>Biliary colic</u> • Severe intermittent RUQ/epigastric pain • Exacerbated by fatty food <u>Cholecystitis</u> • Continuous RUQ/epigastric pain • Murphy's +ve • Tenderness and guarding RUQ <u>CBD stones</u> • Jaundice • RUQ pain	• Severe epigastric/central pain • Radiating to back • Relieved by sitting forwards • Vomiting	• Epigastric pain • Related to meals	• Elderly • LIF pain • Pyrexia • Diarrhoea common	• Vomiting + abdominal pain + no bowel motions	• Increasing iliac fossa/pelvic pain • Around 6 weeks pregnant/not using contraception • May have spotting
Classical examination	• No movement with respiration • Guarding • Firm, peritonitic abdomen • Rebound and percussion tenderness • Severe pain to light palpation	• Hypotension • Peritonitis • Expansile mass	• Soft non-tender abdomen • May be renal angle tenderness	• Tender RIF • Worse at McBurney's point • Guarding/local peritonitis • Rovsing's +ve	<u>Cholangitis</u> • Jaundice • Fever/rigors • RUQ pain	• Epigastric tenderness • Tachycardia • Fever • Shock • Grey-Turner's and Cullen's signs (rare)	• Tender epigastrium • Soft abdomen	• Tender LIF • Guarding/local peritonitis • PR (confirm no malignancy/abscess)	• Distended, tender abdomen • Tinkling bowel sounds	• Tenderness RIF/LIF • Guarding • Adnexal tenderness • Cervical excitation
Standard investigations	• Bloods (including FBC, U&E, LFT, CRP, amylase, INR, G&S) + blood culture if pyrexia • Urine dip ± culture • βHCG (if female)									
Specific investigations	• Erect CXR (if any suspicion) • <u>Urgent CT abdomen/pelvis</u> (help determine cause)	• Bedside USS if freely available • CT angiography	• X-ray KUB • CT KUB	• None if very likely • USS abdomen/pelvis if gynaecological differentials	• Abdominal USS • CT if percutaneous biliary drainage or cholecystostomy required	• Amylase/lipase 3x upper limit of normal range (but not always) • No imaging needed to confirm if very likely e.g. amylase >1000 (300-1000 could be due to other causes e.g. cholecystitis, perf) • CT abdomen if uncertainty • Apache II/Glasgow score • Confirm cause ↘USS abdomen (exclude gallstones in all) ↘Triglycerides ↘Immunoglobulins	• OGD ± biopsy	• CT abdomen/pelvis (if needed)	• AXR • Then CT abdomen/pelvis • Gastrografin study may be used in SBO	• Serum βHCG + trend • Transvaginal USS
General management	• IV fluids, consider catheter and NG tube • Analgesia (paracetamol IV/PO, codeine PO, tramadol PO, morphine IV/IM/SC) and anti-emetics • VTE prophylaxis (anti-embolism stockings + LMWH unless theatre planned <2 hours) • If may require surgery: ↘NBM ↘Check INR and G&S ↘Stop anticoagulants/antiplatelets/diabetic medications									
Management	• 2 wide-bore IV cannulas • <u>Urgent surgical repair</u> • Consider patient comorbidities and chance of survival	• 2 wide-bore IV cannulas • Aim for permissive hypotension (SBP 100) • Activate 'massive haemorrhage protocol' e.g. 10 units • <u>Urgent open repair</u> (/endovascular aneurysm repair if stable)	• Diclofenac analgesia • IV fluids/hydration • Antibiotics if infection • Removal ↘<1cm – smooth muscle relaxants (e.g. tamsulosin) ↘>1cm – uteroscopy/ESWL ↘>2cm in renal pelvis – percutaneous nephrolithotomy • Ureteric stent/nephrostomy if obstruction	• Urgent laparoscopy/appendicectomy	<u>Biliary colic</u> • Outpatient cholecystectomy • Analgesia and fat-free diet <u>Cholecystitis</u> • Antibiotics • Cholecystectomy (hot if mild, after 6 weeks if not) <u>Common bile duct stone</u> • Continuous IV fluids • ERCP <u>Cholangitis</u> • IV antibiotics • Treat cause	• Supportive management • Aggressive fluid resuscitation with Hartmann's solution e.g. 1L every 4h (third space sequestration) – titrate to UO • NBM until nausea/pain improve (enteric feeding if prolonged) • No antibiotics unless proven infection, gas on CT or raised procalcitonin • Treat cause/stop causative medications • ICU may be required	• Proton pump inhibitor (IV/PO) • H. Pylori eradication (if +ve)	• Clear fluids only initially, then gradually build up over 2-3 days • Antibiotics	• NBM • Wide-bore NG tube (free drainage) • IV fluid hydration • Laparoscopy/laparotomy (if complete or non-resolving partial obstruction)	• 2 wide-bore IV cannulas • Laparoscopic salpingostomy/salpingectomy (or methotrexate if uncomplicated) • Anti-D prophylaxis (if required)

UPPER GI BLEED MANAGEMENT

ABCDE MANAGEMENT

- Follow usual ABCDE approach
    - IV fluid resuscitation (aim for systolic blood pressure ~100)
    - In massive blood loss, transfuse blood, FFP and platelets as per local massive haemorrhage protocol
    - Blood transfusion if Hb <7g/L in variceal bleed or <8g/L in non-variceal bleed
    - The patient must be haemodynamically stable before endoscopy

> **Include in assessment**
>
> - **Examination**: ensure you look for signs of common causes (e.g. chronic/decompensated liver disease) and do PR exam (for melaena)
> - **Bloods**: G&S/crossmatch, FBC (blood loss), U&Es (↑urea in GI bleeds), LFTs (varices risk), clotting (coagulopathy common in liver disease), glucose
> - **Catheterise** (monitor UO)
> - **CXR and AXR** once stable (e.g. for aspiration, obstruction)
> - **OGD**
> - **Observations**: check regularly

SPECIFIC TREATMENT

- **Acute variceal bleed** (suggested by history/signs of chronic liver disease):
    - Terlipressin (splanchnic vasoconstrictor that reduces portal blood flow) – *give before endoscopy*
    - Prophylactic IV antibiotics
    - Endoscopic intervention
        - Variceal band ligation
        - Sclerotherapy
    - Other possible interventions
        - Balloon tamponade with Sengstaken-Blakemore tube
- **Non-variceal bleed** (e.g. peptic ulcer, Mallory-Weiss tear, oesophagitis):
    - Endoscopic intervention
        - Adrenaline injection to peptic ulcer
    - Pharmacological intervention
        - IV proton pump inhibitor – *give after endoscopy* (unless haemodynamically unstable)
        - Other treatments used occasionally (e.g. tranexamic acid)
- **In all patients:**
    - Keep NBM
    - Correct any clotting abnormalities
        - ↓Platelets <50x10^9/L: platelet transfusion
        - On warfarin: prothrombin complex concentrate + vitamin K
        - On direct oral anticoagulant: Praxbind for dabigatran; consider prothrombin complex concentrate for others
        - Coagulopathic for other reasons (e.g. in liver cirrhosis): vitamin K ± FFP
        - ↓Fibrinogen <1g/L: cryoprecipitate
    - Stop any antiplatelets or anticoagulants
    - Treat any concurrent issues, e.g. encephalopathy, alcohol withdrawal

SCORING SYSTEMS

- **Glasgow-Blatchford score** (pre-endoscopy): assesses likelihood patient will need intervention (score 0 = manage as outpatient; score ≥1 = manage as inpatient). Takes into account haemoglobin, urea, SBP, sex, HR, presence of melaena, recent syncope, history of liver disease or heart failure (Blatchford et al. 2000).
- **Rockall score** (post-endoscopy): mortality risk assessment (score ≤2 = good prognosis; score >8 = high mortality risk). Takes into account age, shock, comorbidities, diagnosis and evidence of bleeding (Rockall et al. 1996).

PREVENTING FURTHER BLEEDING

Treat the cause/reduce the risk of re-bleeding:
- **Oesophageal varices**
    1. Propranolol (β-blocker that reduces portal venous pressure)
    2. Variceal banding
    3. Transjugular Intrahepatic Portosystemic Shunt Stent (TIPSS) – allows blood to flow out of the portal system into a hepatic vein
    4. Liver transplant
- **Peptic ulcer**
    - Proton pump inhibitor
    - *H. pylori* eradication if +ve
    - Avoid precipitants, e.g. NSAIDs

DIABETIC KETOACIDOSIS (DKA)

In DKA, a relative lack of insulin results in hyperglycaemia as cells are unable to take up glucose – *starvation in the midst of plenty*. This causes cells to switch to a fatty acid metabolism, resulting in the production of acidic ketones.

<table>
<tr><td>Normal values (mmol/L)</td></tr>
<tr><td>Non-diabetic (random) = 4-7.8
Type 1 diabetic = 4-9
Type 2 diabetic = 4-8.5
Hyperglycaemia = >11
Hypoglycaemia = <4
Normal capillary ketones = <0.6</td></tr>
</table>

1. ABCDE

- Follow usual ABCDE approach

2. Confirm diagnosis

- Ensure you include VBG, capillary/urine ketones and glucose measurement
- Confirm diagnosis (all of):
  - **Glucose > 11mmol/L (or known diabetes)**
  - **pH < 7.3 *or* HCO₃⁻ < 15**
  - **Capillary ketones >3mmol/L *or* ++ urinary ketones**

3. Intravenous fluids

NB: dehydration is more lethal than hyperglycaemia.

- 1L saline over 1 hour (or faster if hypotensive) – without potassium
- 1L saline over 2 hours
- 1L saline over 2 hours
- 1L saline over 4 hours
- 1L saline over 4 hours
- 1L saline over 6 hours
- 1L saline over 6 hours

After the 1ˢᵗ litre, add potassium chloride to each litre depending on VBG results:
K+ <4.5mmol/L = 40mmmol KCl
K+ 4.5-5.5mmol/L = 20mmol KCl
K+ > 5.5 = nil

4. Fixed rate insulin infusion

- IV insulin infusion **0.1unit/kg/hour** from 50 units human soluble rapid-acting insulin (e.g. Actrapid) in 50ml 0.9% saline
  NB: maximum rate is 15 units per hour.
- When capillary glucose is <14mmol/L, give 10% IV glucose at 125ml/hour *in addition* to the 0.9% saline – but reduce the saline rate to account for extra fluid. Glucose is used so that insulin can continue to drive more glucose into cells to reduce ketosis and acid production.

5. Investigation to find cause

- History
- Top to tail examination (including for diabetic feet)
- Bloods (FBC, glucose, U&Es, LFTs, osmolality, CRP)
- Blood culture
- MSU
- Chest X-ray

6. Other priorities

- Treat the cause
- Consider intensive care if: ketones >6, HCO₃⁻ < 5/pH<7.1, GCS <12, SBP<90, sats <92% or HR >100/<60
- Continue patient's long-acting insulin throughout and start long-acting insulin (Lantus or Levemir 0.25 units/kg once daily s/c) if it is a new presentation
- Check **VBGs 2-hourly** to assess acid-base balance, potassium and glucose
  - Aim to increase HCO₃⁻ by 3mmol/hour, reduce glucose by 3mmol/hour and reduce ketones by 0.5mmol/L/hour
  - Insulin can be increased by 1 unit/hour if target is not reached
- When the acid-base abnormality is fully corrected (i.e. **pH >7.3**) and **capillary ketones are <0.6mmol/L** (normally takes 24-48 hours) and the patient is eating and drinking, restart their normal insulin regimen at a mealtime
- If abnormal physiology is corrected but the patient is still not eating and drinking, start a variable rate insulin infusion
- Ensure VTE prophylaxis is prescribed
- Consider NG tube (aspiration is a common cause of death)
- Education and medication review

HYPEROSMOLAR HYPERGLYCAEMIC STATE

Hyperglycaemia develops slowly as a result of illness/dehydration and causes hyperosmolarity in the intravascular compartment and severe cellular dehydration. Notably, there is no acidosis/ketones because basal insulin levels allow sufficient cellular glucose uptake. The main dangers are dehydration and a prothrombotic state.

Confirm diagnosis
- Confirm diagnosis
    - Marked hyperglycaemia (≥30mmol/L) without ketosis
    - Serum osmolality ≥320mmol/L
    - Hypovolaemia

Management
- Rehydrate with 0.9% saline (*give fluids at the same rate as in DKA*)
- VTE prophylaxis (high risk of VTE)
- Start IV insulin infusion at 0.05units/kg/hour if glucose is not falling with fluids alone
- Look for cause
- Hold metformin for 2 days (it causes a metabolic acidosis)

HYPERGLYCAEMIA WITHOUT DKA

- Rehydrate if necessary
- STAT dose of rapid-acting (e.g. Novorapid) or short-acting (e.g. Actrapid) insulin dose can be used
    - Type 1: 1 unit decreases blood glucose by 3mmol/L (aim glucose <12mmol/L)
    - Type 2 (more insulin resistant): 0.1unit/kg (aim glucose <14mmol/L)
- Identify and correct cause (and check patient has taken insulin normally)
- Adjust normal insulin regimen as necessary
- Recheck glucose in 1 hour and reassess

HYPOGLYCAEMIA

A dangerous medical emergency!
- **Unconscious**
    - 150ml 10% glucose or 75ml 20% glucose IV STAT (repeat as necessary)
    - Glucagon 1mg IM if no IV access (can only be repeated 1-2 times)
    - Check capillary glucose 10 minutes later, repeat as needed and give long-acting carbohydrate when able to swallow
- **Conscious but cannot swallow**
    - 1.5-2 tubes glucose gel around teeth if mild and patient conscious
    - Check capillary glucose 10 minutes later and give long-acting carbohydrate when able to swallow
- **Can swallow:**
    - 15-30g fast-acting carbohydrate (e.g. 5-7 glucose tablets, 150ml fruit juice/Lucozade)
    - AND long-acting carbohydrates (e.g. biscuits, toast)
- **All:**
    - Correct cause
    - Don't omit insulin/tablets afterwards (risk of rebound hyperglycaemia) – reduce dose instead

---

Common causes of hyperglycaemia

- DKA
- Hyperosmolar hyperglycaemic state
- Sepsis
- Steroids
- Missed hypoglycaemics/insulin
- Pancreatitis
- Dehydration
- Last meal/feeds

Common causes of hypoglycaemia

Not enough going in
- Poor oral intake
- Vomiting

More going out
- Insulin excess/sulfonylureas
- ↓renal function (and hence ↓drug excretion)
- Alcohol
- Abrupt steroid discontinuation

STROKE AND TIA MANAGEMENT

INCLUDE IN ASSESSMENT

- **History**
  - Exact onset/when last well; any change/progression in symptoms; risk factors (e.g. smoking, hypertension, cardiovascular disease, AF)
- **Examination**
  - Full neurological exam
  - Systemic: pulse (AF), heart sounds, carotid bruits, bruising/bleeding
  - Risk factor signs: xanthelasma, corneal arcus

MANAGEMENT ALGORITHM

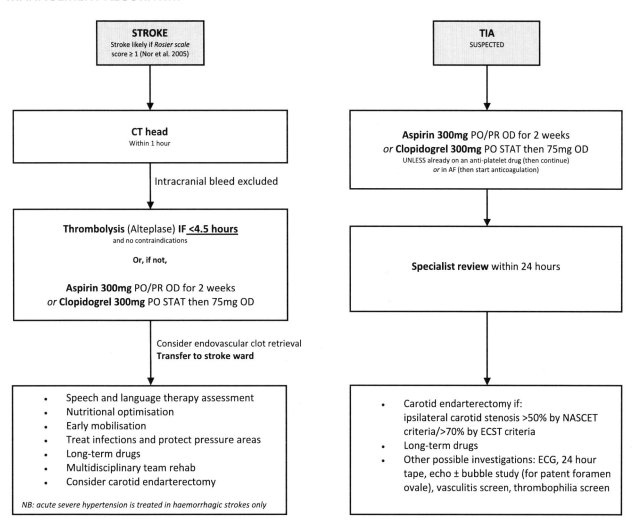

STROKE
Stroke likely if *Rosier scale* score ≥ 1 (Nor et al. 2005)

TIA
SUSPECTED

CT head
Within 1 hour

Intracranial bleed excluded

Thrombolysis (Alteplase) **IF <4.5 hours**
and no contraindications

Or, if not,

Aspirin 300mg PO/PR OD for 2 weeks
or **Clopidogrel 300mg** PO STAT then 75mg OD

Consider endovascular clot retrieval
Transfer to stroke ward

- Speech and language therapy assessment
- Nutritional optimisation
- Early mobilisation
- Treat infections and protect pressure areas
- Long-term drugs
- Multidisciplinary team rehab
- Consider carotid endarterectomy

NB: acute severe hypertension is treated in haemorrhagic strokes only

Aspirin 300mg PO/PR OD for 2 weeks
or **Clopidogrel 300mg** PO STAT then 75mg OD
UNLESS already on an anti-platelet drug (then continue)
or in AF (then start anticoagulation)

Specialist review within 24 hours

- Carotid endarterectomy if:
  ipsilateral carotid stenosis >50% by NASCET criteria/>70% by ECST criteria
- Long-term drugs
- Other possible investigations: ECG, 24 hour tape, echo ± bubble study (for patent foramen ovale), vasculitis screen, thrombophilia screen

LONG-TERM DRUGS

- **Antihypertensives**
- **Clopidogrel 75mg OD** (or anticoagulation if patient is in AF – *but wait 2 weeks after stroke*)
- **Statin** – *but wait 48 hours after stroke*

DVLA advice

- No driving for 4 weeks
- Need to tell DVLA if: HGV driver *or* still having symptoms after 4 weeks *or* complications (seizures, neurosurgery, crescendo TIA)

SEIZURE MANAGEMENT

INITIAL ABCDE-STYLE MANAGEMENT

- Recovery position
- Maintain airway with jaw-thrust
- Consider nasopharyngeal airway if airway concerns (not oropharyngeal airway due to trismus)
- 15L oxygen via non-rebreather mask
- Secure IV access
- Attach monitoring (pulse oximetry, blood pressure, cardiac monitor)

Include in assessment

- **Capillary glucose**
- **Venous blood gas** (to measure lactate and acidosis) and **venous bloods** including FBC, U&Es/Ca^{2+} (look for electrolyte abnormalities), anti-epileptic drug levels, clotting
- **ECG** (look for prolonged QT interval)
- **Further investigations** (if cause unknown):
  - CT/MRI brain (look for any focal lesions or bleed)
  - Electroencephalogram (EEG)
  - Lumbar puncture (if meningitis/ encephalitis suspected)

PHARMACOLOGICAL SEIZURE MANAGEMENT

IF SEIZURE ONGOING, WITHIN:
10 minutes: 4mg lorazepam IV **OR** 10mg diazepam PR
20 minutes: repeat above
30 minutes: phenytoin 18mg/kg IV (max. 2g; at 50mg/minute with cardiac monitoring)
60 minutes: general anaesthesia in intensive care unit

Also: 50ml 50% glucose IV if any suggestion of hypoglycaemia
Also: Pabrinex 2 pairs IV if any suggestion of alcohol abuse

AFTER PATIENT HAS RECOVERED CONSCIOUSNESS

- Post-ictal period may last a few hours
- Find cause
  - Full history
  - Multi-system examination (including full neurological exam)
  - Complete any outstanding investigations above
- Treat cause
- Refer to medical team/neurology or seizure clinic
- Give driving advice and instruct patient to inform DVLA

COMMON CAUSES OF SEIZURES

- **Neurological:** epilepsy (idiopathic or secondary), SOL, meningitis/encephalitis, post-stroke, head trauma, congenital abnormalities/perinatal hypoxia
- **Metabolic:** hypoglycaemia, hyperuricaemia, electrolyte abnormalities
- **Drugs:** overdoses, drugs of abuse, alcohol withdrawal, toxins
- **Febrile convulsion**
- **Eclampsia**

WOUND MANAGEMENT

Include in assessment

• **Who** – age, job, hobbies, hand dominance (if hand/arm involved)
• **What** happened, exact mechanism, force
• **When/where/why** it happened
• Do a thorough wound examination after cleaning, looking for deep structure damage
• Assess for **contamination**
• Check **tendon function**
• Check **neurovascular** status distally
• Check **tetanus vaccination status**
• **X-ray** if any risk of fracture or foreign body

INITIAL APPROACH

- Use an **advanced trauma life support/ABCDE** approach in life-threatening wounds
- Severe haemorrhage may require pressure, elevation and use of a tourniquet or arterial clamp/suture

CLEAN AND DEBRIDE WOUND

- **Clean wound and area** using multiple sterile gauze soaked in sterile saline
- **Anaesthetise:** infiltrate 1% lidocaine subcutaneously around wound edges
- **Mechanical cleansing (debridement):** remove any debris/contamination/foreign bodies/dead tissue. Use sterile gauze soaked in saline to scrub; and forceps and a scalpel to excise tissue if required.
- **Pressure irrigation** (*can omit if wound is clean*): squirt sterile saline into the wound using pressure (from syringe via green needle or from pressure infusion bag via orange cannula)
- **Deep inspection:** thoroughly **re-inspect** the whole of the wound (may need wound edge retraction), look at **deep structures** as able, and ask the patient attempt **full range of movement** to help look for tendon damage
- Perform any further cleansing/irrigation if required – some wounds require more thorough debridement:
  - **Wound debridement under general anaesthesia** is required if large, extensive debris, lots of necrotic skin, dead muscle, contamination, underlying fracture or neurovascular compromise
  - **Urgent surgical exploration** is required if there is any possibility of nerve/vessel/tendon/organ damage

CLOSURE OPTIONS

- **Immediate primary closure:** immediate closure with sutures/clips/Steri-Strips/glue. This is only used if there is negligible skin loss, the wound is clean with no foreign bodies, <12 hours old (<24 hours for face wounds), and the edges come together easily without tension.
- **Delayed primary closure:** wound cleaned thoroughly, then dressed and left open for 48 hours. The wound is then reviewed for signs of infection, swelling and bleeding. If these are absent and the wound edges can be opposed without tension, the wound is sutured closed. This is used for contaminated wounds, contused/bruised wounds, infected wounds, or wounds >12 hours old. Antimicrobial dressings and prophylactic antibiotics should also be used for contaminated/infected wounds.
- **Secondary intention:** allow wound to close by itself, i.e. by granulation, epithelialisation and scarring. This is used for wounds with tissue loss preventing edge approximation, chronic ulcers and partial-thickness burns.
- **Skin grafts:** for significant skin loss (including most full-thickness burns)

OTHER ASPECTS TO MANAGEMENT

Never close a contaminated wound

- Infected or contaminated wounds require **antibiotics**
- Consider **tetanus booster/immunoglobulin** if patient is not up to date with tetanus vaccines (5 total) or high-risk wound
- Consider **rabies immunoglobulin** if high risk wound in high risk area
- **Analgesia**, e.g. Entonox, morphine IV, regional anaesthesia
- If swelling likely – **rest, ice, elevation** for 24 hours
- Select appropriate **dressing** (a primary dressing is placed directly on wound and a secondary dressing is placed over this to provide further protection)
- Consider correcting any factors which may hinder wound healing, e.g. stop smoking/NSAIDs, give nutritional supplements

FOLLOW UP

- Give patient wound advice
- Injured limbs need elevation for 24-48 hours
- Arrange follow-up for: wounds for delayed primary closure (to close), diabetic or immunocompromised patients (to review healing), burns (to look for infection)
- Suture removal:

Head and face	5 days
Upper limb/trunk/abdomen	7 days
Lower limb/diabetic/immunocompromised	10 days

WOUNDS REQUIRING SPECIAL MANAGEMENT

Burns

- **Initial assessment**
    - Test sensation, blanching and check tetanus status
    - Determine the **% body surface area** involved using *rule of 9's* (head 9%, arm 9%, leg 18%, trunk front 18%, trunk back 18%), *palmar surface* (patient's palm and fingers = 0.8%) or a *Lund and Browder chart* (more accurate, especially in children)
    - Classify burn by determining depth:

Classes of burns		
Class	**Characteristics**	**Management**
Superficial	Red and dry, blanches with pressure (like sunburn)	Simple moisturiser/Aloe vera gel
Partial-thickness (superficial/deep) *Need re-epithelialisation ± granulation to heal*	Red and moist, with blisters, does not blanch	*See text below*
Full-thickness	White/grey/scalded, insensate, solid, dry	Skin graft

- **Initial management** for all major burns should begin with an **ABCDE** approach
    - **A**irway burns: call anaesthetist and intubate patient as soon as possible
    - **B**reathing: give all patients 100% oxygen through a humidified non-rebreather mask; nebulisers for smoke inhalation
    - **C**irculation: site 2 large bore cannulas and commence IV fluid resuscitation
        - The *Parkland formula* estimates fluid requirements in 24 hours
            - Fluid requirement (ml) = 4 × total burn surface area (%) × body weight (kg)
            - 50% of this is given in the first 8 hours and 50% in the next 16 hours
            - Children should also be given maintenance fluids
    - **D**isability: check responsiveness, give strong analgesia
    - **E**xposure: examine entire skin and look for other injuries
        - Large area burns: cover with sterile sheets or cling film until specialist review
        - Minor burns: immerse in cool water for 30 minutes (or cover with cool sterile saline soaked towels)
- **Further management of partial-thickness burns**
    - Use systemic (never topical) analgesia if required
    - Cleanse with soap and water, then thoroughly rinse
    - Scrub off any necrotic tissue
    - Dress simple low-exudate burns with multiple layers of low-adherent impregnated tulle gauze. Cover this with a sterile non-adherent absorbent pad dressing and secure with bandages or dressing fixing tape.
    - Review in 48 hours to look for signs of infection
    - Re-dress every 2 days
- **Blisters:** leave intact unless they are open/contaminated (fully debride) or are large/prevent dressing (sterile aspiration)
- **Burns requiring specialist opinion/admission:** full thickness burns (need skin graft); >10-15% body surface area or if elderly/significant comorbidities (risk of significant fluid loss); hands (put in bag with paraffin and keep moving); face (use Vaseline); genitalia/perineum (admit as difficult to dress); burns over major joints; chemical ('irrigate, irrigate, irrigate!'); electrical (spare skin); inhalation injuries (airway risk); circumferential burns (risk of compartment syndrome)

Puncture wounds

- X-ray if any possibility foreign body
- If wound is deep and contaminated, it needs wide debridement in theatre
- If not, use simple debridement and irrigation
- Follow-up is required

Bites

- Cat and human bites are worst
- High risk of tendon injury and joint contamination leading to risk of septic arthritis
- Most require aggressive ± surgical management, often followed by delayed primary closure/healing by secondary intention
- Give antibiotics for 5 days

Others

- **Gunshot wounds** are usually treated with thorough debridement and delayed primary suture
- **Facial injuries** should ideally be sutured by a plastic surgeon– use fine sutures and remove after 2-5 days
- **Crushed tissues** need to be elevated for 7-10 days to reduce swelling prior to closure (risk of compartment syndrome)

LIGAMENT INJURY MANAGEMENT

ANKLE LIGAMENT INJURIES

- Lateral ligament sprain most common
- **Ottawa rules** help decide who needs an X-ray
  - Ankle X-ray if there is pain in the malleolar zone <u>and</u> any of: tenderness over the posterior edge or tip of lateral malleolus; tenderness over the posterior edge or tip of medial malleolus; or inability to weight-bear both immediately after injury and now
  - Foot X-ray if there is pain in the midfoot zone <u>and</u> any of: tenderness over the navicular bone; tenderness over base of 5th metatarsal; or inability to weight-bear both immediately after and now
- **Other examination**
  - Palpate deltoid ligament (medially) and lateral ligament complex (anterior talofibular ligament, calcaneofibular ligament and posterior talofibular ligament)
  - Palpate fibula up to knee (check for associated head of fibula fracture)
  - Squeeze test – squeeze mid-lower leg to test syndesmosis (positive test is pain at syndesmosis, requires urgent orthopaedic assessment if not intact)
  - Test weight-bearing (4 steps)
  - If the patient is not in too much pain
    - Anterior drawer test (hold foot still and push lower leg anteriorly and posteriorly) – tests talofibular ligament
    - Tilt test (invert foot at ankle and compare to other side) – tests lateral ligament complex, bias towards calcaneofibular ligament
  - + distal neurovascular exam (check peroneal and sural nerves)
- **Generic management**
  - Acutely, apply an ice pack for 20 minutes
  - Give patient crutches, analgesia and advice
  - Advice:
    - NSAIDs
    - **RICE**: **R**est, **I**ce (20 minutes four times a day), **C**ompression (elastic bandage) and **E**levation for 24 hours
    - Then mobilise and weight-bear as able (walking on it will hurt but not harm)
    - Try to fully weight-bear on it for ~2 minutes twice a day for a month (e.g. while cleaning teeth)
    - Physio if not better in 1-2 weeks
- **Specific management:**

Grading of ankle ligament injuries and their management			
Grade	Definition	Clinical findings	Specific management
1	Ligament stretch with microscopic tearing	Local tenderness, minimal swelling, no joint instability	Elastic compression bandage (for 2 weeks) *Heals in 2-4 weeks*
2	Ligament stretch with partial tearing	Local tenderness, oedema, ecchymosis, partial loss of joint motion but definite end point	Stirrup splint (for 4 weeks) *Heals in 4-12 weeks*
3	Complete rupture of ligament	Marked swelling, severe pain, gross ankle instability	Aircast boot (for 6 weeks) May require surgical repair *Heals in 3-6 months*

KNEE LIGAMENT INJURIES

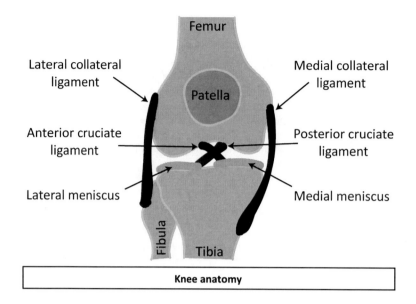

Lateral collateral ligament

Medial collateral ligament

Femur

Patella

Anterior cruciate ligament

Posterior cruciate ligament

Lateral meniscus

Medial meniscus

Fibula

Tibia

| Knee anatomy |

Knee ligament injuries		
Structure damaged	**Mechanism**	**Symptoms**
Cruciate ligaments	**Anterior:** forced flexion, hyperextension of knee (e.g. during tackle) or rotation injury to extended knee **Posterior:** tibia forced backwards, e.g. fall on object or against dashboard in road traffic accident *May hear 'pop'*	Knee collapses when put weight on it Immediate pain Difficulty weight-bearing Rapidly forming haemarthrosis
Collateral ligaments	**Medial:** blow to lateral side of knee **Lateral:** blow to medial side of knee (check peroneal nerve) *Lateral ligament injuries are uncommon*	Pain on inner/outer knee Immediate pain Difficulty weight-bearing May have symptoms of instability (if high grade injury)
Meniscus tears	Rotational injury to flexed knee	Immediate pain Difficulty weight-bearing Slowly forming effusion Clicking and locking (locking limiting extension)

- **Ottawa rules** help decide who needs a knee X-ray: age >55; inability to weight-bear both immediately after injury and now; isolated patella tenderness; head of fibula tenderness; or inability to flex to 90°
- **Knee examination** may be difficult due to swelling and patients may need to return for full examination after 1 week
- **General management**
  - Acutely, apply an ice pack for 20 minutes
  - Give patient crutches, analgesia and advice
  - Advice:
    - NSAIDs
    - **RICE:** **R**est, **I**ce (20 minutes four times a day), **C**ompression (elastic bandage) and **E**levation for 24 hours
    - Then mobilise and weight-bear as able (walking on it will hurt but not harm)
    - Try to fully weight-bear on it for ~ 2 minutes twice a day for a month (e.g. while cleaning teeth)
    - Physio if not better in 1-2 weeks
- **Specific management**:

Grading of knee ligament injuries and their management			
Grade	**Definition**	**Clinical findings**	**Specific management**
1	Ligament stretch with microscopic tearing	Knee stable on clinical testing	Elastic or wool & crepe bandage (for 2 weeks) *Heals in 2-4 weeks*
2	Ligament stretch with partial tearing	Laxity but definite end point	Knee brace (for 4 weeks, or until no laxity on examination) *Heals in 4-12 weeks*
3	Complete rupture of ligament	Joint opens >1cm	Medial/lateral collateral ligament: knee brace (for 6-12 weeks or until no laxity on examination) Anterior/posterior cruciate ligament: cast and surgical reconstruction
Meniscus	Damage to menisci	Knee gives way, clicks and locks	Arthroscopic repair if locked knee or knee is no better in 2 weeks

FRACTURE MANAGEMENT

Fracture management stages include (**4 R's**):

1. **R**esuscitate
2. **R**educe (if displaced) – may be done by open reduction, closed manipulation or traction
3. **R**etain (to maintain position while healing occurs) – by internal fixation, external fixation or conservative methods
4. **R**ehabilitate

> **Include in assessment**
>
> • **Who** – age, job, hobbies, hand dominance (if hand/arm involved)
> • **What** happened, exact mechanism, force
> • **When/where/why** it happened (was it the result of another problem, e.g. collapse?)
> • Examine for **other injuries**
> • Check **neurovascular** status distally
> • Look for **complications**, e.g. compartment syndrome
> • Include **social history** and smoking (delays bone healing)

 ## RESUSCITATE

- **Advanced trauma life support** in life-threatening wounds
- **Look for other injuries** (don't get distracted by one obvious injury!) – does the cervical spine need to be immobilised?

 ## REDUCE (IF DISPLACED)

- **Open reduction** – *when anatomical (perfect) reduction is required (e.g. for intra-articular fractures) or associated neurovascular damage*
- **Closed manipulation** (may be done in emergency department or require general anaesthesia) – *for extra-articular fractures where adequate and acceptable reduction can be achieved*
- **Traction** (to aid reduction, analgesia and in patients who are unsuitable for anaesthesia)

RETAIN (TO MAINTAIN REDUCED POSITION WHILE CALLUS FORMS IN ~6 WEEKS)

- **External fixation** – *required for: contaminated open wounds, severe open fractures, severe associated soft tissue injury*
- **Internal fixation** – *required for: comminuted or displaced fractures, intra-articular fractures, bones not able to be reduced by other methods, associated joint incongruity*
    - Intramedullary
        - Intramedullary nail – for long bone fractures (femur/tibia/humerus)
        - K-wires (stainless steel pins which can be inserted percutaneously to hold bone fragments together; can be used as temporary fixation for ~4 weeks) – for fracture fragments or for intramedullary fixation of small bones
    - Extramedullary
        - Plates and screws – to bridge comminuted fractures, compress simple fractures around joints, support areas of thin cortex or secure tension side of fracture
- **Conservative immobilisation** – *can be used for **most fractures without above properties**, and also to stabilise fractures temporarily in case of delay before reduction/fixation*
    - Splints and casts
        - Splint (non-circumferential immobiliser), e.g. plaster backslab, fibreglass backslab, aluminium/wire/heat-mouldable plastic splints
        - Cast (circumferential immobiliser), e.g. fibreglass cast, full plaster cast
    - Brace (supportive device that allows continued function)
    - Sustained traction:
        - Collar and cuff arm sling
        - Skin traction (adhesive strappings around parts of limb distil and proximal to fracture, and weight traction applied to each in opposite directions)
        - Traction splint
        - Skeletal traction (pins passed through bone to provide point of traction)

NB: femur and tibia/fibula shaft fractures can be managed conservatively but are usually managed with intramedullary nailing to reduce time non-weight-bearing.

> *If using splint/cast:*
>
> ### *In acute fractures: use a splint or backslab (to allow for swelling)*
> ### *1 week post-injury: change to a full circumferential cast (for better immobilisation)*

R REHABILITATE

- **Physiotherapy** to regain function
- Consider weight-bearing status of affected lower limb
  - o Non-weight-bearing (leg must not touch floor) – *for ~6 weeks in conservatively managed unstable fractures and after fixation with plates*
  - o Toe-touch weight-bearing (toe may touch floor to balance but not support any weight)
  - o Partial weight-bearing (<50% body weight)
  - o Weight-bear as tolerated
  - o Full weight-bearing – *after intramedullary nails, external fixations, joint replacements*

May progress through these stages with X-Ray monitoring in some potentially unstable fractures

OTHER ASPECTS TO MANAGEMENT

- **For swelling, RIE: Rest, Ice, Elevation**
- **Smoking cessation** – delays bone healing
- **Analgesia** (but avoid NSAIDs – they interfere with bone healing)
- **Antibiotic prophylaxis** for open fractures
- **VTE prophylaxis**
- **Treat the cause of the fracture if necessary**, e.g. osteoporosis, fall etc.

COMPLICATIONS

- **Immediate:** haemorrhage, arterial damage, surrounding structure damage (e.g. tendons, nerves), fat embolus
- **Early (few weeks):** wound/prosthesis infection, loss of position/fixation, VTE, chest infection, compartment syndrome
- **Late (months-years):** malunion, non-union, delayed union, osteoarthritis, avascular necrosis

NB: compartment syndrome is a rise in pressure in a myofascial compartment. It causes pain out of proportion to the injury and is exacerbated by passive stretching of the muscles within the compartment. The treatment is urgent fasciotomy.

OTHER POINTS

- **Timings**
  - o Callus forms in <u>6 weeks</u> – temporary fixations (e.g. traction, cast, external fixations, K-wires) removed at this stage
  - o Full fracture healing in <u>12 weeks</u>
  - o Generally, lower limb bones take twice as long to fully heal as upper limb bones, and young children's bones heal twice as fast as adult's bones
- **Repeat X-rays** are performed post-operatively or after cast application
- Fractures with a fragment at risk of **avascular necrosis** due to retrograde blood supply:
  - o Head of femur
  - o Waist of scaphoid
  - o Neck of talus

6 weeks
The Orthopaedic
Unit of Time

Management of common fractures	
Clavicle	Broad arm sling or polysling
Proximal humerus	Collar and cuff sling (applies traction)
Mid-humerus	Collar and cuff sling + U-slab cast, or functional brace
Distal humerus	Above elbow backslab/cast
Colles' fracture	Closed manipulation under haematoma block then Colles' backslab/cast (below elbow backslab/cast with wrist flexed and ulnar deviated) applied
Scaphoid	Futuro splint ± thumb extension, or thumb spica splint/cast if definite fracture
Neck of femur (intracapsular)	Displaced >60 years → total hip replacement/hemiarthroplasty Undisplaced/displaced <60 years → cannulated screws
Neck of femur (extracapsular)	Intertrochanteric → dynamic hip screw/gamma nail Subtrochanteric → intramedullary nail
Femur/tibia shaft	Intramedullary nail
Lateral malleolus (Weber A)	Below knee backslab/cast or aircast boot or stirrup brace (full weight-bearing)
Bimalleolar, trimalleolar or lateral malleolar fractures that disrupt the syndesmosis (i.e. Weber C and some Weber B)	Surgical fixation

SEPSIS MANAGEMENT

Sepsis is an infection with a systemic response.

IDENTIFYING A PATIENT WITH SEPSIS

- Think about it in any patient who has a suspected infection
- It is a **clinical judgement** as to whether a patient has sepsis
- They must have a **suspected infection** (e.g. symptoms, fever, feeling unwell) <u>and</u> a **systemic response** (i.e. abnormalities of physiological parameters/altered mental state)
- **Risk factors** = very young, frail/elderly, recent surgery/trauma (<6weeks), impaired immunity (illness or immunosuppression), indwelling catheters/lines, IV drug use, breaks in skin integrity
- **Lactate** correlates with severity (<2mmol/L = mild; 2-4mmol/L = moderate; >4mmol/L = severe)

Include in assessment

- **Observations**
- **Sepsis signs** (capillary refill, skin temp, pulse etc.)
- **Look for infection sources** (multi-system exam; iatrogenic sources, e.g. surgical wounds, drains, cannulas, lines; exposure e.g. look at skin, joints etc.)
- **Investigations**: to find source (septic screen) and to look for complications/organ dysfunction
  - Bloods (especially look at Hb, WCC/neutrophils, Platelets, INR, bilirubin) + VBG (<u>lactate</u>)
  - Blood cultures
  - Capillary glucose
  - Urine dip and culture any other fluids
  - CXR
  - Other relevant imaging (e.g. CT abdomen if possibility of surgical collection)

Parameters suggesting risk of severe illness/death from sepsis (any criteria) Produced using NICE 'NG51 sepsis: recognition, diagnosis and early management' 2016		
	HIGH RISK	**MODERATE TO HIGH RISK**
Mental status	Objective altered metal state	History of altered mental state/behaviour or deterioration of functional ability
Respiratory rate	≥25 (or new oxygen requirement)	>20
Heart rate	>130	>90
Systolic blood pressure	≤90 (or >40 below normal)	≤100
Urine output	<0.5ml/kg/hour (or no urine in >18 hours)	<1ml/kg/hour (or no urine in >12 hours)
Others	Cyanosis or mottled/ashen appearance	Impaired immunity (illness or immunosuppression)
	Non-blanching rash	Recent surgery/trauma (<6w)
		Temperature <36°C
		Signs of potential infection

End organ dysfunction due to sepsis			
System	**Condition**	**Signs**	**Management**
Respiratory	Acute respiratory distress syndrome	Impaired oxygenation, tachypnoea, infiltrates on CXR	Mechanical ventilation
Cardiovascular	Myocardial dysfunction/failure, hypovolaemia, septic shock	Persistent hypotension (SBP<90)	Inotropes/vasopressors
Kidneys	Acute kidney injury	Urine output <0.5ml/kg/hour or creatinine >50% baseline	Haemodialysis if required
Liver	Liver dysfunction	Bilirubin ≥35µmol/L and ALP/ALT >2x normal	No specific treatment
Coagulation	Coagulopathy/disseminated intravascular coagulation	Thrombocytopenia, prolonged PT, low fibrinogen, high D-dimer	Blood products (red cells, platelets, FFP, cryoprecipitate)
Nervous system	Encephalopathy	New confusion/↓GCS	No specific treatment

NB: septic shock is sepsis with refractive hypotension despite adequate fluid resuscitation.

MANAGEMENT

Sepsis Six – within 1 hour!

- **3 IN:**
  - **Oxygen**
  - **Fluids** (adequate fluid resuscitation is normally 20-30ml/kg quickly, e.g. over 30-60 minutes – use 0.9% saline/Hartmann's solution)
  - **Antibiotics**
    - Choice depends on hospital protocol
    - Target source of infection if clear
    - Broad-spectrum if source unclear
- **3 OUT:**
  - **Blood cultures**
  - **Lactate and Hb**
  - **Catheterise** (to measure urine output, i.e. renal end-organ dysfunction)

Other aspects to management

- Use an ABCDE approach (*see notes on ABCDE management p172*)
- Some sources may require surgery (abdominal collections, joints, necrosis)
- Support organ failure (may require ICU, e.g. for vasopressors, intubation, or dialysis)
- If patient is still hypotensive despite adequate fluid resuscitation (30ml/kg), they need vasopressors

POST-OPERATIVE COMPLICATIONS

GENERAL COMPLICATIONS

Immediate
- Anaesthetic complications (e.g. arrhythmia, hypo-/hypertension, hyperthermia, breathing problems, MI/stroke, allergy, teeth/lip/tongue damage)
- Haemorrhage – *often not obvious externally* (*monitor drains, observations, FBC/haematocrit*)

Early
- Fluid depletion
- Electrolyte imbalances
- Local infection (wound/surgical site) or systemic infection (chest/UTI/sepsis)
- Fluid collections
- Atelectasis
- DVT/PE
- Wound break down
- Anastomotic break down
- Bed sores

Operation-specific complications	
Operation	**Specific complications**
General surgery	
Gastrectomy	Dumping syndrome Malabsorption Anastomotic ulcer Peptic ulcers/gastric cancer Small intestinal bacterial overgrowth Abdominal fullness/gas bloating
Small and large bowel operations	Ileus Anastomotic leaks (typically present 5-10 days post-operatively but can be up to 21 days) Stoma retraction Intra-abdominal collections Pre-sacral plexus damage Adhesions/intestinal obstruction Damage to other local structures, e.g. kidneys, ureters, bladder
Cholecystectomy	Common bile duct injury/bile leak
Biliary	Common bile duct injury/bile leak Common bile duct stricture Anastomotic leak Bleeding into biliary tree (jaundice) Pancreatitis
Cardiothoracic	
CABG/stenting	Reperfusion arrhythmias Post-operative acute coronary syndrome Often need inotropes post-operatively; these may reduce organ perfusion elsewhere
Vascular	
Grafts/stents/bypass procedures	Failure of graft, haemorrhage/haematoma, infection, re-thrombosis, limb or organ ischaemia Arteriovenous fistula Cholesterol embolism (e.g. trash foot) Arteriopaths are at high risk of: ACS, stroke, PE Contrast complications, e.g. anaphylaxis, renal injury
Endocrine	
Thyroidectomy	Airway obstruction secondary to haemorrhage – requires urgent opening of thyroidectomy wound Hypocalcaemia (damage to parathyroid glands) Recurrent laryngeal nerve damage
Parotidectomy	Facial nerve damage
Trauma and Orthopaedic	
Any orthopaedic operation	Infection of prosthesis Loss of position/failure of fixation Non-union, malunion, delayed union Neurovascular injury Compartment syndrome
Total hip arthroplasty	Sciatic nerve damage, dislocation, leg length difference, loosening, wear, need for revision surgery
Urology	
Cystoscopy/transurethral resection of the prostate	High risk of UTI Transurethral resection of the prostate syndrome (absorption of irrigation fluid causing hyponatraemia) Impotence/retrograde ejaculation External sphincter damage (incontinence) Urethral stricture
Other	
Endovascular surgery	Retroperitoneal haemorrhage
Lymph node dissection (e.g. axillary nodes in breast cancer surgery)	Lymphoedema
Neck dissection (e.g. branchial cyst excision)	Cranial nerve damage (11, 12)

ASSESSING AN UNWELL POST-OPERATIVE PATIENT

General tips
- Use an **ABCDE approach** (*see notes on ABCDE management p172*)
- Consider the operation, pre-operative fitness and post-operative progress
- Think about specific risks associated with the operation
- Special attention should be given to operative site, newly placed drains and their contents

NB: pain, operative stress and inflammation may be confounding factors when assessing a patient with deranged physiological parameters, but it is important to exclude more serious underlying causes.

Pyrexia
- Assess in conjunction with other **physiological parameters** (heart rate, blood pressure, respiratory rate)
- **Sepsis** is the most common cause but operative intervention causes an inflammatory response in itself and may result in low grade pyrexia
- Surgical patients are at particular risk of **chest infections** due to suboptimal ventilation causing basal atelectasis. But consider other sources of sepsis, such as UTIs.
- The timing of the pyrexia may give a clue to the underlying diagnosis:

Causes of post-operative fever (5 W's)		
Category	**Days post-op**	**Causes**
Wind	<2	Atelectasis, pneumonia
Water	2-4	UTI
Wound	5-7	Wound infection, infected post-operative collections
Walking	8-10	Venous thromboembolism
Wonder drugs	Any time	Transfusion/drug reactions (e.g. serotonin syndrome)

Hypotension
- There should be two aims in assessing a patient with hypotension, identifying a cause and assessing for organ dysfunction
- Causes may include:
    - **Decreased intravascular volume:** long operations and evaporative fluid losses, third space fluid losses, haemorrhage and poor oral intake should all be considered
    - **Pump failure (cardiogenic shock):** surgical stress increases the risk of MI (typically occur 48 hours post-operatively). Fluid overload and heart failure should also be considered.
    - **Sepsis and anaphylaxis**
    - **Sympathetic shock:** patients with epidural analgesia and a high block (T5 and above) can lose sympathetic outflow causing vasodilation and cardiogenic shock – assess epidural blocks using cold sprays. Spinal anaesthetics in elderly patients may contribute to loss of sympathetic tone and hypotension.
- Clinical signs of poor perfusion include: delayed capillary refill time, cold peripheries, tachycardia
- Specific evidence of organ dysfunction should be sought: ABG for lactate, assessment of urine output (should be >0.5ml/kg/hour), confusion

Respiratory difficulties
- Respiratory problems are common in surgical patients
    - **Respiratory tract infections:** post-operative patients are high-risk due to immobility, poor inspiratory effort due to pain and basal atelectasis
    - **Pulmonary embolism:** both surgery and underlying pathologies such as cancers and sepsis increase VTE risk
    - **Pulmonary oedema:** large fluid shifts, hypoalbuminaemia and cardiac dysfunction predispose to this
- Assessment of respiratory difficulties should include: assessment of fluid state (clinical hydration status, JVP, urine output), assessment of calves for DVTs, investigation for infection (e.g. bloods, CXR) and ABG

Low urine output
- An acceptable urine output as a rule is considered to be >0.5ml/kg/hour
- Consider the causes of renal failure
    - **Pre-renal:** most common; usually due to volume depletion but may also be caused by inadequate cardiac output
    - **Renal:** may be secondary to nephrotoxic drugs (e.g. aminoglycosides, metformin)
    - **Post-renal:** may be due to prostatic hypertrophy or raised intra-abdominal pressures causing compression of ureters
- An assessment of the patient with low urine output should include a fluid status assessment (with care to look at fluid losses from drains and 3rd space losses into the bowel or tissues), a medicines review, and a catheter examination/bladder scan

A systemic type I (IgE mediated) life-threatening hypersensitivity reaction.

Immediately get help, call medical emergency team on 2222 (tell switchboard it is a medical emergency and the location) and **remove allergen**.

AIRWAY

- Secure airway
- **Adrenaline 0.5mg IM** (0.5ml of 1:1000)**:** may be repeated at 5 minute intervals
  NB: the injections come as 1ml, so dispose of 0.5ml before injecting.

> **Adrenaline 0.5mg IM**
> (0.5ml of 1:1000)

BREATHING

- Attach **15L/minute oxygen** via a non-rebreather mask
- If wheeze, give salbutamol 5mg NEB

CIRCULATION

- Secure IV access (2 large-bore IV cannulas)
- **IV fluids** 500-1000ml 0.9% saline/Hartmann's solution STAT fluid challenge initially (may need up to 4-8L IV fluids – give as fast as needed and titrate to BP)
- **Hydrocortisone 200mg IV**
- **Chlorpheniramine 10mg IV**
- Apply 3-lead cardiac monitoring

FURTHER SHORT-TERM MANAGEMENT

- If the patient is not improving rapidly, seek anaesthetic/intensive care input
- Admit for observation (at least 6 hours post-adrenaline because biphasic reactions can occur)
- Continue prednisolone 30-40mg OD PO (3-5 day course)
- Continue chlorpheniramine 4mg QDS PO if itching
- Monitor ECG
- Further IV fluids if required
- Document event and allergy
- Consider taking mast cell tryptase to confirm anaphylaxis (must be done ASAP)

LONGER-TERM MANAGEMENT

- Educate patient
- Teach about self-injected adrenaline (Epipen)
- Medic alert bracelet
- Refer to allergy clinic ± skin prick tests to identify allergens if unknown
- Clinical incident form if given allergic antibiotic

RAPID TRANQUILISATION OF AGITATED PATIENT AT RISK TO SELF/OTHERS

ENSURE SAFETY OF PATIENT AND OTHERS
- Try to calm patient down
- Move patient to a safe place (or move other patients and staff)
- Call security to be in background and intervene if needed

TRY ALTERNATIVE MANAGEMENT FIRST
- Turn on the lights
- Give them their hearing aid if needed
- Explain where they are, the time and ascertain their concerns
- See if a relative can come in or has any advice

RAPID TRANQUILISATION PROTOCOL

Only to be used as a last resort if an agitated patient is <u>at risk to themselves or others</u>

Lorazepam 1-2mg PO/IM
OR **Haloperidol** 2-5mg PO/IM

Notes
- Use oral route if possible (always offer)
- **Half doses in elderly or renal failure**
- Haloperidol is contraindicated in Parkinson's disease, Lewy body dementia, alcohol withdrawal, heart problems (ideally see ECG and check QT interval is not prolonged first)
- Ensure procyclidine 5-10mg IM/IV is available if using haloperidol to counteract dystonia if needed

Repeating doses
- Repeat at 30-60 minute intervals if required, up to 3 times
- Oral therapy takes 45-60 minutes to take effect; IM therapy takes 30 minutes
- If it fails, call anaesthetist/intensive care team for sedation

Observations
- Every 30 minutes in light sedation (normal functioning)
- Every 15 minutes in deep sedation (reduced GCS)

DOCUMENT
- Clearly document why you had to do it!

This page is intentionally left blank

CHAPTER 5: CLINICAL PROCEDURES

PERIPHERAL VENEPUNCTURE

INTRODUCTION

- **W**ash hands; **I**ntroduce self; **P**atient's name, DOB and wrist band; **E**xplain procedure and obtain consent
- Check for allergies (including chlorhexidine)
- Ask preferred (or non-dominant) arm

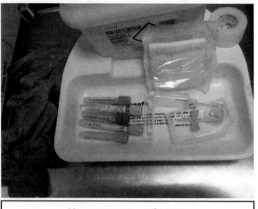

Venepuncture equipment

PREPARATION

- Wash hands
- Clean tray
- Gather equipment around tray (think through what you need in order)
    - Gloves
    - Tourniquet
    - Alcohol 70%/chlorhexidine 2% skin-cleansing wipe
    - Green *21G* Vacutainer needle (standard or butterfly)
    - Vacutainer holder
    - Required blood tubes (in order of draw order)
        - Light blue – clotting
        - Yellow   – U&Es and everything else
        - Purple   – FBC
        - Pink   – group and save
        - Grey   – glucose
      NB: yellow tube <u>must</u> be taken before purple tube which contains K+ EDTA that will produce a pseudo-hyperkalaemia)
    - Sterile gauze
    - Tape
- Wash hands
- Open packets and place neatly in tray, keeping items in plastic parts of packets (without touching the instruments themselves)
- Attach Vacutainer holder to end of needle/butterfly
- Return to patient (with tray and a sharps bin)

PROCEDURE

Vein identification
- Wash hands
- Expose arm and place a pillow beneath it
- Place tourniquet around patient's arm 4-5 finger widths above intended venepuncture site (antecubital fossa is usually the easiest)
  NB: if you are using the back of the hand, you must use a butterfly needle.
- Identify a suitable vein (i.e. one you can <u>feel</u>, not necessarily one you can see)
  NB: take sufficient time to find the best vein – this is the main determinant of whether you will be successful or not.
- Remove tourniquet

Venepuncture
- Wash hands
- Put on gloves
- Sterilise area using skin-cleansing wipe (clean for 30 seconds, then allow to air-dry for 30 seconds)
- Re-apply tourniquet
- Anchor the skin distally with your non-dominant hand and insert the needle (bevel up) at **10-30˚** with your dominant hand

Use your dominant hand to hold the butterfly wings/Vacutainer steady on the patient's arm. Then use your non-dominant hand to:
- Fill blood bottles in correct order of draw, inverting them after filling
- Remove tourniquet after removing the last bottle
- Place gauze loosely over the puncture site while you remove the needle. Then apply pressure to the gauze once the needle is fully removed.
- Put the needle immediately in the sharps bin
- Maintain pressure over the gauze until bleeding has stopped, then tape the gauze down over puncture site

TO COMPLETE

- Thank patient and restore clothing
- Discard waste and clean tray; then discard gloves; wash hands
- Fill in blood bottle labels, put in bags with printed request forms, send to lab
- Document procedure and tests requested in patient's notes

ATTAINING A VENOUS BLOOD SAMPLE FOR BLOOD CULTURE

INTRODUCTION
- **W**ash hands; **I**ntroduce self; **P**atient's name, DOB and wrist band; **E**xplain procedure and obtain consent
- Check for allergies (including chlorhexidine)
- Ask preferred (or non-dominant) arm

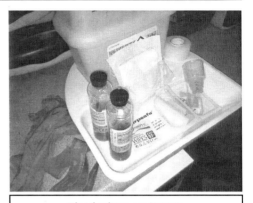

Blood culture equipment

PREPARATION
- Wash hands thoroughly with soap and water
- Put on apron
- Clean a trolley
- Clean tray thoroughly inside and out, clean sharps bin and place on trolley
- Gather equipment around tray (think through what you need in order)
  - Gloves
  - Tourniquet
  - Alcohol 70%/chlorhexidine 2% skin-cleansing wipe
  - Alcohol 70%/chlorhexidine 2% device disinfection wipe
  - Green *21G* Vacutainer butterfly needle
  - Large Vacutainer holder
  - Blood culture bottles (aerobic and anaerobic) – *CHECK DATE AND MARK 10ML*
  - Sterile gauze
  - Tape
- Wash hands
- Open packets and place neatly in tray, keeping items in plastic parts of packets (without touching the instruments themselves)
- Place Vacutainer holder on end of butterfly tubing
- Return to patient (with tray and sharps bin)

PROCEDURE
Vein identification
- Wash hands
- Expose arm and place a pillow beneath it
- Place tourniquet around patient's arm 4-5 finger widths above intended venepuncture site (antecubital fossa is usually the easiest)
- Identify a suitable vein (i.e. one you can feel, not necessarily one you can see). *NB: take sufficient time to find the best vein – this is the main determinant of whether you will be successful or not.*
- Remove tourniquet

Taking blood culture
- Wash hands
- Put on gloves
- Sterilise area using skin-cleansing wipe (clean for 30 seconds, then allow to air-dry for 30 seconds)
- Remove caps of blood culture bottles and clean tops with device disinfection wipe
- Re-apply tourniquet
- Anchor the skin distally with your non-dominant hand and insert the needle at **10-30° to the skin** with your dominant hand

Use your dominant hand to hold the butterfly wings steady on the patient's arm. Then use your non-dominant hand to:
- Fill blood culture bottles (minimum requirement is 10ml) and invert them after filling. Fill the aerobic bottle first then anaerobic bottle to avoid getting air from the tube in the anaerobic bottle.
- Remove tourniquet after removing the last bottle
- Place gauze loosely over the puncture site while you remove the needle. Then apply pressure to the gauze once the needle is fully removed.
- Put the needle immediately in the sharps bin
- Maintain pressure over the gauze until bleeding has stopped, then tape the gauze down over puncture site

TO COMPLETE
- Thank patient and restore clothing
- Discard waste and clean tray; then discard gloves and apron; wash hands
- Fill in blood bottles, put in bags with printed request forms, send to lab
- Document procedure and tests requested in patient's notes

PERIPHERAL VENOUS CANNULATION

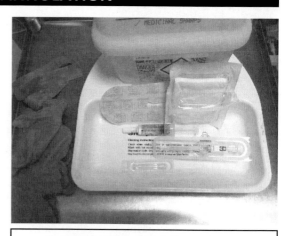

INTRODUCTION

- **W**ash hands; **I**ntroduce self; **P**atient's name, DOB and wrist band; **E**xplain procedure and obtain consent
- Check for allergies (including chlorhexidine)
- Ask preferred (or non-dominant) arm

Peripheral venous cannulation equipment

PREPARATION

- Wash hands
- Clean tray
- Gather equipment around tray (think through what you need in order)
    - Gloves x 2
    - Disposable tourniquet
    - Alcohol 70%/chlorhexidine 2% skin-cleansing wipe
    - Cannula (use a pink *20G* cannula unless patient needs a wider-bore cannula for urgent fluid resuscitation)
    - Sterile gauze
    - Cannula dressing
    - Pre-prepared saline flush (or 10ml 0.9% saline + 10ml syringe + green *21G* drawing-up needle) – *CHECK DATE*
    - Cannula IV extension set (+ alcohol 70%/chlorhexidine 2% device disinfection wipe)
    - Tape
- Wash hands
- Open packets and place neatly in tray, keeping items in plastic parts of packets (without touching the instruments themselves)
- If flush is not pre-prepared:
    - Wash hands, put on apron and 1st pair of gloves
    - Put needle on 10ml syringe and draw up the 10ml 0.9% saline (holding the saline bottle upside down)
    - Remove needle (to sharps bin), expel air and place back into syringe packet
    - Place in tray
- Priming cannula IV extension set
    - Wash hands, put on apron and 1st pair of gloves (or leave on previous ones if you had to prepare flush)
    - Prime cannula IV extension set by flushing 1ml saline flush in to each lumen
    - Lock all lumens and place cannula IV extension set and flush back into packets
    - Place in tray
    - Discard waste; then discard gloves and apron; wash hands
- Return to patient (with tray and a sharps bin)

PROCEDURE

Vein identification
- Wash hands
- Expose arm and place a pillow beneath it
- Place tourniquet around patient's arm 4-5 finger widths above intended cannulation site (dorsum of hand/antecubital fossa/forearm)
- Identify a suitable vein (i.e. one you can <u>feel</u>, not necessarily one you can see). *NB: take sufficient time to find the best vein – this is the main determinant of whether you will be successful or not.*
- Remove tourniquet

Cannulation
- Wash hands
- Put on gloves
- Sterilise area using skin-cleansing wipe (clean for 30 seconds, then allow to air-dry for 30 seconds)
- Re-apply tourniquet
- Anchor the skin distally with your non-dominant hand and insert the cannula at **10-30° to the skin** with your dominant hand
- When flashback is observed, advance a further 2mm into the vein (to ensure the cannula tubing is in the vein and not just the needle tip)
- Hold the end of the introducer needle steady with your non-dominant hand while fully advancing the cannula tubing into the vein without the introducer needle

Now keep your dominant hand on the cannula (with the needle still partially in) while resting against the patient's arm to keep it steady. Occlude the vein proximal to the cannula with your dominant hand's middle finger. While doing this, use your non-dominant hand to:

- Remove tourniquet
- Place gauze underneath the cannula opening
- Remove the needle fully and immediately drop it in the sharps bin
- Attach the cannula IV extension set on the end of the cannula
- Remove gauze and clean any spilt blood

Securing:

- Remove the two steristrips from the cannula dressing and stick them on the wings of the cannula
- Apply the rest of the dressing
- If the dressing has a third sticky strip for filling in the date and time, do this and stick it on top

Flushing:

- Holding the proximal part of the administration ports of the cannula IV extension set, clean the ports with the device disinfection wipe, unlock the lumens, slowly flush ~5mls 0.9% saline in each lumen (in pulsating manner) and then lock the lumens

TO COMPLETE

- Thank patient and restore clothing
- Discard waste and clean tray; then discard gloves and apron; wash hands
- Complete a peripheral cannula observation chart (or document with time, date, cannula size, site used and your role in notes)

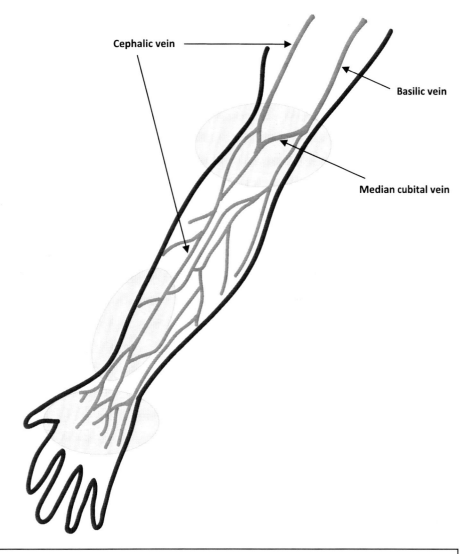

Cephalic vein

Basilic vein

Median cubital vein

Upper limb veins:
common cannulation sites (dorsum of hand, forearm and antecubital fossa) are highlighted

ARTERIAL BLOOD GAS SAMPLING

INTRODUCTION
- <u>W</u>ash hands; <u>I</u>ntroduce self; <u>P</u>atient's name, DOB and wrist band; <u>E</u>xplain procedure and obtain consent
- Check for allergies (including chlorhexidine)
- Ask preferred (or non-dominant) arm

PREPARATION
- Wash hands
- Clean tray
- Gather equipment around tray (think through what you need in order)
  - Gloves
  - Alcohol 70%/chlorhexidine 2% skin-cleansing wipe
  - Arterial blood gas kit
    - Heparinised 1-3ml syringe with *23G* needle
    - Rubber cube or needle cover
    - Cap for syringe
  - Sterile gauze
  - Tape
- Wash hands
- Open packets and place neatly in tray, keeping items in plastic parts of packets (without touching the instruments themselves)
- Put needle on syringe if not already attached
- Return to patient

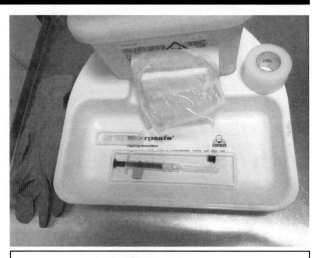

Arterial blood gas equipment

PROCEDURE

<u>Modified Allen's test</u>
- Wash hands
- Expose wrist and place a pillow beneath it
- Perform modified Allen's test
  - With patient's palm facing upwards, occlude both radial and ulnar arteries
  - Ask patient to open and close hand until the palm becomes pale, then ask them to hold it open
  - Release the ulnar artery and time how long the hand takes to reperfuse (i.e. become pink again)
  - If ≤10 seconds, continue with ABG

<u>Sampling</u>
- Firmly hyper-extend the patient's wrist (ask them, or hold it down yourself)
- Palpate radial artery with index and middle fingers
- Wash hands
- Put on gloves
- Sterilise area using skin-cleansing wipe (clean for 30 seconds, then allow to air-dry for 30 seconds)
- Expel air from the heparinised syringe (only necessary for some ABG kits)
- With the index and middle fingers of your non-dominant hand, re-palpate the artery just <u>proximal to</u> the point of insertion
- Holding the bevel of the needle as close to your non-dominant hand's fingers as possible (without touching them), insert the needle (bevel up) into the site of pulsation, at **45° to the skin**
- When blood enters the syringe, hold it still while it self-fills (no need to aspirate)
- Place gauze loosely over the puncture site while you remove the needle. Then apply pressure to the gauze once the needle is fully removed.
- Secure needle with rubber block or needle cover
- Maintain pressure over the gauze for 5 minutes. Check it has stopped bleeding before taping down the gauze.

TO COMPLETE
- Thank patient and restore clothing
- Remove the needle from the syringe and dispose of it in the sharps bin
- Put the cap on the end of the syringe and expel the air
- Discard waste and clean tray; then discard gloves; wash hands
- Label the sample and take it to the blood gas machine or call the porters to collect it on ice
- Document procedure and results in patient's notes with the patient's FiO_2 and temperature

SUTURING TECHNIQUE

GENERAL PRINCIPLES

- Equipment

  Dominant hand — o Needle-holder
  - o Scissors

  Non-dominant hand — o Non-toothed forceps – used to bring the needle out from the other side of the wound
  - o Toothed forceps – used to manipulate skin if needed

- Holding instruments
  - o Hold the needle-holder and scissors with thumb and ring finger in the holes, middle finger on the side and index finger on the top; hold the forceps like a pen
  - o Use your **dominant hand** to grip the needle with the needle-holder
    - ▪ Position of needle within needle-holder teeth: the needle should be grasped at a right angle, two thirds of the way from the tip, facing medially, with the needle tip pointing upwards
  - o Use your **non-dominant hand** mainly to bring the needle out from the other side of the wound using the non-toothed forceps. You can also use it to hold the needle directly if desired, or hold the toothed forceps to manipulate skin.
  - o The needle should be held in the needle-holder to enter skin; the non-toothed forceps should be used to bring the needle out of the centre/other side of the wound, before transferring it back to the needle-holder for more suturing.
  - o When tying an instrumental knot, the needle can be held by the non-toothed forceps (in your non-dominant hand) or your non-dominant hand's fingers directly

- Placing sutures
  - o Suture so the skin edges are slightly everted (it is the dermis-dermis contact that allows healing)
  - o Do constrict the tissue
  - o In general, most sutures are placed 5mm wide from each wound edge and 5mm apart (except for face – 2-3mm wide and 3-5mm apart)
  - o Note, in order to ensure the final sutures are 5mm wide from each wound edge, you will need to place them a bit wider because the skin will compress when the sutures are tied
  - o Where possible, enter the side of the wound opposite and farthest from you (so you are bringing the needle towards yourself)

- Deep, gaping wounds will need deep absorbable sutures placed before closing the skin

- Sharp safety
  - o If you hold the needle directly, ensure you only hold the distal end and never bring the needle out of the skin with your fingers to avoid risk of sharp injury
  - o When finished, clamp the sharp part of the needle longitudinally inside the needle-holder to safely dispose of it

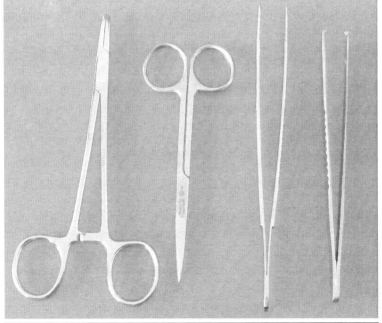

Left to right: needle-holder, scissors, non-toothed forceps, toothed forceps

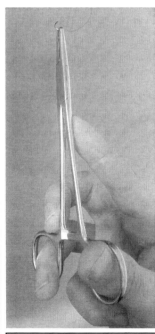

Holding needle-holder

215

TECHNIQUES OVERVIEW

<u>Suture techniques</u>
- Interrupted sutures (several individually tied sutures) – *permits precise opposition of wound edges; can be used anywhere; best if you are worried about the cleanliness of the wound*
    - Interrupted over-and-over suture – most commonly used
    - Interrupted vertical mattress suture – mattress sutures are useful if wound edges are difficult to evert
    - Interrupted horizontal mattress suture
- Continuous sutures (one continuous suture to close wound) – *permits closer approximation of wound edges; prevents passage of bodily fluids (including blood); evenly distributes tension; wound must be clean and it must be easy to oppose edges; not commonly used for skin*
    - Continuous over-and-over suture
    - Continuous interlocking suture
    - Continuous everting mattress suture
- Special sutures
    - Intracutaneous (subcuticular) suture – creates inconspicuous wound
    - Tendon suture
    - Cervical suture

<u>Knot-tying techniques</u>
- Instrument ties – most commonly used
- Two-handed
- One-handed

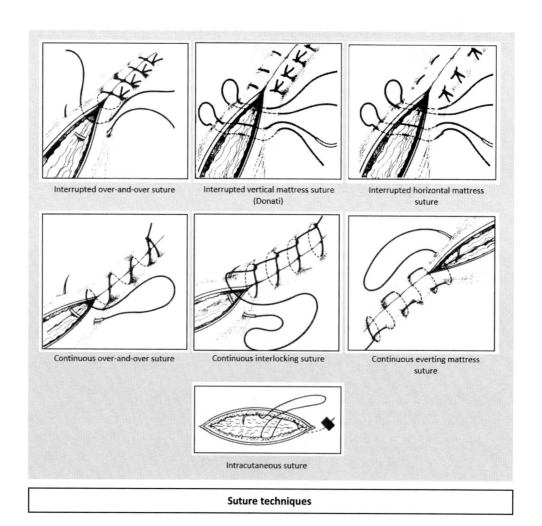

Interrupted over-and-over suture

Interrupted vertical mattress suture (Donati)

Interrupted horizontal mattress suture

Continuous over-and-over suture

Continuous interlocking suture

Continuous everting mattress suture

Intracutaneous suture

Suture techniques

INTERRUPTED OVER-AND-OVER SUTURE

This is the most common technique for closing skin using non-absorbable sutures.

- Start in the middle of a linear wound, or at the corners of a jagged wound
- Enter the skin at a right angle, about 5mm wide of the edge of the wound, on the side farthest from you
- Then go about 5mm deep into the subcutaneous tissues before coming out of the centre of the wound (optional – usually done for the first sutures but not as the wound edges become closer together)
- If you came out of the centre, enter the subcutaneous tissues of the other side of the wound about 5mm deep
- Come out of the skin on the opposite side of the wound at a 90° angle about 5mm wide of the wound edge
- Pull most of the thread through the wound, leaving enough distally to tie a knot
- Tie knot and cut ends (*as below*)
- Start the process again for the other sutures – place sutures about 5mm apart

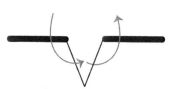

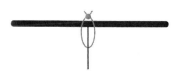

Over and over suture

INSTRUMENTAL KNOT-TYING

This is the most common knot-tying technique.

- Pull most of the thread through the wound, leaving enough distally to tie a knot
- Using your non-dominant hand, hold the needle with your fingers or with the non-toothed forceps (like when you brought it out of the wound edge)
- Twist the needle end of the suture around the shaft of the needle-holder in your dominant hand
- **2 throws away:** do this twice away from you first, then tie knot by gripping the other end of the suture with the needle holder's teeth and pulling this through the loops. Then tighten the knot by pulling each end in opposite directions.
- **1 throw towards:** repeat the process but twist the needle end of the suture in the <u>opposite direction</u> around the needle-holder and only once
- **1 throw away:** repeat the process, twisting the needle end of the suture in the <u>original direction</u> around the needle-holder once
- Cut ends about 5-10mm from knot
- Ensure knots are pulled to one side of the wound rather than left overlying the centre (they may get stuck in the granulation tissue and become difficult to remove)

REMOVAL TIMES

Face	3-5 days
Limbs/trunk/abdomen/scalp	7 days
High tension/diabetic/immunocompromised	10-14 days

Types of sutures for skin

<u>Size</u>
- 3-0 (thick) – foot, over big joints, scalp
- 4-0 (medium) – hand, body, limbs
- 5-0 (fine) – face
- 6-0 (very fine) – child's face, delicate structures

<u>Materials</u>
Non-absorbable – for superficial sutures
- Novafil™ (synthetic monofilament polybutester)
- Nylon e.g. Ethilon™, Dermalon™, Monosof™ (synthetic monofilament polyamide)
- Prolene™ (synthetic monofilament polypropylene)

Absorbable – for deep sutures
- *Vicryl™ (synthetic polyfilament polyglactin)
- Monocryl™ (synthetic monofilament polyglecaprone)

Polyfilaments are stronger but cause more inflammation and infection

<u>Needles</u>
- Curved cutting needle – sharp tip and sharp edges, used for skin

· INTERMITTENT INTRAVENOUS INFUSION

INTRODUCTION

- **W**ash hands; **I**ntroduce self; **P**atient's name, DOB and wrist band; **E**xplain procedure and obtain consent
- Cannula check: check when inserted, for signs of phlebitis and any pain
- Allergy check: check for allergies with patient and on drug chart
- Prescription check: check the prescription drug and dose, and confirm the name and DOB are correct (check with patient and their wristband)

DRUG PREPARATION

NB: if infusing fluids without drug additives, skip this stage.

- Look up drug in *Injectable Medicines* book. Determine:
  - Volume of sterile water/saline required to reconstitute drug (if it is in powder form)
  - Type and volume of infusion fluid
  - Infusion rate
- Wash hands
- Clean tray
- Gather equipment around tray (think through what you need in order)
  - Gloves
  - Apron
  - Drug vial – *CHECK DATE, DOSE, PRESCRIPTION AND ALLERGIES*
    - + if drug is in powder form: vial of sterile water/saline *for reconstituting drug – CHECK DATE*
  - Syringe
  - 2x green *21G* needles *for drawing-up and injecting into bag*
  - 'Drugs added to this infusion' sticker
  - Saline/dextrose infusion bag – *CHECK DATE*
- Wash hands
- Open packets and place neatly in tray, keeping items in plastic parts of packets (without touching the instruments themselves)
- Wash hands
- Put on gloves and apron
- If the drug is in powder form:
  - Snap top off sterile water/saline vial
  - Put drawing-up needle on syringe, hold sterile water/saline vial upside-down and draw up required amount for reconstitution (plus a bit extra)
  - Expel air and some water to leave the exact amount needed for reconstitution
  - Flick top off drug vial
  - Insert the needle and inject the sterile water/saline. Twist the vial back and forth on end of needle until drug powder is fully dissolved.
- If the drug is in liquid form:
  - Put drawing-up needle on syringe and fill with approximately the same volume of air as in the drug vial *if drug vial contains a vacuum*
  - Flick top off drug vial
  - Insert needle into the vial, and inject the air into the airspace *if drug vial contains a vacuum* (stops a vacuum forming)
- Draw up drug solution while vial is upside-down
- Remove and replace the needle on the end of the syringe filled with the drug solution (put old one directly in sharps bin), expel the air, and inject the drug solution directly into the infusion bag
- Invert bag a few times to mix
- Fill in the details on the yellow sticker and stick it on the back of the infusion bag (expiry depends on drug, but is usually 24 hours)
- Dispose of sharps in sharps bin
- Discard waste and clean tray; then discard gloves and apron; wash hands

---

INFUSION PREPARATION

- Wash hands
- Clean tray (in and out)
- Gather equipment around tray (think through what you need in order)
  - Gloves x 2
  - Apron
  - Giving set
  - Infusion bag (with or without drug in) – *CHECK DATE*
  - Sterile gauze
  - Alcohol 70%/chlorhexidine 2% device disinfection wipe
  - Pre-prepared saline flush (or 10ml 0.9% saline + 10ml syringe + green needle + bung) – *CHECK DATE*
- Wash hands

- Open packets and place neatly in tray, keeping items in plastic parts of packets (without touching the instruments themselves)
- Wash hands
- Put on 1st pair of gloves and apron (2nd if prepared drug)
- <u>If</u> flush is not pre-prepared:
    - Put green needle on syringe, hold saline upside-down and draw up 10ml saline
    - Dispose of needle in sharps bin
    - Expel air from syringe and place back into syringe packet in tray
- Preparing the giving set
    - Close roller clamp on giving set
    - Remove twist cap from infusion bag
    - Insert giving set spike into infusion bag
    - Hang infusion bag up on a drip stand, squeeze chamber on giving set until it is just under half full
    - Fully open roller clamp and allow fluid to run all the way down the tubing
    - Close roller clamp and put bag with attached set back into tray
    NB: This should all be done without touching the parts of equipment which will come into direct contact with the infusion fluid or patient – the 'key parts'.
- Discard waste; then discard gloves and apron; wash hands
- Walk to patient

PROCEDURE

- Wash hands
- Put on 2nd pair of gloves (3rd if prepared drug)
- If no cannula IV extension set on cannula:
    - Place gauze under back of cannula
    - Open back port of cannula while occluding the vein proximally
    - Clean cannula back port with device disinfection wipe
- If cannula IV extension set on cannula:
    - Holding the proximal part of the administration port of the cannula IV extension set, clean the port with the device disinfection wipe
    - Unlock port
- Slowly flush 5-10mls flush 0.9% saline through the cannula back port/cannula IV extension set slowly (in a pulsating manner)
- Take cap off the giving set's luer connector
- Attach it to the cannula's back port/IV extension set
- Hang up the infusion bag on the patient's drip stand
- Open the giving set's roller clamp and adjust to give the correct amount of *drops per minute* (time it):

> **Drops per minute = total drops in bag / infusion time (minutes)**
> *where:* Total drops in bag = bag volume (ml) x drops per ml (usually 20 but depends on giving set)

e.g. a 1L (1000ml) bag of normal saline is prescribed over 8 hours (480 minutes). The giving set runs fluid through at 20 drops per ml and so the total drops in the bag are 1000 x 20, which is 20,000. To run the infusion over 8 hours, the rate required in drops per minute is 20,000 / 480, which is 42 drops per minute. This is approximately 10 drops in 15 seconds (42 / 4), and the giving set clamp can be adjusted to give that rate.

TO COMPLETE

- Thank patient and restore clothing
- Discard waste and clean tray; then discard gloves; wash hands
- Sign on the drug chart that the drug has been administered
- Re-check flow rate regularly
- Return when finished: remove giving set and flush cannula

INTRAVENOUS INJECTION

Intravenous injections are administered directly into the blood via a vein. They do not need to be absorbed and have an immediate action.

INTRODUCTION

- **W**ash hands; **I**ntroduce self; **P**atient's name, DOB and wrist band; **E**xplain procedure and obtain consent
- Cannula check: check when inserted, for signs of phlebitis and any pain
- Allergy check: check for allergies with patient and on drug chart
- Prescription check: check the prescription drug and dose, and confirm the name and DOB are correct (check with patient and their wristband)
- Look up drug in *Injectable Medicines* book to determine volume of sterile water/saline required to reconstitute drug (if it is in powder form) and injection rate

PREPARATION

- Wash hands
- Clean tray
- Gather equipment around tray (think through what you need in order)
    - Gloves (+ extra pair and apron if you need to draw up drug/flush)
    - Drug – *CHECK DATE, DOSE, PRESCRIPTION AND ALLERGIES*
        - + if drug is in liquid form: green *21G* needle and syringe *for drawing-up*
        - + if drug is in powder form: green *21G* needle, syringe and vial of sterile water/saline *for reconstituting drug and drawing-up* – CHECK DATE
    - Alcohol 70%/chlorhexidine 2% device disinfection wipe
        - + if cannula does not have cannula IV extension set: sterile gauze and replacement bung
    - 2 x pre-prepared saline flushes (or 2 x: 10ml 0.9% saline + 10ml syringe + green *21G* needle) – *CHECK DATE*
- Wash hands
- Open packets and place neatly in tray, keeping items in plastic parts of packets (without touching the instruments themselves)
- If flushes are not pre-prepared:
    - Wash hands, put on apron and extra pair of gloves
    - Snap top off 0.9% saline
    - Put green needle on syringe, hold saline upside-down and draw up 10ml saline
    - Dispose of needle in sharps bin
    - Expel air from syringe and place back into syringe packet in tray
    - Repeat the process for second flush
    - Discard waste; then discard gloves and apron; wash hands (if not drawing up drug)
- If the drug is in powder form:
    - Wash hands, put on apron and extra pair of gloves (or leave on previous ones if you had to prepare flush)
    - Snap top off sterile water/saline vial
    - Put drawing-up needle on syringe, hold sterile water/saline vial upside-down and draw up required amount for reconstitution (plus a bit extra)
    - Expel air and some water from syringe to leave the exact amount needed for reconstitution
    - Flick top off drug vial
    - Insert needle and inject the sterile water/saline. Twist the vial back and forth on end of needle until drug powder is fully dissolved.
    - Draw up drug solution while the vial is upside-down
    - Remove and dispose of drawing-up needle in sharps bin
    - Expel air from syringe and place back into syringe packet in tray
    - Discard waste; then discard gloves and apron; wash hands
- If the drug is in liquid form:
    - Wash hands, put on apron and extra pair of gloves (or leave on previous ones if you had to prepare flush)
    - Put drawing-up needle on syringe and fill with approximately the same volume of air as in the drug vial *if drug vial contains a vacuum*
    - Flick/snap top off drug vial
    - Insert needle into the vial, and inject the air into the airspace *if drug vial contains a vacuum*
    - Draw up drug solution while the vial is upside-down
    - Dispose of drawing-up needle in sharps bin
    - Expel air from syringe and place back into syringe packet in tray
    - Discard waste; then discard gloves and apron; wash hands
- Walk to patient

PROCEDURE

- Wash hands
- Put on gloves
- If no cannula IV extension set on cannula:
    - Place gauze under back of cannula
    - Open back port of cannula while occluding the vein proximally
    - Clean cannula back port with device disinfection wipe
- If cannula IV extension set on cannula:
    - Holding the proximal part of the administration port of the cannula IV extension set, clean the port with the device disinfection wipe
    - Unlock port
- Flush 5-10mls flush 0.9% saline through the cannula's back port/IV extension set slowly (in a pulsating manner)
- Administer drug at rate stated in *Injectable Medicines* book
- Administer 2nd 5-10ml flush through the cannula's back port/IV extension set slowly (in a pulsating manner)
- If no cannula IV extension set, place new cannula back port bung; if using cannula IV extension set, lock lumen

TO COMPLETE

- Thank patient and restore clothing
- Discard waste and clean tray; then discard gloves; wash hands
- Sign on the drug chart that the drug has been administered

INTRAMUSCULAR INJECTION

Intramuscular injections are administered to the muscle fascia. This has a good blood supply and hence a faster rate of absorption than the subcutaneous route but also allows a reasonably prolonged action.

INTRODUCTION

- **W**ash hands; **I**ntroduce self; **P**atient's name, DOB and wrist band; **E**xplain procedure and obtain consent
- Allergy check: check for allergies with patient and on drug chart
- Prescription check: check the prescription drug and dose, and confirm the name and DOB are correct (check with patient and their wristband)
- Look up drug in *Injectable Medicines* book to determine volume of sterile water/saline required to reconstitute drug (if it is in powder form)

PREPARATION

- Wash hands
- Clean tray
- Gather equipment around tray (think through what you need in order)
    - Gloves (+ extra pair and apron if you need to draw up drug)
    - Drug – *CHECK DATE, DOSE, PRESCRIPTION AND ALLERGIES*
        - + if drug is in liquid form: green *21G* needle and syringe *for drawing-up*
        - + if drug is in powder form: green *21G* needle, syringe and vial of sterile water/saline *for reconstituting drug and drawing-up – CHECK DATE*
    - Alcohol 70%/chlorhexidine 2% skin-cleansing wipe – *optional*
    - **Blue 25mm 23G needle** *for injection* (or orange *25mm 25G* for babies/infants)
    - Sterile gauze
    - Tape
- Wash hands
- Open packets and place neatly in tray, keeping items in plastic parts of packets (without touching the instruments themselves)
- If the drug is in powder form:
    - Wash hands, put on apron and extra pair of gloves
    - Snap top off sterile water/saline vial
    - Put drawing-up needle on syringe, hold sterile water/saline vial upside-down and draw up required amount for reconstitution (plus a bit extra)
    - Expel air and some water to leave the exact amount needed for reconstitution
    - Flick top off drug vial
    - Insert needle and inject the sterile water/saline. Twist the vial back and forth on end of needle until drug powder is fully dissolved.

- o Draw up drug solution while the vial is upside-down
- o Remove and dispose of drawing-up needle in sharps bin and replace with injection needle (leave sheath on)
- o Expel air from syringe and place back into syringe packet in tray
- o Discard waste; then discard gloves and apron; wash hands
- If the drug is in liquid form:
  - o Wash hands, put on apron and extra pair of gloves
  - o Put drawing-up needle on syringe and fill with approximately the same volume of air as in the drug vial *if drug vial contains a vacuum*
  - o Flick/snap top off drug vial
  - o Insert the needle into the vial, and inject the air into the airspace *if drug vial contains a vacuum*
  - o Draw up drug solution while the vial is upside-down
  - o Remove and dispose of drawing-up needle in sharps bin and replace with injection needle (leave sheath on)
  - o Expel air from syringe and place back into syringe packet in tray
  - o Discard waste; then discard gloves and apron; wash hands
- Walk to patient (with tray and sharps bin)

PROCEDURE

Exposure
- Wash hands
- Expose injection site:
  - o **Mid-deltoid:** inject (from laterally) into **middle third of the deltoid region** (3 fingerbreadths down from acromion)
  - o **Vastus lateralis:** inject (from laterally) into the upper part of the **middle third of thigh**
  - o **Dorsogluteal:** inject (from posteriorly) into upper outer part of the **upper outer quadrant of the buttock** (to avoid sciatic nerve)

In children: use deltoid if >12 months; use vastus lateralis if <12months; do not use gluteus maximus in infants as sciatic nerve not fixed. Ask parent to hold child securely in cuddle position (child sideways on knee) or straddle position (child facing towards parent straddled on their lap).

Injection
- Wash hands
- Put on gloves
- Sterilise area using skin-cleansing wipe (clean for 30 seconds, then allow to air-dry for 30 seconds) – *optional*
- With the thumb and index finger of your non-dominant hand, **stretch the skin** at the injection site
- Holding the syringe (like a dart) between the thumb, index and middle fingers of your dominant hand, quickly insert the needle at a **right angle** to the skin
- Using your dominant hand to securely hold the syringe in place (resting against the patient), use your non-dominant hand to:
  - o Pull back on the top of the syringe (to confirm you are not in a blood vessel) – *optional*
  - o Slowly, inject the drug
- Gently but briskly remove the needle and immediately dispose of it (with syringe) in the sharps bin
- Wipe the injection site and press over it firmly with gauze, before applying tape

TO COMPLETE

- Thank patient and restore clothing
- Discard waste and clean tray; then discard gloves; wash hands
- Sign on the drug chart that the drug has been administered

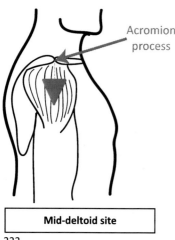

Mid-deltoid site

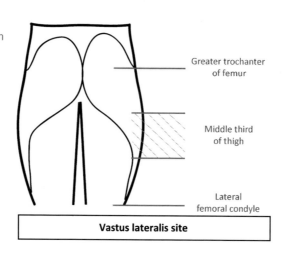

Vastus lateralis site

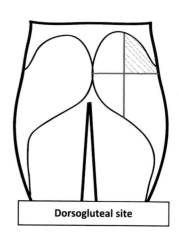

Dorsogluteal site

SUBCUTANEOUS INJECTION

Subcutaneous injections are administered in to the subcutaneous adipose tissue below the dermis. This allows a slow and more sustained rate of absorption. Many drugs can be given by this route, including insulin and heparin.

INTRODUCTION

- **W**ash hands; **I**ntroduce self; **P**atient's name, DOB and wrist band; **E**xplain procedure and obtain consent
- Allergy check: check for allergies with patient and on drug chart
- Prescription check: check the prescription drug and dose, and confirm the name and DOB are correct (check with patient and their wristband)
- Look up drug in *Injectable Medicines* book to determine volume of sterile water/saline required to reconstitute drug (if it is in powder form)

PREPARATION

- Wash hands
- Clean tray
- Gather equipment around tray (think through what you need in order)
    - Gloves (+ extra pair and apron if you need to draw up drug)
    - Drug – *CHECK DATE, DOSE, PRESCRIPTION AND ALLERGIES*
        - + if drug is in liquid form: green *21G* needle and syringe *for drawing-up*
        - + if drug is in powder form: green *21G* needle, syringe and vial of sterile water/saline *for reconstituting drug and drawing-up – CHECK DATE*
    - Alcohol 70%/chlorhexidine 2% skin-cleansing wipe – *optional*
    - **Orange *16mm 25G* needle** *for injection*
    - Sterile gauze
    - Tape
- Wash hands
- Open packets and place neatly in tray, keeping items in plastic parts of packets (without touching the instruments themselves)
- If the drug is in powder form:
    - Wash hands, put on apron and extra pair of gloves
    - Snap top off sterile water/saline vial
    - Put drawing-up needle on syringe, hold sterile water/saline vial upside-down and draw up required amount for reconstitution (plus a bit extra)
    - Expel air and some water to leave the exact amount needed for reconstitution
    - Flick top off drug vial
    - Insert needle and inject the sterile water/saline. Twist the vial back and forth on end of needle until drug powder is fully dissolved.
    - Draw up drug solution while the vial is upside-down
    - Remove and dispose of drawing-up needle in sharps bin and replace with injection needle (leave sheath on)
    - Expel air from syringe and place back into syringe packet in tray
    - Discard waste; then discard gloves and apron; wash hands
- If the drug is in liquid form:
    - Wash hands, put on apron and extra pair of gloves
    - Put drawing-up needle on syringe and fill with approximately the same volume of air as in the drug vial *if drug vial contains a vacuum*
    - Flick/snap top off drug vial
    - Insert the needle into the vial, and inject the air into the airspace *if drug vial contains a vacuum*
    - Draw up drug solution while the vial is upside-down
    - Remove and dispose of drawing-up needle in sharps bin and replace with injection needle (leave sheath on)
    - Expel air from syringe and place back into syringe packet in tray
    - Discard waste; then discard gloves and apron; wash hands
- Walk to patient (with tray and sharps bin)

PROCEDURE

<u>Exposure</u>
- Wash hands
- Expose injection site (upper outer **arms**, upper outer **thighs** or **central abdomen** avoiding area around umbilicus)
- Support the limb with pillows if necessary

<u>Injection</u>
- Wash hands
- Put on gloves

- Sterilise area using skin-cleansing wipe (clean for 30 seconds, then allow to air-dry for 30 seconds) – *optional*
- With the thumb and index finger of your non-dominant hand, **pinch a 5cm fold of skin** at the injection site
- Holding the syringe (like a dart) between the thumb, index and middle fingers of your dominant hand, insert the needle into the subcutaneous tissue at **45°**, then release the pinch
- Using your dominant hand to securely hold the syringe in place (against the patient), use your non-dominant hand to:
  - Pull back on the top of the syringe (to confirm you are not in a blood vessel) – *optional*
  - Slowly, inject the drug
- Gently but briskly remove the needle and immediately dispose of it (with syringe) in the sharps bin
- Wipe the injection site and press over it firmly with gauze, before applying tape

NB: some purpose-made subcutaneous injection needles are very short (≤8mm), e.g. insulin or LMWH needles - these should be inserted at 90°.

TO COMPLETE
- Thank patient and restore clothing
- Discard waste and clean tray; then discard gloves; wash hands
- Sign on the drug chart that the drug has been administered

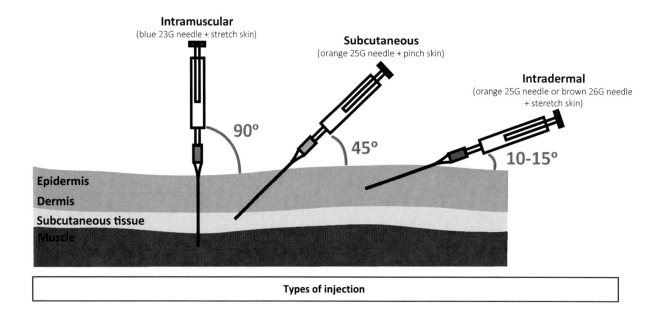

Types of injection

INTRADERMAL INJECTION

Intradermal injections are administered into the dermis, which it just below the epidermis. This injection is the most superficial and has the longest absorption time. Intradermal injections may be used for sensitivity tests (such as allergy testing or tuberculin skin test) or for local anaesthesia.

INTRODUCTION
- **W**ash hands; **I**ntroduce self; **P**atient's name, DOB and wrist band; **E**xplain procedure and obtain consent
- Allergy check: check for allergies with patient and on drug chart
- Prescription check: check the prescription drug and dose, and confirm the name and DOB are correct (check with patient and their wristband)
- Look up drug in *Injectable Medicines* book to determine volume of sterile water/saline required to reconstitute drug (if it is in powder form)

PREPARATION

- Wash hands
- Clean tray
- Gather equipment around tray (think through what you need in order)
  - Gloves (+ extra pair and apron if you need to draw up drug)
  - Drug – *CHECK DATE, DOSE, PRESCRIPTION AND ALLERGIES*
    - + if drug is in liquid form: green *21G* needle and syringe *for drawing-up*
    - + if drug is in powder form: green *21G* needle, syringe and vial of sterile water/saline *for reconstituting drug and drawing-up – CHECK DATE*
  - Alcohol 70%/chlorhexidine 2% skin-cleansing wipe – *optional*
  - **Orange *16mm 25G* needle or brown *26G* needle** *for injection*
  - Sterile gauze
  - Tape
- Wash hands
- Open packets and place neatly in tray, keeping items in plastic parts of packets (without touching the instruments themselves)
- <u>If</u> the drug is in powder form:
  - Wash hands, put on apron and extra pair of gloves
  - Snap top off sterile water/saline vial
  - Put drawing-up needle on syringe, hold sterile water/saline vial upside-down and draw up required amount for reconstitution (plus a bit extra)
  - Expel air and some water to leave the exact amount needed for reconstitution
  - Flick top off drug vial
  - Insert needle and inject the sterile water/saline. Twist the vial back and forth on end of needle until drug powder is fully dissolved.
  - Draw up drug solution while the vial is upside-down
  - Remove and dispose of drawing-up needle in sharps bin and replace with injection needle (leave sheath on)
  - Expel air from syringe and place back into syringe packet in tray
  - Discard waste; then discard gloves and apron; wash hands
- <u>If</u> the drug is in liquid form:
  - Wash hands, put on apron and extra pair of gloves
  - Put drawing-up needle on syringe and fill with approximately the same volume of air as in the drug vial *if drug vial contains a vacuum*
  - Flick/snap top off drug vial
  - Insert the needle into the vial, and inject the air into the airspace *if drug vial contains a vacuum*
  - Draw up drug solution while the vial is upside-down
  - Remove and dispose of drawing-up needle in sharps bin and replace with injection needle (leave sheath on)
  - Expel air from syringe and place back into syringe packet in tray
  - Discard waste; then discard gloves and apron; wash hands
- Walk to patient (with tray and sharps bin)

PROCEDURE

<u>Exposure</u>
- Wash hands
- Expose injection site
- Support the limb with pillows if necessary

<u>Injection</u>
- Wash hands
- Put on gloves
- Sterilise area using skin-cleansing wipe (clean for 30 seconds, then allow to air-dry for 30 seconds) – *optional*
- With the thumb and index finger of your non-dominant, **stretch the skin** at the injection site
- Holding the syringe (like a dart) between the thumb, index and middle fingers of your dominant hand, insert the needle into the dermis at an **acute angle (10-15˚)**
- Using your dominant hand to securely hold the syringe in place (resting against the patient), use your non-dominant hand to slowly inject the drug, watching a wheal form (no need to aspirate prior to injecting)
- Gently but briskly remove the needle and immediately dispose of it (with syringe) in the sharps bin
- Wipe the injection site gently with gauze (don't rub or apply pressure because medication will disperse)

TO COMPLETE

- Thank patient and restore clothing
- Discard waste and clean tray; then discard gloves; wash hands
- Sign on the drug chart that the drug has been administered

BLOOD TRANSFUSION

INTRODUCTION

- **W**ash hands; **I**ntroduce self; ask **P**atient's name, DOB and check wristband; **E**xplain:
    - Reason for transfusion
    - Benefits
    - Risks
        - Viral infections (HIV: 1 in 6.5 million; hepatitis B: 1 in 1.3 million; hepatitis C: 1 in 28 million; variant Creutzfeldt-Jakob disease: 4 isolated cases)
        - Bacterial infection (contamination)
        - Transfusion reactions (*see next page*)
    - Will never be able to donate blood again
- Gain consent

REQUESTING BLOOD PRODUCTS

- Take a blood sample (pink tube) and fill in all details by hand at patient's bedside (cross-referencing with the patient and their wristband)
- Complete a blood transfusion crossmatch request form
- Include all details:
    - Patient (full name, DOB, sex, hospital number, address/NHS number)
    - Transfusion (indication, Hb if known, blood product required, number of units, special requirements, e.g. CMV negative or irradiated)
    - Doctor (name, signature)
    - Date and ward
- Send the form with the blood tube to the haematology laboratory
- Complete a blood transfusion prescription form (each unit prescribed separately)
    - Demographic details
    - Units prescribed
    - Infusion rate:
        - Packed red cells: normally 1 unit over 2-3 hours (maximum 4 hours)
        - Fresh frozen plasma (FFP): 30 minutes
        - Platelet concentrate: 30 minutes
        - Cryoprecipitate: 30 minutes
- Consider prescribing 40mg furosemide IV/PO with each/every other unit if patient is at risk of fluid overload

SETTING UP THE BLOOD TRANSFUSION

- Follow the notes on *administering an intravenous infusion p218*
- Additionally you must:
    - Check the blood unit
        - Any leaks
        - Any haemolysis (pink plasma)
        - Any clots
        - Red colour
    - With a colleague, check the details on the blood unit against the following:
        - Transfusion slip
        - Patient
        - Patient's wristband
    - Route the giving set line through a blood-warmer if patient has undergone surgery, has cold agglutinins, requires large volumes, a rapid transfusion, or exchange transfusion
    - Request nursing observations at 0, 15, 30 minutes and then hourly, and at the end of the transfusion. Ask to be informed of any problems.
    - Document in notes

Indications for red cell concentrates

- Haemoglobin <70 g/L (or <80g/L if elderly/cardiovascular/respiratory disease)
- Significant blood loss (>1.5L or >30% blood volume)
- Symptomatic anaemia (myocardial ischemia, orthostatic hypotension or tachycardia)
- Acute sickle cell crisis (stroke prevention)

Indications for platelet concentrate

- Platelets <10x10^9/L in bone marrow failure (or <20 x10^9/L if septic)
- Platelets <50x10^9/L if undergoing surgery or actively bleeding
- Acquired/inherited platelet dysfunction (but not TTP/HUS/HIT)
- Disseminated intravascular coagulation + haemorrhage
- Other rarer platelet disorders

Indications for fresh frozen plasma (FFP)

- Disseminated intravascular coagulation + haemorrhage
- Massive haemorrhage
- Coagulation factor replacement (if specific factor concentrate unavailable)
- Immediate warfarin reversal (if prothrombin complex concentrate not available)
- Liver disease-related bleeding

Indications for cryoprecipitate

Used if fibrinogen is low (<1g/L) and there is active bleeding, e.g. in:

- Disseminated intravascular coagulation
- Liver disease

Indications for CMV seronegative components

Used for patients at risk of severe CMV disease:

- Pregnant women
- Neonates/intrauterine transfusions

Indications for irradiated components

Used to prevent transfusion-associated graft vs. host disease:

- Congenital immune deficiencies
- Hodgkin lymphoma
- Bone marrow or stem cell transplant recipients
- Patients who have had purine analogues or anti-T cell monoclonal antibodies
- Directed donations from families
- Exchange transfusions
- Neonates/intrauterine transfusions

FOLLOW-UP

- Consider taking a post-transfusion blood sample
  - Red cell concentrates: FBC 6 hours after or the next day. *NB: one unit should increase haemoglobin concentration by approximately 10g/L.*
  - Platelet concentrates: FBC 30 minutes after. *NB: one transfusion should increase platelet count by 30-60x10^9/L.*
  - FFP: coagulation screen 30 minutes after

BLOOD TRANSFUSION REACTIONS

- Most transfusion reactions occur **within 15 minutes**
- For all reactions (except febrile reaction), **STOP the transfusion**, maintain IV access with saline and call consultant haematologist
- Consider:
  - FBC, U&Es, lactate dehydrogenase, repeat compatibility testing, direct antiglobulin test, serum haptoglobin coagulation screen and D-dimer (for disseminated intravascular coagulation)
  - Blood cultures
  - Venous blood gas

Types of transfusion reaction			
Reaction	**Clinical features**	**Management**	**Notes**
Non-haemolytic febrile transfusion reaction (alloimmunised recipient produces cytokines due to donor leukocytes/HLA antigens)	•Shivering, <u>fever</u>, ± headache, nausea, flushing, tachycardia •Usually 30-60 minutes after starting transfusion	•Slow transfusion •Monitor frequently •Paracetamol	•Most common reaction (1 in 8 patients) •The patient is HOT, but <u>WELL</u> (unlike other causes)
Acute haemolytic reaction /ABO incompatibility (IgM mediated)	•Fever, hypotension •<u>Agitation</u>, <u>flushing</u>, abdominal/chest pain, bleeding/ disseminated intravascular coagulation/renal failure •Occurs within minutes of starting transfusion	•Stop transfusion •Supportive management •ABCDE	•The patient is <u>SICK</u> •Both cause fever + hypotension •Differentiate by agitation/flushing vs. rigors
Bacterial contamination	•Fever, hypotension •<u>Rigors</u> (→ septic shock)	•Stop transfusion •**Treat as sepsis** ↘Broad spectrum antibiotics	
Delayed haemolytic reaction	•Anaemia,, jaundice, haemoglobinuria • Usually 4-8 days (but potentially up to 4 weeks) after transfusion	•Investigations •Monitor renal function •Specific treatment rarely required	
Transfusion-related acute lung injury (TRALI)	•Acute respiratory distress syndrome •Dyspnoea, cough, CXR white-out •Occurs <6 (usually about 2) hours after transfusion	•Stop transfusion if ongoing •Supportive care •ABCDE •Oxygen •ICU	•Symptoms similar • TRALI more likely if severe or no history of LVF •Overload more likely if LVF history present

Fluid overload	•Dyspnoea, hypoxia, tachycardia, increased JVP, basal crepitations	•Stop transfusion
		•**Treat as acute LVF**
		  ↘Furosemide
		  ↘Oxygen	

Anaphylaxis (IgA mediated)	•Bronchospasm, cyanosis, hypotension, soft tissue swelling	•Stop transfusion
		•**Treat as anaphylaxis**
		  ↘IM adrenaline
		  ↘Maintain airway
		  ↘Call anaesthetist	

Allergic reactions (plasma protein incompatibility)	•Urticaria and itch	•Stop or slow transfusion depending on severity •Chlorpheniramine	•<u>Rarely severe</u>

ADMINISTERING NEBULISED MEDICATION

INTRODUCTION

- **W**ash hands; **I**ntroduce self; **P**atient's name, DOB and wrist band; **E**xplain procedure and obtain consent
- Allergy check: check for allergies with patient and on drug chart
- Prescription check: check the prescription drug and dose, and confirm the name and DOB are correct (check with patient and their wristband)

PREPARATION

- Wash hands
- Gather equipment (think through what you need in order)
  - Mouthpiece or facemask
  - Nebuliser
  - Tubing
  - Drug nebule – *CHECK DATE, DOSE, PRESCRIPTION AND ALLERGIES*
  - Nebuliser compressor machine or compressed air/oxygen supply
- Assemble the nebuliser and tubing
- Attach mouthpiece
- Wash hands
- Put on gloves
- Open the nebuliser drug chamber (just below the mouthpiece)
- Squeeze the drug nebule to pour it into the chamber
- Close the nebuliser drug chamber
- Discard waste; then discard gloves; wash hands
- Walk to patient

PROCEDURE

- Wash hands
- Give the mouthpiece or facemask to the patient
  - Mouthpiece: lips should create a seal around it
  - Facemask: should fit well around patient's face
- Connect the nebuliser tubing to the compressor machine or compressed air/oxygen supply (flow 6-8L/minute)
- Ask the patient to breathe in and out normally
- When nebule has fully nebulised, turn off compressor or compressed air/oxygen supply and remove mouthpiece or facemask from patient

TO COMPLETE

- Thank patient
- Discard waste; then discard gloves; wash hands
- Sign on the drug chart that the drug has been administered

CERVICAL SMEAR

INTRODUCTION

- **W**ash hands; **I**ntroduce self; ask **P**atient's name and what they like to be called; **E**xplain examination, why it's necessary, and obtain consent
- Get a **chaperone**
- Explain smear programme
- Explain procedure
    - Be impersonal, e.g. 'It will involve placing a small plastic tube inside the vagina to look at the cervix.'
    - 'It shouldn't be painful, but if at any point you are uncomfortable or want to stop, just say so. One of the nurses will also be present to ensure you are comfortable and act as a chaperone.'
    - Patient should be lying flat in lithotomy position but remain covered initially: 'You will need to undress from the waist down, put your heels together and bring them as close to your bottom as possible, then flop your knees down outwards.'
- Before starting, ask about: last menstrual period, intra-menstrual bleeding, discharge, contraception, last smear
- Ask if the patient needs the toilet before the procedure
- Position the patient so you are on their right side if possible

NB: keep talking to and reassuring the patient, using their name throughout.

GATHER EQUIPMENT

- Gloves and apron
- Speculum
- Cervical smear brush
- Cervical smear sample bottle
- Wash tray and place equipment inside in partially open packets

NB: ensure you also have suitable lighting and a source of warm tap water

PERFORMING THE SMEAR

- Put on gloves and apron
- Inspect the vulva for any obvious abnormalities
- If required, use warm water to lubricate the speculum (lubrication jelly is generally avoided because it can alter the results)
- Warn the patient prior to insertion
- Part labia and insert the speculum with the screw sideways
- Rotate speculum as you advance it so that the screw is facing upwards. Open speculum and tighten screw when resistance is met.
- Hold it in place with your left hand so it doesn't slide out
- Direct light to visualise cervix – look for discharge, erosions, ulcerations, growths, cervicitis, blood, polyps, ectropion
- Use your right hand to open the sample bottle and place it in your left hand (which is also holding the speculum)
- Take the smear using your right hand. Place the centre piece of the brush in the endocervical canal and **rotate the brush 5 times (360°) clockwise** in the endocervix and then remove.
- Depending on type of brush, either snap off the head into the sample bottle or twirl the brush in the liquid inside the sample bottle 10 times
- Replace the lid and return sample bottle to tray
- Close speculum blades (but not fully to avoid pinching vaginal wall)
- Remove speculum while rotating it back sideways

TO COMPLETE

- Thank patient, give them a tissue and restore clothing
- Fill in the sample bottle and request form details
    - Name, DOB, hospital/clinic number, address, GP name and address
    - Date of test, last smear and last menstrual period
    - Reason for smear (e.g. routine recall, first smear, previous abnormal test etc.)
    - Sampling device
    - Condition (pregnant, postnatal, any intra-uterine devices, taking hormones)
    - Appearance of cervix
    - Clinical details
- Document in patient's notes
- Advise patient results will take approximately 2 weeks and will be sent by letter

GYNAECOLOGICAL SWABS

INTRODUCTION

- **W**ash hands; **I**ntroduce self; ask **P**atient's name and what they like to be called; **E**xplain examination, why it's necessary, and obtain consent
- Get a **chaperone**
- Explain procedure
  - Be impersonal, e.g. 'It will involve placing a small plastic tube inside the vagina.'
  - 'It shouldn't be painful, but if at any point you are uncomfortable or want to stop, just say so. One of the nurses will also be present to ensure you are comfortable and act as a chaperone.'
  - Patient should be lying flat in lithotomy position but remain covered initially: 'You will need to undress from the waist down, put your heels together and bring them as close to your bottom as possible, then flop your knees down outwards.'
- Before starting, ask about: last menstrual period, intra-menstrual bleeding, discharge, contraception, last smear
- Ask if the patient needs the toilet before the procedure
- Position the patient so you are on their right side if possible

NB: keep talking to and reassuring the patient, using their name throughout.

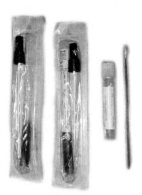

Charcoal and
***Chlamydia* swabs**

GATHER EQUIPMENT

- Gloves and apron
- Lubricating gel
- Speculum
- Swabs as required by local protocol (double swabs most commonly used now)
  - **'Double swabs':** nucleic acid amplification test (NAAT) swab (*endocervical*), charcoal media swab (*high-vaginal*)
  - **'Triple swabs':** charcoal media swabs x 2 (*high-vaginal and endocervical*), Chlamydia swab (*endocervical*)
- Wash tray and place equipment inside in partially open packets

PERFORMING THE SWABS

- Put on gloves and apron
- Warm the speculum if necessary with warm water
- Lubricate the sides of the speculum (not the tip because this may alter results) and warn the patient prior to inserting
- Part the labia and insert the speculum with the screw sideways
- Rotate speculum as you advance it so that the screw is facing upwards. Open speculum and tighten screw when resistance is met.
- Hold it in place with your left hand so it doesn't slide out
- Direct light to visualise cervix – look for discharge, erosions, ulcerations, growths, cervicitis, blood, polyps, ectropion
- To take each swab in turn:
  - Use your right hand to pick up the swab's sample tube and place this in your left hand (also holding the speculum). Remove the lid and put this back in the tray for the meantime.
  - Take the swab with your right hand
  - Place the used swab back in its tube (held your left hand), tighten the lid and place back in the tray
- If taking double swabs:
  - **Endocervical NAAT swab** (*Chlamydia, Gonorrhoea ± Trichomonas*): place tip in endocervix and rotate for 10 seconds
  - **High-vaginal charcoal media swab** (*Bacterial vaginosis, Candida, group B Streptococcus, Trichomonas*): place tip in the posterior fornix and rotate for 10 seconds
- If taking triple swabs:
  - **High-vaginal charcoal media swab** (*Bacterial vaginosis, Candida,* group B *Streptococcus, Trichomonas*): place tip in the posterior fornix and rotate for 10 seconds
  - **Endocervical charcoal media swab** (*Gonorrhoea*): place tip in endocervix and do one full 360° sweep (not rotation)
  - **Endocervical *Chlamydia* swab**: scrub endocervical region in and out for 10-30 seconds. Once done break off bottom half into its sample tube.
- Close speculum blades (but not fully to avoid pinching vaginal wall)
- Remove speculum while rotating it back sideways

TO COMPLETE

- Thank patient, give them a tissue and restore clothing
- Fill in the sample and request form details and send to lab
- Document in patient's notes
- Advise patient results will take approximately 1-2 weeks and they will have to come in to get the results (or they can get them by text if in a sexual health clinic setting)

ENT AND WOUND SWABS

INTRODUCTION

- **W**ash hands; **I**ntroduce self; ask **P**atient's name and DOB; **E**xplain procedure and obtain consent

GATHER EQUIPMENT

- Swabs – *CHECK EXPIRY*
  - Black = general bacteriology (can also be used for MRSA)
  - Red = MRSA
  - Green = viral
  - Orange = ear
  - Blue = pernasal for pertussis
- Sterile saline (if taking swab of dry area, e.g. nose, skin)
- Tongue depressor and torch (if taking throat swab)
- Wash tray and place swab inside in partially open packets
- Put on gloves and apron

PERFORMING THE SWABS

- **Ear swab**
  - Place swab in outer ear
  - Rotate to collect secretions
- **Nasal swab**
  - Patient should sit with head tilted backwards
  - Moisten end of swab with sterile saline
  - Insert the swab vertically into the anterior nares (approximately 2cm)
  - Rotate swab against anterior nasal mucosa
  - Repeat on other side using the same swab
- **Throat swab**
  - Patient should sit with head tilted backwards and light shining into open mouth
  - Ask them to stick out their tongue while you depress it with a tongue depressor
  - Quickly but lightly rub the swab over tonsillar fossa/lesion/exudate
  NB: patient may gag during procedure.
- **Wound/skin swab**
  - Expose site
  - Moisten end of swab with sterile saline if the area is dry
  - Roll swab along moist or purulent area
- **MRSA screening**
  - Groin: gently roll moistened swab back and forth against skin on both sides of groin
  - Nasal: *as per nasal swab above*

TO COMPLETE

- Place swab into container without touching anything else
- Thank patient
- Discard waste and clean tray; then discard gloves and apron; wash hands
- Fill in the samples and request form details
  - Name, DOB, hospital/clinic number, address, GP name and address
  - Specimen site
  - Clinical details
- Send to lab
- Document in patient's notes

URETHRAL CATHETERISATION

INTRODUCTION

- **W**ash hands; **I**ntroduce self; **P**atient's name, DOB and wrist band; **E**xplain procedure and obtain consent
- Get a **chaperone**
- Ask patient to remove clothing from waist down and lie on bed (but ask them to cover up with a sheet until you are ready)
- Position patient so you can perform the procedure from their right side if possible

PREPARATION

- Wash hands and put on apron
- Clean trolley
- Gather equipment on bottom shelf of trolley (think through what you need in order):
  - Sterile catheterisation pack (kits vary – add anything which is not in there)
    - 2 pairs of sterile gloves
    - Sterile drape with hole in centre *to extend sterile field*
    - Sterile gauze
    - Sterile cotton wool balls
    - Waste bag
    - Sterile bowl
  - Sterile anaesthetic lubrication jelly in pre-filled syringe
  - Catheter (usually start with 12 French gauge; use a larger size, e.g. 14/16 French gauge, if prostatic hyperplasia) with 10ml sterile water to inflate catheter balloon – *CHECK DATE AND KEEP PACKET STICKER FOR PATIENT'S NOTES*
  - Equipment to be kept outside the sterile field
    - Incontinence pad *for spillage*
    - Catheter drainage bag with tubing
    - Sterile water sachets
- Walk to patient
- Wash hands
- Open sterile catheterisation pack on top shelf to make a sterile field
- Use the tweezers if present to arrange the equipment in the pack on the sterile field (and then discard)
- Pick up the waste bag from the sterile field without touching anything else and tape to the side of the trolley
- Open other sterile equipment packets (without touching the instruments) and drop them onto the sterile field
- Pour the water sachets into the sterile bowl
- Ensure a catheter collection bag is ready on a stand/hook by the bedside (does not need to be in sterile field)

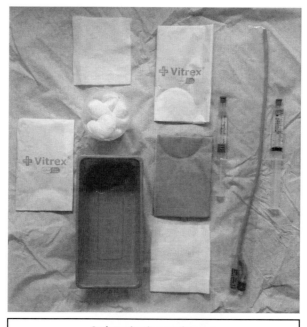

Catheterisation equipment

232

PROCEDURE

<u>Positioning and exposure</u>
- Expose patient and position them supine with extended legs if male, or in lithotomy position if female
- Place incontinence pad under the patient's buttocks and thighs

<u>Part 1 – cleaning</u>
- Wash hands and apply the 1st pair of sterile gloves

Using your left hand <u>only</u> to handle genitalia, and keeping your right hand sterile to handle sterile equipment:
- If male, hold penis in sling with gauze and retract foreskin using your left hand.
  If female, use your left hand to part the labia.
- Wet the cotton wool balls and, with your right hand, clean around the urethral meatus. Do one downward stroke only per cotton wool ball and then discard. Do one stroke down each side and one stroke down the middle.
- Remove and discard gloves

<u>Part 2 – catheterising</u>
- Wash hands and apply the 2nd pair of sterile gloves
- Keeping hands sterile, place the sterile drape over the patient (with the hole over their genitalia)

Using your left hand <u>only</u> to handle genitalia, and keeping your right hand sterile to handle sterile equipment:
- If male, hold penis in sling with gauze using your left hand.
  If female, use your left hand to part the labia.
- Insert the nozzle of the lubrication jelly syringe into the urethra and slowly expel the contents into the urethra
- Wait 3-5 minutes for the anaesthetic to take effect
- Using your sterile right hand, remove both ends of the plastic sleeve covering catheter
- Place the bowl near the patient's genitalia and allow the lower end of the catheter/sleeve to sit in the bowl (to collect urine)
- Using a non-touch technique (i.e. only touching the catheter's plastic sleeve), advance the catheter into the urethra with your right hand
- Once the catheter is <u>fully</u> inserted, check urine is flowing and then:
  - Slowly inflate the catheter balloon with 10ml sterile water (checking there is no pain)
  - Attach the drainage bag tube
- Retract catheter until you encounter resistance of balloon at top of urethra
- Reposition the foreskin if male (never forget!)
- Clean away any rubbish and ensure there is no residual urine spilt on the patient
- Help the patient get dressed
- Discard all waste and clean trolley, then remove and discard your gloves and apron

TO COMPLETE

- Thank patient and advise them on catheter care
- Check urine is flowing from the catheter and note residual volume
- Remove a urine sample for analysis if required
- Document in patient's notes and fill out urinary catheter insertion chart (catheter label, size, indication, volume of water in balloon, complications, residual volume, urinalysis results, if sample sent to lab, date and time, signature)

NASOGASTRIC TUBE INSERTION

INTRODUCTION

- **W**ash hands; **I**ntroduce self; **P**atient's name, DOB and wrist band; **E**xplain procedure and obtain consent
    - Risks: sores around nose/tape, tube misplacement (into lungs), aspiration/pneumonia, discomfort/irritation
    - Contraindications: oesophageal varices, base of skull fracture, recent epistaxis, maxillofacial disorders
- Warn patient it will be uncomfortable and ask them to raise their hand if they want to stop
- Advise the patient they must swallow when asked

PREPARATION

- Wash hands and put on apron
- Clean tray inside and out
- Gather equipment around tray (think through what you need in order)
    - Gloves
    - Vomit bowl
    - Cup of water with a straw (if patient is able/safe to swallow)
    - Nasogastric tube
        - Fine-bore feeding tube (usually 6-8 French gauge): made of polyurethane (lasts 6-8 weeks), used for feeding
        - Wide-bore Ryle's tube (usually 14-16 French gauge): made of polyvinyl chloride (lasts 7-10 days), used for drainage
    - Lubrication jelly
    - 50ml syringe (to aspirate)
    - 10ml syringe filled with normal saline (to flush)
    - pH paper strip
    - Tape (to stick down)
- Wash hands
- Open packets and place neatly in tray, keeping items in plastic parts of packets (without touching the instruments themselves)
- Return to patient

PROCEDURE

Preparation
- Wash hands
- Sit patient straight upright (head in normal position)
- Ask patient to blow their nose
- Measure from the patient's tip of nose → ear lobe → xiphisternum in centimetres with the nasogastric tube (it has measurements on it). Then add 10cm and remember the total.
- Give patient cup of water with a straw

Insertion
- Wash hands
- Put on gloves
- Lubricate the tip of the tube
- Gently push the tube into the nostril aiming posteriorly as close to horizontal as possible
- The patient will gag when the tube reaches the back of their throat
- Ask them to swallow and then keep swallowing. Push the tube down fast when they are swallowing.
- Continue advancing the tube until the memorised measurement is reached
- Confirm correct placement (i.e. in the stomach, not the lungs) by one of two possible methods (in order of preference):
    - Aspirate gastric contents and drop onto pH paper (pH should be ≤5.5). If you cannot aspirate, try asking the patient to lie on their left for 30 minutes and then try again.
    - Order a chest x-ray
        - NG must pass vertically down the oesophagus (transecting carina) in the midline to below the diaphragm
        - NG must not follow the course of either of the main bronchi below the carina
        - Tip of the NG tube must be visible at least 10cm beyond the gastro-oesophageal junction below diaphragm
- Remove tube guidewire – *present in fine-bore feeding tubes only.*
  NB: never try to replace guidewire after removing.
- Tape tube down at nose and over ear
- Flush with saline

TO COMPLETE

- Thank patient and restore clothing; discard waste and clean tray, then discard gloves, and wash hands; document procedure and aspirate pH

Other points
- Check the pH is ≤5.5 and flush the tube before every feed
- Daily care: check skin around tubing, clean around nose, flush tube
- Drugs are put down separately – you cannot give enteric coated/slow release drugs via NG
- To remove: Inject 10ml air down tube and gently remove

NASOPHARYNGEAL AIRWAY

- Flexible rubber tube which goes through the nose and ends at base of tongue (an *adjunct* to help keep airway open)
- An oxygen mask or bag-mask ventilation can be applied over the top if needed
- **Function:** prevents tongue covering epiglottis in patients with reduced GCS. It is better tolerated than oropharyngeal airways in more alert patients.
- **Size:** 7mm diameter for most adults; length should be similar to distance between tip of nose and earlobe
- **Insertion technique:**
  - Lubricate the nasopharyngeal airway with water-soluble jelly
  - Insert into the nostril (preferably right) vertically along the floor of the nose with a slight twisting action (aim towards the back of the opposite eyeball)
  - Confirm airway patency

OROPHARYNGEAL AIRWAY (GUEDEL)

- Rigid plastic tube which sits along top of oral cavity and ends at base of tongue (an *adjunct* to help keep airway open)
- An oxygen mask or bag-mask ventilation can be applied over the top if needed
- **Function:** prevents tongue covering epiglottis in patients with reduced GCS
- **Size:** should be similar to distance between the incisors and the angle of jaw; size 3 (orange) for medium adult
- **Insertion technique:**
  - Ensure no foreign bodies in the mouth
  - Lubricate the oropharyngeal airway
  - Insert into the mouth upside-down (reduces risk of pushing tongue back) – do not continue if patient gags
  - Once tip is around the hard-soft palate junction, rotate 180° and advance the rest of the way
  - Confirm airway patency

SUPRAGLOTTIC AIRWAY (LARYNGEAL MASK AIRWAY, LMA; OR I-GEL)

- Flexible plastic tube with a cuff on the end which sits over top of larynx. Provides some protection against aspiration but does not fully secure airway and can only withstand a small amount of positive pressure ventilation.
- Can be attached to ventilation bag in respiratory arrest; or, during surgery, to ventilator which allows spontaneous ventilation ± low-level positive pressure ventilation supplementation
- **Function:** *airway protection* during anaesthetic for surgery (if no risk of aspiration and a muscle relaxant is not required); respiratory arrest; if endotracheal intubation is indicated but fails, or the clinician is not trained in intubation
- **Size:** 4 for average adult (3 for small adult, 5 for big adult)
- **Gather equipment**
  - Supraglottic airway
  - 50ml syringe for cuff inflation (LMA only)
  - Water-soluble lubricating jelly
  - Tape
  - Suction
  - Ventilation bag
  - Ventilation face mask (will be required if insertion fails)
  - Oxygen supply and tubing
  - Monitoring: end-tidal CO_2 monitor, pulse oximeter, cardiac monitor, blood pressure cuff
  - Medications for awake patients (hypnotic and analgesia)
- **Insertion technique:**
  - Give medications if required
  - Test cuff by inflating and deflating it using 50ml syringe (LMA only)
  - Lubricate outer cuff
  - Position patient – neck flexed to 15°, head extended on neck (i.e. chin anteriorly), no lateral deviation
  - Standing behind the patient, hold the tube like a pen and insert into the mouth (cuff opening inferiorly), sliding the outer cuff along the palate
  - Push back over tongue until it reaches the posterior pharyngeal wall
  - Apply pressure to force it backwards and downwards until it reaches the back of the hypopharynx
  - The teeth should be between the two black lines on the airway
  - Inflate the cuff using the 50ml syringe (LMA only)
    - *Air required (ml) = (LMA size – 1) x 10*
  - Attach ventilation bag/machine and ventilate (~10 breaths/minute) with high concentration oxygen. Observe chest expansion and auscultate to confirm correct placement.
  - Consider applying end-tidal CO_2 monitor to confirm placement and then secure with bandage or tape

ENDOTRACHEAL TUBE

- Flexible plastic tube with cuff on end which sits inside the trachea (fully secures airway – gold standard)
- Attached to ventilation bag/machine
- **Function:** *ventilation* during anaesthetic for surgery (if muscle relaxant is required, long case, abdominal surgery, or if head positioning may be required); if patient cannot protect their airway (GCS <8, aspiration risk, muscle relaxation); potential airway obstruction (airway burns, epiglottitis, neck haematoma); inadequate ventilation/oxygenation (e.g. COPD, head injury, acute respiratory distress syndrome)
- **Rapid sequence induction intubation** = procedural variant using rapid anaesthetisation with cricoid pressure to prevent aspiration while airway is quickly secured – used for patients at risk of aspiration, e.g. non-fasted patients
- **Size:** 7.5-8mm diameter for men, 7mm diameter for women
- **Gather equipment**
    - Laryngoscope (check size – the blade should reach between the lips and larynx – size 4 for most patients), turn on light
    - Cuffed endotracheal tube
    - 10ml syringe for cuff inflation
    - Tape
    - Suction
    - Ventilation bag
    - Ventilation face mask
    - Oxygen supply and tubing
    - Monitoring: end-tidal CO_2 monitor, pulse oximeter, cardiac monitor, blood pressure cuff
    - Medications for awake patients (hypnotic, analgesia and short-acting muscle relaxant)
- **Laryngoscope technique:**
    - Give medications if required
    - Pre-oxygenate patient with high flow oxygen for 3-5 minutes
    - Position patient – neck flexed to 15°, head extended on neck (i.e. chin anteriorly), no lateral deviation
    - Stand behind the head of the patient
    - Open mouth and inspect: remove any dentures/debris, suction any secretions
    - Holding laryngoscope in left hand, insert it looking down its length
    - Passing the tongue
        - Slide down right side of mouth until the tonsils are seen
        - Now move it to the left to push the tongue centrally until the uvula is seen
    - Advance over the base of the tongue until the epiglottis is seen
- **Insertion technique:**
    - Apply traction to the long axis of the laryngoscope handle (this lifts the epiglottis so that the V-shaped glottis can be seen)
    - Insert the endotracheal tube via the groove of the laryngoscope so that the cuff passes the vocal cords (male 22-24cm, female 20-22cm)
    - Remove laryngoscope and use syringe to inflate the tube's cuff with the minimum amount of air required for an effective seal
    - Attach ventilation bag/machine and ventilate (~10 breaths/minute) with high concentration oxygen. Observe chest expansion and auscultate to confirm correct placement.
    - Consider applying end-tidal CO_2 monitor to confirm placement
    - Secure the endotracheal tube with tape

NB: if it takes more than 30 seconds, remove all equipment and ventilate patient with a bag-mask and high flow oxygen until ready to reattempt intubation.

TRACHEOSTOMY

- Surgical hole made in trachea, through which a tracheostomy tube is passed
- Attached to ventilation bag/machine
- **Function:** a *tracheostomy* is performed for long-term ventilation in intensive care
- *NB: a needle or surgical cricothyroidotomy is different and is used in the emergency setting when an acute upper airway obstruction is preventing endotracheal intubation*

Sedation, paralysis, ventilation

- If a patient has had a muscle relaxant they _need_ to be ventilated
- Otherwise the need for ventilation/supplementation of breathing depends on the *degree* of sedation (a low amount of sedation can allow spontaneous ventilation)
- Patients need to be sedated to a certain degree to allow intubation
- A short-acting muscle relaxant helps endotracheal intubation

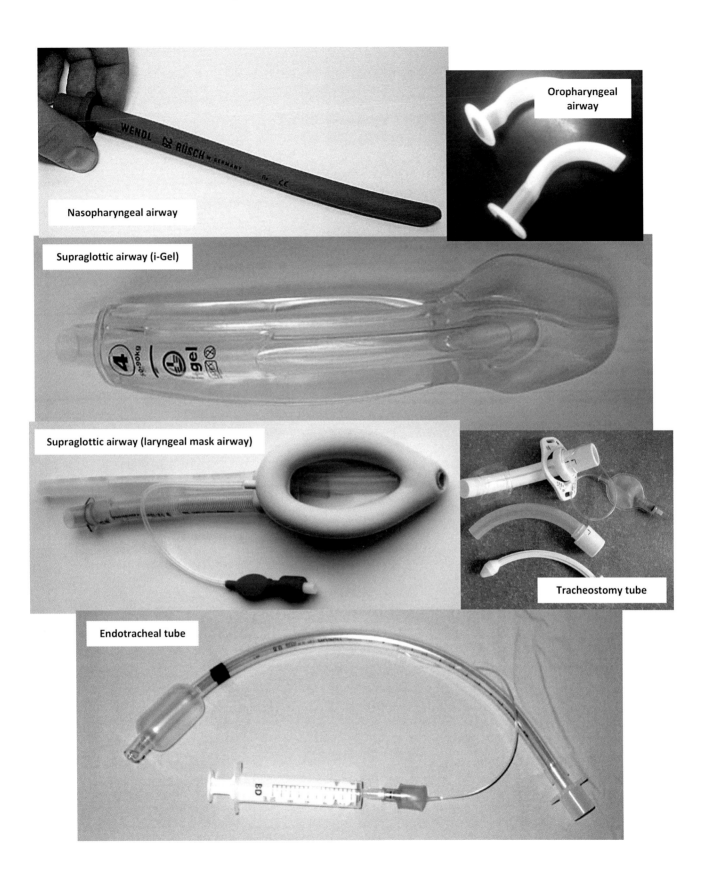

Nasopharyngeal airway

Oropharyngeal airway

Supraglottic airway (i-Gel)

Supraglottic airway (laryngeal mask airway)

Tracheostomy tube

Endotracheal tube

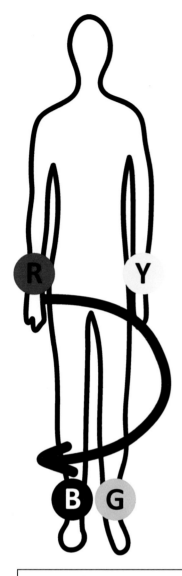

R ide

Y our

G reen

B icycle

Limb lead positioning

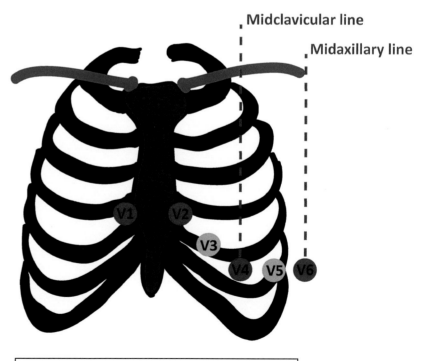

Midclavicular line

Midaxillary line

Chest lead positioning

INTRODUCTION

- **W**ash hands; **I**ntroduce self; **P**atient's name, DOB and wrist band; **E**xplain procedure and obtain consent
- **Chaperone** if female patient
- Lie patient flat, expose chest
- If needed, shave skin or wipe with alcohol wipe

APPLY LEADS

- Apply **limb leads** (clockwise from right arm: **Ride Your Green Bicycle**)

Red	Right arm, just proximal to wrist
Yellow	Left arm, just proximal to wrist
Green	Left leg, just proximal to ankle
Black	Right leg, just proximal to ankle

- Apply the **chest leads**

V1	4th intercostal space, right sternal edge
V2	4th intercostal space, left sternal edge
V3	Equidistant between V2 and V4
V4	5th intercostal space, midclavicular line
V5	Anterior axillary line in same horizontal plane as V4
V6	Midaxillary line in same horizontal plane as V4 and V5

NB: if female, electrodes should go under breast (not on it).

USING THE MACHINE

- Calibrate ECG machine to: speed = 25mm/s; voltage = 10mm/mV
- Enter the patient details (name, DOB, hospital number, sex etc.) and ECG details (date, time)
- When ready, ask the patient to stay as still as possible and not speak
- Press the button to begin the trace ('auto')
- Check the printed trace to ensure:
  - Calibration is correct (paper speed 25mm/s; 1mV calibration deflection is 2 large squares in height)
  - All leads are working
  - Clear traces can be seen

TO COMPLETE

- Remove the leads and stickers
- Thank patient and restore clothing
- Label the ECG if the patient's details are not printed
- Document procedure in patient's notes

MID-STREAM URINE (MSU) SAMPLE COLLECTION

- **W**ash hands; **I**ntroduce self; ask **P**atient's name, DOB and what they like to be called; **E**xplain procedure and obtain consent
- Explaining procedure
    - Patient must wash hands and genitals prior to sample collection
    - Before passing urine, men must retract foreskin and women part labia
    - Patient must urinate into the container you give them
    - **However,** only the <u>middle part</u> of the urine stream should be collected, i.e. they must pass the first part of the stream into the toilet, then collect the sample, then pass the rest of the urine into the toilet
    - They must not touch the inside of the container and must replace the lid as soon as the sample is in the collection pot
    - They should then place it in the bag you provide and bring it back
- Label the urine container and lab sample collection bag and give them to the patient
- Ask them to return after they have obtained the sample
- Thank patient
- Perform dipstick testing on urine if required (*see below*)
- Send the collected sample in the labelled collection bag to the lab for MC&S if required. Advise patient when to return for the result (usually 2-3 days).

URINE DIPSTICK

- Collect MSU (*as above*)
- Wash hands
- Put on gloves and apron
- Check patient details on the sample are correct
- Note the features of the urine
    - **Odour**
        - Sweet: DKA/glycosuria
        - Pungent: infection
        - Ammonia-type smell: alkaline urine
    - **Discolouration**
        - Red: haematuria/haemoglobinuria/myoglobinuria, porphyria, beetroot, drugs (rifampicin)
        - Brown: bile pigments, myoglobin, methaemoglobin, drugs (levodopa, metronidazole, antimalarials, nitrofurantoin)
        - Green/blue: Pseudomonas UTI, biliverdin, drugs (amitriptyline, methylene blue, propofol)
        - Orange: bile pigments, drugs (phenothiazines)
    - **Cloudiness:** pus, pyuria, alkaline urine phosphate crystals
    - **Sedimentation**
- Check the date on the urine dipstick container, remove a dipstick and close container
- Open the urine sample pot with one hand
- Dip the dipstick into the sample so all of the coloured squares are immersed
- Remove the dipstick and hold it horizontally
- Close the urine sample pot
- Use a stopwatch/clock to keep time and read the relevant squares at the correct times
- Discard the urine sample in the hazardous waste bin or send it to the lab for MC&S if required
- Wash hands
- Record results in the patient's notes
- Interpret the result (*see interpretation notes on urinalysis p278*)
- Suggest further investigations you would do after a full history (if any abnormal findings)

24-HOUR URINE SAMPLE COLLECTION

This may be taken to test for: catecholamines/metanephrines (*phaeochromocytoma*), free cortisol (*Cushing's syndrome*), 5-HIAA (*carcinoid*), sodium/calcium/oxalate/uric acid/citrate (*renal stone assessment*), protein (*nephrotic syndrome*).

- **W**ash hands; **I**ntroduce self; ask **P**atient's name, DOB and what they like to be called; **E**xplain procedure and obtain consent
- Explaining procedure
    - When you wake up tomorrow, go to the toilet and empty your bladder fully
    - Note the time (e.g. Wednesday, 7am)
    - Collect <u>all</u> of the rest of your urine for the next 24 hours in the large urine container provided
    - Collect the last urine exactly 24 hours after starting (e.g. Thursday, 7am)
    - When it is finished, you must take the container to the hospital's laboratory desk within 24 hours
- Label the urine container and give it to the patient
- Thank patient and advise them when to return for the result

BLOOD PRESSURE MEASUREMENT

INTRODUCTION
- **W**ash hands; **I**ntroduce self; ask **P**atient's name, DOB and what they like to be called; **E**xplain procedure and obtain consent
- Ensure the patient has been seated for 5 minutes
- Ask them to try to relax and not speak or move during the measurement

EQUIPMENT
- Sphygmomanometer – identify the correct cuff size for the patient
- Stethoscope

PREPARATION
- Expose the patient's arm and remove tight-fitting clothing
- Apply the sphygmomanometer cuff
  - The bladder should encircle at least 80% of the arm circumference
  - The bladder must be placed over the mid-upper arm
  - The artery arrow marker (or mid-point of the cuff bladder) should be placed above the brachial artery pulsation
- Ensure the patient is seated comfortably at rest with back supported and legs not crossed
- Support their forearm horizontally on a surface <u>at the level of their heart</u>

SYSTOLIC BLOOD PRESSURE ESTIMATION
- Palpate their brachial pulse (above the antecubital fossa) with index and middle finger
- While palpating the brachial pulse, inflate the blood pressure cuff until the pulse disappears
- **Systolic blood pressure estimate** = the sphygmomanometer pressure when the brachial artery pulsation can no longer be palpated
- Deflate the sphygmomanometer cuff quickly by fully opening the valve

MEASUREMENT
- Palpate their brachial pulse (above the antecubital fossa) with index and middle finger to identify and remember the point of maximal pulsation
- Inflate the sphygmomanometer to 30mmHg above the *systolic blood pressure estimate*
- Place the diaphragm or bell of the stethoscope over the point of maximal pulsation of the brachial artery
- Slowly deflate the sphygmomanometer cuff (2-3mmHg/s)
  - **Systolic blood pressure** = the sphygmomanometer pressure at which the first Korotkoff sound is heard (<u>not</u> when the sphygmomanometer dial starts to pulsate – ignore this)
  - **Diastolic blood pressure** = the sphygmomanometer pressure when the Korotkoff sounds disappear
- When the diastolic pressure has been identified, quickly deflate the sphygmomanometer cuff by fully opening the valve

TO COMPLETE
- Remove the sphygmomanometer cuff
- Thank patient and ask them to get dressed
- Document procedure and result in patient's notes

Hypertension grades	Hypertension investigation	Hypertension drug treatment
Stage 1: ≥140/90 in clinic + average ≥135/85 at home **Stage 2**: ≥160/100 in clinic + average ≥150/95 at home **Severe**: systolic ≥180 or diastolic ≥110 in clinic	Urine dipstick for protein 12 lead ECG (check for left ventricular hypertrophy) Blood glucose, U&Es, lipid profile	1. **<55 years** → ACE inhibitor **>55 years or Afro-Caribbean** → Ca^{2+} channel blocker
Hypertension history and exam History: renal disease, stroke, IHD Exam: renal bruits, radio-femoral delay, retinopathy	BP ≥180 /110 → immediate treatment BP≥140/90 → ambulatory or home blood pressure monitoring ⬊Average <135/85 → routine review ⬊Average ≥135/85 → treat (lifestyle ± drugs)	2. ACE inhibitor + Ca^{2+} channel blocker 3. Add thiazide-like diuretic (i.e. chlorthalidone or indapamide) 4. Add spironolactone or α- or β-blocker

Produced using NICE 'CG127 Hypertension in adults: diagnosis and management' 2011 (updated 2016)

PEAK FLOW MEASUREMENT

The peak expiratory flow rate or *peak flow* is a measurement of the maximum speed of expiration, starting from full lung inflation. It is a useful aid for assessing the degree of large airway obstruction.

PROCEDURE

- **W**ash hands; **I**ntroduce self; ask **P**atient's name, DOB and what they like to be called; **E**xplain
- Explain peak flow measures the maximum speed of expiration
- Give patient specific details of what they should do:
  - Stand or sit upright
  - Set the meter dial to zero
  - Hold the meter horizontally and ensure they are not touching the dial
  - Take a deep breath in to full capacity
  - Place lips tightly around the cardboard tube to form a tight seal
  - Blow out as hard and as fast possible (it measures the first puff, so they do not need to expire fully)
- Demonstrate for them with a different cardboard tube
- Observe them doing it and comment on any mistakes
- Ask patient to perform test three times at one minute intervals

TO COMPLETE

- Thank patient and ask if they have any questions
- Bin the cardboard tube
- Document in the notes the best of the three readings (in litres/minute)

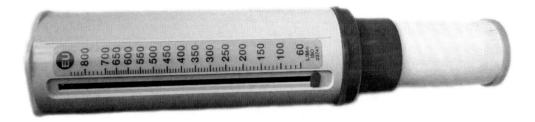

Peak flow meter

CAPILLARY GLUCOSE MEASUREMENT

INTRODUCTION
- **W**ash hands; **I**ntroduce self; **P**atient's name, DOB and wrist band; **E**xplain procedure and obtain consent
- Ask the patient to wash their hands prior to the procedure with soap and water

PREPARATION
- Wash hands
- Clean tray
- Place equipment in tray (think through what you need in order)
    - Gloves
    - Lancet/puncture system
    - Glucometer (calibrate glucometer with calibration fluid if necessary)
    - Glucometer test strip (insert into glucometer and turn glucometer on)
    - Sterile gauze
    - Tape
- Return to patient (with tray and a sharps bin)

PROCEDURE
- Wash hands
- Place patient's hands on a pillow
- Choose lateral/medial border of any finger pulp
- Put on gloves
- Pierce skin with lancet on lateral/medial border of finger pulp
- Discard lancet into sharps bin
- Wipe off the first drop of blood from the puncture site with gauze
- Massage the finger from proximal to distal (to encourage blood flow)
- When a second, large drop of blood accumulates, apply the golden part of the test strip (in the groove at the distal end) to the side of the drop of blood until the glucometer beeps
- Place gauze over the puncture site and apply pressure until it has stopped bleeding
- Tape gauze down over puncture site if needed

TO COMPLETE
- Thank patient
- Discard test strip/waste and clean tray, then discard gloves and wash hands
- Record the capillary glucose reading in the patient's notes

SURGICAL SCRUB

- Gather equipment
  - Surgical mask – put this on now (you should already have a surgical hat on)
  - Sterile gown pack (contains 2 towels and a gown)
  - Sterile gloves
  - Sterile brush/sponge (with nail pick inside)
- Prepare equipment
  - Open outer packaging of gown pack and drop pack onto clean surface
  - Unfold the sterile inner packaging of gown pack (touching only the corners of the packet) over a surface to create a sterile field
  - Open the outer packaging of the gloves and drop them into the sterile field
- Open the sponge packet and leave inside its container by the sink
- From now on, keep your hands elevated above your elbows

Wash hands and forearms (1 minute)
- Turn taps on
- Rinse hands and forearms
- Apply 3 doses of scrub solution to hands (using elbows to dispense it)
- Wash hands and forearms for 1 minute
- Rinse off scrub solution (keeping hands higher than elbows)

↓

Clean nails (1 minute)
- Apply scrub solution to hands and forearms
- Use nail pick to clean each nail in turn (rinse pick after each nail)
- Rinse hands and forearm
- Apply water and scrub solution to brush (using elbows to dispense it)
- Scrub nails
- Rinse off scrub solution (keeping hands higher than elbows)

↓

Wash hands and forearms again (3 minutes)
- Apply 3 doses of scrub solution to hands (using elbows to dispense it)
- Wash hands very thoroughly and then down to forearms (but not down as far as the first wash)
- Rinse off scrub solution (keeping hands higher than elbows)
- Turn off the taps using your elbows

↓

Dry arms
- Use a separate sterile towel for each arm (from scrub gown pack)
- Start at fingers and work down to elbows (dabbing to dry), then discard towel

↓

Apply gown
- Place hands in sleeve pockets on either side of gown
- Raise your arms high and step backward so the gown falls open in the air
- Slide your arms into the sleeves (but ensure your hands remain inside the cuffs)
- Hold your arms up in the air and ask a colleague to tie the back of the gown

↓

Put on gloves
- Open the sterile inner packaging of the gloves using the cuffs of your gown
- Using your right hand (inside the gown cuff), place left glove over left cuff with your left palm facing upwards
- Open your left hand into the glove leaving the cuff around your wrist (inside the glove)
- Repeat on other side

↓

Secure the gown
- Hand the card attached to the gown's right tie to a colleague
- Ask them to hold it while you turn around 360° (left)
- Pull the strap away from the card they are holding so it detaches
- Tie the strap to the other strap in a bow to secure the gown

CHAPTER 6: INTERPRETATION

ECG INTERPRETATION

1 small square = 40 milliseconds
1 big square = 200 milliseconds

INTRODUCTION

- **Patient** name, DOB, any symptoms (e.g. chest pain)
- **ECG date and time** and which in series
- Check **calibration**
  - Standard paper speed: 25mm/s
  - Standard voltage calibration: 10mm/mV (1mV deflection at start/end of trace should be 2 large squares in height)

RATE AND RHYTHM

Use rhythm strip

- **Rate**: calculate by dividing 300 by number of large squares between R peaks **OR**, if irregular, total R waves on ECG multiplied by 6 (ECG is 10 seconds long)
  - Sinus bradycardia <60 (*physical fitness, hypothermia, hypothyroidism, sinoatrial node disease, β-blockers/digoxin*)
  - Sinus tachycardia >100 (*exercise/pain/anxiety, pregnancy, anaemia, PE, hypovolaemia, fever/sepsis, thyrotoxicosis*)
- **Rhythm**
  1. Regularity: mark four R wave peaks on a plain piece of paper and move it along the trace to compare regularity against subsequent R waves (*irregular: AF, ectopics, 2nd degree heart block, sinus arrhythmia, atrial flutter with variable block*)
  2. Sinus rhythm or not? Look for a normal P wave before each QRS complex (***no clear P waves and irregular QRS** = AF; **saw-tooth baseline** = atrial flutter; **narrow complex tachycardia with abnormal or no discernible P waves** = supraventricular tachycardia; **broad complex tachycardia with no P waves** = VF, VT or rarely SVT/AF with BBB/pre-excitation; **bradycardia with no P waves** = sinoatrial arrest with junctional or ventricular escape rhythm; **P waves present but without constant PR interval** = 2nd degree/complete heart block*)

AXIS

Use leads I and II

- Short method: QRS is normally predominantly positive in leads I and II, i.e. both point upwards
  - If QRS is predominantly positive in lead I and negative in lead II (i.e. pointing away from each other), there is <u>left</u> axis deviation – Leaving each other = Left axis (*more electricity going to left due to: LV hypertrophy, left anterior hemiblock, LBBB, inferior MI, Wolff-Parkinson-White syndrome, VT*)
  - If the QRS is predominantly negative in lead I and positive in lead II (i.e. pointing towards each other), there is <u>right</u> axis deviation – Reaching towards each other = Right axis (*more electricity going to right due to: tall and thin body type, RV hypertrophy (e.g. in PE, lung disease), left posterior hemiblock, lateral MI, Wolff-Parkinson-White syndrome*)

P WAVE

Use rhythm strip

- **Height:** should be ≤2 small squares (*increased in right atrial enlargement, e.g. caused by pulmonary hypertension*)
- **Morphology**
  - Bifid (looks like an 'm') = P mitrale (*left atrial enlargement – classically caused by mitral stenosis*)
  - Peaked = P pulmonale (*right atrial enlargement – classically in lung disease*)

PR INTERVAL

Use rhythm strip

- **Length:** should be 3-5 small squares
  - Decreased: accessory conduction pathway (*look for delta wave in Wolff–Parkinson–White syndrome*)
  - Increased in AV node block (*'heart block'*)
    - 1st degree heart block: PR >5 small squares and regular
    - 2nd degree heart block
      - Mobitz type 1 (Wenckebach): PR progressively elongates until there is failure of conduction of an atrial beat (then the cycle repeats)
      - Mobitz type 2: constant PR interval in the conducted beats but some of the P waves are not conducted
      - 2nd degree heart block with 2:1/3:1/4:1 block: alternate conducted and non-conducted atrial beats (P:QRS)
    - Complete heart block: complete dissociation between P waves and QRS complexes. Normal atrial beats are not conducted to ventricles, which results in the ventricles self-depolarising at a much slower rate (a 'ventricular escape rhythm').

Causes of heart block

- *Increased vagal tone/athletes*
- *Electrolyte disturbances*
- *Inferior MI*
- *AV-blocking drugs (β-blockers, Ca²⁺ blockers, digoxin, amiodarone)*
- *Conduction system fibrosis*
- *Inflammatory conditions (myocarditis/rheumatic fever)*
- *Autoimmune conditions (SLE/systemic sclerosis)*
- *Infiltrative conditions (amyloid/ haemochromatosis)*

Cardiac conduction circuit

SA node
AV node
Bundle of His
RBB
LBB
Anterior fascicle
Posterior fascicle

QRS COMPLEX

Check in all leads
- **Q wave:** note that small Q waves (<1 small square wide and <2 small squares deep) are **normal in I, aVL and V6** (LV leads) due to septal depolarisation
  - o Pathological Q waves (*established/previous full thickness MI*)

Use chest leads
- **R wave progression:** QRS complexes should progress from mostly negative in V1 (i.e. dominant S) to mostly positive in V6 (i.e. dominant R). Normally the 'transition point' (i.e. the lead where R and S are equal) is V3/4.
  - o 'Clockwise rotation' i.e. transition point after V4 (*right ventricular dilatation, usually caused by chronic lung disease*)
  - o Dominant R wave in V1/2 (*right ventricular hypertrophy, posterior MI*)

Use rhythm strip (and V1 and V6 if prolonged)
- **Length** <3 small squares
  - o Increased = bundle branch block
    - ▪ <u>R</u>BBB: QRS in V1 has **M** (RSR') pattern and QRS in V6 has **W** pattern – **Ma<u>rr</u>oW** (*may be caused by: right ventricular hypertrophy/cor pulmonale, PE, atrial septal defect, ischaemic disease, cardiomyopathy*)
    - ▪ <u>L</u>BBB: QRS in V1 has **W** pattern and QRS in V6 has **M** pattern – **Wi<u>lli</u>aM** (*may be caused by: aortic stenosis, ischaemic disease, hypertension, anterior MI, cardiomyopathy, conduction system fibrosis, ↑K⁺*)
    - ▪ NB: the W pattern is often not fully developed; the RSR' pattern may be seen with a normal QRS length – this is partial (incomplete) bundle branch block and is of no clinical significance

Use V1 and V5/V6
- **Height:** look for ventricular hypertrophy
  - o S wave depth in V1 + tallest R wave in V5/6 = >7 big squares (*left ventricular hypertrophy, e.g. hypertension, AS, AR, MR, coarctation of aorta, hypertrophic obstructive cardiomyopathy*)
  - o Dominant R wave in V1 + dominant S wave in V5/6 (*right ventricular hypertrophy, e.g. pulmonary hypertension, MS, PE*). If this is present, look for other signs too, e.g. T wave inversion in right chest leads (V1-V3) and right axis deviation.

ST SEGMENT

Check in all leads – ST-elevation/depression is measured from the 'J point' (start of ST segment)
- **Elevation** ≥1 small square (*infarction; or pericarditis or tamponade if in every lead*)
- **Depression** ≥0.5 small square (*ischaemia; or reciprocal change in posterior MI*)
- **Morphology** – ST segment is normally upwardly concave
  - o Convex or straight ST-elevation (*infarction*)
  - o Concave ST-elevation (*usually other causes, e.g. early repolarisation, LVH*)
  - o Saddled ST-elevation (*pericarditis, tamponade*)
  - o Downward sloping ST/'reverse tick' (*digoxin toxicity*)

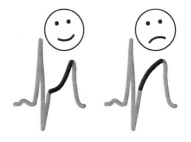

ST-elevation morphology
Upwardly concave (left) and upwardly convex (right)

T WAVE

Check in all leads
- **Inversion:** note it can be **normal in III, aVR and V1** (right leads) due to the angle from which they view the heart (also in V2-3 in Afro-Caribbean patients). It's almost always inverted in aVR.
  - o Causes: ischaemia/post-MI, PE, right/left ventricular hypertrophy (*right chest or lateral leads respectively*), bundle branch block, digoxin treatment
- **Morphology**
  - o Tented (*hyperkalaemia*) or flat (*hypokalaemia*)
  - o Biphasic (*ischaemia → up then down; hypokalaemia → down then up*)

ECG lead changes by infarct territory		
	Leads	**Artery**
Inferior	II, III, aVF	Right coronary
Anteroseptal	V1-V4	Left anterior descending
Anterolateral	V4-V5, I, aVL	Left anterior descending or left circumflex
Lateral	I, aVL ± V5-6	Left circumflex
Posterior	Dominant R wave V1-2, horizontal ST↓ V1-3	Left circumflex or right coronary

OTHER THINGS

Use rhythm strip
- **Corrected QT interval (QT$_c$):** usually <450ms. It may be calculated by the ECG machine; if not, an online calculator can be used. It is likely prolonged if T waves extend beyond midpoint of RR interval. An increased QT$_c$ interval predisposes to polymorphic VT.
  - o Causes of increased QT$_c$ interval: congenital syndromes, anti-psychotics, sotalol/amiodarone, tricyclic antidepressants, macrolides, hypokalaemia/hypomagnesaemia/hypocalcaemia
- **U waves** – *can be normal or seen in hypokalaemia, hypothermia, or with antiarrhythmics*

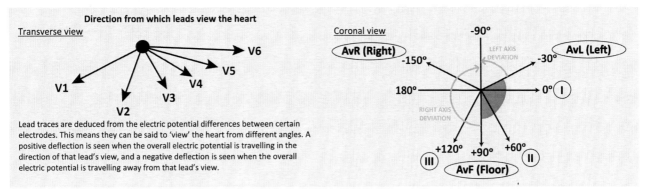

Direction from which leads view the heart

Transverse view

Coronal view

Lead traces are deduced from the electric potential differences between certain electrodes. This means they can be said to 'view' the heart from different angles. A positive deflection is seen when the overall electric potential is travelling in the direction of that lead's view, and a negative deflection is seen when the overall electric potential is travelling away from that lead's view.

COMMON ECG PATHOLOGIES

Rhythm abnormalities
- **AF/flutter**
    - **AF**: irregular without P waves
    - **Atrial flutter**: saw-tooth baseline (fluttering P waves) – *may be regular with 2:1, 3:1 or 4:1 block, or irregular with variable block*
- **Supraventricular tachycardias**
    - **Atrial tachycardia**: regular with abnormal P waves
    - **AV <u>nodal</u> re-entry tachycardia/AV re-entry tachycardia**: regular, usually without discernible P waves
- **VT**: regular, organised wavy line (broad complex tachycardia is VT until proven otherwise) – *MAY BE PULSED VT OR PULSELESS VT*
- **Polymorphic VT (*Torsades de pointes*)**: VT with varying amplitude
- **VF**: random wavy line with no discernible P waves or QRS complexes – *NO PULSE!*
- **Asystole**: flat line – *NO PULSE!*
- **Atrial ectopic**: narrow QRS ± preceding abnormal P wave (resets the P wave cycle)
- **Ventricular ectopic**: abnormal broad QRS at abnormal time (usually followed by compensatory pause)
- **Ventricular bigeminy (regular ventricular ectopics)**: abnormal premature ventricular complexes after every normal complex

Perfusion abnormalities
- **Infarction**: ST-elevation (first change), T wave inversion, pathological Q waves (signify full thickness MI and develop 8-12 hours after ST-elevation if myocardium is not reperfused)
- **STEMI criteria**: ST-elevation in >2 small squares in 2 adjacent chest leads <u>or</u> ST-elevation > 1 small square in 2 adjacent limb leads <u>or</u> new LBBB
- **Ischaemia**: ST-depression, new T wave inversion
- **Posterior (wall of LV) infarction**: dominant R wave in V1/2 with horizontal ST-depression V1-3.
  NB: Q waves can only be seen by placing the chest leads on the patient's back.
- **Previous infarcts**: T wave inversion (persists weeks to months), pathological Q waves (permanent)

Hypertrophy
- **Left ventricular hypertrophy** = left axis deviation, dominant S wave in V1, tall R wave (>5 big squares in V5/6), T wave inversion in lateral leads. *Sokolow-Lyon voltage criteria: S depth in V1 + tallest R wave height in V5/6 = >7 big squares.*
- **Right ventricular hypertrophy** = right axis deviation, dominant R wave in V1, dominant S wave in V5/6, T wave inversion in right/inferior chest leads (V1-3, II, III, aVF)

Fascicular blocks
- Any of the three conduction paths after the bundle of His can become blocked (*see conduction circuit image p246*)
    1. Right bundle branch → RBBB pattern
    2. Anterior fascicle of left bundle branch (i.e. left anterior hemiblock) → marked left axis deviation
    3. Posterior fascicle of left bundle branch (i.e. left posterior hemiblock; rare) → marked right axis deviation
- **Bifascicular block** is RBBB + left anterior/posterior hemiblock → RBBB + left/right axis deviation
- **Trifascicular block** is RBBB + left anterior hemiblock + left posterior hemiblock
    - **'Incomplete'** may be either of these patterns:
        1. Fixed block of 2 fascicles + delayed conduction in remaining fascicle = bifascicular block + 1st/2nd degree heart block
        2. Fixed block of 1 fascicle + intermittent failure of other 2 = RBBB + alternating left anterior/posterior hemiblock
    - **'Complete'** → complete heart block (escape rhythm shows signs of bifascicular block)
  NB: bifascicular block with 1st degree heart block is the most common pattern referred to as 'trifascicular block'.

Metabolic
- **Hyperkalaemia**: wide flat P waves, wide bizarre QRS, tall tented T waves
- **Hypokalaemia**: prolonged PR, depressed ST, flattened/inverted T waves, prominent U wave
- **Hypercalcaemia**: short QT interval
- **Hypocalcaemia**: prolonged QT interval

Genetic conditions
- **Wolff-Parkinson-White syndrome**: slurred upstroke into the QRS complex (delta wave), short PR interval, QRS complexes may be slightly broad, dominant R wave in V1 (if accessory pathway is left-sided, i.e. type A)/dominant S wave in V1 (if accessory pathway is right-sided, i.e. type B)
- **Hypertrophic cardiomyopathy** = left ventricular hypertrophy signs + <u>dramatic</u> T wave inversion in lateral leads (maximal in V4 rather than V6)

Other conditions
- **PE – possible changes**: tachycardia, right axis deviation, RA enlargement (i.e. P pulmonale), RBBB, RV dilation (i.e. dominant R in V1), RV strain (i.e. T wave inversion in right chest and inferior leads)
  NB: the 'classical' $S_1Q_3T_3$ pattern (prominent S wave in lead I, and Q wave and inverted T wave in lead III) is uncommon
- **Pericarditis**: PR depression, saddle-shaped ST-elevation

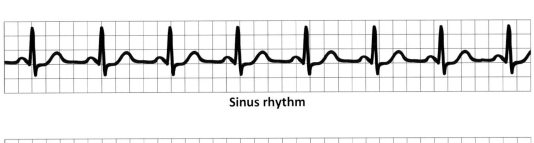

Sinus rhythm

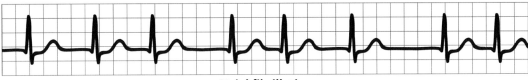

Atrial fibrillation

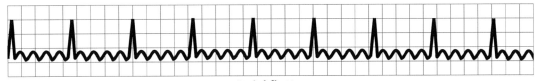

Atrial flutter

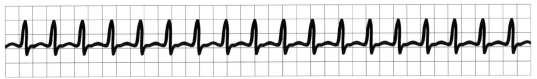

Supraventricular tachycardia (SVT)

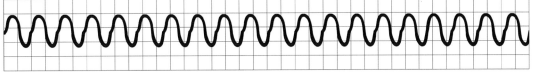

Ventricular tachycardia (VT)

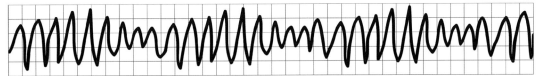

Polymorphic ventricular tachycardia (torsades de pointes)

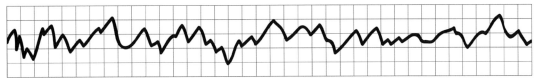

Ventricular fibrillation (VF)

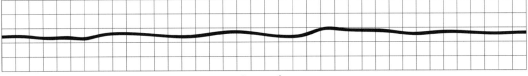

Asystole

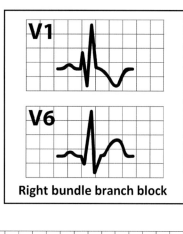

Right bundle branch block

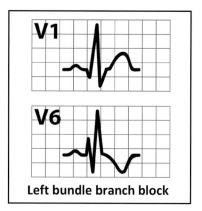

Left bundle branch block

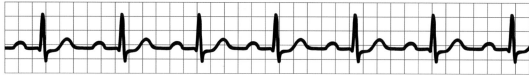

First degree heart block

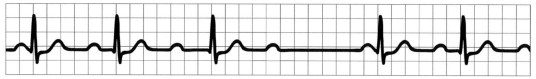

Mobitz type 1 second degree heart block (Wenckebach)

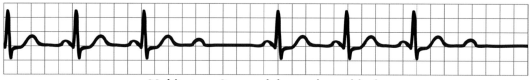

Mobitz type 2 second degree heart block

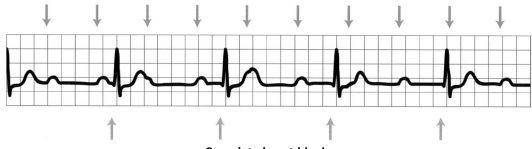

Complete heart block

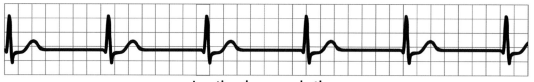

Junctional escape rhythm

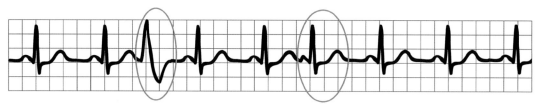

Ventricular ectopic (left) and atrial ectopic (right)

SPIROMETRY

BASIC SPIROMETRY PROCEDURE

- **W**ash hands; **I**ntroduce self; **P**atient's name and DOB; **E**xplain procedure and obtain consent
- Obtain patient details: sex, age, height, ethnic origin (to work out predicted values)
- Check that their current condition is stable
- Attach a clean mouthpiece to the spirometer
- Ensure patient is seated upright and apply nose clip
- Measure FEV_1 and FVC
  - Ask them to take a deep breath in to full capacity
  - Place their lips around the mouthpiece forming a tight seal
  - Breathe out as hard and fast as possible through their mouth
  - Encourage them to keep exhaling until their lungs feel empty
  - Repeat 2 more times
- Measure VC
  - Ask them to take a deep breath in to full capacity
  - Place their lips around the mouthpiece forming a tight seal
  - Breathe out steadily at a comfortable pace
  - Encourage them to keep exhaling until their lungs feel empty
  - Repeat 2 more times
- Calculate % of predicted values:

$$\% \text{ predicted} = \frac{\text{Best patient reading}}{\text{Predicted value}} \times 100$$

- Calculate the FEV_1/FVC ratio:

$$FEV_1/FVC \text{ ratio} = \frac{\text{Best } FEV_1 \text{ reading}}{\text{Best FVC reading}}$$

- Thank the patient and document results

Key

Major values
- FEV_1 = forced expiratory volume in 1 second
- FEV = forced expiratory volume
- VC = vital capacity
- FVC = forced vital capacity

Special values
- T_LCO (sometimes called D_LCO) = transfer capacity of lung for CO
- KCO = transfer coefficient, i.e. diffusing capacity of the lung *per unit volume* (**KCO = Korrected**)

Other values
- TLC = total lung capacity
- RV = residual volume
- FRV = functional residual volume

BACKGROUND PHYSIOLOGY

Spirometry graph measurements

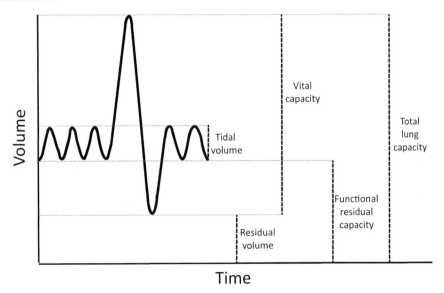

Obstructive vs. Restrictive disorders

- **Obstructive diseases** such as **asthma and COPD** result in obstructed airways. This creates <u>airway resistance to expiratory flow</u>, so the patient struggles to get air out quickly and has a decreased FEV_1. A smaller FEV_1 also results in a smaller FEV_1/FVC ratio.
  NB: an obstructive pattern due to asthma will show reversibility following administration of a bronchodilator such as salbutamol.
- **Restrictive diseases** such as **pulmonary fibrosis/interstitial lung disease, obesity, neuromuscular and chest/spine deformities** <u>restrict lung expansion</u>, reducing the amount of air the lungs can hold (the vital capacity). This means the patient has a lower FVC. As there is decreased compliance and elasticity, it is also harder for the lungs to force air out quickly, resulting in a decreased FEV_1. As both the FEV_1 and the FVC have decreased, the FEV_1/FVC ratio remains near normal.

BASIC VALUE INTERPRETATION

Summary of basic spirometry interpretation		
	Obstructive	**Restrictive**
FEV₁	↓ (<80%)	
FVC	N (>80%)	↓ (<80%)
FEV1/FVC ratio	↓ (<0.7)	N or ↑ (0.7-0.8) (>0.8)

1. What is the FEV_1? (<80% predicted = lung disease)
- **FEV_1** = volume expelled in the first second of forced expiration (calculated as % of predicted value)
- **Physiology:** FEV_1 is reduced in obstructive disorders because there is airway resistance to expiratory flow. It is also reduced in restrictive disorders because there is decreased compliance and elasticity, so the lungs cannot force air out quickly.
- **Results**
  - FEV_1 <80% predicted = lung disease
  - FEV_1 >80% predicted = normal = no lung disease (breathlessness due to another cause, e.g. PE, vasculitis)
- **Other points:** FEV_1 is also used to grade severity of COPD into mild (≥80%), moderate (50-80%), severe (30-50%), or very severe (<30%). Asthma is not usually diagnosed with spirometry (as tests are often normal when the patient is asymptomatic). However, reversibility of >12% of FEV_1 with a bronchodilator may suggest the diagnosis. Asthma is usually diagnosed clinically or with serial peak flow demonstrating >20% diurnal variation.

2. What is the FVC? (<80% predicted = restrictive lung disease)
- **FVC** = total volume expelled without time limit from maximal inspiration to <u>forced</u> maximal expiration (calculated as % of predicted value)
- **Physiology:** FVC is reduced in restrictive disorders because there is reduced lung expansion, so the volume the lungs can hold is smaller. In obstructive disorders, there is airway resistance to expiratory flow, but a normal volume of air in the lungs, so the FVC is normal.
- **Results:** FVC <80% predicted = restrictive disorder (FVC is normal in obstructive disorders)
- **Other points:** VC = non-forced total volume expelled without time limit from maximal inspiration to maximal expiration (calculated as % of predicted value). The value will be similar to the FVC, which is more commonly used.

3. What is the FEV_1/FVC ratio?
- **FEV_1/FVC ratio** = proportional volume breathed out in first second compared to the whole breath (normally 0.7-0.8)
- **Physiology:** This is calculated by dividing the FEV_1 value by the FVC value. It is low in obstructive disorders because the FEV_1 is low and the FVC is normal (as above). It is normal or high in restrictive disorders because the FEV_1 is low and the FVC is proportionally as low or lower.
- **Results**
  - FEV_1/FVC ratio <0.7 = obstructive
  - FEV_1/FVC ratio 0.7-0.8 = normal or restrictive
  - FEV_1/FVC ratio >0.8 = restrictive (if FVC more affected than FEV_1)

ADVANCED VALUE INTERPRETATION

Lung volume (TLC and residual volume)
- **TLC =** total volume of air inside the lungs, including the VC (maximal volume that can be breathed in and out) and the residual volume (the volume left inside the airways after maximal expiration)
- **Results**
  - TLC is low in restrictive disorders (as described above)
  - TLC may be high in emphysema because reduced elasticity causes hyperinflation and so results in a high RV. In this situation, the proportion of TLC comprised by the residual volume (the 'RV%TLC') will also increase.

Diffusion (T_LCO and KCO)
- **T_LCO** = total diffusing capacity of lung. To measure the T_LCO, the patient inspires a fixed amount of carbon monoxide in a single breath. The quantity expired again is then calculated to determine how much has diffused into the blood.
- **KCO** = T_LCO/alveolar volume = diffusing capacity of lung <u>per unit volume</u> (i.e. as above but corrected for lung volume)
- **Results:** a low T_LCO may be due to:
  - Pulmonary vascular bed abnormalities (e.g. pulmonary embolism, pulmonary hypertension)
    - KCO is also low (because diffusion per unit alveolar volume is also affected)
  - Alveolar destruction (e.g. interstitial lung disease, emphysema)
    - KCO is also low (because diffusion per unit alveolar volume is also affected)
  - Reduced alveolar volume (e.g. pneumonectomy)
    - KCO is normal (because KCO corrects for alveolar volume)
  - Incomplete alveolar expansion (i.e. restrictive disorders)
    - KCO is normal (because KCO corrects for alveolar volume)
- **Other points:** in the rare circumstance that both are raised, this suggests intra-alveolar haemorrhage (e.g. Granulomatosis with polyangiitis or Goodpasture syndrome)

GRAPH INTERPRETATION

Volume-time graph

The graph plots the total volume of air expired by time, from full inspiration until full expiration.
- Normal – rapid increase in volume of air expired initially, then curve forms a plateau
- Obstructive – prolonged increase (because air cannot be expired as quickly due to airway resistance) but ends at the same point because the FVC is normal
- Restrictive – rapid increase as normal, but curve forms a plateau much sooner (because total air volume in lungs is smaller)

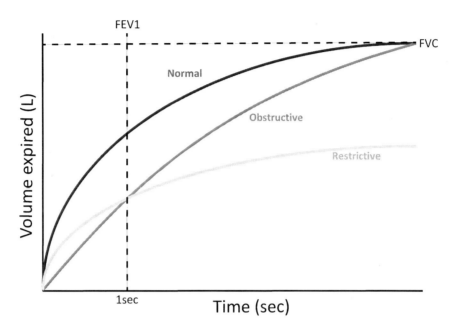

Flow-volume curve

The graph plots the expiratory flow rate (in litres per second) versus the volume expired (in litres), from full inspiration until full expiration, when air flow stops.
- **Normal:** rapid increase in flow rate, then gradual decrease until the end of expiration
- **Obstructive:** decreased peak expiratory flow rate with steeper reduction in flow rate after it peaks creating a characteristic dip in the curve (worst in emphysema, due to small airway collapse)
- **Restrictive:** curve is normal in shape but smaller due to proportionally reduced flow rates (total volume of lungs is restricted)

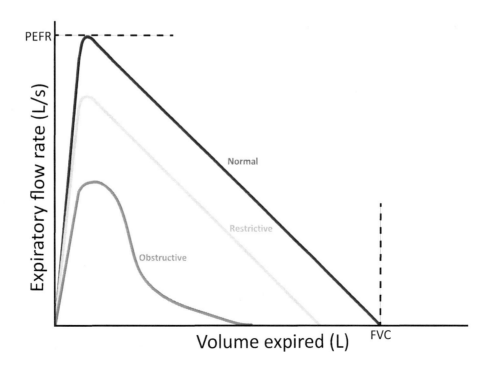

A partogram is used to monitor the active phase of the first stage of labour.

INTRODUCTION

- **P**atient: name, DOB, age, parity, allergies, blood group, haemoglobin level
- **P**regnancy: expected delivery date, preferences/action plans/risks, gestation
- **P**artogram: date and time

OBSERVATIONS DURING PARTOGRAM

- Heart rates performed <u>every 30 minutes</u>; other maternal observations performed <u>every 4 hours</u>
- Look at:
  - Fetal heart rate (*if between 100 and 180, may indicate fetal distress – CTG monitoring should be started, oxygen given and oxytocin stopped*)
  - Maternal observations
    - Pulse
    - Blood pressure
    - Temperature (↑ = *chorioamnionitis, UTI, group B streptococcal infection*)
    - Urinalysis (*protein = pre-eclampsia/liquor contamination; glucose = diabetes; ketones = starvation; blood = UTI/obstructed labour*)
- Look at observations and trends
  - Note responses to fluids/drugs given

CONTRACTIONS

- Noted over <u>every hour</u>
- Assess:
  - Frequency per 10 minutes (*aim by 2nd stage is: 3-5 strong, 1 minute contractions in 10 minutes*)
  - Strength
  - Regularity
- Determine the trend

CERVICAL DILATION

- PV exam performed <u>every 4 hours</u>
- Cervical dilation (*aim: 1cm/hour primiparous, 2cm/hour multiparous; alert line: 1cm/2 hours if primiparous, 1cm/hour if multiparous; if there is delay, oxytocin may be considered*)
- Determine progress through labour
  - Note responses to oxytocin

HEAD DESCENT

- PV exam performed <u>every 4 hours</u>
- Assess:
  - Fifths palpable per abdomen
  - Station of presenting part (*measured relative to ischial spines, -1cm = 1cm above ischial spines*)
  - Position, moulding and caput
    - Position: orientation of fetal head, assessed during PV exams, by feeling fontanelles/sutures
    - Moulding: extent of overlapping of fetal skull bones (*excess moulding may suggest cephalopelvic disproportion and C-section may be indicated*)
    - Caput: swelling of presenting part
- Assess progress through labour
  - Note responses to oxytocin

LIQUOR

- Noted <u>every hour</u>
- Assess if liquor is intact, clear (*membrane rupture*), bloody (*placental abruption*), or if meconium is present (*fetal distress – CTG and fetal blood sampling should be performed*)
- Note when changes occurred

FINAL BIRTH DETAILS

- Note times of the following:
  - Onset of labour
  - Rupture of membranes
  - Active 2nd stage
  - Delivery of fetus
  - Delivery of placenta
- Mechanism of delivery, e.g. normal vaginal delivery, instrumental vaginal delivery, C-section
- Position of occiput
- *APGAR score* at 1 and 5 minutes to evaluate the wellbeing of the baby after delivery (Apgar et al. 1953)
  - Score takes into account **A**ppearance, **P**ulse, **G**rimacing, **A**ctivity and **R**espiration
  - If total score is <7, baby needs oxygen and specialist paediatric input
- Estimated blood loss

SUMMARY

- Summarise
- Identify causes for slow progression
  - **P**assenger: cephalopelvic disproportion, fetal malpresentation (e.g. persistent occipito-posterior position)
  - **P**assage: fibroids, cervical stenosis, narrow mid-pelvis
  - **P**ower: primary uterine inertia
- Note if/when and why oxytocin was given, and the response

Example partogram

CHEST RADIOGRAPH INTERPRETATION

INTRODUCTION
- Patient: name, DOB, hospital number, age, sex
- Previous films for comparison

RADIOGRAPH DETAIL
- Date
- Type (anteroposterior or posteroanterior; erect or supine)
- Adequacy (**RIPE**)
    - **R**otation: medial borders of clavicles should be equidistant from nearest spinous process
    - **I**nspiration: at least 5-6 anterior ribs should be visible above diaphragm
    - **P**icture area: lung apices and costodiaphragmatic recesses should be visible; scapulae should be out of the way
    - **E**xposure: vertebral bodies should be just visible through the lower part of the cardiac shadow (overexposure = too black; underexposure = too white)

INTERPRETATION (**ABCDE**)
Briefly mention obvious abnormalities first

Airway
- **Tracheal deviation** (*away from a pneumothorax or large effusion; towards a collapse*)

Breathing
- **Lung fields** (compare in thirds) – *see notes on analysing lung field abnormalities on following page*
    - Air (*pneumothorax*)
    - Fluid (*effusion*)
    - Consolidation (*e.g. due to infection*)
    - Lobar collapse
    - Lesions (*e.g. malignancy, abscesses*)
- **Pleura:** look for pleural thickening (pleura not normally visible), and at lung borders for a pneumothorax
- **Hilar region:** look for lymphadenopathy, masses (*malignancy*), calcification, bilateral enlargement (*sarcoidosis*)

Circulation
- **Heart size:** should be <50% thorax diameter on PA film (*cardiomegaly suggests heart failure*)
- **Heart position** (*may be displaced if there is lobar collapse or a large effusion*)
- **Heart shape and borders** (right border = right atrium; left border = left ventricle)
- **Great vessels:** the aortic knuckle should be visible
- **Mediastinal width:** should be <8cm on PA film (*widening may indicate aortic dissection*)

Diaphragm
- **Position and shape:** right usually slightly higher due to liver (*flat in COPD*)
- **Costophrenic angles** (*blunting indicates effusion*)
- **Air below diaphragm** (*abdominal viscus perforation*)

Extra things
- **Bones:** trace around ribs for fractures if clinically suspicious
- **Soft tissues:** look for swelling, subcutaneous air, masses, calcification of aorta

TO COMPLETE
- 'To complete my analysis, I would examine previous films and ascertain the clinical history.'
- Summarise and suggest differentials

ANALYSING LUNG FIELD ABNORMALITIES

Background knowledge
- Four densities to note on a chest radiograph:
  - **Bone**
  - **Soft tissue**
  - **Fat**
  - **Air**

  White ↑ / Black ↓
- Wherever a density changes, a *silhouette* will be seen
- Consolidated/unaffected lobes may be identified by determining if consolidation is contiguous with:
  - Diaphragm = lower lobes
  - Cardiac border = middle lobe (right)/lingula (left)

Describing the abnormality
- Density
  - Bone/soft tissue/fat/air density
  - Uniform (i.e. same shade throughout) or non-uniform (i.e. blotchy)
- Radiograph position
  - Left or right
  - Zone
    - Upper (above 2nd anterior rib)
    - Mid (between 2nd and 4th anterior rib)
    - Lower (lower than 4th anterior rib)
- Anatomical position (lung parenchyma/pleural space)
- Size
- Borders

For example: 'There is a non-uniform soft tissue density in the left lower zone. Anatomically, this is in the lower lobe because the left hemi-diaphragm is not visible.'

Diagnosing the abnormality
- Consolidation
  - **Non-uniform** soft tissue density (i.e. blotchy white)
  - 'Air bronchogram' = visible bronchioles penetrating the consolidated areas (hence, it cannot be collapsed)
- Collapse
  - **Uniform** soft tissue density (i.e. pure white)
  - Affected lobe is smaller
  - Other structures move towards it into empty space (e.g. heart, other lung lobes, trachea)
- Effusion
  - **Uniform** soft tissue density (i.e. pure white)
  - Meniscus sign
  - Fluid at lung bases if erect or along posterior thorax if supine
- Pneumothorax
  - Normal lung lobes, but they are partially deflated
  - Uniform air density (usually at top if erect)
  - Seen better on an expiration film
  - Look very carefully around pleura!

Differentials
- Collapse vs. consolidation
  - Collapse is uniform soft tissue density, consolidation is non-uniform
  - It is lobar consolidation if there is an air bronchogram
- Effusion vs. collapse
  - Both uniform with density of soft tissue
  - Follow a clear border laterally and look for a meniscus (effusion)
  - Surrounding structures
    - Pulled **towards** collapse
    - Pushed **away** from an effusion

Common cardiorespiratory conditions with multiple abnormalities
- COPD: hyperinflation (>8 anterior ribs visible), flat hemi-diaphragms, decreased lung markings, black lesions (bullae), prominent hila
- Heart failure (**ABCDE**): **A**lveolar shadowing ('bat's wings' sign), **B**-lines (interstitial oedema), **C**ardiomegaly, **D**iversion of blood to upper lobe, **E**ffusion

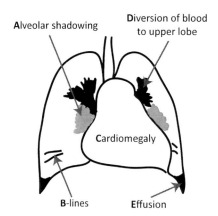

Alveolar shadowing / **D**iversion of blood to upper lobe / Cardiomegaly / **B**-lines / Effusion

CXR changes in heart failure

ABDOMINAL RADIOGRAPH INTERPRETATION

INTRODUCTION
- Patient: name, DOB, hospital number, age, sex
- Previous films for comparison

3-6-9 rule
Upper limits of normal bowel diameters

3cm = small bowel
6cm = large bowel
9cm = caecum and sigmoid

RADIOGRAPH DETAIL
- Date
- Type (supine, upright, lateral decubitus)
- Adequacy
  - Area (diaphragm to pelvis)
  - Rotation
  - Penetration

INTERPRETATION (BOB)
Briefly mention obvious abnormalities first.

B **Bowel**
- **Small bowel**
  - Identify by: central position; plicae circulares/valvulae conniventes (mucosal folds that cross the **whole width** of the bowel)
  - Should be <3cm in diameter (*enlarged in small bowel obstruction*)
- **Large bowel**
  - Identify by: peripheral position; faecal contents; haustra (pouches that protrude into the lumen)
  - Should be <6cm in diameter (*enlarged in large bowel obstruction*)
- **Faeces** (mottled appearance)
- **Gas** (normal in fundus and large bowel only): extra-luminal gas indicates perforation; check for gas in rectum if bowel obstruction suspected (presence makes complete obstruction less likely)
- **Fluid levels** seen in perforation/infection

O **Other organs**
- **Soft tissue shadows** (<u>may</u> be seen)
  - Liver
  - Spleen
  - Kidneys
  - Gallbladder
  - Psoas shadow (*lost in retroperitoneal inflammation or ascites*)
- **Calcification** of pancreas (*chronic pancreatitis*), abdominal aorta (*atherosclerosis*) or renal stones/gallstones

B **Bones**
- Spine and pelvis: Paget's disease (cotton wool lytic/sclerotic pattern); metastasis (lytic/sclerotic lesions); osteoarthritis (loss of joint space, osteophytes, subchondral sclerosis/cysts); vertebral fractures

TO COMPLETE
- 'To complete my analysis, I would examine previous films and ascertain the clinical history.'
- 'If there is any suspicion of perforation, I would request an erect chest x-ray to look for air under the diaphragm.'
- Summarise and suggest differentials

COMMON PATHOLOGY
- **Small bowel obstruction:** small bowel distension >3cm, no gas in large bowel, fluid levels if erect
- **Large bowel obstruction:** large bowel distension >6cm
- **Toxic megacolon:** colonic dilatation without obstruction, associated with colitis
- **Volvulus:** twisting of bowel on its mesentery, causing *coffee-bean* appearance if sigmoid volvulus or 'fetal' appearance if caecal
- **Chronic pancreatitis:** pancreatic calcification
- **Urinary stones**
- **Pneumoperitoneum** (due to viscus perforation or recent surgery): Rigler's double wall sign – both sides of bowel wall visible due to air outside the bowel

MUSCULOSKELETAL RADIOGRAPH INTERPRETATION

INTRODUCTION
- Patient: name, DOB, hospital number, age, sex
- Previous films
- Other orientations (need AP <u>and</u> another view – usually lateral)

RADIOGRAPH DETAILS
- Date
- Type (AP, lateral, other view)
- Area of body (including left/right)
- Adequacy
  - Area: ideally need joint above and below
  - Rotation
  - Penetration (exposure)

Only one view is one view too few

INTERPRETATION (ABCS)
Briefly mention obvious abnormalities first.

A — Alignment
- Joints and bones – *look for dislocation or subluxation*

B — Bones
- Trace around cortex looking for fractures – *see notes on describing fractures below*
- Bone fragments
- Texture of bone between cortex

C — Cartilage
- Joint spaces
- Disruption of joint contours
- Signs of osteo-/rheumatoid/psoriatic arthritis, gout/pseudogout

S — Soft tissues
- Disruption
- Swelling
- Foreign bodies or calcification

DESCRIBING FRACTURES
<u>System for describing a fracture (SOD)</u>

Site
- Bone
- Intra-/extra-articular
- Position (proximal/middle/distal third)

Obliquity
- Completeness (complete, incomplete)
- Direction (transverse, oblique, spiral)
- Skin penetration (open, closed)
- Condition of bone (comminuted, segmental, multiple, impacted)

Displacement
- Translation (% of bone diameter) – *anterior/posterior or medial/lateral*
- Angulation (°) – *anterior/posterior or medial/lateral*
- Rotation (°)
- Length distraction/shortening

For example: 'There is an extra-articular fracture of the distal third of the right tibia. It is a complete transverse fracture. The fracture is closed. It is non-displaced.'

GLOSSARY OF TERMS

Completeness	
Complete	Bone broken along the whole of its width
Incomplete	Bone cracked but ends not separated
Direction	
Transverse	Straight break at a right-angle to the long axis of the bone
Spiral	Corkscrew type fracture due to rotation injury
Oblique	Straight break through a bone but at an angle – *rare*
Surrounding structural damage	
Simple	Isolated bone damage, i.e. no significant soft tissue damage
Complex	Significant soft tissue damage
Closed	Skin is intact
Open/compound	Broken bone protrudes through the skin
Condition of bone	
Stable	Likely to stay in a sound position during healing
Unstable	Likely to change position
Comminuted	More than two detached bone fragments
Segmental	Multiple complete fractures creating an isolated bone fragment
Multifragmentary	Several fracture lines or fragments
Impacted	Break ends are compressed together
Stress	Small crack in a bone
Greenstick	Incomplete fracture of one side of the bone resulting in bending of the bone – *usually in children*

COMMON JOINT PATHOLOGY

- Osteoarthritis (**LOSS**)
  - o **L**oss of joint space
  - o **O**steophytes
  - o **S**ubchondral cysts
  - o **S**ubchondral sclerosis
- Rheumatoid arthritis
  - o Loss of joint space
  - o Periarticular osteopenia
  - o Juxta-articular (marginal) erosions – *classic*
  - o Soft tissue swelling
- Psoriatic arthritis
  - o Central erosions (→ 'pencil in cup' appearance)
- Gout
  - o Punched out lesions in bone (periarticular tophi)
- Pseudogout
  - o Chondrocalcinosis

COMMON RADIOGRAPHS

Shoulder
- **Anterior dislocation of glenohumeral joint:** seen on AP view as humeral head lying directly below coracoid process
- **Posterior dislocation of glenohumeral joint** (rare, but sometimes occurs during epileptic fit): humeral head looks like a lightbulb on AP view; seen clearly on apical oblique and scapula Y views, where humeral head is posterior to glenoid
- **Proximal humeral fracture**
- **Clavicle fracture:** occurs due to fall onto shoulder/out-stretched hand or direct trauma
- **Acromioclavicular joint** dislocation/subluxation

<u>Wrist</u>

- Distal radius fracture
  - **Colles' fracture:** distal radius fracture with dorsal angulation
  - **Smith's fracture:** distal radius fracture with volar angulation
  - **Barton's fracture:** intra-articular distal radius fracture
- **Scaphoid fracture:** scaphoid views should be requested if suspected (clinical signs: 1. anatomical snuffbox tenderness, 2. scaphoid tubercle tenderness, 3. thumb telescoping tenderness). However, fractures are often not visible on X-rays until 10 days after injury. If there is clinical suspicion, treat as a fracture and repeat X-ray in 10 days. Scaphoid fractures are important because of the risk of avascular necrosis due to retrograde blood supply.

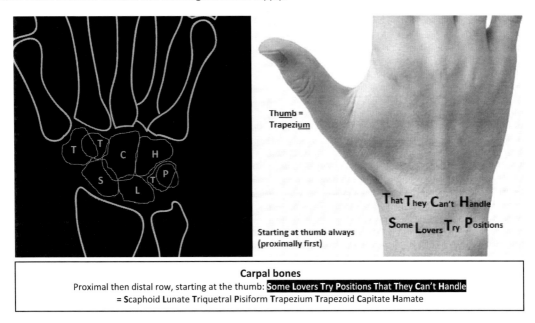

Carpal bones
Proximal then distal row, starting at the thumb: Some Lovers Try Positions That They Can't Handle
= Scaphoid Lunate Triquetral Pisiform Trapezium Trapezoid Capitate Hamate

<u>Pelvis and hip</u>

- **Neck of femur fracture:** elderly patient after fall; may be a white line (impacted) or a black line (displaced); intracapsular fractures carry risk of avascular necrosis
- **Pubic ramus fracture:** elderly patient after fall
- **Femoral head dislocation:** occurs commonly after total hip replacement and in major trauma
- Children and adolescents with hip pain
  - **Perthes disease:** 5-10 years; signified by increased density and decreased size of epiphysis
  - **Slipped upper femoral epiphysis (SUFE):** 10-15 years; seen best on lateral radiograph

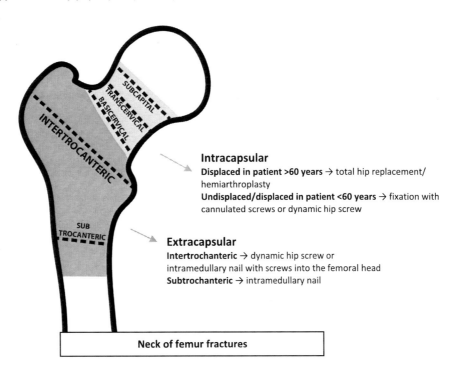

Intracapsular
Displaced in patient >60 years → total hip replacement/ hemiarthroplasty
Undisplaced/displaced in patient <60 years → fixation with cannulated screws or dynamic hip screw

Extracapsular
Intertrochanteric → dynamic hip screw or intramedullary nail with screws into the femoral head
Subtrochanteric → intramedullary nail

Neck of femur fractures

ARTERIAL BLOOD GAS INTERPRETATION

Remember: $H_2O + CO_2 \leftrightarrow H_2CO_3 \leftrightarrow HCO_3^- + H^+$

1
ASSESS OXYGENATION
- **Hypoxaemic?** (i.e. Is the PaO₂ <11kPa?)
- Is there impaired **oxygenation?**
  - ○ Oxygenation takes into account the percentage of oxygen the patient is on (the *fraction of inspired oxygen* or FiO₂)
  - ○ PaO₂ should be approximately 10kPa less than the FiO₂ percentage

---

RESPIRATORY FAILURE

Type 1 = 1 gas abnormal ($\downarrow O_2$)
Type 2 = 2 gases abnormal ($\downarrow O_2 + \uparrow CO_2$)

2
DETERMINE PH STATUS
- Acidosis (pH↓)
- Alkalosis (pH↑)

3
DETERMINE RESPIRATORY COMPONENT (PaCO₂)
- Respiratory acidosis (pH↓, PaCO₂↑)
- Respiratory alkalosis (pH↑, PaCO₂↓)

NB: if the PaCO₂ doesn't fit with the pH, ignore it until step 5.

4
DETERMINE THE METABOLIC COMPONENT (HCO₃⁻ OR BE)
- Metabolic acidosis (pH↓, HCO₃⁻↓)
- Metabolic alkalosis (pH↑, HCO₃⁻↑)

NB: if the HCO₃⁻ doesn't fit with the pH, ignore it until step 5.

5
COMBINE
- **Primary disturbance**: you know this from the above steps
  NB: both the respiratory and metabolic components may have fitted with the pH, i.e. a mixed respiratory and metabolic acidosis/alkalosis.
- **Compensation**: If either the respiratory/metabolic component did not fit with the pH, there is 'compensation'
  - ○ Acidosis may be compensated by:
    - ▪ Respiratory compensation: increasing respiratory rate to blow off CO₂ (will result in ↓CO₂)
    - ▪ Metabolic compensation: increased bicarbonate reabsorption by kidney (will result in ↑HCO₃⁻)
  - ○ Alkalosis may be compensated by:
    - ▪ Respiratory compensation: decreasing respiratory rate to retain CO₂ (will result in ↑CO₂)
    - ▪ Metabolic compensation: decreased bicarbonate reabsorption by kidney (will result in ↓HCO₃⁻)

  Partial compensation = pH not quite back to normal yet; full compensation = pH normal (you cannot over-compensate)

NB: metabolic compensation by the kidneys takes a few days, whereas respiratory compensation is fast.

CAUSES OF ACID-BASE MISMATCH

Causes of acid-base mismatch		
	Acidosis	**Alkalosis**
Respiratory	**Hypoventilation** in: - Obstructive lung disease (COPD, severe asthma attack) - Central nervous system depression → decreased respiratory drive - Neuromuscular (obesity, Guillain-Barré, myasthenia gravis)	**Hyperventilation** in: - Anxiety - Pain - Hypoxia - Acute pulmonary insult (e.g. PE, pneumonia, asthma attack, pulmonary oedema)

Metabolic	Check anion gap = $Na^+ - (Cl^- + HCO_3^-)$
	
	Normal = 3-11
	
	INCREASED ANION GAP = new acid added to body (**MUDPILES**: **M**ethanol, **U**raemia, **D**KA, **P**ropylene glycol, **I**ron/isoniazid, **L**actate, **E**thylene glycol, **S**alicylates)
	
	NORMAL ANION GAP = retaining H^+ (renal failure, renal tubular acidosis, Addison's) or losing HCO_3^- (diarrhoea)
		Acid loss may be:
		
		- **Chloride (saline) responsive:** gastric loss (vomiting), diuretics
		  Urine chloride < 10mEq/L
		- **Chloride (saline) resistant:** hyperaldosteronism, hypokalaemia
		  Urine chloride > 20mEq/L

CAUSES OF RESPIRATORY FAILURE

TYPE 1 = 1 gas abnormal = $\downarrow O_2$, normal CO_2
Most commonly occurs due to:

- **Impaired diffusion**; *causes include: pneumonia, acute respiratory distress syndrome, pulmonary fibrosis*
- **Ventilation-perfusion (V/Q) mismatch**
  - **Low V/Q:** areas of lung are perfused with deoxygenated blood but not ventilated with oxygen (i.e. airway obstruction). *Causes include: mucus plug in asthma/COPD, airway collapse in emphysema.*
  - **High V/Q:** areas of lung are ventilated with oxygen but not perfused with deoxygenated blood (i.e. blood flow obstruction). *Typically caused by: PE.*

CO_2 is normal in type 1 respiratory failure because areas of lung which *are* perfused and ventilated can blow off extra CO_2 with increased ventilation. Hence, low CO_2 in these areas makes up for high CO_2 in the area of V/Q mismatch, making overall CO_2 normal. Extra oxygen, on the other hand, cannot be absorbed (without giving a higher oxygen concentration) because diffusion of oxygen across the alveolar membrane is already maximal in normal circumstances.

TYPE 2 = 2 gases abnormal = $\downarrow O_2$, $\uparrow CO_2$
Occurs due to alveolar hypoventilation. This means oxygen cannot get into alveoli and carbon dioxide cannot get out.
Causes include: obstructive lung diseases (e.g. COPD), central nervous system depression (decreased respiratory drive), neuromuscular disease.

LACTIC ACIDOSIS

- **Lactic acid =** a product of anaerobic metabolism
- Types of lactic acidosis
  - **TYPE 1 (hypoxic)** = due to hypoxaemia (e.g. respiratory failure) or tissue hypoperfusion (e.g. LVF, local ischaemia)
  - **TYPE 2 (non-hypoxic) =** due to systemic disease (e.g. sepsis, hepatic/renal failure, diabetes), drugs/toxins (e.g. metformin, paracetamol, alcohols), or inborn errors of metabolism
- **Lactate dehydrogenase** = an enzyme involved in the anaerobic metabolism pathway (increased in tissue breakdown/turnover, e.g. muscle trauma, MI, stroke, haemolysis, cancer, acute pancreatitis, HIV, meningitis/encephalitis)

Common ABG patterns					
Situation	pH	CO_2	HCO_3^-	O_2	Details
Hyperventilation	↑	↓	N	↑	Respiratory alkalosis (lungs in overdrive)
Stable chronic COPD	N	↑	↑	↓	Fully compensated respiratory acidosis + type 2 respiratory failure (reliant on hypoxic drive)
Acute COPD exacerbation	↓	↑↑	↑	↓↓	Partially compensated respiratory acidosis + type 2 respiratory failure
Stable asthmatic	N	N	N	N	
Asthma exacerbation	↑	↓	N	N/↑	Respiratory alkalosis (wheeze → anxiety → hyperventilation)
Decreased respiratory drive (e.g. CNS depression, neuromuscular disease)	↓	↑	N	↓	Respiratory acidosis + type 2 respiratory failure (lungs stop ventilating)
Pulmonary fibrosis	N	N	N	↓	Isolated type 1 respiratory failure (despite hypoxia, there is no increase in respiratory rate, likely due to chronic hypoxic desensitisation)
PE	↑	↓	N	↓	Type 1 respiratory failure ± respiratory alkalosis (hypoxia drives an increase in respiratory rate, which allows perfused areas to excrete excess CO_2 to compensate but not absorb extra oxygen)

NB: respiratory alkalosis ΔΔ = hyperventilation (↑O_2), asthma exacerbation (normal O_2), PE (↓O_2).

RED BLOOD CELLS

Constituents of the red cell count

Most important

- **Haemoglobin (Hb):** *concentration* of haemoglobin within the blood. Hb is the protein in red blood cells which carries oxygen. It is the first value you should look at. Low haemoglobin = 'anaemia'.
- **Mean corpuscular volume (MCV):** mean *volume* of the red blood cells ('-cytic'). This is the main method used to classify anaemia (macrocytic = large cells; normocytic = normal cells; microcytic = small cells).
- **Reticulocyte count:** proportion of red blood cells that are immature. The proportion is increased in blood loss and haemolytic anaemia because the bone marrow works harder to replace lost cells.
- **Red cell count (RCC):** the *concentration* of red blood cells within the blood
  - It may be increased due to: reduced plasma volume (e.g. dehydration), or increased red blood cell production (e.g. polycythaemia rubra vera)
  - It may be decreased due to: increased plasma volume (e.g. pregnancy), or reduced red blood cell production/red blood cell loss (e.g. bone marrow failure, bleeding, anaemias)
- **Haematocrit (HCT)/packed cell volume (PCV):** *percentage* of the total volume of blood accounted for by red blood cells. Causes of abnormalities are similar to the RCC but the haematocrit is based on volume so is also affected by the red cell volume (MCV).
- **Mean corpuscular haemoglobin (MCH)/haemoglobin concentration (MCHC):** the mean *quantity*/*concentration* of haemoglobin within the red bloods cells. This affects the colour of the cells ('-chromic': hypochromic = pale; normochromic = normal red).
  - Most normocytic and macrocytic anaemias are normochromic
  - Most microcytic anaemias are hypochromic (except anaemia of chronic disease)
- **Red blood cell distribution width (RDW):** measure of the variation of red blood cell volumes. It is used in conjunction with MCV to determine if anaemia is due to a mixed cause or a single cause. Raised red cell distribution width = 'anisocytosis'.

Anaemia

Anaemia = a reduced concentration of haemoglobin within the blood.

Other relevant tests

- **WCC and platelet count:** if both are also abnormal, a bone marrow cause is likely
- **Reticulocyte count:** if raised, the cause is blood loss or haemolytic anaemia
- **Mean corpuscular volume (MCV):**

Causes of anaemia by MCV		
Microcytic (TAILS)	**Normocytic**	**Macrocytic**
Thalassaemia	Acute blood loss	Megaloblastic
Anaemia of chronic disease	Haemolytic anaemia	↓B$_{12}$
Iron deficiency (most)	Renal failure (↓erythropoietin)	↓folate
Lead poisoning		Drug-induced
Sideroblastic anaemia		Non-megaloblastic
		Alcohol
		Reticulocytosis
		Liver disease
Chronic disease		Pregnancy
		Hypothyroidism
		Bone marrow failure (aplastic anaemia, myelodysplasia, leukaemia, myelofibrosis)

Tests for specific causes

- **Haematinics:** B$_{12}$, folate and ferritin (*NB: ferritin is also an acute phase protein so may be falsely elevated due inflammation*)
- **Iron studies:** *see table below*
- **TFTs**
- **Bilirubin** (unconjugated bilirubin is raised in haemolysis)
- **Blood film ± bone marrow biopsy** (if bone marrow cause/sideroblastic anaemia suspected)
- **Hb electrophoresis** (if haemoglobinopathy suspected)

Iron studies			
Test	**Meaning**	**Result in iron deficiency**	**Result in anaemia of chronic disease**
Ferritin	Intracellular iron store	↓	N/↑
Iron	Serum iron level	↓	↓
Transferrin	Main iron transport protein in the serum *(upregulated when overall iron stores are low)*	↑	N/↓
Total iron binding capacity	Indirect measurement of transferrin	↑	N/↓
Transferrin saturation	Proportion of transferrin with iron bound to it	↓	↓
Soluble transferrin receptor	Receptors produced by cells in order to take up transferrin-iron complexes *(increased when cells are low in iron)*	↑	N

Commonest causes

- **Iron-deficiency anaemia**
  - Physiology: iron is found in meats and fish as haem iron, and in cereals, green vegetables and beans as non-haem iron. In humans, $2/3$ is stored as haem, $2/9$ as ferritin and $1/9$ as haemosiderin.
  - Causes:
    - Chronic blood loss (from GI tract, e.g. malignancy/inflammation/ulcers/varices/haemorrhoids; or menorrhagia)
    - ↑ demand (pregnancy, growth)
    - ↓ absorption (coeliac disease, gastrectomy, achlorhydria)   *Check urea (↑ in upper GI bleeding)*
    - Poor intake
  - Investigations if no clear cause: OGD + colonoscopy, coeliac screen
  - Treatment: treat cause, iron supplementation (infusion/ferrous sulphate/fumarate tablets), transfusion if Hb<70
- **B$_{12}$-deficiency anaemia**
  - Physiology: vitamin B$_{12}$ is found in meat and dairy products. The stomach produces *intrinsic factor* which binds to B$_{12}$, allowing it to be absorbed in the *terminal ileum*. Body stores last up to 4 years.
  - Causes: pernicious anaemia/atrophic gastritis, malabsorption (e.g. after gastrectomy or terminal ileal disease/resection), strict veganism, chronic alcoholism, drugs (proton pump inhibitors, metformin)
  - Investigations for pernicious anaemia: parietal cell antibodies, intrinsic factor antibodies, Schilling's test (rarely used)
  - Treatment: treat cause; hydroxocobalamin (B$_{12}$) injections 3-monthly, or oral vitamin B$_{12}$ may be used if dietary deficiency
- **Folate-deficiency anaemia**
  - Physiology: folate is found in green vegetables and fortified cereals. Body stores only last 4 months and deficiency develops earlier in malabsorption/pregnancy.
  - Causes:
    - Dietary (alcoholism, neglect, poor diet)
    - ↑ requirements (pregnancy, haematopoiesis)
    - Malabsorption in small bowel (coeliac disease, pancreatic insufficiency, Crohn's disease, tropical sprue)
    - Drugs that interfere with metabolism (phenytoin, methotrexate, trimethoprim)
  - Treatment: treat cause, oral folic acid supplements

  NB: in coexistent B12 and folate deficiency, always treat B12 first to prevent subacute combined degeneration of the cord. (Treat in alphabetical order!)
- **Anaemia of chronic disease** – *see iron studies table on previous page*
  - Physiology: inflammatory cytokines reduce the ability of bone marrow to respond to erythropoietin, leading to anaemia. They also reduce cellular iron release, which reduces the serum iron level and also results in lower transferrin saturation. Ferritin (intracellular iron store) is still normal/high, and transferrin and cellular soluble transferrin receptors are not upregulated because overall body iron stores are normal.
  - Causes: any chronic disease
  - Treatment: treat cause, transfuse if Hb<70
- **Haemolytic anaemia**
  - Physiology:
    - Normally, red cells are destroyed extravascularly by macrophages with the following effects:
      1. Hb → globulin (which is broken down into amino acids) + haem (which is broken down into bilirubin)
      2. Bilirubin is then conjugated by the liver (a rate-limited process), and released as bile into the bowel, where it is converted to urobilinogen
      3. Some urobilinogen is passed in stool; the rest is reabsorbed and excreted in urine as urinary urobilinogen
    - However, if red cells are destroyed intravascularly (pathological), free Hb follows one of three pathways:
      - Some binds to haptoglobin (and is removed by liver)
      - Some is filtered by the glomerulus and passed as haemoglobinuria or haemosiderinuria
      - Some is oxidised to methaemoglobin which dissociates into globin + ferriheme (most ferriheme then binds to albumin → methaemalbuminaemia)
  - Inherited causes:
    - Haemoglobinopathies: sickle cell, thalassaemia
    - Membrane defects: hereditary spherocytosis, elliptocytosis
    - Enzyme defects: G6PD deficiency, pyruvate kinase deficiency
  - Acquired causes:
    - Immune-mediated: autoimmune haemolytic anaemia, drug-induced haemolytic anaemia (e.g. due to cephalosporins, penicillins, levofloxacin, dapsone, levodopa), alloimmune haemolytic anaemia
    - Non-immune-mediated: disseminated intravascular coagulation*, thrombotic thrombocytopenic purpura*, haemolytic uraemic syndrome*, physical damage (e.g. by metallic valves), toxins (e.g. lead/uraemia/drugs), malaria, paroxysmal nocturnal haemoglobinuria
  - Investigations to confirm haemolysis:
    - Increased Hb breakdown: ↑ unconjugated bilirubin, ↑ lactate dehydrogenase (from red cells), ↑ urinary urobilinogen (on urine dipstick)
    - Increased Hb production: ↑ reticulocytes
    - Intravascular haemolysis: ↓ free haptoglobin, haemoglobinuria (on urine microscopy), ↑ urinary haemosiderin, red cell fragments on blood film
  - Investigations to find cause:
    - Blood film: sickle cells, schistocytes (microangiopathic haemolytic anaemia*), inclusion bodies (malaria), spherocytes/elliptocytes (hereditary spherocytosis/elliptocytosis), Heinz bodies (G6PD), bite/blister cells (G6PD), distorted prickle cells (pyruvate kinase deficiency)
    - Direct antiglobulin/'Coombs' test (for autoimmune haemolytic anaemia)
    - Osmotic fragility testing (for membrane abnormalities)
    - Hb electrophoresis (for haemoglobinopathies)
    - Enzyme assays (for enzyme defects)

*Microangiopathic hemolytic anemia** is a subtype of haemolytic anaemia, due by haemolysis in small blood vessels (causes starred above). It is characterised by schistocytes on blood film.

Polycythaemia

Polycythaemia = increased volume percentage of red blood cells within the blood.

<u>Causes</u>
- **Relative polycythaemia** (i.e. ↓ plasma volume)
    - Acute dehydration
    - Chronic (associated with obesity, hypertension, alcohol excess, smoking)
- **Absolute polycythaemia** (i.e. ↑ red blood cells)
    - Primary = polycythaemia rubra vera
    - Secondary = due to increased erythropoietin because of chronic hypoxia (e.g. COPD, altitude, congenital cyanotic heart disease) or erythropoietin-secreting tumours (e.g. renal cell carcinoma)

<u>Investigations</u>
- **WCC and platelet count** (both also raised in primary absolute polycythaemia, but not in secondary absolute polycythaemia)
- **Erythropoietin level**
- If polycythaemia rubra vera suspected: request JAK-2 mutation testing and consider bone marrow biopsy

WHITE BLOOD CELLS

Causes of deranged white cell count			
	Constituents of the white cell count	**High**	**Low**
Lymphoid	**Lymphocyte count**	Viral infection (especially infectious mononucleosis) Chronic infections Chronic lymphocytic leukaemia Other leukaemias Lymphomas	Viral infection HIV Post-chemotherapy Bone marrow failure (e.g. in leukaemia/lymphoma) Whole body radiation Myelodysplastic syndrome
Myeloid	**Neutrophil count**	Bacterial infection Inflammation (e.g. RA, IBD, vasculitis) Necrosis Corticosteroids Malignancy/myeloproliferative disorder Stress (trauma, surgery, burns) Chronic myeloid leukaemia	Post-chemotherapy Drugs causing agranulocytosis (**4C's: C**arbamazepine, **C**lozapine, **C**olchicine, **C**arbimazole) Viral infection Hypersplenism Bone marrow failure (e.g. in leukaemia/lymphoma) Immune disorders (Felty's syndrome, SLE, HIV) Autoimmune neutropaenia Myelodysplastic syndrome
	Monocyte count	Some infections (TB, malaria, typhoid, infective endocarditis) Autoimmune diseases Leukaemias/Hodgkin's disease Chronic inflammation Chronic myeloid leukaemia Myeloproliferative disorders Malignancy	Acute infections Corticosteroids Some leukaemias Post-chemotherapy
	Eosinophil count	Allergic disorders Parasitic infections Drug reactions Connective tissue disorders Malignancy (e.g. Hodgkin's disease)	N/A
	Basophil count	Some leukaemias/lymphomas IgE mediated hypersensitivity Inflammatory disorders (e.g. RA, UC) Myeloproliferative disorders Viral infection Chronic myeloid leukaemia	N/A

PLATELETS

Thrombocytopenia

Causes
- **Decreased production:** bone marrow infiltration, aplastic anaemia, megaloblastic anaemia, myelosuppression
- **Increased destruction/consumption**
  - **Non-immune:** disseminated intravascular coagulation (DIC), thrombotic thrombocytopenic purpura (TTP), haemolytic uraemic syndrome (HUS), heparin induced thrombocytopenia (HIT), sequestration in hypersplenism (including portal hypertension, e.g. in liver disease)
  - **Primary immune:** idiopathic thrombocytopenic purpura (ITP)
  - **Secondary immune:** SLE, chronic lymphocytic leukaemia, viruses, drugs, alloimmune

Possible investigations
- **Blood film ± bone marrow biopsy**
- **Infection screen**, e.g. HIV, hepatitis C
- **LFTs** (liver dysfunction can also cause thrombocytopenia)
- **Lactate dehydrogenase** (increased in haemolysis and lymphoproliferative disorders)
- **Serum vitamin B$_{12}$** and **folate**
- **Coagulation screen** including fibrinogen and D-dimer (if disseminated intravascular coagulation suspected)
- **Acute phase proteins** (look for evidence of infection)

Treatment
- Treat cause, for example:
  - ITP: observation, or corticosteroids ± IVIg ± platelet concentrate transfusion (if bleeding)
  - TTP: plasmapheresis + corticosteroids ± FFP ± rituximab
  - HUS: supportive ± dialysis ± plasmapheresis
  - HIT: stop heparin, use non-heparin anticoagulant
- Give platelet concentrate transfusion if platelets <10x10^9/L, or if <50x10^9/L and bleeding (although not for TTP/HUS/HIT – increases thrombosis)
- Splenectomy may be considered

Thrombocytosis

Causes
- **Primary:** essential thrombocythaemia, other myeloproliferative disorders
- **Secondary (reactive):** bleeding, inflammation, infection, malignancy, post-splenectomy

Possible investigations
- **Blood film ± bone marrow biopsy**
- **Acute phase proteins** (look for evidence of infection)
- **JAK2 mutation** (myeloproliferative diseases)
- **Ferritin** (to look for chronic bleeding)

Treatment
- Aspirin (to prevent thromboembolic disease)
- Hydroxycarbamide (if primary cause)

PANCYTOPENIA

Causes
- **Bone marrow infiltration:** acute leukaemia, myeloma, lymphoma, myelofibrosis, metastatic carcinoma, TB
- **Myelosuppression:** drugs (e.g. chemotherapy, herbal, some antibiotics), lead, irradiation, infection (e.g. HIV, parvovirus B19, sepsis)
- **Impaired haematopoiesis:** vitamin B12/folate deficiency, aplastic anaemia, myelodysplastic syndrome
- **Peripheral destruction of blood cells:** hypersplenism, paroxysmal nocturnal haemoglobinuria, autoimmune disorders

Possible investigations
- **Blood film ± bone marrow biopsy**
- **Lactate dehydrogenase** (increased in haemolysis and lymphoproliferative disorders)
- **Serum vitamin B$_{12}$** and **folate**
- **Reticulocytes**
- **Electrophoresis and immunoglobulins** (myeloma)
- **Viral serology** (HIV/EBV/CMV/Parvovirus)
- **Autoimmune profile**
- **Serum direct antiglobulin test**

INTERPRETATION OF UREA AND ELECTROLYTES

UREA AND CREATININE

Physiology
Creatinine
- Creatine is a substance produced primarily by the liver
- Creatine is phosphorylated to creatine phosphate, which is used as an energy store for muscles
- To produce energy, creatine phosphate is broken down to creatine and phosphate, which allows ADP to be converted to ATP
- Creatine is metabolised to the waste product creatinine, which passes to the kidneys where it is excreted
- Changes in serum creatinine concentration are specific for determining kidney injury, but baseline levels depend on muscle mass

Urea
- Ammonia is a toxic waste product produced during amino acid catabolism
- Ammonia is converted to urea in the liver by the 'urea cycle'
- Urea then passes to the kidneys where it is excreted
- Serum urea concentration also rises in kidney injury but it is not specific for this. Other causes of high/low urea include:
    - ↑urea = dehydration, GI bleeding, increased protein breakdown (trauma, infection, malignancy), high protein intake
    - ↓urea = malnutrition, liver disease, pregnancy

Acute kidney injury
Acute kidney injury (AKI) = rise in serum creatinine >50% from baseline, or urine output <0.5ml/kg/hour for 6 hours.
Determine if AKI is pre-renal, renal, or post-renal.

ALL patients need:
- *Urine dipstick (interpreted in context of history)*
- *Bloods: FBC ± haematinics, U&Es, CRP, Ca^{2+}, PO_4^{3-}, PTH*
- *VBG: check for: metabolic acidosis/low bicarbonate (may need weak bicarbonate infusion); and hyperkalaemia*
- *Accurate fluid balance chart (requires catheterisation)*
- *Stopping of any renal-excreted/nephrotoxic drugs*

Pre-renal renal failure (70%) – caused by renal hypoperfusion
- **Causes:** hypovolaemia/sepsis (most common AKI cause), renovascular disease, cardiorenal failure (increased venous pressure reduces renal perfusion pressure)
- **Suggested by:** history, dehydration, hypotension, rise in urea greater than rise in creatinine
- **Investigation:**
    - Hydration status assessment *(see p108)*
    - Renal artery Doppler (if suspect renovascular disease)
- **Treatment:** treat cause (IV fluids in hypovolaemia)
- **Complications:** acute tubular necrosis

Intrinsic renal failure (20%) – caused by renal damage
- **Causes:** acute tubular necrosis (ischaemic or nephrotoxic), acute interstitial nephritis, acute glomerulonephritis
- **Suggested by:** causative drugs, renal hypoperfusion, other glomerulonephritis symptoms, haematuria and proteinuria
- **Investigation:**
    - Urine dipstick
        - blood +++ protein +++ in glomerulonephritis
        - in acute tubular necrosis, urine is usually bland
    - Urine protein/creatinine ratio (to quantify and monitor proteinuria if dipstick is positive for protein; <15mg/mmol = normal; >300mg/mmol = nephrotic)
    NB: urine protein/creatinine ratio (mg/mmol) X 10 ≈ 24 hour protein loss (mg)
    - Possible further tests
        - Nephritic screen (if suspect glomerulonephritis): anti-nuclear antibodies, anti-neutrophil cytoplasmic antibodies, anti-glomerular basement membrane antibody, complement, rheumatoid factor, anti-streptolysin O titre, hepatitis serology, anti-phospholipid antibodies
        - Myeloma screen: protein electrophoresis and serum free light chains
        - Creatinine kinase (if rhabdomyolysis suspected)
        - Renal biopsy (if: unexplained AKI, suspected glomerulonephritis, positive nephritic screen, persistent acute tubular necrosis, or suspected interstitial nephritis)
        - Urgent renal biopsy (if rapidly progressive glomerulonephritis suspected – suggested by rapid loss of kidney function, worsening severe proteinuria/haematuria, and nephritic syndrome)
- **Treatment:**
    - Treat cause
    - Stop causative agent for acute interstitial nephritis
    - Corticosteroids, diuretics and ACE inhibitor may be required for glomerulonephritis
- **Complications:** irreversible renal damage

Post-renal renal failure (10%) – caused by obstruction of the urinary tract
- **Cause:** urinary tract obstruction
  - o Ureters: ureteric calculi, vesico-ureteric reflux, ureteric stricture, tumour (e.g. transitional cell carcinoma), extrinsic compression
  - o Bladder: neurogenic bladder, bladder calculi, tumour (e.g. bladder carcinoma)
  - o Urethra: benign prostatic hypertrophy, prostate cancer, stricture, blocked catheter
- **Suggested by:** history, urea and creatinine raised in equal proportion
- **Investigation:**
  - o Bladder scan
  - o Renal tract USS
- **Treatment:** relieve obstruction (catheter if urethral; nephrostomy if ureteric) and treat cause
- **Complications:** hydronephrosis (can progress to irreversible renal damage)

Dialysis indications in acute kidney injury

Refractory:

A **A**cidosis – *pH<7.1*

E **E**lectrolyte abnormalities (hyperkalaemia, hyponatraemia, hypercalcaemia) – *K^+>6.5 or ECG changes*

I **I**ntoxicants (methanol, lithium, salicylates)

O **O**verload – *acute pulmonary oedema*

U **U**raemia – *urea >60, uraemic pericarditis or encephalopathy*

NB: in chronic kidney disease, regular dialysis is required when the GFR is <15ml/minute.

Chronic kidney disease
Chronic kidney disease = presence of marker of kidney damage (e.g. proteinuria) or decreased GFR for > 3 months

Commonest causes
1. Diabetes (secondary glomerular disease)
2. Chronic hypertension
3. Chronic glomerulonephritis
4. Polycystic kidney disease

Determining cause
- History
- Urine dipstick
- Renal USS
- Renal biopsy if required

Management
- **Manage cause**
- **General measures:** fluid restriction, dietary protein restriction, ACE inhibitor
- **Treat complications:**
  - o Hypertension → antihypertensives
  - o Oedema → fluid restriction ± furosemide
  - o Anaemia → erythropoietin ± iron supplementation
  - o Secondary hyperparathyroidism →
    - ▪ Active vitamin D therapy, e.g. alfacalcidol, calcitriol
    - ▪ Dietary phosphate restriction ± phosphate binders, e.g. calcium edetate/sevelamer
    - ▪ Calcium *if low*, e.g. supplement tablets or use of calcium-based phosphate binder
  - o Acidosis → sodium bicarbonate
  - o Hyperlipidaemia → statin
  - o Hyperkalaemia → dietary potassium restriction
- **Dialysis** (when GFR <15)

SODIUM

Physiology
- Na^+ is an extracellular ion
- H_2O follows solutes due to osmosis (e.g. Na^+, albumin)
- Aldosterone increases Na^+ reabsorption (in exchange for K^+) from the distal convoluted tubule
- Antidiuretic hormone causes reabsorption of H_2O (alone) from the collecting duct

Hyponatraemia → *nausea/vomiting, headache, confusion, seizures, reduced consciousness*
Causes

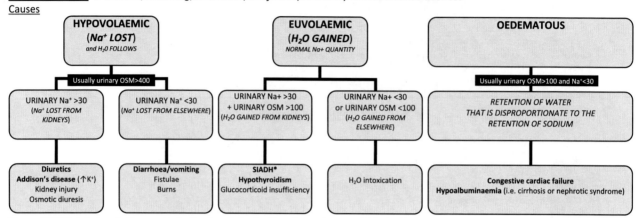

*Causes of SIADH include: drugs (antidepressants, ciprofloxacin, cyclophosphamide, carbamazepine, ecstasy); infection (abscesses, pneumonia, meningitis); neurological (brain haematomas, encephalitis, Guillain-Barré, hydrocephalus); paraneoplastic (especially small cell lung cancer)

Investigations
- Plasma osmolality (to confirm if true hyponatraemia)
  - **Low** = true
  - **Normal** = false ('pseudohyponatraemia' due to high lipids, or high glycine post-operatively)
  - **High** = dilutional (due to high glucose, e.g. hyperosmolar hyperglycaemic state, alcohols or mannitol)
- Urinary sodium and osmolality (to determine whether the problem is occurring in the kidneys or elsewhere)
- Specific tests to confirm specific causes, for example:
  - **Addison's disease:** Synacthen (synthetic ACTH) test, or 9am cortisol screening test
  - **SIADH:** confirmed by combination of low plasma osmolality (<275) and high urine osmolality (>100); investigate cause
  - **Hypothyroidism:** TFTs

Management
- Treat cause
- Sodium correction
  - **Seizures/coma:** consider 3% hypertonic saline with ICU input (e.g. 150ml over 15 minutes, repeated if necessary)
  - **Hypovolaemic:** replace lost fluid with 0.9% saline/Hartmann's solution – *slowly if chronic, e.g. 1L over 12 hours*
  - **Euvolaemic:** correct cause
  - **If SIADH or oedematous:** fluid restrict to 1 litre/day (excess H_2O causes dilutional hyponatraemia); consider demeclocycline for fluid restriction-resistant SIADH; diuretics for heart failure

NB: correct chronic hyponatraemia slowly (risk of osmotic change causing central pontine demyelination).

Hypernatraemia → *thirst, confusion, muscle twitching/spasms*
Causes
- **Euvolaemic** = iatrogenic (e.g. excess IV sodium-containing fluids, sodium-containing drugs)
- **Hypovolaemic**
  - **Producing small volumes of concentrated urine (*normal response to hypovolaemia*)**
    - Dehydration
  - **Not producing small volumes of concentrated urine (*abnormal response to hypovolaemia*)**
    - Diabetes insipidus = urine osmolality <750 + serum osmolality >300 (*kidneys not reabsorbing sufficient H_2O*)
    - Osmotic diuresis, e.g. DKA (*kidneys losing H_2O and solutes*)

Investigation
- Urine and serum osmolality
- Fluid deprivation test to confirm diabetes insipidus

Management
- Treat cause
- Sodium correction
  - **Most patients:** 5% dextrose – *slowly if chronic, e.g. 1L over 12 hours*
  - **Signs of volume depletion** (e.g. orthostatic hypotension): replace lost fluid with 0.9% saline/Hartmann's solution

NB: correct chronic hypernatraemia slowly (risk of osmotic change causing central pontine demyelination).

POTASSIUM

Physiology
- K⁺ is 90% intracellular
- Insulin and catecholamines increase cellular K⁺ uptake by stimulating cellular Na⁺(out)/K⁺(in) ATPase pumps
- Aldosterone increases renal K⁺ excretion by stimulating Na⁺(out)/K⁺(in) ATPase pumps in the distal convoluted tubule
- Acidosis decreases cellular K⁺ uptake by inhibiting cellular Na⁺(in)/H⁺(out) exchangers. This results in a fall in intracellular Na⁺ levels and consequently in the activity of Na⁺(out)/K⁺(in) ATPase pumps.
- Alkalosis increases cellular K⁺ uptake by the opposite mechanism

Hypokalaemia → *arrhythmias, tremor, muscle weakness/cramps, constipation*
Causes
- **Increased renal loss**
  - Diuretics (except potassium-sparing diuretics)
  - Endocrinological (steroids, Cushing's syndrome, hyperaldosteronism)
  - Renal tubular acidosis
  - Hypomagnesaemia
- **Intestinal loss**
  - Intestinal fluid loss (vomiting/diarrhoea)
- **Increased cellular uptake**
  - Salbutamol
  - Insulin
  - Alkalosis

Management
- **>2.5mmol/L:** potassium supplements (e.g. Sando-K 2 tablets TDS x ³/₇), or 20-40mmol potassium chloride in each litre IV fluids
- **<2.5mmol/L:** 40mmol/L potassium chloride in 1L 0.9% saline over 4-6 hours (**NEVER** give >10mmol/hour K⁺ outside ICU)
- Treat cause

Hyperkalaemia → *arrhythmias, lethargy, muscle weakness*
Causes
- **Reduced renal excretion**
  - Acute/chronic kidney injury
  - Drugs (potassium-sparing diuretics, ACE inhibitors, NSAIDs)
  - Aldosterone deficiency (Addison's disease)
- **Excess K⁺ load**
  - Iatrogenic
  - Massive blood transfusion
- **Release from intracellular fluid**
  - Acidosis
  - Tissue breakdown, e.g. rhabdomyolysis, haemolysis, tumour lysis syndrome, burns, crush injury

NB: may be due to pseudohyperkalaemia (haemolysis/EDTA-contaminated sample).

Management
- **Acute management**
  1. ECG and 3-lead cardiac monitoring
     - Changes: flat wide P waves, wide bizarre QRS, tall tented T waves
  2. Calcium gluconate: **10**ml **10**% IV over **10** minutes
     - Protects myocytes (required if K⁺ > 6.5mmol/l or if there are ECG changes)
     - Works in minutes – check ECG changes resolved; if not, repeat dose every 10 minutes up to 50ml
     - Lasts 30-60 minutes
  3. Actrapid insulin: **10** units in 250ml **10**% dextrose IV over 30 minutes
     - Temporarily shifts potassium into cells
     - Check capillary glucose before, during and after
     - Gradually decreases potassium
     - Lasts 60 minutes
     - Check K⁺ has normalised after 2 hours (dose can be repeated if not)
     - Nebulised salbutamol may be used in addition for similar but lesser effect – lasts 2 hours
  4. Calcium resonium
     - Works slowly
     - Only treatment that actually <u>removes</u> potassium from body
     - May start with this if only moderate hyperkalaemia, i.e. K⁺ < 5.9mmol/L
     - Give with regular lactulose (causes constipation)
- **Consider haemodialysis** if above fails (also consider sodium bicarbonate in severe acidosis)
- **Treat cause**

CALCIUM

Physiology

- Arrows indicate movement of calcium under influence of vitamin D and PTH:

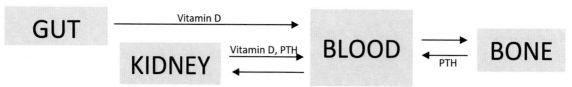

- PTH should increase in response to hypocalcaemia due to hormonal feedback
- Always look at the *corrected* calcium value, which is adjusted for albumin

Hypocalcaemia → `CATs go numb`: *Convulsions, Arrhythmias, Tetany, numb**ness** (periorbital, hands, feet)*

Causes

- **PTH deficiency (↑PO_4^{3-}, ↓PTH)**
  - Hypoparathyroidism
  - Hypomagnesaemia (magnesium is required for PTH secretion)
  - Cinacalcet
- **Vitamin D deficiency**
- **Increased deposition in bones**   ⎤ (↓PO_4^{3-}, ↑PTH)
  - Bisphosphonates
- **Other causes (↑PO_4^{3-}, ↑PTH)**
  - Chronic kidney disease (inability to hydroxylate 25-OH vitamin D and calcium binding to retained phosphate)
  - Pseudohypoparathyroidism (resistance to PTH)
  - Rhabdomyolysis/tumour lysis syndrome (calcium binds to high phosphate)

Investigation

- **Initial tests**
  - Renal function
  - PTH
  - Phosphate, magnesium

Management

- **Severe (<1.9mmol/L or symptomatic):** calcium gluconate 10ml 10% IV over 10 minutes – may be repeated until asymptomatic and can be followed by an infusion if required (50ml 10% calcium gluconate in 500ml 0.9% saline over 12 hours)
- **Mild (>1.9mmol/L and asymptomatic):** calcium supplements (e.g. Sandocal or Calcichew 1000mg BD)
- **Treat cause:** in severe vitamin D deficiency, load with 50,000 units colecalciferol once weekly for 8 weeks; in mild vitamin D deficiency, give 800 units once daily long-term; or, if calcium and vitamin D deficient, give Adcal-D3 long-term; in CKD-associated vitamin D deficiency, use alfacalcidol (1-α hydroxycholecalciferol) instead because the kidney disease impairs the terminal hydroxylation required for vitamin D synthesis.

Hypercalcaemia → *'painful bones, renal stones, abdominal groans, and psychic moans'*

Causes

- **PTH excess**
  - Primary hyperparathyroidism (↑PTH) or tertiary hyperparathyroidism (↑↑↑PTH)
  - Ectopic PTH/PTH-related peptide secretion (e.g. squamous cell lung cancer)
- **Vitamin D excess**
  - Excessive vitamin D intake
  - Sarcoidosis
- **Increased release from bones**
  - Bony metastasis (↑ALP)
  - Myeloma (normal ALP)
  - Thyrotoxicosis (mechanism unknown)
- **Other causes**
  - Drugs that decrease renal excretion (e.g. thiazide diuretics)

NB: dehydration is also a common cause. (Urea and albumin also likely raised.)

Investigation

Investigate for cause if not clear:

- Initial tests: renal function, ALP, PTH, phosphate
- Myeloma screen (if myeloma suspected)
- Serum ACE (if sarcoidosis suspected)
- Isotope bone scan (if bony metastasis suspected)

Management

- Treat cause
- Replace fluid deficit and keep patient very well hydrated (e.g. continuous 0.9% saline at 1L over 4-6 hours)
- If severe (>3.5mmol/L or symptomatic – a medical emergency): also bisphosphonate, e.g. IV zoledronic acid 4mg depending on severity and renal function (one-off dose which takes around 3 days to work fully)

MAGNESIUM

Hypomagnesaemia → *lethargy, muscle weakness/cramps, tremors, arrhythmias, seizures*

Causes
- **Reduced intake**
    - o   Poor nutritional intake
    - o   Malabsorption
    - o   Alcoholism
- **Excess loss**
    - o   GI loss, e.g. severe diarrhoea, vomiting, NG losses, proton pump inhibitors
    - o   Renal loss, e.g. ketoacidosis, renal tubular diseases, hyperaldosteronism, diuretics, aminoglycosides

NB: hypomagnesaemia can cause hypokalaemia (magnesium normally inhibits renal potassium excretion) and hypocalcaemia (magnesium is required for PTH secretion and sensitivity)

Management
- **PO:** magnesium aspartate 1 sachet (10mmol) BD x $^3/_7$
- **IV:** 5grams (20mmol) magnesium in 500ml 0.9% saline over 5 hours
- Correct hypomagnesaemia <u>before</u> concurrent hypokalaemia and hypocalcaemia if possible

PHOSPHATE

Hypophosphataemia → *lethargy, muscle weakness, change in mental state*

Causes
- **Reduced intake/absorption**
    - o   Vitamin D deficiency
    - o   Poor nutrition/malabsorption/alcoholism
- **Shift into intracellular space**
    - o   Refeeding syndrome (phosphate required to produce ATP from ADP)
    - o   Insulin therapy
    - o   Alkalosis
- **Excess renal loss**
    - o   Primary hyperparathyroidism
    - o   Renal tubular diseases

Management
- **PO:** Phosphate-Sandoz 2 tablets TDS x $^3/_7$
- **IV:** Phosphate Polyfusor (50mmol in 500ml), 100-300ml over 12-24 hours depending on severity and patient weight <u>or</u> sodium glycerophosphate 10mmol in 500ml 0.9% saline over 12 hours
- Do not give if hypercalcaemic or oliguric

INTERPRETATION OF LIVER FUNCTION TESTS

PATTERNS

- **Acute hepatitic picture**: ALT/AST in 1000s, ALP mildly raised
- **Chronic hepatitic picture**: ALT/AST in 100s
- **Cholestatic (obstructive) picture**: ALP significantly raised, ALT/AST mildly raised, ↑bilirubin
- **Alcoholic**: ↑γGT, ↑mean corpuscular volume, AST/ALT mildly elevated (AST>ALT), ↑bilirubin in acute alcoholic hepatitis (may be disproportionate to ALT/AST)
- **Cirrhosis/chronic liver disease**: liver enzymes may be normal, ↓albumin, ↑coagulation tests

LIVER ENZYMES

Enzymes leak from damaged liver cells and therefore they reflect liver injury (not function).

Aminotransferases – alanine aminotransferase (ALT) and aspartate aminotransferase (AST)

- ALT sources: specific to liver
- AST sources: liver, heart, skeletal muscle, kidneys, pancreas
- **Marked increase (>1000)**:
  1. Toxin-/drug-induced hepatitis (e.g. paracetamol)
  2. Acute viral hepatitis (Hep A/B/E, EBV, CMV)
  3. Liver ischaemia
- **Modest increase (300-500)**: chronic viral/alcoholic/autoimmune hepatitis, biliary obstruction
- **Mild increase (<300)**: cirrhosis, non-alcoholic fatty liver disease, hepatocellular carcinoma, haemochromatosis/Wilson's
- Ratio of ALT:AST
  - ALT>AST: chronic liver disease
  - AST>ALT: + in established cirrhosis, ++ in alcoholic liver disease

Alkaline phosphatase (ALP)

- Main sources: biliary ducts, bone (Paget's disease, bony metastasis, fractures, osteomalacia, renal bone disease)
- Lesser sources: placenta (pregnancy), small intestine (fatty meals), kidneys (chronic kidney disease)
- γGT can be used to help determine if ALP is of hepatic origin; and isoenzyme analysis can confirm
- **Marked increase (>4x normal)**: cholestasis (e.g. gallstones, primary biliary cholangitis, primary sclerosing cholangitis, pancreatic cancer, drugs)
- **Moderate increase (<3x normal)**: hepatitis, cirrhosis, infiltration (e.g. hepatocellular carcinoma, liver abscess etc.)

Gamma-glutamyltransferase (γGT)

- **Mirrors ALP** so can be used to confirm if a rise in ALP is of hepatic origin
- Raised with alcohol abuse and enzyme-inducing drugs

BILIRUBIN

Extravascular haemolysis results in breakdown of Hb → globulin (further broken down into amino acids) + haem (further broken down into bilirubin). This unconjugated bilirubin is then conjugated by the liver so it can be excreted in bile.

- **Unconjugated hyperbilirubinaemia**: increased indirect bilirubin (_unconjugated = indirect_)
  - Increased red blood cell breakdown (haemolytic anaemia)
  - Impaired hepatic uptake (drugs, heart failure)
  - Impaired conjugation (Gilbert's syndrome, physiological neonatal jaundice)
- **Conjugated hyperbilirubinaemia**: increased direct bilirubin (_direct = directly related to the liver_)
  - Hepatocellular dysfunction (liver disease)
  - Impaired hepatic secretion (cholestasis)

Split bilirubin fractions	
	Direct bilirubin fraction
Normal fraction	20-50%
Unconjugated hyperbilirubinaemia	<20%
Conjugated hyperbilirubinaemia	>50%

FUNCTIONAL LIVER TESTS

Albumin

Albumin makes up more than half of the total protein in the blood. The remainder is made up by globulins (other blood proteins) which include α1-globulins (α1-antitrypsin), α2-globulins (α2-macroglobulin, haptoglobin), β-globulins (complement, transferrin), and γ-globulins (immunoglobulins). Albumin is synthesised by the liver and has a half-life of around **20 days**. Hence, changes in levels happen over weeks.

- ↓albumin + ↓protein = advanced cirrhosis, alcoholism, protein malnutrition, chronic inflammation, renal/gut/skin loss
- ↓albumin + normal protein = infection (albumin is a negative acute phase protein)
- ↓albumin + ↑protein = myeloma, chronic inflammation/autoimmune conditions, acute infection, Waldenström's macroglobulinaemia

Prothrombin time/INR

PT/INR depend on clotting factors and fibrinogen which are synthesised by the liver. Some clotting factors have short half-lives (e.g. 6-8 hours) so changes can occur rapidly.

- Raised PT/INR: liver disease (with impaired function), vitamin K deficiency, consumptive coagulopathy (e.g. disseminated intravascular coagulation)

OTHER TESTS

FBC clues

- Anaemia = GI bleeding
- Macrocytosis = alcohol
- Thrombocytopenia = effect of alcohol on bone marrow, hypersplenism, liver cirrhosis or disseminated intravascular coagulation

FURTHER INVESTIGATIONS TO FIND CAUSE

Blood tests

- Viral
  - Viral hepatitides: hepatitis A IgM, hepatitis B surface antigen, hepatitis C IgG, hepatitis E IgM
  - CMV serology
  - EBV serology
- Autoimmune liver screen
  - Anti-smooth muscle (*autoimmune hepatitis type 1*)
  - Anti-mitochondrial (*primary biliary cholangitis*)
  - Anti-liver-kidney microsomal (*autoimmune hepatitis type 2, hepatitis C/D, drug-induced hepatitis*)
  - Anti-nuclear (*autoimmune hepatitis type 1, SLE*)
- Tumour markers – *if cirrhosis/weight loss*
  - α- fetoprotein (*hepatocellular carcinoma*)
- Infiltrative
  - Ferritin and transferrin saturation (*haemochromatosis*) – *but be aware ferritin is also an acute phase protein*
  - Serum copper and caeruloplasmin ± 24-hour urinary copper (*Wilson's disease*)
  - Fasting glucose and lipids (*fatty liver disease*)
- Metabolic
  - $α_1$-antitrypsin (*$α_1$-antitrypsin deficiency*)
  - Immunoglobulins and protein electrophoresis (*IgM raised in primary biliary cholangitis, IgA raised in alcoholic liver disease, IgG raised in autoimmune hepatitis*)
  - Tissue transglutaminase antibody (*coeliac disease*)
- Toxins
  - Paracetamol level (*paracetamol overdose*)

Imaging

- Abdominal ultrasound: first line imaging (quick and cheap) that is useful for determining liver texture, size and presence of any gallstones or cholecystitis
- Abdominal CT: can confirm pancreatitis or tumour
- Elastography: grades liver fibrosis in chronic liver disease non-invasively
- Magnetic resonance cholangiopancreatography: to look for duct disease/stones if ultrasound normal

Procedures

- Ascitic tap: if ascites present
- Liver biopsy (CT-guided usually, but done trans-jugular if there is ascites or coagulopathy)

SOME NON-HEPATIC CAUSES OF DERRANGED LFTS

In addition to any described above:

- Drugs
  - **Hepatitis**: tuberculosis antibiotics (rifampicin/isoniazid/pyrazinamide), sodium valproate, methotrexate, methyldopa, amiodarone, statins, paracetamol, phenytoin, ketoconazole/fluconazole, nitrofurantoin, sulfonylureas/sulfonamides
  - **Cholestasis**: **c**o-amoxiclav (may be delayed/severe), **c**larithromycin/erythromycin, **c**arbamazepine, **c**hlorpromazine, **c**ontraceptives, flu**c**loxacillin, sulfonylureas/sulfonamides
- Right heart failure
- Sepsis
- Coeliac disease
- Haemolysis
- Hyperthyroidism
- Right lower lobe pneumonia

INTERPRETATION OF COAGULATION SCREEN

BACKGROUND KNOWLEDGE

- Haemostasis process:

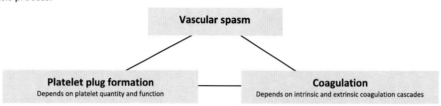

- Coagulation cascade:

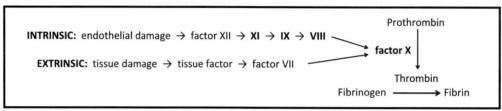

- Clot dissolution:

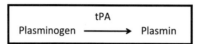

- Natural anticoagulants: proteins C and S (inactivate factors V and VIII); antithrombin (inactivates many clotting factors)
- Vitamin K dependent clotting factors: II, VII, IX, X (+ proteins C and S)
- Most coagulation factors are synthesised by the liver

NB: when an 'a' is placed after the clotting factor number (e.g. 'factor Xa'), it means it is in its activated form.

TESTS

<u>Basic</u>

- **PT and INR = *EXTRINSIC***
  - Tissue factor is added to blood in the laboratory to activate the <u>extrinsic</u> pathway. Clotting time (PT) is measured in seconds (normal usually = 12-13). However, the PT may vary depending on the reagent used, so the laboratory can use the PT to calculate the *INR* to standardise results (normal = 0.8-1.2).
  - **WEPT** – **W**arfarin **E**xtrinsic **P**rothrombin **T**ime
  - Only factor VII is involved in the extrinsic pathway, before the common pathway. Isolated factor VII deficiencies are rare, so PT/INR is only really affected by globally reduced clotting factor synthesis or increased consumption:
    - Warfarin/vitamin K deficiency
    - Liver disease
    - Disseminated intravascular coagulation
- **APTT = *INTRINSIC***
  - A contact activator is added to blood in the laboratory to activate the <u>intrinsic</u> pathway. Clotting time (APTT) is measured in seconds (normal usually = 30-50). The APTT can be divided by the mean normal value to calculate the *APTT ratio* if required.
  - The APTT involves similar clotting factors to the extrinsic pathway PLUS others (VIII, IX, XI) so is affected by:
    - Warfarin/vitamin K deficiency
    - Liver disease ⎤ Like the extrinsic pathway
    - Disseminated intravascular coagulation ⎦
    - PLUS anything which affects factor VIII (haemophilia A/von Willebrand disease), factor IX (haemophilia B), or factor XI (haemophilia C)

    NB: factor XII is also involved in the intrinsic pathway but isolated deficiencies are rare.
    NB: anti-phospholipid syndrome is a common cause of a misleadingly prolonged APTT, due to antibody-mediated inactivation of the phospholipid added in the laboratory to activate the intrinsic pathway.
- **Bleeding time = *PLATELET FUNCTION***
  - Involves making an incision in the patient's skin and timing how long it takes to stop bleeding
  - Measures platelet plug formation so *only affected by conditions involving platelet quantity/function*
  - Rarely used in practice
- **Fibrinogen**
  - Fibrinogen is a clotting factor involved in the final stage of coagulation
  - The fibrinogen level reflects the blood's clotting ability (low = increased bleeding risk; high = may increase clotting)
  - Low levels are due to increased consumption (e.g. disseminated intravascular coagulation) or decreased production (e.g. liver disease, malnutrition)
  - Fibrinogen is an acute phase protein and high levels may be due to: inflammation, malignancy, trauma, or infection

Other relevant tests
- **Full blood count:** to check platelet count and other haematological abnormalities
- **Liver function tests:** to exclude liver function abnormalities as a cause for clotting problems
- **Albumin:** gives an indication of nutrition, e.g. a high INR (with no clear cause) and a low albumin suggest vitamin K deficiency
- **D-dimer/fibrin degradation products:** tests the level of fibrin degradation products suggesting recent clot formation (e.g. DVT, PE, disseminated intravascular coagulation etc.)

Advanced tests
- **Anti-phospholipid antibodies** (e.g. anti-cardiolipin, lupus anticoagulant) – to look for anti-phospholipid syndrome
- **Factor assays ± factor inhibitor antibodies** (e.g. factors VIII, IX, XI) – the level of individual clotting factors may be tested to look for common deficiencies (e.g. haemophilia A, B, C respectively)

IMPORTANT CONDITIONS

- Factor synthesis problems
  - **Vitamin K deficiency:** vitamin K is a fat-soluble vitamin so may be deficient if there is fat malabsorption (e.g. in biliary obstruction – check LFTs) or a simple dietary deficiency. Deficiency leads to reduced synthesis of vitamin K dependent clotting factors (2, 7, 9, 10) and so affects both intrinsic and extrinsic pathways. If due to dietary deficiency, treat with oral vitamin K (phytomenadione) 5-10mg OD for 3 days; if due to fat malabsorption, give IV vitamin K or oral menadiol (a water-soluble vitamin K derivative).
  - **Liver failure:** the liver synthesises most clotting factors so liver failure can result in a global deficiency, affecting both intrinsic and extrinsic pathways. Platelets may also be reduced due to hypersplenism. Liver-related coagulopathy is difficult to manage and is mainly supportive (e.g. FFP, cryoprecipitate, platelet transfusions as required). Vitamin K may be given if deficiency is suspected.
- Consumption
  - **Disseminated intravascular coagulation:** in severe systemic illness, dying cells release procoagulants, resulting in fibrin generation, which can occlude small vessels. This process consumes platelets and clotting factors, resulting in bleeding elsewhere. Blood tests reveal thrombocytopenia; increased PT/INR and APTT; low fibrinogen; and raised D-dimer and fibrin degradation products. Treat the cause and give supportive therapies (e.g. blood, platelets, FFP, cryoprecipitate).
- Drugs
  - **Warfarin (vitamin K antagonist):** reduces synthesis of vitamin K dependent clotting factors (II, VII, IX, X) and so affects both intrinsic and extrinsic pathways. Its effect is monitored using INR, which is a measure of the extrinsic pathway. It can be reversed using prothrombin complex concentrate and vitamin K.
  - **Heparin:** heparin is an anticoagulant that increases antithrombin activity by enhancing its binding to factor Xa and thrombin. Types of heparin that are commonly used include:
    - Subcutaneous LMWH (e.g. enoxaparin): most commonly used for prophylactic and therapeutic anticoagulation. LMWH consists of only short chain heparins, so most of its activity is mediated by inhibition of factor Xa. Its effects are therefore more predictable than those of standard (unfractionated) heparin. Monitoring is not routinely required, but its effect can be measured by anti-factor Xa assay.
    - IV or subcutaneous unfractionated (standard) heparin: consists of heparin chains with a variety of molecular lengths. Its effect on the coagulation cascade is therefore more wide-ranging and less predictable.
      - Subcutaneous therapy may be used for prophylactic anticoagulation in patients with reduced renal function, since unfractionated heparin is predominantly cleared by the liver, whereas LMWH is not.
      - IV heparin has a short half life and stops working after 4 hours. It can therefore be used for therapeutic anticoagulation peri-operatively, or if there is significant risk of bleeding. It must be monitored regularly, using the APTT ratio, and dose-adjusted according to hospital guidelines.
    Both types of heparin can be reversed with protamine sulphate if required.
- Deficiencies
  - **Haemophilia A** (factor VIII deficiency), **B** (factor IX deficiency), **C** (factor XI deficiency): clinical features depend on levels of affected factor but characteristically include haemarthroses and muscle haematomas
  - **Von Willebrand disease:** deficiency of von Willebrand factor, which is involved in platelet aggregation and adhesion, and binds to factor VIII to prevent its destruction. Von Willebrand disease produces a platelet disorder picture of bleeding (petechiae, menorrhagia, contact bleeding, e.g. from gums).
- Autoimmune
  - **Anti-phospholipid syndrome:** anti-phospholipid antibodies (anti-cardiolipin and lupus anticoagulant) react against proteins that bind to plasma membrane phospholipids, resulting in arterial and venous thrombosis. Anti-phospholipid syndrome misleadingly causes a prolonged APTT because the antibodies inactivate the phospholipid added to activate the intrinsic pathway during the laboratory measurement of APTT.

Differentiating common bleeding disorders			
	Haemophilia A	**Von Willebrand disease**	**Vitamin K deficiency**
Bleeding time	N Because platelets not affected	↑ Because vWF is mainly involved in platelet adhesion	N Because platelets not affected
PT/INR	N Because factor VIII is not involved in the extrinsic pathway	N Because vWF is mainly involved in platelet adhesion	↑ Because vitamin K dependent clotting factors are used in the extrinsic pathway
APTT	↑ Because factor VIII is involved in the intrinsic pathway	↑/N Because vWF binds factor VIII to prevent its destruction	↑ Because vitamin K dependent clotting factors are used in the intrinsic pathway
Factor VIIIc Pro-coagulant activity of factor VIII	↓↓ Because factor VIII is deficient	↓ Because vWF binds factor VIII to prevent its destruction	N Because factor VIII is not vitamin K dependent
Von Willebrand factor (vWF)	N Because vWF is not affected	↓ Because vWF is deficient	N Because vWF is not affected

URINALYSIS

ODOUR

- **Sweet:** DKA/glycosuria
- **Pungent:** infection
- **Ammonia-type smell:** alkaline urine

APPEARANCE/TURBIDITY

- **Discolouration**
    - **Red:** haematuria/haemoglobinuria/myoglobinuria, porphyria, beetroot, drugs (rifampicin)
    - **Brown:** bile pigments, myoglobin, methaemoglobin, drugs (levodopa, metronidazole, antimalarials, nitrofurantoin)
    - **Green/blue:** Pseudomonas UTI, biliverdin, drugs (amitriptyline, methylene blue, propofol)
    - **Orange:** bile pigments, drugs (phenothiazines)
- **Cloudiness:** pus, pyuria, alkaline urine phosphate crystals
- **Sedimentation**

URINE DIPSTICK ANALYSIS

	Interpretation of urine dipstick results		
Test	**Meaning**	**Interpretation of abnormal result**	**Possible further investigations**
Specific gravity	Indicates the amount of solutes dissolved in the urine	Increased (i.e. concentrated urine) Dehydration, SIADH, heart failure/renal artery stenosis (decreased renal perfusion), proteinuria Decreased (i.e. dilute urine) •Inability to concentrate urine, e.g. diabetes insipidus, renal failure •Excess hydration, e.g. psychogenic polydipsia	•U&Es
pH	Indicates the acidity of the urine	Alkaline •Systemic: alkalosis, vegetarian/low carb diet •Local: UTI, renal tubular acidosis Acidic •Systemic: acidosis, diarrhoea, starvation •Acidic diet (high protein, cranberry)	•Urine culture •VBG
Blood	May be: haematuria (i.e. red blood cells), haemoglobinuria or myoglobinuria	Haematuria ONNIT = Obstruction (calculi), Neoplasm (transitional cell carcinoma/renal cell carcinoma/prostate), Nephritic syndrome (e.g. due to glomerulonephritis), Inflammation (UTI), Trauma Haemoglobinuria Intravascular haemolysis, e.g. paroxysmal nocturnal haemoglobinuria, malaria, sickle cell crisis, severe burns, autoimmune haemolytic anaemia, haemolytic uraemic syndrome, etc. Myoglobinuria Rhabdomyolysis	•Urine culture •Urine microscopy (look for red cells to determine if cause is haematuria or haemoglobinuria/myoglobinuria) •FBC, U&Es, coagulation screen, CRP •Antistreptolysin O + complement if suspect post-streptococcal glomerulonephritis •CT KUB + cystoscopy (if suspect malignancy /calculi) •CK and haemolytic screen if no red cells seen on microscopy
Protein	Increased protein production or decreased renal reabsorption	•Decreased renal reabsorption: nephrotic syndrome, glomerulonephritis, renovascular disease, interstitial nephritis, pre-eclampsia •Increased serum protein: myeloma (Bence-Jones protein) •Local infection: UTI NB: false negative results may occur if urine is very dilute or acidic; false positives may occur if concentrated or alkaline.	•MSU protein-creatinine ratio to quantify and monitor proteinuria if dipstick protein +ve (<0.2 normal, >3.5 nephrotic) •Urine culture •Renal function tests •Serum protein and albumin
Leukocyte esterase	If raised, indicates white blood cells in urine (pyuria)	UTI NB: false positive results may occur in vaginal discharge.	•Urine culture
Nitrites	Indicates presence of Gram-negative bacteria due to conversion of nitrates	Gram-negative UTI NB: false negative results may occur in decreased bladder incubation time or in acidic urine	•Urine culture
Ketones	Indicates fatty acid metabolism	Starvation/low carb diet, diabetes/DKA, alcoholism, pregnancy, hyperthyroidism NB: false negative results may occur if dehydrated or on levodopa/ sodium valproate.	•Blood/capillary glucose measurements •VBG
Glucose	Hyperglycaemia or decreased renal reabsorption	•Hyperglycaemia: diabetes mellitus, Cushing's disease, acromegaly •Renal glycosuria: pregnancy, renal tubular disease, drugs (e.g. SGLT-2 inhibitors)	•Blood/capillary glucose measurements •Renal function tests •Dexamethasone suppression test
Bilirubin	Indicates conjugated bilirubinaemia (unconjugated bilirubin is water insoluble and so not excreted in urine)	•Conjugated hyperbilirubinaemia: bile duct obstruction, liver disease NB: false negative results may occur if urine exposed to UV light.	•Liver function tests
Urobilinogen	Bilirubin is conjugated by the liver and enters the bowel in bile. It is then converted to urobilinogen, some of which is passed in stool; some is reabsorbed and recirculated to the liver; and some is reabsorbed excreted in urine (as trace urinary urobilinogen).	Increased •Increased bilirubin turnover: haemolytic anaemia •Liver disease Decreased Bile duct obstruction NB: false positive results may occur if ↑urinary nitrites.	•Evidence of haemolysis: ↑unconjugated bilirubin, ↑lactate dehydrogenase (from red cells), ↑reticulocytes, ↓free haptoglobin •Cause of haemolysis: blood film, direct antiglobulin (Coombs) test, osmotic fragility testing, Hb electrophoresis, enzyme assays •Liver function tests

CHAPTER 7: PRESCRIBING

Oxygen comes out of a wall tap/canister at 100% concentration, but you can adjust the *flow rate* on the tap/dial (0-15L/minute). Different delivery devices tolerate different flow rates. The FiO_2 (percentage of oxygen delivery) is determined by the flow rate and delivery device.

NASAL CANNULA

Delivers 24-30%. Comfortable. Flow rate 1-4L/minute. *Used for mild hypoxia and use in non-acute wards.*

HUDSON SIMPLE FACE MASK

Delivers 30-40%. Flow rate 5-10L/minute. *Delivers slightly more oxygen than a nasal cannula but the precise FiO_2 cannot be determined so a Venturi mask is often used instead.*

VENTURI (AIR ENTRAPMENT) MASK

Delivers 24-60%. Oxygen delivery depends on mask: this is marked on the side of the mask, along with the appropriate flow rate setting. *Often used in patients with COPD/type 2 respiratory failure so you know the precise FiO_2 you are delivering.*

Types of Venturi mask		
Colour	Flow rate (L/min)	Oxygen delivery (%)
Blue	2-4	24
White	4-6	28
Yellow	8-10	35
Red	10-12	40
Green	12-15	60

NON-REBREATHER MASK

Delivers 85-90% with 15L/minute flow rate. Mask with a reservoir bag and valve which stops almost all rebreathing. *Used for acutely unwell hypoxic patients.*

HIGH FLOW NASAL OXYGEN (OPTIFLOW)

Delivers up to 100% with up to 60L/minute flow rate. The very high flow rate also creates a small positive airway pressure effect similar to CPAP. *Used in type 1 respiratory failure as an alternative to CPAP or a non-rebreather mask.*

NON-INVASIVE VENTILATION Delivers up to 100%

CPAP (continuous positive airway pressure): air/oxygen delivered through a tight-fitting mask at constant positive pressure to keep alveoli open. *Used in type 1 respiratory failure (e.g. due to sleep apnoea or acute LVF).*
BiPAP (bi-level positive airway pressure): same system but with a high positive pressure on inspiration and a lower positive pressure on expiration. *Used in type 2 respiratory failure with respiratory acidosis or exhaustion (e.g. due to COPD or neuromuscular diseases).*

INVASIVE VENTILATION

Delivers up to 100%. A ventilation bag or machine is attached to an artificial airway to ventilate lungs. *Used in intensive care and theatre.*

General points
- **Intubate if GCS ≤ 8** (airway is not protected)
- Aim for oxygen saturations of **94-98%** in non-COPD patients, and **88-92%** in COPD patients and those known to retain CO_2
- If oxygen therapy is maximal and oxygen levels continue to drop, involve seniors and/or intensive care for consideration of non-invasive or invasive ventilation
- Do an ABG on any patient with oxygen saturations of <92%
- Humidified oxygen helps secretions and prevents mucosal drying if prolonged high-concentration oxygen therapy is required

CO_2 retainers
- Breathing is normally driven by CO_2 levels. However, 'CO_2 retainers' are desensitised to hypercapnia, relying instead on hypoxia to stimulate their respiratory drive. The aim of acute oxygen therapy in these patients is to provide enough oxygen but not so much that it depresses their respiratory drive (as this will increase CO_2 levels and worsen respiratory acidosis).
- Conditions which can lead to CO_2 retention include: severe obstructive lung disease (approximately 10% of COPD patients) and severe restrictive lung diseases (e.g. neuromuscular, severe kyphoscoliosis, severe obesity)
- Generally, start on 24-28% (via Venturi mask) if no ABG result. However, if they need oxygen (e.g. they are in respiratory distress or dangerously hypoxic) then you <u>must</u> give high flow oxygen initially – *hypoxia will kill faster than hypercapnia*
- Perform baseline ABG (preferably on room air):
  - Hypoxaemia with hypercapnia ($PaCO_2$ > 5.3kPa) = hypoxic drive likely → continue FiO_2 24-28% initially
  - Hypoxaemia without hypercapnia ($PaCO_2$ < 5.3kPa) = hypoxic drive less likely → can try higher flow rate of oxygen
- If significant hypoxaemia continues, try gradual increments in oxygen therapy, repeating ABG 30 minutes after each adjustment
  - Hypercapnia and <u>acidosis</u> worsening → reduce oxygen and consider non-invasive ventilation if still hypoxic
  - Hypercapnia and <u>acidosis</u> stable or improving → can increase oxygen further if needed
- If you cannot achieve oxygen saturations of 88-92% without depressing respiratory drive and causing hypercapnic acidosis, the patient needs non-invasive ventilation (BiPAP)

ADULT INTRAVENOUS FLUIDS

BACKGROUND KNOWLEDGE

Fluid compartments (e.g. in 70kg patient)

INTRVASCULAR	INTERSTITIAL	INTRACELLULAR
Plasma	Between cells, lymphatics, body cavities, cerebrospinal fluid	Inside cells
$1/_9$ (5L)	$2/_9$ (9L)	$2/_3$ (28L)

Normal maintenance requirements if NBM

Depends on the patient's weight:

		(e.g. for an average 70kg patient over 24 hours):
H_2O:	1.5ml/kg/hour	(2.5L)
Na^+:	1-2mmol/kg/day	(70-140mmol)
K^+:	0.5-1mmol/kg/day	(35-70mmol)

NB: urine output should be >0.5ml/kg/hour   (>35ml/hour)

You should memorise all of these values – they are important for working out intravenous fluid prescriptions

Types of intravenous fluids

Contents of intravenous fluids (mmol/L)					
Class	Fluid	Na⁺	Cl⁻	K⁺	Other contents
NORMAL PLASMA		135-145	100-110	3.5-5.0	
Crystalloid	5% Dextrose	0	0	0-40*	50g glucose (170 kcal)
	Dextrose-saline 4%/0.18%	30	30	0-40*	40g glucose (130 kcal)
	Hartmann's solution	131	111	5	29mmol/L lactate (metabolises into HCO³⁻)
	0.9% saline	154	154	0-40*	-
Colloid	Gelofusine	154	120	0	-
* there are pre-prepared versions of 5% dextrose, dextrose-saline and 0.9% saline with potassium (20 or 40mmol/L).					

Small volume stays in intravascular space

5% dextrose: this is given instead of pure water. The glucose is present to maintain initial osmolality but is quickly used up and plays no role thereafter (the calorific content is negligible). It is used as part of a maintenance fluid regimen, when water is required without electrolytes. It is of no use in treating hypovolaemia because it is not physiological (i.e. similar to plasma) and distributes widely across all fluid compartments. Administering too much, too quickly can cause hyponatraemia.

Dextrose-saline: this is a good choice for maintenance fluids because, when given alone at the correct maintenance rate (i.e. at 1.5ml/kg/hour), it will provide approximately the correct sodium requirement over 24 hours. Because the sodium content is much lower than that of plasma, however, it is of no use in treating hypovolaemia. Administering too much, too quickly can cause hyponatraemia.

Hartmann's solution: this is the most physiological fluid and so is very good for replacing plasma loss, e.g. GI losses or during surgery. However, this does not mean it is good for normal maintenance fluids alone, as 3L Hartmann's solution over 24 hours would give three times too much sodium and not enough potassium.
NB: Hartmann's solution is also known as Ringer's lactate solution, and similar solutions are available, such as Plasmalyte.

Larger volume stays in intravascular space

0.9% saline: this is much more physiological than dextrose as it contains sodium chloride, but is not as physiological as Hartmann's solution because it contains a greater concentration than plasma. Also, be warned: too much chloride will cause hyperchloraemic acidosis and also renal vasoconstriction. Too much sodium places a massive load on the kidneys.

Colloids: these contain large molecules which stay in the intravascular space and create an osmotic gradient. However, they are not commonly used because they are not as inert as crystalloids and can have side effects such as anaphylaxis and renal failure. Types include starches (Voluven/Volulyte), gelatins (Gelofusine), and albumins.

NB: fluids are given intravenously and so enter the intravascular space. However, depending on the osmolality, the fluid will be distributed across the various fluid compartments (intravascular, interstitial, intracellular) to different extents, as above. The aim of fluid resuscitation in hypovolaemic patients is to expand the intravascular volume by administering fluids that stay in the intravascular space, such as Hartmann's solution, 0.9% saline and colloids.

CHOOSING A FLUID REGIMEN

Overall fluid requirements = maintenance fluids + replacement of fluid losses

The different components of the above formula should be considered separately because each may need a different fluid prescribed. When prescribing fluids, you need to be clear about what type of fluid you are prescribing, how much of it, and why. The type and quantity of *maintenance fluid* is based on the patient's fluid and electrolyte requirements (dependent on their weight), and the type and quantity of *replacement fluid* is based on the type and quantity of fluid lost. You will usually be giving fluids for **either** maintenance **or** replacement rather than both – but you need to be clear in your own head what you are doing!

MAINTENANCE FLUIDS

The type of fluid does not matter provided that, over 24 hours, it approximately matches the patient's weight requirements of **water, sodium and potassium**. Calculate how much of all of these are needed and choose fluids which match these requirements closest. By convention, bags are given over multiples of 2 hours.

Note, there are problems with the **traditional fluid regimen of '1 salty + 2 sweet'**:

> 1L saline 0.9% + 20mmol potassium chloride (over 8 hours)
> 1L dextrose 5% + 20mmol potassium chloride (over 8 hours)
> 1L dextrose 5% + 20mmol potassium chloride (over 8 hours)

This gives 3L H_2O, 154mmol Na^+ and 60mmol K^+. This is only acceptable for a very large patient because it provides about 0.5L more water and more sodium than is required for an average patient. The fluids you give should <u>always</u> reflect the patient's weight. Thus for a 70kg patient, maintenance regimens need to provide approximately 2.5L fluid, 70-140mmol Na^+, and 35-70mmol K^+). Example prescriptions therefore include:

- 1L dextrose-saline with 20mmol K^+ (over 10 hours) + 1L dextrose-saline with 20mmol K^+ (over 10 hours) + 500ml dextrose-saline (over 4 hours)
- 500ml saline 0.9% with 20mmol K^+ (over 6 hours) + 1L dextrose 5% with 20mmol K^+ (over 10 hours) + 1L dextrose 5% with 20mmol K^+ (over 8 hours)
- 1L Hartmann's solution (over 10 hours) + 1L 5% dextrose with 40mmol K^+ (over 8 hours) + 500ml 5% dextrose with 20mmol K^+ (over 6 hours)

Other points:

- **Always check the U&Es before prescribing any fluids** and adjust the regimen as necessary for any electrolyte abnormalities
- Only give maintenance fluids if the patient cannot drink enough. Oral/NG-tube fluids are safer because they do not require a cannula and are much less likely to cause fluid overload or electrolyte abnormalities.
- If a patient is drinking some fluids but not enough, you need to calculate their fluid intake and top it up with IV/NG fluids

REPLACEMENT OF FLUID LOSSES

Two components of this need to be considered:
1. Pre-existing fluid deficit (replaced using STAT boluses)
2. Ongoing losses (prescribe fluids to replace future losses as they are likely to occur)

Fluid losses should be replaced with fluids which have a similar electrolyte content to the fluid that has been lost. The main types of fluid loss and what they should be replaced with are:

- Extracellular fluid/volume depletion, e.g. due to diarrhoea and vomiting, NG aspirates, stomas, burns, pancreatitis, sepsis: this should be replaced with a fluid similar to extracellular fluid, which is similar to plasma (e.g. Hartmann's solution or 0.9% saline). *NB: if a patient needs a lot of sodium-rich fluid resuscitation, Hartmann's solution is preferred to 0.9% saline because it contains less chloride (too much chloride causes a hyperchloraemic acidosis).*
- Dehydration/total water loss, e.g. due to poor intake: should be replaced by normal maintenance-type fluids (e.g. dextrose-saline). However, if these patients are hypotensive and need a fluid bolus, use Hartmann's solution or 0.9% saline, because a larger volume will stay in the intravascular space.
- Blood loss: should be replaced with blood. If the patient continues to bleed, they may also need other products, e.g. FFP/platelets to stop the bleeding rather than just replace the lost red cells.

WARNINGS: DO NOT use maintenance regimens to correct plasma or blood loss because this can cause a dangerous hyponatraemia. DO NOT give potassium at a rate greater than 10mmol/hour.

Pre-existing fluid deficit

The quantity of fluid replacement depends on your estimate of the fluid deficit. Determine the approximate deficit and the cause by:

- The history
- Observations, fluid balance chart and hydration status examination
- U&Es: but be aware this is a measurement of plasma levels and may not represent total body stores (because homeostasis mechanisms keep plasma levels within a certain range)

Classes of shock		
Shock class	Fluid lost	Signs
1	0.75L (15%)	Minimal, mild tachycardia
2	0.75-1.5L (15-30%)	Moderate tachycardia, prolonged capillary refill
3	1.5-2L (30-40%)	Severe tachycardia and hypotension, confusion
4	>2L (>40%)	Critical tachycardia and hypotension

Fluid resuscitation to replace pre-existing deficits is delivered in **STAT boluses**. 500ml 0.9% saline/Hartmann's solution is a good choice. You must reassess the patient's fluid status (including blood pressure and urine output) after each bolus to guide further fluid resuscitation. If they require large fluid volumes, also regularly assess for signs of fluid overload (e.g. raised JVP, increasing oxygen requirements, peripheral/pulmonary oedema).

For acutely hypotensive patients when you are unsure of the exact cause or quantity of fluid loss, unless you suspect heart failure, give a fluid challenge and then assess the response:

- ↘respond fully: just prescribe fluids for future losses/maintenance
- ↘respond and become hypotensive again: give more resuscitation fluids (amount depends on patient but usually around 20ml/kg quickly)
- ↘no response: patient may be very depleted (give lots of fluids), or in heart failure (don't give any more fluids) – assess clinically and look for signs of fluid overload such as raised JVP and pulmonary/peripheral oedema

WARNING: be cautious if the patient has a history of heart failure history and use only 250ml fluid challenges. Bear in mind heart failure patients may normally run hypotensive. If there are signs of heart failure, DO NOT give fluids – ask for senior advice because diuretics or inotropes may be required.

Ongoing losses
You must estimate these and aim to prescribe a regimen to replace them as they occur with a type of fluid similar in electrolyte content to what is being lost.

SPECIAL SITUATIONS

Post-operatively
K^+ stores are mostly intracellular and serum levels can increase due to cell lysis during surgery. Hence, if K^+ is over 4.5mmol/L post-operatively, omit it from your fluid prescription for 24 hours. If K^+ is normal/low, you can give some, e.g. 40mmol in 24 hours.

Some centres advise against using 0.9% saline post-operatively because surgery can trigger endocrinological sodium retention mechanisms, and because sodium-containing substances are often given in theatre (e.g. colloids, Hartmann's solution and IV antibiotics). Too much sodium chloride can result in oedema, hyperchloraemic acidosis, increased kidney load, increased post-operative complications, and GI problems. Dextrose-saline contains less sodium chloride and so is often recommended instead.

Sepsis
Sepsis causes intravascular depletion due to plasma loss through leaky capillaries and vasodilation. Replace fluid with Hartmann's solution or 0.9% saline, but avoid too much chloride (i.e. 0.9% saline) if large quantities of fluid are required (risk of hyperchloraemic acidosis). Monitor response carefully – remember patients may need vasopressors to maintain blood pressure and reduce peripheral fluid losses.

Heart failure
Heart failure patients are prone to fluid overload and pulmonary oedema. Be attentive to their fluid balance and remember they may normally run hypotensive. If overload develops, start fluid restriction, furosemide, a low sodium diet, and record daily weights. There is no logic in giving furosemide together with fluids.

If a patient is at risk of LVF and has low SBP and urine output, you <u>must</u> examine the patient because there are two opposite explanations for this clinical picture:
1. Dehydration: they may simply be fluid deplete (treatment = fluids)
2. Worsening fluid overload: they may be fluid overloaded, which causes a low SBP, cardiorenal failure, and a low urine output (treatment = diuresis, which will reduce high venous pressure and improve LVF, increase SBP, and improve renal function and urine output)

Liver failure
Excess Na^+ may cause ascites so use 5% dextrose unless they are acutely hypotensive.

Acute kidney injury
Avoid potassium.

Severe chronic kidney disease
Avoid excess fluid, sodium and potassium as the kidneys cannot excrete them.

Alcoholic
Give Pabrinex before giving dextrose. It can precipitate Korsakoff syndrome.

Brain haemorrhage
Avoid dextrose as this can cause osmotic haematoma swelling. ***Dextrose Destroys the brain if there's a bleed!*** Saline is best.

Risk of re-feeding syndrome
Avoid dextrose where possible because it can precipitate re-feeding syndrome.

Electrolyte imbalances
See interpretation notes on U&Es p268.

Acute bleeding/trauma
In actively bleeding patients, fluid and blood product resuscitation is important; however, replacing fluid too aggressively may increase bleeding. For this reason, a less than normal blood pressure is often accepted – 'permissive hypotension'.

ONLY give fluids if your patient REALLY needs them – they can be dangerous

ADULT NUTRITION

BACKGROUND KNOWLEDGE

Normal requirements for hospital patients
Dependent on patient weight:

> **Energy: 30kcal/kg/day**
> **Protein: 0.8-1g/kg/day**
> **Fluid: 30-35ml/kg/day**

e.g. for an average 70kg patient over 24 hours: energy 2100kcal, protein 56-70g, fluid 2.1-2.45L

Assessing nutritional status
- *Malnutrition Universal Screening Tool* (*MUST*) *score*: 0 = low risk; 1 = medium risk (observe); 2 or more = high risk (treat). Scoring takes into account BMI, unplanned weight loss, and whether patient is acutely ill and has had/will have no nutritional intake for >5 days (Elia et al. 2003)
- BMI
- History
- Nutritional status exam *(see p109)*
- Bloods: haemoglobin, electrolytes (including Mg^{2+}, PO_4^{3-}, Ca^{2+}), LFTs (including albumin), haematinics (B_{12}, folate, ferritin)

Foods
- Meals should ideally contain 650-850kcal
- A food guide should be used to calculate energy and protein intake

ORAL SUPPLEMENTS

Nutritional drinks
Quantity required is determined by calculating the difference between the patient's daily calorie requirement and their intake.

Nutritional drinks contents (reference table)				
	Energy (kcal)	**Carbohydrate (g)**	**Protein (g)**	**Fat (g)**
Fortisip Extra (200ml milkshake)	320	36	20	11
Fortisip Compact (125ml milkshake) – similar contents in smaller volume	300	37	12	12
Fortisip Multi Fibre (200ml milkshake) – with 5g fibre to help bowel function	300	37	12	12
Fortijuice (200ml juice) – *avoid in diabetes (contains sugar)*	300	67	8	0
Nestlé Resource Energy (200ml milkshake)	300	42	11	10
Nestlé Build Up soup (49g sachet)	200	27	7	6.9
Nutricia PreOp (200ml clear drink) – 2 taken 2 hours pre-op for major elective operations	100	25	0	0

Additional micronutrients to consider
- Vitamin supplements
  - Sanatogen multivitamin tablets
  - Oral Vitamin B Compound Strong + thiamine
  - Pabrinex (IV equivalent of oral Vitamin B Compound Strong + thiamine) – use IV for first 3 days before changing to oral if patient has anorexia nervosa or chronic alcoholism
- Electrolyte supplements (replace if low)
  - Potassium
  - Phosphate
  - Magnesium

ENTERIC FEEDS

Required when oral intake is likely to be absent for >5-7 days and gut is functioning

Administration methods
- Fine-bore nasogastric (NG) tube – for short-term use
- Nasojejunal (NJ) tube – if problems with gastric reflux or delayed gastric emptying
- Percutaneous gastrostomy/jejunostomy tube – for longer-term feeding, i.e. >4-6 weeks, or if there is a mechanical swallowing obstruction
- May be inserted:
  - Endoscopically: percutaneous endoscopic gastrostomy/ jejunostomy (PEG/J) – *most*
  - Radiologically: radiologically inserted gastrostomy (RIG) – *if patient cannot swallow*
  - Surgically – *if having other surgery, tube may be placed at the same time*

Matching requirements
- Most feeds contain **1 kcal/ml** and are nutritionally complete (hence, 30 ml/kg/day will match requirements, but start at <10 ml/kg/day in patients at risk of re-feeding syndrome)
- Reduce feed if they are also eating (deduct their oral intake of calories)
- Exact feed choice is influenced by nutritional requirements, absorption/motility abnormalities, diarrhoeal loss, and presence of liver/renal failure

Types of feed
- Polymeric feeds (polypeptides), e.g. Nutrison, Nutrison Multifibre – most commonly used
- Pre-digested feeds (small peptides) – better absorbed, for maldigestive patients, patients with short gut or pancreatic insufficiency
- Disease-specific and pharmaco-nutrient feeds – for liver/renal failure patients

Administration options
- Boluses (e.g. 200-400ml over 15-60 minutes at regular intervals) – more physiological but can cause *dumping syndrome*
- Intermittent infusion (breaks of 6 or more hours depending on requirements) – most commonly used
- Continuous infusion – used for very ill patients

Giving drugs via enteric tubes
- Use solutions where possible
- Some tablets can be crushed and some capsules can be opened (check with pharmacist)
- Tablets which cannot be crushed: modified release tablets, enteric coated tablets

PARENTERAL NUTRITION

Parenteral nutrition may be required in intestinal failure (acute or chronic) and is given via central venous line
- Parenteral nutrition (PN) – if also feeding patient by other methods
- Total parenteral nutrition (TPN) – only IV feeding

RE-FEEDING SYNDROME

- Feeding malnourished patients can cause an insulin surge and activation of cellular membrane pumps. This can drop various serum electrolyte levels (especially K^+, PO_4^{3-}, Mg^{2+}), which can lead to arrhythmias and death.
- Risk factors: low BMI, weight loss >15% over 3-6 months, poor intake for >10 days, low electrolytes, alcohol excess
- In anyone who is at risk:
  - Start feeding at ~ **10 kcal/kg/day** (5 kcal/kg/day if very malnourished) and build up gradually
  - Check K^+, PO_4^{3-}, Mg^{2+} at least daily at first
  - Give supplements
    - Pabrinex (convert to oral Vitamin B Compound Strong and thiamine after 3 days)
    - Electrolytes as required
- Management
  - Continue low level of feed
  - Replace all low electrolytes IV (K^+, PO_4^{3-}, Mg^{2+})

COMMONLY PRESCRIBED DRUGS IN HOSPITAL

EMERGENCIES
You __must__ know these:
CARDIAC ARREST: DC shock 150J biphasic, **adrenaline** 1mg IV (10ml of 1 in 10,000), **amiodarone** 300mg IV (if shockable rhythm)
ANAPHYLAXIS: adrenaline 0.5mg IM (0.5ml of 1 in 1000), **hydrocortisone** 200mg IV, **chlorpheniramine** 10mg IV
SEIZURE: lorazepam 4mg IV (or if no IV access, **diazepam** 10mg PR)
HYPOGLYCAEMIA: 10% glucose 150ml IV or **20% glucose** 75ml IV (repeat as needed), or **glucagon** 1mg IM (if no IV access)
HYPERKALAEMIA: 10% calcium gluconate 10ml IV over 5 minutes **THEN 10% glucose** 250ml IV **with 10 units Actrapid insulin added** over 30 minutes
BRADYCARDIA: atropine 500mcg IV (repeat every 3-5 minutes to maximum of 3mg if needed)
SVT: adenosine 6mg IV (can be followed by 12mg, then another 12mg if unsuccessful)
NB: must be given as a bolus and flushed quickly via a large vein.
VT (without adverse signs): amiodarone 300mg IV over 20-60 minutes
RAPID TRANQUILISATION OF AGITATED PATIENT AT RISK TO SELF/OTHERS: lorazepam 1-2mg PO/IM or **haloperidol** 2-5mg PO/IM
Tranquilisation notes: use oral where possible; give half dose in elderly or renal failure; haloperidol is contraindicated in Parkinson's disease, Lewy body dementia and alcohol withdrawal

ANALGESIA

ANALGESIC LADDER: *1. Non-opioid (paracetamol or NSAID), 2. Weak opioid (e.g. codeine) ± non-opioid, 3. Strong opioid (e.g. morphine) ± non-opioid*

Paracetamol 1 gram PO/IV, PRN 4-6 hourly (max. 4 grams), or QDS
Ibuprofen 400mg PO, QDS (*contraindicated if gastritis history*)
Co-codamol 8/500 or 30/500 2 tablets PO, PRN 4-6 hourly (max. 8 tablets), or QDS
Dihydrocodeine 30mg PO, PRN 4-6 hourly (max. 120mg), or QDS
Tramadol 50-100mg PO, PRN 4-6 hourly (max. 400mg), or QDS
Morphine sulphate oral solution (Oramorph) 10mg/5ml 5-10ml PO, PRN 2 hourly (*reduce dosing interval or use alternative in renal impairment*)
Morphine 1-10mg IV/IM/SC, PRN 4 hourly (max. 60mg; *reduce dosing interval or use alternative in renal impairment*)
Morphine sulphate modified release tablets (Zomorph/MST) 10-60mg PO, 12-hourly
Morphine patient-controlled analgesia 1-5mg IV bolus, 5-10 minute lockout (start with a 1mg bolus, 5 minute lockout)
▼ **Fentanyl patient-controlled analgesia** 10-50micrograms IV bolus, 5-10 minute lockout (start with a 10 microgram bolus, 5 minute lockout)

Opioid conversions
IV morphine = 3 x stronger than oral morphine
Subcutaneous morphine = 2 x stronger than oral morphine
Oxycodone = 2 x stronger than morphine (if same administration route)
Fentanyl patch: 24 hour oral morphine dose (in mg) ÷ 3 = fentanyl patch dose in mcg/hour (*safe in renal impairment*)
Buprenorphine patch: 24 hour oral morphine dose (in mg) ÷ 2.3 = buprenorphine patch dose in mcg/hour
Subcutaneous alfentanyl = 30 x stronger than oral morphine (*safe in renal impairment*)

Concept of background and breakthrough analgesia
For patients with ongoing severe pain, you should prescribe regular *background* (long-acting) analgesia with PRN *breakthrough* (short-acting) analgesia. The initial dose of background analgesia should be equivalent to the average dose of PRN analgesia they are currently needing over 24 hours. Breakthrough analgesia should be about $^1/_6$ the dose of the total background analgesia dose. Prescribe this 4-hourly PRN. For example, if a patient has been needing 60mg Oramorph a day, convert them to 30mg MST BD, and also prescribe 10mg Oramorph PRN 4-hourly for breakthrough pain.

Subcutaneous PRN medications in palliative patients (all PRN 1-2 hourly)
Morphine 2.5mg (max. 20mg/24 hours)	- for **pain** and SOB (*use alternative in renal failure, e.g. fentanyl/oxycodone*)
Hyoscine butylbromide 20mg (max. 120mg/24 hours)	- for bronchial **secretions**
Haloperidol 0.5-1.5mg (max. 5mg/24 hours)	- for **nausea** and vomiting
Midazolam 5mg (max. 20mg/24 hours)	- for **anxiety** and agitation (*reduce dose in renal failure*)

Subcutaneous syringe driver in palliative patient (all over 24 hours)
Tailor to patient's symptoms – content options include:
Morphine 10-20mg	- for **pain** and breathlessness (*use alternative in renal failure, e.g. fentanyl/oxycodone*)
Hyoscine butylbromide 40-120mg	- for bronchial **secretions**
Midazolam 20-100mg	- for **confusion** without hallucinations (*reduce dose in renal failure*)
Haloperidol 2.5-10mg	- for **nausea** and vomiting; or **confusion** with hallucinations
Cyclizine 75-150mg	- for **nausea** and vomiting
Levomepromazine 6.25-100mg	- for **nausea** and vomiting (*2nd line*)

NUTRITIONAL SUPPLEMENTS

Fortisip Compact Extra 125ml PO, BD/TDS/QDS
Sanatogen A-Z Complete tablets 1 tablet PO, OD
Thiamine 100mg PO, BD
Vitamin B Compound Strong 2 tablets PO, BD

CONSTIPATION

Senna 7.5-15mg PO, ON (*stimulant laxative – first line for acute and opiate constipation*)
Macrogol oral powder (Movicol) 1-2 sachets PO, OD/BD/TDS (*osmotic laxative – for faecal impaction*)
Ispaghula husk (Fybogel) 1 sachet PO, BD (*bulk forming laxative – first line for chronic constipation, elderly patients and pregnant patients*)
Magnesium hydroxide 30-45ml PO, ON (*osmotic laxative – often used for post-operative patients*)
Glycerol 4g suppository 1 suppository PR, STAT (*stimulant laxative*)
Phosphate enema 1 enema PR, STAT (*osmotic laxative*)

NAUSEA/VOMITING

Cyclizine 50mg IV/IM/PO, PRN 6-8 hourly (max. 150mg)
Ondansetron 4mg IV/IM/PO, PRN 4-6 hourly (max. 16mg) – *can cause QT prolongation*
Metoclopramide 10mg IV/PO TDS (*anti-dopaminergic SEs, so give for maximum of 5 days and avoid if young/Parkinson's/dyskinesias*)

SLEEPING TABLETS

Zopiclone 7.5mg PO (3.75mg if elderly), ON (*caution in renal failure*)
Temazepam 10mg PO, ON (*caution in renal failure*)

WHEEZE

Salbutamol 2.5-5mg NEB, PRN 4-6 hourly (max. 20mg) – *can be given more frequently if required*
Ipratropium bromide 250-500micrograms NEB, PRN 4-6 hourly (max. 2mg)
Prednisolone 40mg PO, OD

CORRECTING ELECTROLYTES

Hypokalaemia
Mild (>2.5mmol/L): Sando-K 2 tablets TDS x $^3/_7$, or add 20-40mmol/L potassium chloride to each litre of IV fluids
Severe (<2.5mmol/L or ECG changes): 40mmol/L potassium chloride in 1L 0.9% saline over 4-6 hours (**NEVER** >10mmol/hour K$^+$ outside ICU)

Hyperkalaemia
1. ECG and cardiac monitoring
2. Calcium gluconate 10ml 10% IV over 10 minutes
3. Actrapid insulin 10 units in 250ml 10% glucose IV over 30 minutes ± *salbutamol nebs*
4. Calcium resonium 15g sachet TDS (with laxatives)

Hypocalcaemia
Mild (>1.9mmol/L and asymptomatic): calcium (e.g. Sandocal or Calcichew) 1000mg BD + vitamin D if deficient
Severe (<1.9mmol/L or symptomatic): calcium gluconate 10ml 10% IV over 10 minutes – *can be repeated until asymptomatic and usually needs to be followed by an infusion (50ml 10% calcium gluconate in 500ml 0.9% saline over 12 hours)*

Hypercalcaemia
Replace fluid deficit with 0.9% saline and keep patient very well hydrated (continuous IV fluids)
If severe (>3.5mmol/L or symptomatic): also bisphosphonate, e.g. zoledronic acid 4mg IV depending on severity and renal function (one-off dose)

Hypomagnesaemia
PO: magnesium aspartate 1 sachet (10mmol) BD x $^3/_7$
IV: 5grams (20mmol) magnesium sulphate in 500ml 0.9% saline over 5 hours

Hypophosphataemia
PO: Phosphate-Sandoz 2 tablets TDS x $^3/_7$
IV: Phosphate Polyfusor (50mmol in 500ml) 100-300ml over 12-24 hours depending on weight and severity *OR* sodium glycerophosphate 10mmol in 500ml 0.9% saline over 12 hours

COMMONLY PRESCRIBED DRUGS IN COMMUNITY

ANTI-HYPERTENSIVES

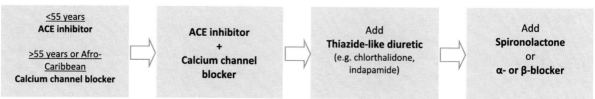

<55 years **ACE inhibitor** **>55 years or Afro-Caribbean** **Calcium channel blocker**	**ACE inhibitor** **+** **Calcium channel blocker**	**Add** **Thiazide-like diuretic** (e.g. chlorthalidone, indapamide)	**Add** **Spironolactone** or **α- or β-blocker**

Produced using NICE 'CG127 Hypertension in adults: diagnosis and management' 2011 (updated 2016)

ORAL HYPOGLYCAEMICS

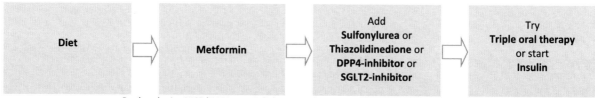

Diet	**Metformin**	**Add** **Sulfonylurea or** **Thiazolidinedione or** **DPP4-inhibitor or** **SGLT2-inhibitor**	**Try** **Triple oral therapy** or start **Insulin**

Produced using NICE 'NG28 type 2 diabetes in adults: management' 2015 (updated 2016)

Types of oral hypoglycaemics

Drug class	Drug name	Mechanism	Side effects	Contraindications
First line				
Biguanides *Taken with meals*	Metformin	↑insulin sensitivity and ↓gluconeogenesis	•GI disturbance •Weight loss •Lactic acidosis •Metallic taste	•**GFR<30** (or creatinine >150) •Low BMI
Second line				
Sulfonylureas *Taken before meals*	Gliclazide, Glibenclamide	↑β-cell insulin secretion	•Hypoglycaemia •Weight gain	•**GFR<15** •Patients at risk of hypos
Thiazolidinedione (*glitazones*)	Pioglitazone	PPARγ agonist → increases fat/muscle glucose uptake	•Fluid retention •Fractures ('glita*zones* and broken *bones*') •Hepatotoxic •Weight gain	•Hepatic impairment •Heart failure •History of bladder cancer or uninvestigated haematuria
DPP-4 inhibitors (*gliptins*)	Linagliptin, Alogliptin, Sitagliptin	Inhibits DPP4 which breaks down GLP-1 (a hormone released by the gut to ↑insulin after food)	•Pancreatitis has been reported •GI disturbance	
SGLT2 inhibitors (*flozins*)	Empagliflozin, Dapagliflozin, Canagliflozin	Increase urinary glucose excretion	•UTIs/thrush •Ketoacidosis •May ↑ risk of amputations	•**GFR <60**
Third line				
GLP-1 agonists *Subcutaneous*	Exenatide, Liraglutide	Mimics GLP-1 (a hormone released by the gut to ↑insulin after food)	•GI disturbance and indigestion •Pancreatitis •Weight loss	•**GFR <30** •History of pancreatitis •Severe gastrointestinal disease
Meglitinide	-glinides, e.g. Repaglinide, Nateglinide	Closes ATP-dependent K+ channels of β-cells → insulin release pre-meal	•Hypoglycaemia •Weight gain	•Patients at risk of hypos

NB: only metformin and insulin are known to be safe in pregnancy; all drugs should be temporarily discontinued in ketoacidosis; metformin should be temporarily discontinued in lactic acidosis, perioperatively, and if using iodinated contrast agents.
NB: aim HbA1c 48-58mmol/mol

ASTHMA LADDER

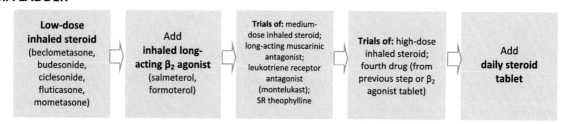

Low-dose inhaled steroid (beclometasone, budesonide, ciclesonide, fluticasone, mometasone)	**Add inhaled long-acting β₂ agonist** (salmeterol, formoterol)	**Trials of:** medium-dose inhaled steroid; long-acting muscarinic antagonist; leukotriene receptor antagonist (montelukast); SR theophylline	**Trials of:** high-dose inhaled steroid; fourth drug (from previous step or β₂ agonist tablet)	**Add daily steroid tablet**

PLUS **Inhaled short-acting β₂ agonist** (salbutamol) PRN for all patients

Produced using British Thoracic Society/Scottish Intercollegiate Guidelines Network 'Guideline for the management of asthma' 2016

COPD LADDER

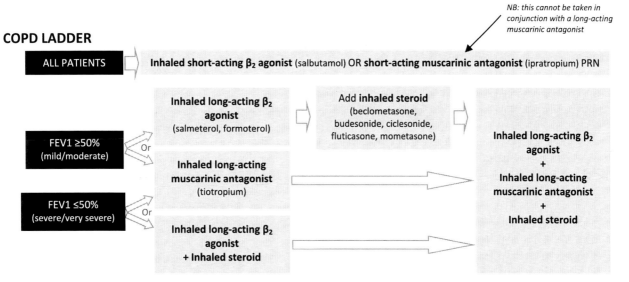

NB: this cannot be taken in conjunction with a long-acting muscarinic antagonist

ALL PATIENTS → Inhaled short-acting β₂ agonist (salbutamol) OR **short-acting muscarinic antagonist** (ipratropium) PRN

FEV1 ≥50% (mild/moderate)

Or

FEV1 ≤50% (severe/very severe)

Inhaled long-acting β₂ agonist (salmeterol, formoterol)

Inhaled long-acting muscarinic antagonist (tiotropium)

Inhaled long-acting β₂ agonist + Inhaled steroid

Add **inhaled steroid** (beclometasone, budesonide, ciclesonide, fluticasone, mometasone)

Inhaled long-acting β₂ agonist + Inhaled long-acting muscarinic antagonist + Inhaled steroid

Produced using NICE 'CG101 chronic obstructive pulmonary disease in over 16s: diagnosis and management' 2010

Combination inhalers
Seretide = salmeterol + fluticasone
Symbicort = formoterol + budesonide
Fostair = formoterol + beclometasone

Abbreviations
LABA = long-acting β₂ agonist
LAMA = long-acting muscarinic antagonist
ICS = inhaled corticosteroid

HORMONE REPLACEMENT THERAPY

- Routes of administration
  - Systemic: oral or transdermal (oestrogen/combined patches, oestrogen implant, or oestrogen gel) – *progesterone must still be taken separately at relevant time for women with a uterus on transdermal oestrogen-only preparations*
  - Vaginal oestrogen (for urogenital atrophy): tablet, cream, pessary, or vaginal ring
- Types of systemic therapy
  - **No uterus → oestrogen-only HRT** (oral or transdermal)
  - **Uterus**
    - **Perimenopausal → cyclical HRT** (oestrogen every day, but oestrogen and progesterone given together for 14 days to cause bleed at the end of every menstrual cycle ('monthly') if still having regular periods, or every 13 weeks ('three-monthly') if having irregular periods)
    - **Post-menopausal (i.e. no periods for >1 year or been on cyclical HRT for >1 year) → continuous HRT** (continuous combined oestrogen and progesterone – no bleed)

Contraindications: undiagnosed PV bleeding, pregnancy/breastfeeding, oestrogen-dependent cancer, active liver disease, uncontrolled hypertension, history of breast cancer, history of venous thromboembolism, recent stroke/MI/angina
Side effects: vaginal bleeding, premenstrual syndrome, breast tenderness, leg cramps, nausea/bloating
Long-term risks: increased VTE risk (except transdermal preparations), increased stroke risk, increased breast cancer risk with time, increased ovarian cancer risk if used >5 years, increased endometrial cancer risk (but only with unopposed oestrogen), coronary artery disease (if started >10 years after menopause)

ANTIDEPRESSANTS

Types of antidepressants				
Drug class	Drug name	Mechanism	Side effects	Notes
Selective serotonin reuptake inhibitors (SSRIs) *First line*	Fluoxetine, Citalopram, Paroxetine, Sertraline	Increase availability of extracellular neurotransmitter serotonin by limiting its reabsorption by presynaptic cell	• Sexual dysfunction • Withdrawal • Insomnia • Hyponatraemia • Bleeding	• Safe in overdose • May increase suicide risk
Serotonin-noradrenaline reuptake inhibitors (SNRIs)	Duloxetine, Venlafaxine	Increase availability of extracellular serotonin and noradrenaline by limiting their reabsorption	• Similar to SSRIs • May elevate blood pressure	
5-HT2 receptor antagonists	Mirtazapine	Antagonizes the serotonin 5-HT2 receptors, thereby enhancing serotonin neurotransmission at the 5-HT1 receptor	• Weight gain • Sleepiness • Constipation; dry mouth	
Tricyclic antidepressants (TCAs) *No longer recommended*	Amitriptyline	Block serotonin and noradrenaline transporters resulting in elevation of their synaptic concentrations	• Anticholinergic effects (dry mouth, constipation, blurred vision, urinary retention) • Hyponatraemia	• Dangerous in overdose
Monoamine oxidase inhibitors (MAOIs) *Rarely used*	Moclobemide, Phenelzine, Selegiline	Inhibits monoamine oxidase (an enzyme that oxidises monoamines to inactivate them)	• 3H's: **H**ypertension **H**epatocellular jaundice **H**yperthermia • Many drug and food interactions	• 'Cheese effect': if tyramine-containing foods (e.g. cheeses, cured meats) are ingested while on MAOIs, they may trigger a hypertensive crisis

LIPID-LOWERING DRUGS

Types of lipid lowering drugs					
Drug class	**Drug name**	**Mechanism**	**Indications**	**Side effects**	**Notes**
Statin *First line*	Atorvastatin, Fluvastatin, Pravastatin, Rosuvastatin, Simvastatin	Inhibit HMG-CoA reductase (enzyme involved in hepatic cholesterol synthesis)	•10 year risk of cardiovascular disease (QRISK2 score) of ≥10% •Any vascular disease •Lipid disorder •Type 1 diabetes <u>and</u> >40 years or had diabetes >10 years or nephropathy or cardiovascular risk factors •Chronic kidney disease	•Myalgia and rhabdomyolysis •Hepatotoxicity and increased liver enzymes	•Most effective at lowering LDL-cholesterol (but less effective than fibrates at reducing triglyceride levels)
Ezetimibe *Second line*	Ezetimibe	Decreases cholesterol absorption in small intestine	•Statin not tolerated or contraindicated (2nd line) •In conjunction with statin if statin fails to control total cholesterol or LDL-cholesterol	•Headache •Diarrhoea (steatorrhoea)	•Can be used with statins
Fibrates *Third line (or first for isolated triglyceridaemia)*	Bezafibrate, Ciprofibrate, Fenofibrate, Gemfibrozil	Activate PPARα transcription factors, which regulate lipid metabolism in the liver	•Isolated triglyceridaemia (>10mmol/L) •Hypercholesterolaemia if statin not tolerated or contraindicated (3rd line)	•GI disturbance •Myalgia and rhabdomyolysis	•Most effective at reducing triglyceride levels •Not to be used with statins

HEART FAILURE

- Core medications
  - ACE inhibitor (<u>or</u> angiotensin receptor blocker <u>or</u> angiotensin receptor-neprilysin inhibitor)
  - β-blocker
  - Diuretic (e.g. furosemide, bumetanide) *if peripheral/pulmonary oedema*
- Other medications: add aldosterone antagonist (e.g. spironolactone, eplerenone) *if uncontrolled with core treatments*; add ivabradine *if in sinus rhythm ≥70 bpm despite maximum β-blocker dose*

ANTICOAGULANTS

See notes on anticoagulants p294

ANALGESIC LADDER

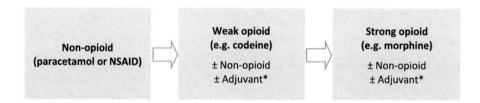

*Adjuvants = drugs to calm fears and anxiety

Produced using World Health Organisation 'Cancer pain ladder for adults' accessed 2017

BACTERIA – BACKGROUND KNOWLEDGE

	Gram positive		Gram negative	
Cocci	**Staphylococcus** (clusters and catalase +ve) ↘Coagulase +ve (*aureus*) – skin infections, pneumonia, endocarditis, abscess formation ↘Coagulase -ve (*epidermidis, saprophyticus*) CONS = Contaminants (unless foreign bodies present) **Streptococcus** (strips and catalase -ve) ↘α-haemolytic, *i.e. partially lyse RBCs* -pneumoniae – pneumonia, meningitis, URTIs, invasive -viridans group (*mitis, mutans, salivarius, sanguinis, anginosus*) – endocarditis, dental ↘β-haemolytic, i.e. completely lyse RBCs -Group A *Strep* (*pyogenes*) – skin infections, Rh fever, scarlet fever, 'strep throat', post-strep GN, erysipelas, necrotising fasciitis, strep toxic shock -Group B *Strep* (*agalactiae*) – vaginal colonisation, neonatal infections ↘Non-haemolytic -Group D *Strep* (*bovis, equinus*) – bacteraemia -Enterococcus (*faecium, faecalis*) –UTIs, bacteraemia, endocarditis, diverticulitis -α-haemolytic / -Group A β-haemolytic / -Group B β-haemolytic B=Baby		**Diplococci** **Neisseria** ↘*meningitidis* – meningitis ↘*gonorrhoeae* –gonorrhoea, conjunctivitis, pharyngitis, disseminated infection, arthritis **Moraxella** ↘*catarrhalis* –URTIs, chronic lung disease exacerbations, pneumonia	

	Gram positive	Enteric		Non-enteric
Rods (bacilli)	**Big and spore-forming** **Clostridium** (anaerobic) ↘*difficile* – colitis ↘*tetani* – tetanus ↘*perfringens* – gas gangrene ↘*botulinum* – botulism **Bacillus** ↘*anthracis* – anthrax (infected animal/product spores → cutaneous: black ulcer, lymphadenopathy, fever; lung: pneumonia; or GI: haematemesis/diarrhoea) ↘*cereus* – gastroenteritis (risk = improperly refrigerated rice) **Small and non-spore-forming** **Listeria** ↘*monocytogenes* – gastroenteritis, septicaemia, meningitis, encephalitis, pneumonia, neonatal, endocarditis (risks = soft cheeses, unpasteurized milk, meats) **Corynebacterium** ↘*diphtheriae* – diphtheria, colonisation	ENTEROBACTERIACEAE **Long** **E. coli** – UTIs, gastroenteritis, neonatal meningitis **Klebsiella** – pneumonia, UTIs **Enterobacter** – LRTIs, UTIs, skin, intra-abdominal, endocarditis **Citrobacter** – UTIs }Aerobic glucose + lactose-fermenting ('COLIFORMS' – normal bowel flora) **Salmonella** – gastroenteritis, typhoid **Shigella** – gastroenteritis/dysentery **Proteus** – UTIs, nosocomial **Yersinia** – yersiniosis (diarrhoeal illness), plague }Aerobic glucose only-fermenting **Serratia** – nosocomial infections **Pseudomonas** – pneumonia, UTIs, sepsis, necrotising enterocolitis, wound }Aerobic non-fermenting **Bacteroides** – intra-abdominal }Anaerobic **Curved** **Vibrio** ↘*cholerae* – cholera (dysentery) **Campylobacter** (microaerophilic) ↘*jejuni* – gastroenteritis (raw meat) **Helicobacter** ↘*pylori* – gastritis		**Coccobacilli** **Haemophilus** ↘*influenzae* – pneumonia, meningitis, epiglottitis **Bordetella** ↘*pertussis* – Whooping cough **Gardnerella** ↘*vaginalis* – bacterial vaginosis **Acinetobacter** – nosocomial infections **Legionella** ↘*pneumophilia* – Legionnaires' disease (water tanks/air conditioners → atypical pneumonia) **Coxiella** ↘*burnetii* – Q fever (livestock → flu-like illness, pneumonia, granulomatous hepatitis, endocarditis) **Brucella** – brucellosis (unpasteurized milk → long flu-like illness) **Pasteurella** – pasteurellosis (cat bite → septic phlegmon) **Francisella** – tularaemia (tick/deer fly bite → ulcer at site of entry, fever/sepsis, lymphadenopathy)
Spirochaetes		**Treponema** ↘*pallidum* – syphilis **Borrelia** ↘*burgdorferi* – Lyme disease **Leptospira** – leptospirosis (spread by rodents)		
Branching filamentous growth	**Actinomyces** (anaerobic) – head and neck swellings, thoracic infection, abscesses, bowel **Nocardia** (partially acid-fast) – pneumonia/cavitation, endocarditis, brain abscess, cellulitis			
Pleomorphic		**Chlamydia** ↘*trachomatis* – cervicitis/urethritis ↘*psittaci* – psittacosis/pneumonia (spread by birds) **Rickettsia** – typhus, rickettsialpox, Boutonneuse fever, African tick bite fever, Rocky Mountain spotted fever (all tick-borne)		
Unique cell wall	**Mycobacterium** (acid-fast) ↘*tuberculosis* – TB			
No cell wall	**Mycoplasma** – pneumonia			

ANTIBIOTICS

Targets: Target DNA · Target protein synthesis · Target cell wall

Spectrum arrow: Gram Positive → Gram Negative

β-lactams: β-lactam ring lodges in bacterial cell wall

Class	Subclass	Antibiotic	Enterococcus	MRSA	Staphylococcus aureus (MSSA)	Streptococcus	Neisseria meningitidis	Haemophilus	E. coli and coliforms	β-lactamases which confer resistance*	Pseudomonas	Anaerobes (except C. diff)	Atypical pneumonias
β-lactams — Penicillins	Penicillins	Flucloxacillin *(Large molecule so not affected by β-lactamases)*			+++								
		Benzylpenicillin			*Staph secretes penicillinase (a β-lactamase that destroys the β-lactam ring of penicillin)*	+++	++			Penicillinase *(also: ESBL, Amp C, carbapenemase)*			
		Amoxicillin/Ampicillin	++ *(Not all)*			++++	++	++	+ *(Many resistant)*	*(also: ESBL, Amp C, carbapenemase)*			
		Co-Amoxiclav (Amoxicillin + β-lactamase inhibitor)			+++	+		+++	+			++	
		Tazocin (Piperacillin + β-lactamase inhibitor)			+++	+++		+++	+++	Amp C *(also: Amp C, carbapenemase; ESBL variable)*	+++	++	
	Carbapenems	Meropenem			+++	+++		+++	+++	Carbapenemase / *Variable: ESBL, carbapenemase*	+++	++	
	2nd gen Cephalosporins	Cefuroxime			+++	+++	+ *(Cefuroxime does not penetrate BBB)*	++					
	3rd gen Cephalosporins	Ceftriaxone/Cefotaxime			+++	+++	++++	+++	+++	ESBL *(also: Amp C, carbapenemase)*	+		
	4th gen Cephalosporins	Cefepime *(not used in UK)*									+ *(Ceftazidime is used for Pseudomonas only (best agent))*		
Glycopeptides *(Inhibit peptidoglycan links in cell wall)*		Vancomycin/Teicoplanin	+++ *(Some strains resistant (VRE))*	+++	+++	++						+	
Aminoglycosides *(Inhibit 30S ribosomal subunit)*		Gentamicin	+	+		++		++	+++	*Some cross-resistance by ESBL and carbapenemase*	+++	+ *(Aminoglycosides use oxygen-dependent active transport)*	
Tetracyclines *(Inhibit 30S ribosomal subunit)*		Doxycycline	+	++	++	++	+/-	++	+/-	*Some cross-resistance by ESBL and carbapenemase*		++	++
Lincosamides *(Inhibit 50S ribosomal subunit)*		Clindamycin		++	++	++						++	
Macrolides *(Inhibit 50S ribosomal subunit)*		Erythromycin/Clarithromycin/Azithromycin (gram -ve)			++	++		++	+/-				+++
Misc. *(Inhibit 50S ribosomal subunit)*		Chloramphenicol		+	+	++	++	++	++			++	
Fluoroquinolones *(Inhibit DNA gyrase)*		Ciprofloxacin	++	+	+	++	++	+++	+++	*Some cross-resistance by ESBL and carbapenemase*	++		+++
Misc. *(Inhibit DNA)*		Metronidazole										+++	
		Trimethoprim		+ *(Not alone)*			++	+	++				
		Co-trimoxazole (sulfamethoxazole + trimethoprim)		++	++			++	++	*Some cross-resistance by ESBL and carbapenemase*			
		Nitrofurantoin	++						++				

β-lactamase types (rods): Penicillinase — + (Pseudomonas); Amp C — +++ (Pseudomonas); ESBL — +++ (Pseudomonas); Carbapenemase — +++ (Pseudomonas). *Penicillinase (also: ESBL, Amp C, carbapenemase)* · *(also: Amp C, carbapenemase; ESBL variable)* · *ESBL (also: Amp C, carbapenemase)*

MRSA is resistant to β-lactams due to modification of penicillin-binding protein

Atypical pneumonias: Legionella (Gram -ve coccobacilli), Mycoplasma (no cell wall)

Anaerobes: Clostridium (Gram +ve rod), Bacteroides (Gram -ve rod)

*β-lactamase resistance: β-lactamases are enzymes produced by some bacteria which break down the β-lactam ring of certain β-lactam antibiotics and cause resistance.

Penicillinase is produced by several bacteria, most notably Staphylococcus; the other β-lactamases (ESBL, Amp C, carbapenemase) are mainly produced by some members of the enterobacteriaceae group.

Coliforms (lactose-fermenting enterobacteriaceae): E. coli, Enterobacter, Klebsiella, Citrobacter

Other important bacteria to know antibiotics for: Mycobacterium; Clostridium difficile; Chlamydia

COVERAGE NEEDED

Community-acquired pneumonia
- *Streptococcus pneumoniae*
- *Haemophilus influenzae* (if not vaccinated)
- Atypicals

If immunocompromised (e.g. malnourished, alcoholic, diabetic, on long-term steroids), also: *Staphylococcus aureus*, coliforms, TB
If severely immunosuppressed (e.g. HIV with CD4 <200, transplant recipient), also: *Pneumocystis carinii, Cryptococcus, CMV, Varicella zoster* virus, influenza, fungal infections

Hospital-acquired pneumonia
- *Staphylococcus aureus* (including MRSA)
- Anaerobes
- Coliforms
- *Pseudomonas*

Colonising bacteria in chronic respiratory diseases (may or may not cause infections/exacerbations)
- *Streptococcus pneumoniae*
- *Haemophilus influenzae*
- *Moraxella catarrhalis*
- *Staphylococcus aureus*
- *Pseudomonas*

In cystic fibrosis, also: *Burkholderia cepacia*

Upper respiratory tract infections
- *Streptococcus pneumoniae*
- *Streptococcus pyogenes*
- *Haemophilus influenzae*
- *Moraxella catarrhalis*

Cavitating pneumonia
- *Streptococcus pneumoniae*
- *Staphylococcus aureus*
- *Klebsiella*
- TB
- Anaerobes

Intra-abdominal (including biliary)
Normal bowel flora:
- Anaerobes, e.g. *Bacteroides*
- Coliforms
- *Enterococcus*

Gastroenteritis/diarrhoea
→ ceftriaxone/ciprofloxacin/azithromycin
- *Salmonella enteritidis*
- *Shigella*
- *Campylobacter*
- *Escherichia coli* (enterotoxic)

Less common: *Yersinia enterocolitica, Bacillus cereus, Staphylococcus aureus*
If risk factors, also: *Clostridium difficile, Vibrio cholerae, Salmonella typhi*
If dysentery: *Shigella, Vibrio cholerae,* amoebiasis
Don't forget viral, parasitic and non-infectious causes!

Skin/joints/bone
- *Staphylococcus aureus*
- *Streptococcus pyogenes*

For wound/ulcer infections or severe/necrotising cellulitis, also: anaerobes
For burns, also: anaerobes, *Pseudomonas*
For post-surgical wounds, also: Gram negative bacilli (e.g. *E. coli, Klebsiella, Pseudomonas*), Enterococci, MRSA, CONS
NB. wound-colonising bacteria (i.e. bacteria present in exudate without necessarily causing infection) include: coliforms, Enterococcus, *anaerobes*

Meningitis
- *Neisseria meningitidis* (meningococcal)
- *Streptococcus pneumoniae* (pneumococcal)
- *Haemophilus influenzae* (if not vaccinated)
- *Listeria* (if >65 years or immunocompromised)

If neonatal: group B *Streptococcus, E. coli*/coliforms, *Listeria* (rare)

Urine
1. *Escherichia coli*
2. *Staphylococcus saprophyticus*
3. Non-*E. Coli* enterobacteriaceae (*Klebsiella, Enterobacter, Proteus*), *Pseudomonas*, Enterococci, Staphylococci (*CONS/aureus*)

Less common organisms (3) are associated with: catheters, hospitals, structural abnormalities and instrumentation

Infective endocarditis
- *Viridans* group *Streptococci* and other *Streptococci* (e.g. *bovis*)
- *Enterococci*
- *Staphylococcus aureus* and coagulase-negative *Staphylococci* (e.g. *epidermidis*)
- *Coxiella burnetii*
- HACEK organisms

Surgical prophylaxis
- Need to cover skin ± intra-abdominal organisms

Sepsis of unknown origin
- Need to cover skin, chest, urine, intra-abdominal organisms

BACKGROUND KNOWLEDGE

- Haemostasis process:

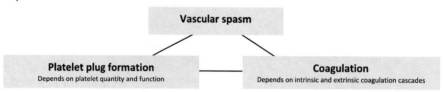

- Coagulation cascade:

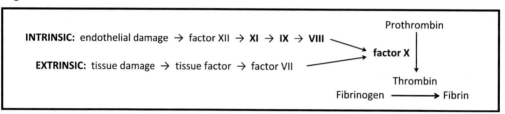

- Clot dissolution:

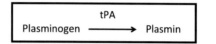

- Natural anticoagulants: proteins C and S (inactivate factors V and VIII); antithrombin (inactivates many clotting factors)
- Vitamin K dependent clotting factors: II, VII, IX, X (+ proteins C and S)
- Tests
  - **PT and INR** = *EXTRINSIC*: tissue factor is added to blood in the laboratory to activate the extrinsic pathway. Clotting time (PT) is measured in seconds (normal usually = 12-13). However, the PT may vary depending on the reagent used, so the laboratory can use the PT to calculate the INR to standardise results (normal = 0.8-1.2).
  WEPT: Warfarin Extrinsic Prothrombin Time
  - **APTT** = *INTRINSIC*: a contact activator is added to blood in the laboratory to activate the intrinsic pathway. Clotting time (APTT) is measured in seconds (normal usually = 30-50). The APTT can be divided by the mean normal value to calculate the APTT ratio if required.

ANTICOAGULANTS

Types of anticoagulants						
	Action	**Monitoring**	**Reversal**	**Common uses**	**Advantages**	**Disadvantages**
Oral anticoagulants						
Vitamin K antagonist *Warfarin*	Reduces the synthesis of vitamin K dependent clotting factors	INR	•Vitamin K •Prothrombin complex concentrate	•AF (including valvular AF) •VTE •Metallic heart valves	•Reversible	•Regular INRs required •Risk of under-/over-coagulation •Interactions
Direct thrombin inhibitor (-tran's) *Dabigatran*	Inhibits thrombin	None	Praxbind	•AF (non-valvular) •VTE	•Quick onset/offset •No monitoring required	•Renally cleared
Direct factor Xa inhibitors (-xaban's) *Rivaroxaban, apixaban, edoxaban*	Inhibit factor Xa (the active form of factor X) directly	None	None (but prothrombin complex concentrate may be tried)	•Post-op VTE prophylaxis		•Irreversible •Renally cleared
IV and S/C anticoagulants						
Unfractionated heparin (IV infusion or S/C)	Anticoagulant that increases antithrombin activity by enhancing its binding to factor Xa and thrombin	APTT ratio used to monitor infusion Anti-factor Xa assay may also be used	Stop infusion Protamine sulphate	•Perioperatively in patients requiring full anticoagulation for a high risk indication (e.g. metallic heart valve)	•Very fast onset •Very fast reversal by stopping infusion •S/C unfractionated heparin may be used in patients with renal impairment instead of LMWH	•Regular APTT ratios required for infusion •Complex to manage •Risk of under-/over-coagulation
Low molecular weight heparin S/C *Enoxaparin*	Consists of only short chain heparins so most of its activity is mediated by inhibition of factor Xa	Anti-factor Xa assay (if required)	Protamine sulphate	•VTE •VTE prophylaxis •AF •ACS	•More predictable effect than unfractionated heparin so routine monitoring is not required •Safe in pregnancy	•Renally cleared
Indirect factor Xa inhibitor S/C *Fondaparinux*	Synthetic anticoagulant derived from the antithrombin binding region of heparin, which indirectly inhibits factor Xa	Anti-factor Xa assay (if required)	None	•ACS •VTE •VTE prophylaxis	•Safer in ACS than LMWH •Lower risk of heparin-induced thrombocytopenia	•Renally cleared •Irreversible

(left margin: Direct oral anticoagulants)

INSULIN PRESCRIBING

TYPES OF INSULIN

- **Rapid-acting** (*given at start of meal*)
  - Novorapid (Aspart)
  - Humalog (Lispro)
  - Apidra (Glulisine)
- **Short-acting** (*given 30 minutes before a meal*)
  - Actrapid
  - Humulin **S**
- **Intermediate-acting** (*usually given once/twice daily or as part of mix*)
  - Humulin **I**
  - Insulatard
  - Insuman basal
- **Long-acting** (*usually given once daily*)
  - Levemir (Detemir)
  - Lantus (Glargine)
  - Tresiba (Degludec)

Normal values (mmol/L)

Non-diabetic (random) = 3.5-7.8
Type 1 diabetic = 4-9
Type 2 diabetic = 4-8.5
Hyperglycaemia = >11
Hypoglycaemia = <4

Mixtures (for twice daily pre-mixed regimens)

<u>Intermediate + short</u> (*given 30 minutes before breakfast and dinner*)
- Humulin M3 (*30% short-acting*)
- Insuman comb 15 or 25 or 50 (*15/25/50% short-acting respectively*)

<u>Intermediate + rapid</u> (*given at start of breakfast and dinner*)
- NovoMix 30 (*30% rapid-acting*)
- Humalog Mix 25 or 50 (*25/50% rapid-acting respectively*)

REGIMENS

- **Basal bolus regimen** (basal long-acting insulin given at night with rapid-acting insulin given before every meal):

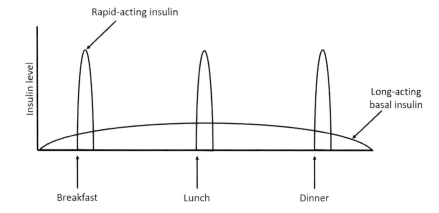

Most common type 1 regimen

- **Twice daily pre-mixed regimen** (mixed intermediate-acting and short-/rapid-acting insulin given twice daily, before breakfast and before dinner):

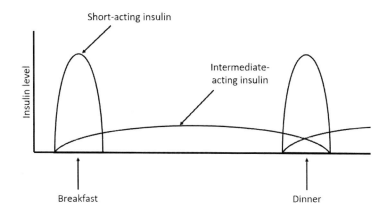

Most common type 2 regimen

- **Intermediate insulin once/twice daily** may also be used in type 2 diabetes to supplement oral hypoglycaemics and aid glycaemic control in the day (OM), at night/in morning (ON) or both (BD)

ADJUSTING INSULIN REGIMENS (IN RESPONSE TO GLUCOSE LEVELS)

- Review the capillary glucose monitoring chart and work out the <u>pattern of variation in glucose levels</u> in relation to meals (readings are usually taken before meals)
- Use common sense – if a patient is eating less, the insulin dose will need to be reduced; on the other hand, certain conditions may require it to be increased *(see box)*
- Adjusting a **basal bolus regimen**:
  - Levels high/low before breakfast (or in night) → increase/decrease bedtime long-acting insulin
  - Levels high/low before lunch or dinner or bed → increase/decrease rapid-acting insulin given with meal <u>before</u>
- Adjusting a **twice daily pre-mixed/intermediate regimen**:
  - Levels high/low before bed <u>and</u> before breakfast → increase/decrease evening insulin
  - Levels high/low before lunch <u>and</u> before evening meal → increase/decrease morning insulin
- Adjusting a **once daily morning regimen**:
  - Levels high/low before lunch <u>and</u> evening meal → increase/decrease insulin
- Adjusting a **once daily evening regimen**:
  - Levels high/low before breakfast → increase/decrease insulin
- Doses are usually adjusted by approximately 10% depending on how abnormal the glucose levels are. Capillary glucose levels must then be closely monitored and dose-adjusted as required (it's partly trial and error).
- Remember, hypoglycaemia is more dangerous than hyperglycaemia
- If you cannot get on top of it, ask the diabetes team for help (insulin type may need changing)

Changes in insulin requirements

Increased requirement
- DKA/hyperosmolar hyperglycaemic state
- Sepsis
- Illness
- Steroids
- Pancreatitis
- Dehydration

Decreased requirement
- Reduced calorific intake
- Exercise
- Reduced renal function (may reduce drug excretion)
- Alcohol

INSULIN PUMPS

- Insulin pumps continuously infuse a basal rate of rapid-/short-acting insulin subcutaneously
  - The rate can be changed depending on requirements (e.g. during exercise, diet or capillary glucose level)
  - A button is pressed to give an insulin bolus at the start of a meal
- If patients are nil by mouth, the pump should be set to continue basal rate insulin but no boluses should be given. (5% dextrose infusion can be given and their basal rate adjusted accordingly – they do not need a variable rate insulin infusion.)

VARIABLE RATE INSULIN INFUSION (FORMERLY CALLED 'SLIDING SCALE')

NB: This is different to a fixed rate insulin infusion, as used in DKA.
- Used for diabetic patients who are nil by mouth, e.g. perioperatively
- The capillary glucose is checked 1-2 hourly and the rate of insulin infusion is modified according to a predetermined protocol
- Continuous IV fluids containing glucose <u>must</u> be given alongside to maintain patient glucose levels and hydration
- **Starting** a variable rate insulin infusion:
  - Most hospitals have a variable rate insulin infusion chart which just needs a signature
  - Continuous IV fluids also need prescribing as below
  - If the patient is taking long-acting insulin, this should be continued throughout (but short-/rapid-acting insulin must be suspended)
- **During** a variable rate insulin infusion:
  - Continuous IV fluids, for example:
    - Surgical patients: 5% glucose/0.45% saline/0.15% KCl at 80ml/hour
    - Medical patients: 5% glucose (1L with 20mmol KCl) at 100ml/hour (unless capillary glucose is >15mmol/L, in which case give 0.9% saline until it returns to <15mmol/L)
  - Check plasma Na^+ and K^+ daily
  - Re-sign the variable rate insulin infusion chart daily
  - The protocol's infusion rates can be modified if the patient is particularly insulin-resistant/sensitive
- **Stopping** a variable rate insulin infusion: confirm patient is eating and drinking and ensure the patient has received their long-acting insulin. (If not, a proportionate dose should be given at least 1 hour before stopping.) Give their usual mixed/rapid-acting insulin with meal and wait 30 minutes before stopping the variable rate insulin infusion. Monitor capillary glucose QDS for at least 24 hours.

INSULIN PRESCRIBING RULES

- Use insulin prescription chart if available (write **'insulin as per insulin prescription chart'** at relevant times on main chart)
- You must write **'UNITS'** (do not abbreviate to 'U')
- Specify the **brand name** and indicate the **device** the patient uses (e.g. disposable pen, vial, pen cartridge)
- Write **'pre-breakfast/lunch/dinner'** rather than times if the insulin must be taken before meals
- Ensure you corroborate their prescription if unsure of a dose – never estimate!

DRUG UNITS AND CALCULATIONS

UNIT CONVERSIONS

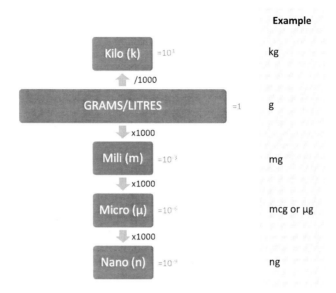

Example

NB: prior to performing calculations, always convert all values the same units.

DRUG DILUTIONS AND CONCENTRATIONS

- **Ratios** = unit of solute *to* units of solvent **or** grams of solvent in mls of solution (because 1g = 1ml)

> Ratio = grams of drug in mls of solution

e.g. 1:10,000 adrenaline = 1 unit adrenaline to every 10,000 units saline **or** 1g adrenaline in every 10,000ml saline

- **% solutions** = grams of solvent per 100ml solute (because 1ml = 1g)

> % = grams of drug per 100ml of solution

e.g. 0.01% adrenaline = 0.01g adrenaline per 100ml saline (or 1g adrenaline per 10,000ml)

- **Moles** = weight (g)/molecular mass (u)
  Where molecular mass is the total of the atomic masses of each atom in the molecule (individual atom's atomic masses are shown in the periodic table)

> Moles = weight (g) / molecular mass (u)

e.g. magnesium's atomic mass is 24 and there is only one atom of magnesium in Mg^{2+}, so the molecular mass is 24. Hence, using the above formula, 1 mole of magnesium is 24g.

- **Molarity (M)** = number of moles of a chemical in 1L of solution

> Molar (M) = moles per litre

e.g. 1 molar solution of magnesium consists of 24g magnesium dissolved in 1L water

WEIGHT-DOSAGE CALCULATIONS

> Dose required (mg) = weight-dosage (mg/kg) x weight (kg)

e.g. the weight-dosage of a phenytoin infusion in status epilepticus is 18mg/kg and the patient weighs 80kg. The dose required is therefore 18 x 80, which is 1440mg.

INFUSION RATE CALCULATIONS

Infusion time/rate

> Infusion time (minutes) = total dose required (mg) / drug rate required (mg/min)

e.g. the infusion rate of phenytoin in status epilepticus is 50mg/minute and the total dose required for an 80kg patient is 1.44g (1440mg). The infusion time is therefore 1440 / 50, which is 29 minutes.

> Infusion rate (ml/hour) = dose rate (mg/hour) / concentration (mg/ml)

e.g. a 5g (5000mg) magnesium infusion is prescribed to run at 1g/hour (1000mg/hour). The 500ml infusion bag contains magnesium at a concentration of 10mg/ml. The infusion rate is therefore 1000 / 10, which is 100ml/hour.

Infusion set drop rate

> Drops per minute = total drops in bag / infusion time (minutes)
> *where:* Total drops in bag = bag volume (ml) x drops per ml (usually 20 but depends on giving set)

e.g. a 1L (1000ml) bag of normal saline is prescribed over 8 hours (480 minutes). The giving set runs fluid through at 20 drops per ml and so the total drops in the bag are 1000 x 20, which is 20,000. To run the infusion over 8 hours, the rate required in drops per minute is 20,000 / 480, which is 42 drops per minute. This is approximately 10 drops in 15 seconds (42 / 4), and the giving set clamp can be adjusted to give that rate.

NUMBER OF TABLETS/LIQUIDS NEEDED

Calculate first

What you need to give (number of tablets or ml) = dose you want / dose of what you've got (dose **per tab** or dose **per ml**)

> What you need to give = dose you want / dose of what you have

e.g. you want to give 40mg prednisolone. Only 5mg tablets are available. The amount you need to give is therefore 40 / 5, which is 8 tablets.

HOSPITAL INPATIENT PRESCRIPTIONS

SECTIONS OF THE DRUG CHART

- **Patient details:** hospital number, name, age, DOB, weight, consultant, ward, chart date, chart number, allergies
- **Once only drugs:** for drugs to be given once only at a certain time/date
- **Regular prescriptions**
- **As required (PRN) medications:** for medications only to be given if the patient requests them/complains, e.g. analgesia, anti-emetics etc.
- **Oxygen**
- **Fluids**

Abbreviations	
Routes	
PO	Oral
IV	Intravenous
IM	Intramuscular
PR/PV	Rectally/vaginally
INH	Inhaled
NEB	Nebulised
SC	Subcutaneous
TOP	Topically
	One (tablet/dose)
	Two (tablets/doses)
Timings	
OD	Once daily
OM/mane	Once daily in morning
ON/nocte	Once daily in evening
BD	Twice daily
TDS	3 times daily
QDS	4 times daily
X-hourly/X*	Doses X hours apart (exactly)
PRN	As required
STAT	Immediately

GENERAL POINTS

- **Review dates** for antibiotics should be 48 hours (because this is when culture results should be back). All medications should be reviewed weekly.
- **Allergy box** must be filled out with all (not just drug) allergies, with details of reactions in brackets. The box should also be signed and dated.
- **Times** must be written in 24 hour format (00:00)
- The total dose should be indicated, i.e. if the patient needs 2 x 500mg tablets, put 1g in the dose
- When stopping a drug, cross it through neatly, and sign and date
- If a drug needs to be omitted on a certain date, note this in the comments and cross through like this:

	11/12/12	12/12/12	13/12/12	14/12/12	15/12/12	16/12/12	17/12/12	18/12/12	19/12/12
09:00									
13:00									
17:00									
21:00									

- If re-writing a chart, include all of the original start dates

CHOOSING PRESCRIPTION TIMES

- **BD:** circle/tick the two intended times (usually latest and earliest times)
- **TDS:** circle/tick three times throughout the day as spaced out as possible. If there are 4 possible times on the drug chart, it usually does not matter which middle time you choose, unless the medication needs to be taken at mealtimes (e.g. hypoglycaemics).
- **8-HOURLY:** must be 8 hours apart, so cross out printed times and write in new ones so they fall 8 hours apart
- **QDS:** circle/tick four times throughout the day as spaced out as possible
- **PRN:** in the PRN section of the chart, 'frequency' is the maximum frequency (i.e. don't write 'PRN,' write, for example, '4-hourly')
- **OD:** circle/tick the first dose time of the day (unless it is to be given at night, e.g. statin or sleeping medication)
- **ON:** circle/tick the last dose time of the day

TIPS FOR PRESCRIBING STATIONS

- Order of station:
  1. Fill in **patient details**
  2. Check **allergies** and fill in allergies box
  3. Prescribe **antibiotics** (checking for allergies)
     WARNING: many antibiotics contain penicillin, e.g. amoxicillin, flucloxacillin, ampicillin, co-amoxiclav/Augmentin, Tazocin
  4. Prescribe other **new medications**
  5. Say 'Normally, I would now check drug **interactions**. Would you like me to do that now or go on to write up the regular medications?' (Always check interactions if prescribing any drugs with a narrow therapeutic range, or enzyme-inducers/inhibitors)
  6. Prescribe **regular medications** last
- The time is usually short so be as quick as you can
- If you do not know the length of an antibiotic course, say you would call microbiology to confirm while writing the usual duration: IV antibiotics 5 days; oral antibiotics 7 days

RULES FOR ALL PRESCRIPTIONS

<u>Pen</u>
- Write in **black, capital letters**

<u>Units</u>
- For doses less than 1 gram, write in milligrams; and for doses less than 1 milligram, write in micrograms
- For volumes, use millilitres (ml), not cubic centimetres or cc
- Do not abbreviate:
  - **Micrograms**
  - **Nanograms**
  - **Units**

<u>Drug names</u>
- Use **generic drug names** (not brand names), except for:
  - Inhalers
  - Insulin
  - Psychiatric drugs
  - Epilepsy drugs
  - Modified release products
  - 5-aminosalicylic acids
  - Narrow therapeutic range drugs (**G**uys **W**ith **L**arge **D**ongles **T**otally **M**ake **P**erfect **I**nternet **C**onnections)
    - **G**entamicin
    - **W**arfarin
    - **L**ithium
    - **D**igoxin
    - **T**heophylline
    - **M**ethotrexate
    - **P**henytoin
    - **I**nsulin
    - **C**iclosporin

    In these cases, write the generic name first, then the brand name in brackets afterwards.

<u>Special case prescriptions</u>
- **PRN prescriptions**
  - Include the minimum dose interval and maximum total daily amount, e.g. 'DRUG: Tramadol. DOSE: 100mg. FREQUENCY: as required every 6 hours (maximum 400mg in 24 hours)'
- **Solutions**
  - Write the drug and concentration in the drug box, and how many ml are to be taken in the dose box. e.g. 'DRUG: Oramorph 5mg/5ml. DOSE: 5ml'
- **Inhalers**
  - Write the inhaler and puff content in the drug box, and how many puffs are to be taken in the dose box, e.g. 'DRUG: Salbutamol 100 micrograms. DOSE: 2 Puffs'
- **Combined drugs**
  - Write the combination specifics in the drug box, and how many tablets are to be taken in the dose box, e.g. DRUG: Co-Codamol 8/500. DOSE: 2 Tablets'
- **Complex analgesia**
  - You should prescribe background analgesia regularly and breakthrough analgesia PRN ($1/6^{th}$ of the regular dose, repeated up to 4-hourly)
- **Oxygen**
  - Include the target saturations
- **Fluids**
  - Include the fluid, volume, additives, and flow rate

<u>Controlled drugs</u>
- **Outpatient controlled drug prescriptions**
  - Must be handwritten in indelible ink
  - Include patient's name and address
  - Drug, strength, and formulation (e.g. tablets, capsules, liquid etc.)
  - Dose and frequency, e.g. '5 mg up to 2-hourly as required for pain'
  - Total <u>quantity</u> must be spelled out as well as given in numerals, e.g. 'supply 20 (twenty) tablets'

SECTIONS OF THE PRESCRIPTION

- **Top (patient details)**
  - Name
  - Address
  - Age (in years and months if <5 years)
  - Date of birth
- **Middle (medication details)**
  - Drug prescription blank box
- **Bottom (prescriber details)**
  - Prescriber's signature
  - Date
  - Prescriber's name and address (usually pre-printed)

Abbreviations	
Routes	
PO	Oral
IV	Intravenous
IM	Intramuscular
PR/PV	Rectally/vaginally
INH	Inhaled
NEB	Nebulised
SC	Subcutaneous
TOP	Topically
⊤	One (tablet/dose)
⊤⊤	Two (tablets/doses)
Timings	
OD	Once daily
OM/mane	Once daily in morning
ON/nocte	Once daily in evening
BD	Twice daily
TDS	3 times daily
QDS	4 times daily
X-hourly/X°	Doses X hours apart (exactly)
PRN	As required
STAT	Immediately

FILLING IN THE DRUG PRESCRIPTION BOX

Divide into 3 lines:

1. **DRUG**: include strength (e.g. 40mg) and preparation (e.g. tablets)
2. **DOSING INSTRUCTIONS**: write patient-friendly dose in numbers (e.g. '1 tablet') followed by frequency in words (e.g. 'four times a day') — Included on drug sticker
3. **QUANTITY**: write quantity to be dispensed in numbers (e.g. '28 tablets')

Examples of outpatient prescriptions		
Drug	**Dosing instructions**	**Quantity**
Simvastatin 40mg tablets	1 tablet once a day at night	28 tablets
Co-codamol 8/500 tablets	2 tablets as required every 4-6 hours (maximum 8 tablets in 24 hours)	28 tablets
Flucloxacillin 250mg capsules	2 capsules four times a day	20 capsules
Clobetasone butyrate 0.05% ointment	Apply thinly twice a day to affected area for 2 weeks	30g tube
Beclometasone 100micrograms/puff inhaler	2 puffs twice a day	1 inhaler
Diamorphine 30mg injection ampoules	60 mg by subcutaneous infusion over 24 hours	6 (six) ampoules

GENERAL POINTS

- If you want anything extra to be on the drug label, write it in inverted commas, e.g. 'strong painkiller'
- Cross out any unused space in the prescription box

MONITORING NARROW THERAPEUTIC RANGE DRUGS

The therapeutic range of drugs is a concentration range that is high enough to ensure they work but not so high that they cause adverse effects. Some drugs have a particularly narrow therapeutic range and need close monitoring because a small increase in concentration can result in serious toxicity.

Guys With Large Dongles Totally Make Perfect Internet Connections

	Toxicity	Monitor	Starting drug	Subsequent monitoring/dosing	Adjusting dose
			Monitoring of commonly used narrow therapeutic range drugs		
Gentamicin	Ototoxicity Renal failure	Gentamicin level	•Give loading dose 5mg/kg (ideal body weight) •Check level 6-14 hours later •Use Urban and Craig nomogram to determine dosing interval	Check level (6-14 hours post-dose) every 1-3 days depending on stability (increase monitoring frequency if renal function changes) *Reference: Urban and Craig nomogram*	Adjust dosing interval as per Urban and Craig nomogram
Vancomycin		Vancomycin level	•Give initial loading dose (dependent on weight) •Select maintenance <u>dose and interval</u> from hospital dosing table (dependent on creatinine clearance) •Check a pre-dose (trough) level prior to the third dose, give the dose regardless, and then check the level prior to the next dose •If level is too high/low, adjust the dose and interval to next level down/up in dosing table respectively	Check pre-dose (trough) level every 3 days if renal function is stable *Reference range: pre-dose level = 10-15mg/L*	<u>Level too high</u> Adjust dose and interval to next level down in dosing table <u>Level too low</u> Adjust dose and interval to next level up in dosing table
Warfarin	Bleeding	INR	•Start concomitantly with treatment dose LMWH if immediate therapeutic effect required (stop LMWH when INR in range and after at least 5 days of dual therapy) •Start 5mg each evening •Check INR on days 3, 4 and 5 – hospital warfarin dosing charts tell you how to adjust the dose depending on the INR	Monitor in anticoagulant clinic – intervals depend on INR stability *Target INR for most indications = 2-3 Metallic aortic valve = 2.5-3.5 Metallic mitral valve = 3-4*	Adjust dose depending on INR
Lithium	Tremor Coma Renal failure	Lithium level + TFTs, LFTs, U&Es	•Check level (12 hours post-dose) after 5 days •Then check weekly until level has been stable for 4 weeks	Check levels every 3 months *Reference range (12 hours post-dose) = 0.4-0.8mmol/L*	Adjust dose (check compliance if low)
Digoxin	GI disturbance Xanthopsia Arrhythmias	Digoxin level *Also check for hypokalaemia (increases toxicity)*	•500mcg loading dose given with cardiac and BP monitoring •Similar dose given 6 hours later •Maintenance dose (62.5-250mcg OD – use lower dose if elderly/in renal failure) is started 24 hours after the first loading dose	No routine monitoring required – check level if concerned, e.g. if renal injury, toxicity, poor response or interacting medications *Reference range (6-12 hours post-dose) = 1-2mcg/L*	Adjust dose
Theophylline	Arrhythmias Seizures	Theophylline level	•PO: check levels 5 days after starting, and 3 days after any dose changes (levels are taken 4-6 hours post-dose) •IV infusion: check levels 4-6 hours after starting, then daily	Check level 3 days after any dose changes *Reference range = 10-20mcg/ml*	Adjust dose
Methotrexate	Myelosuppression Liver toxicity Renal failure	FBC LFTs U&Es	•Monitor before starting, then every 2 weeks until stabilised •Start at 10-15mg/week with 5mg folic acid on a different day	Monitor every 2-3 months	Increase gradually by 2.5mg depending on response if no signs of toxicity
Phenytoin	Arrhythmias Cerebellar syndrome	Phenytoin level	•IV loading dose (18mg/kg) given in high-dependency area with cardiac and BP monitoring •Check level 2 hours later •Start normal oral dose 300mg OD •Check levels at 5 and 10 days	No routine monitoring required – check pre-dose (trough) level if suspecting toxicity or non-compliance; otherwise check at 5 and 10 days after dose changes *Reference range = 10-20mg/L*	Adjust dose
Insulin	Hypoglycaemia	Capillary glucose HbA1C	•Decide on regimen and educate patient •Capillary glucose should be checked before each meal and before bed	Review patient regularly with glucose monitoring book and check HbA1C and compliance	*See notes on insulin prescribing p295*
Ciclosporin	Renal failure	Blood-ciclosporin concentration + U&Es, LFTs, FBC	<u>IV</u> •Start as infusion at 2mg/kg over 24 hours •Check levels on days 3 and 5, then twice weekly <u>PO</u> •Start at 2.5mg/kg/day in 2 divided doses •Check pre-dose levels weekly until stable	Monthly pre-dose level *Reference range: 100-300mcg/L*	Adjust dose

COMMON SIDE EFFECTS

GROUPS OF SIDE EFFECTS

- **Anti-cholinergic**: dilated pupils, blurred vision, dry mouth, flushed skin, urinary retention, constipation
  Tricyclic antidepressants, antihistamines, hyoscine, atropine, antipsychotics, incontinence medications
- **Anti-histaminergic**: weight gain, sedation
  Tricyclic antidepressants, anti-psychotics, antihistamines
- **Anti-α-adrenergic**: postural hypotension, sexual dysfunction, nasal congestion, headache
  Tricyclic antidepressants, anti-psychotics, α-blockers
- **Anti-dopaminergic**: extrapyramidal side effects (e.g. tardive dyskinesias, parkinsonism), hyperprolactinaemia (→ galactorrhoea, oligomenorrhea, subfertility), neuroleptic malignant syndrome, oculogyric crisis
  Metoclopramide, anti-psychotics

SIDE EFFECTS TO MEMORISE

- **TB drugs**
  - **R**ifampicin: orange-red tears/urine   + hepatitis
  - **I**soniazid: neuropathy   + hepatitis
  - **P**yrazinamide: -   + hepatitis
  - **E**thambutol: optic neuritis
- **Anti-epileptics**
  - Phenytoin: toxicity (→ cerebellar syndrome), acne, coarse face, gum hypertrophy, hirsutism   + inhibit COCP
  - Carbamazepine: rash, dizziness, hyponatraemia, hair thinning   + inhibit COCP
  - Sodium valproate: tremor, weight gain, hair thinning   + teratogenic (avoid if child-bearing age)
  - Lamotrigine: rash (Stevens-Johnson syndrome)
- **Antidepressants**
  - SSRI (e.g. fluoxetine, citalopram, sertraline): nausea, low libido, withdrawal, insomnia, hyponatraemia
  - Tricyclic antidepressant (e.g. amitriptyline): [anti-cholinergic effects], [anti-histaminergic effects], [anti-α-adrenergic effects], hyponatraemia (SIADH), arrhythmias
  - Monoamine oxidase A inhibitors (e.g. selegiline): **3Hs** – **H**ypertension, **H**epatocellular jaundice, **H**yperthermia
- **Anti-hypertensives**
  - ACE inhibitors: <u>dry cough</u>, postural hypotension, renal failure in renal artery stenosis (check U&Es before and 2 weeks after starting), angioedema of the tongue, hyperkalaemia, profound hypotension when started
  - Ca^{2+} blocker: <u>ankle oedema</u>, headache/flushing/dizziness
  - β-blocker: diabetes risk, impotence, bradycardia, fatigue, cold hands and feet, sleep disturbance
  - α-blocker: [anti-α-adrenergic effects]
- **Diuretics**
  - ALL: dehydration, hypotension, hyperuricaemia, <u>hypokalaemia</u> (except K+ sparing), hyponatraemia, hypomagnesaemia
  - Loop: <u>hypocalcaemia</u> (used in treatment of hypercalcaemia)
  - Thiazide (e.g. indapamide): hypercalcaemia
  - K+ sparing: <u>hyperkalaemia</u>, gynaecomastia
- **DMARDs**
  - Sulfasalazine: myelosuppression, oligospermia, hepatitis, rashes (Stevens-Johnson syndrome, erythema nodosum), renal problems, discoloured urine
  - Gold injections: skin discoloration, nephrotic syndrome/interstitial nephritis, myelosuppression, erythroderma, thrombocytopenia
  - Penicillamine: nephrotic syndrome/interstitial nephritis, myelosuppression, myasthenia, lupus-like syndrome
  - Chloroquine: <u>retinopathy</u>, tinnitus, myopathy
  - Methotrexate: hepatic toxicity, pulmonary toxicity, myelosuppression, mucositis
  - TNF antagonists: infusion reactions (including anaphylaxis), infections (including TB reactivation), autoimmune reactions, blood disorders
  - Cyclophosphamide: haemorrhagic cystitis, myelosuppression, alopecia
- **Hypoglycaemics**
  - Insulin: hypoglycaemia, fat-hypertrophy at injection site, hypokalaemia (used in treatment of hyperkalaemia), weight gain
  - Metformin: <u>weight loss</u>, <u>lactic acidosis</u>, metallic taste, GI disturbance, B_{12} deficiency
  - Sulphonylureas (e.g. gliclazide): <u>hypoglycaemia</u>, weight gain
  - Thiazolidinediones (glitazones, e.g. pioglitazone): fluid retention (→ heart failure, oedema), hepatotoxicity, fractures
  - DPP4 inhibitors (gliptins, e.g. sitagliptin): pancreatitis
  - SGLT2 inhibitors (flozins, e.g. empagliflozin): UTIs/thrush, ketoacidosis, weight loss, may increase risk of amputations

- **Contraception:** *see table on p321*
- **Anti-psychotics**
  - ALL: [anti-dopaminergic effects], [anti-cholinergic effects], [anti-histaminergic effects], [anti-α-adrenergic effects]
  - Clozapine: agranulocytosis
  - Chlorpromazine: cholestatic jaundice
  - Haloperidol: prolonged QT interval, interference with temperature regulation
- **Lithium:** toxicity (tremor/ataxia/dysarthria → coma, convulsions, hypotension), diarrhoea, hypothyroidism, diabetes insipidus
- **Steroids:** diabetes risk, cushingoid appearance, psychosis, osteoporosis, hypokalaemia, hyperglycaemia, infections, leukocytosis, risk of avascular necrosis
- **Azathioprine:** myelosuppression
- **Ciclosporin:** tremor, chronic interstitial nephritis, hypertrichosis, gum hyperplasia, burning sensation in hands/feet
- **Levodopa:** nausea, red urine/other body fluids, postural hypotension, dyskinesias, 'on-off' and 'wearing off' effects
- **Proton pump inhibitor:** tinnitus, GI disturbance, headache, hyponatraemia, hypomagnesaemia
- **Antiarrhythmics**
  - Amiodarone: <u>thyroiditis</u>, <u>pulmonary fibrosis</u>, peripheral neuropathy, myopathy, blue-grey skin pigmentation/photosensitivity, hepatitis, metallic taste
  - Digoxin toxicity: <u>xanthopsia</u> (yellow/orange tinge to vision), GI distress, any arrhythmia
  - Adenosine: flushing, sense of impending doom

DRUGS CAUSING...

Electrolyte imbalances
- **Hypernatraemia:** sodium-containing antibiotics/fluids, sodium bicarbonate, drugs causing diabetes insipidus (e.g. lithium)
- **Hyponatraemia:** <u>antidepressants</u>, <u>diuretics</u>, <u>c</u>hlorpromazine, <u>c</u>arbamazepine, proton pump inhibitors, ACE inhibitors
- **Hyperkalaemia:** <u>K⁺ sparing diuretics</u>, <u>ACE inhibitors</u>/angiotensin receptor blockers, NSAIDs, trimethoprim, ciclosporin/tacrolimus, heparin
- **Hypokalaemia:** <u>salbutamol</u> (used in Tx of hyperkalaemia), <u>insulin</u>, <u>diuretics</u> (except K⁺ sparing), caffeine/theophylline
- **Hypercalcaemia:** <u>thiazide diuretics</u>, lithium
- **Hypocalcaemia:** <u>loop diuretics</u>, <u>bisphosphonates</u>, phenytoin

Organ toxicity
- **Hepatitis:** TB antibiotics (rifampicin/isoniazid/pyrazinamide), sodium valproate, methotrexate, methyldopa, amiodarone, statins, paracetamol, phenytoin, ketoconazole/fluconazole, nitrofurantoin, sulfonylureas/sulfonamides
- **Cholestasis:** <u>c</u>o-amoxiclav (may be delayed/severe), <u>c</u>larithromycin/erythromycin, <u>c</u>arbamazepine, <u>c</u>hlorpromazine, <u>c</u>ontraceptives, flu<u>c</u>loxacillin, sulfonylureas/sulfonamides
- **Pulmonary toxicity/fibrosis:** nitrofurantoin, amiodarone, methotrexate, cyclophosphamide, gold/sulfasalazine, bleomycin
- **Renal failure**
  - Interstitial nephritis: NSAIDS, penicillins/cephalosporins, calcineurin inhibitors (ciclosporin/tacrolimus)
  - Acute tubular necrosis: lithium, contrast, gentamicin, amphotericin B
  - Precipitate renal artery stenosis: ACE inhibitors
  - Glomerular damage: gold, NSAIDs, penicillamine
- **Creatinine rise:** trimethoprim, cimetidine/ranitidine
- **Photosensitivity:** <u>tetracyclines</u>, terbinafine, chlorpromazine, amiodarone (→ blue/grey discoloration), chemo (vincristine), ciprofloxacin, psoralens, retinoids, thiazide diuretics, sulphonylureas
- **Hypothyroidism:** amiodarone, carbimazole, lithium, propylthiouracil, radio-iodine

Other reactions
- **Stevens-Johnson syndrome/erythroderma:** <u>sulphur-based drugs</u> (sulphonamides, sulfonylureas), <u>anti-epileptics</u>, gold, allopurinol, antibiotics
- **Vasculitis:** allopurinol, penicillin, sulphonamides, thiazides, phenytoin, cephalosporins
- **Agranulocytosis:** C's – Carbamazepine, Clozapine, Colchicine, Carbimazole, Cytotoxic agents
- **Gynaecomastia:** DISCO MTV – Digoxin, Isoniazid, Spironolactone, Cimetidine, Oestrogens, Methyldopa/metronidazole, Tricyclic antidepressants, Verapamil
- **Neuropathy:** metronidazole, nitrofurantoin, isoniazid, vincristine, cisplatin, amiodarone, phenytoin
- **Megaloblastic anaemia:** methotrexate, phenytoin, ethanol, trimethoprim, sulfonamides, sodium valproate, metformin, antidepressants
- **Dyskinesia:** dopaminergic drugs (levodopa, bromocriptine), dopamine-blocking drugs (anti-psychotics), antidepressants
- ***Clostridium difficile* risk:** <u>c</u>ephalosporins, <u>c</u>lindamycin, <u>c</u>iprofloxacin, broad spectrum penicillins

DRUG INTERACTIONS

MECHANISMS OF DRUG INTERACTIONS

Drug interaction mechanisms			
Class	Subclass	Details	Examples (index drug + interacting drug)
Pharmacokinetic (ADME)			
Absorption	Gastric pH alterations	Reduced stomach acidity (e.g. by antacids, H2 antagonists or PPIs) can lead to reduced absorption of drugs requiring an acidic environment for absorption	• Ketoconazole + PPI/H2 antagonist (reduced absorption of ketoconazole because it is only ionised at low pH)
	Chelation	Some drugs can react with each other in the GI tract and form complexes which cannot be absorbed	• Tetracyclines/quinolones + cations, e.g. iron, magnesium, calcium (chelation complex cannot be absorbed) • Variety of drugs, e.g. digoxin, levothyroxine, steroids, loop diuretics + cholestyramine (binding and reduced absorption)
	GI motility	Some drugs increase GI motility (e.g. metoclopramide, domperidone) and others decrease it (e.g. antacids, anticholinergics) which can affect the absorption of other drugs	• Slowly absorbed drugs (e.g. modified release/enteric coated preparations) are absorbed less with a quicker GI transit time
	Transporter based	Induction or inhibition of transporter proteins	• Digoxin + rifampicin (rifampicin induces P-gp efflux pump which excretes digoxin into the gut, reducing digoxin levels)
Distribution	Plasma protein-binding displacement	Highly protein-bound drugs (e.g. phenytoin, benzodiazepines, digoxin, NSAIDs, furosemide, warfarin, amiodarone, sulfonylureas/sulfonamides, statins) may displace each other from protein-binding sites, which increases the proportion of the displaced drug in its unbound (active) form	• Warfarin + other highly protein-bound drugs (displacement of warfarin increases INR/bleeding)
	Tissue-binding site displacement	Drugs may displace each other from tissue-binding sites	• Digoxin + quinidine (quinidine displaces digoxin from muscle-binding sites, increasing risk of toxicity)
	Volume of distribution changes	Volume changes in fluid compartments can affect drug concentrations and distribution	• Gentamicin + furosemide (furosemide reduces extracellular volume, which causes increased gentamicin concentration and risk of toxicity)
Metabolism	Phase I – oxidation/reduction/hydrolysis reactions (cytochrome P450 system)	See next page	• Statin + macrolides (macrolides inhibit P450 enzymes which decreases statin elimination, increasing the risk of rhabdomyolysis) • COCP + phenytoin (phenytoin induces P450 enzymes which increases COCP elimination, decreasing its efficacy)
	Phase II – conjugation reactions (other enzymes)	Interactions less clinically significant	N/A
Excretion	Kidneys	There are many mechanisms of renal interactions, e.g. competition for active transport sites, alterations in glomerular filtration, and tubular pH changes	• Metformin + cimetidine (competition for renal tubular clearance) • Digoxin + amiodarone (competition for renal tubular clearance) • Lithium + thiazide (thiazide decreases lithium clearance) • Methotrexate + aspirin (aspirin decreases methotrexate clearance)
	Bile	No drug-drug interactions	N/A
Pharmacodynamic (at receptor level)			
Synergism		Drugs with similar effects (therapeutic or adverse) can have an additive effect when used together	• Multiple serotonergic drugs (serotonin syndrome) • Multiple nephrotoxic drugs (renal damage) • ACE inhibitors + potassium-sparing diuretics (hyperkalaemia) • Metformin + ACE inhibitors (enhanced hypoglycaemic effect) • Amiodarone + quinolones (both block cardiac K^+ channels → prolonged QT interval)
Antagonism		Drugs can have opposite effects and so inhibit each other	• β-blockers + salbutamol • Opioids + naloxone

CYTOCHROME P450 SYSTEM INTERACTIONS

The cytochrome P450 system is a collection of liver enzymes that make up a key pathway for drug metabolism. The system is a major source of important drug interactions.

Cytochrome P450 inducers
Reduce the concentration of drugs metabolised by the cytochrome P450 system.

C	**C**arbamazepine
R	**R**ifampicin
A	b**A**rbiturates
P	**P**henytoin
S	**S**t John's wort
OUT DRUGS	

Cytochrome P450 inhibitors
Increase the concentration of drugs metabolised by the cytochrome P450 system.

Some Certain Silly Compounds Annoyingly Inhibit Enzymes, Grrrrrrr

Sodium valproate

Ciprofloxacin

Sulphonamides

Cimetidine/omeprazole

Antifungals, **A**miodarone

Isoniazid

Erythromycin/clarithromycin

Grapefruit juice

Cytochrome P450 substrates
Drugs metabolised by the P450 system that are affected by cytochrome P450 inducers/inhibitors.

C	**C**iclosporin, **C**arbamazepine, **C**italopram
O	**O**ral contraceptive pill
W	**W**arfarin
P	**P**henytoin, **P**rotease inhibitors
A	**A**cetylcholinesterase inhibitors (e.g. donepezil)
T	**T**heophylline
S	**S**tatins, **S**teroids

HIGH RISK DRUGS

Always look for interactions in the BNF.
- **Narrow therapeutic range drugs**
  - Examples (**Guys With Large Dongles Totally Make Perfect Internet Connections**): **G**entamicin, **W**arfarin, **L**ithium, **D**igoxin, **T**heophylline, **M**ethotrexate, **P**henytoin, **I**nsulin, **C**iclosporin
  - Interactions are particularly important for narrow therapeutic range drugs because small changes in their concentrations can cause severe toxicity
- **Cytochrome P450 inducers/inhibitors**
  - Examples: *see above*
  - Many interactions!
- **Highly protein-bound drugs**
  - Examples (**Protein Bound Drugs Normally Fight When Available Space is Sparse**): **P**henytoin, **B**enzodiazepines, **D**igoxin, **N**SAIDs, **F**urosemide, **W**arfarin, **A**miodarone, **S**ulfonylureas/sulfonamides, **S**tatins
  - Often displace each other from protein binding sites, which increases the proportion of the displaced drug in its unbound (active) form
- **Drugs affecting physiology**
  - Examples: anti-hypertensives, hypoglycaemics, anticoagulants
  - Affect the physiological environment and are more likely to have interactions

DRUGS AND RENAL FAILURE

DRUGS CAUSING RENAL FAILURE

Pre-renal	Acute tubular necrosis	Interstitial nephritis	Glomerular damage
ACE inhibitors Diuretics NSAIDs	Lithium Contrast agents Calcineurin inhibitors Gentamicin Amphoteracin B Cisplatin	NSAIDs Antibiotics, e.g. penicillins, cephalosporins, rifampicin Others (less common): sulfonamides, proton pump inhibitors, diuretics, allopurinol, phenytoin	Gold Penicillamine

DRUGS TO AVOID/DOSE-REDUCE IN RENAL FAILURE

Always look them up in the BNF if there is any renal impairment:
- Drugs that can cause renal failure (*above*)
- Hypoglycaemics
- Drugs which increase potassium (e.g. supplements, potassium-sparing diuretics, ACE inhibitors)
- Antibiotics (e.g. ciprofloxacin, nitrofurantoin, some penicillins, trimethoprim, clarithromycin, teicoplanin)
- Opioids/NSAIDs
- Statins
- β-blockers
- Psychotropics (e.g. lithium, gabapentin, fluoxetine)
- Anticoagulants (direct oral anticoagulants, low molecular weight heparin)
- Many others (e.g. allopurinol, colchicine, digoxin, ranitidine)

This page is intentionally left blank

CHAPTER 8: COMMUNICATION

HOW TO COUNSEL/EXPLAIN TO PATIENTS

HOW TO COUNSEL

- **Beginning**
    - Introduce yourself and explain why you are there
    - Build rapport before launching into the explanation
    - Ask if the patient knows why they are there. Ask them what has happened up to this point.
    - Assess their **prior knowledge** – it is important to find out what they already know
    - Tell them what you plan to talk about, ask if they would find that useful, and check there isn't anything else they want to discuss

- **Middle**
    - Consider using **diagrams** where appropriate
    - **'Chunk and check'**: this is very important – only give small 'chunks' of information at a time, then check their understanding. Pause after each section in case the patient has any questions.
    - Speak slowly and clearly. Listen to the patient and be alert to their concerns.

- **Ending**
    - **Summarise** what you have talked about and make a **plan**
    - Check they've **understood** everything
    - Ideally you should **offer something**, e.g. a leaflet, website address, specialist nurse contact, follow-up appointment

HOW TO STRUCTURE EXPLANATIONS

- **Explaining a disease**
    - Normal anatomy/physiology
    - What the disease is
    - Cause
    - Problems and complications
    - Management

- **Explaining a procedure**
    - Explain what it is
    - Reason for it
    - Details of procedure (before, during, after)
    - Risks and benefits

    If you are also asked to obtain consent: thoroughly check their understanding, get them to weigh up the pros and cons, and ask them why they chose their answer

- **Explaining a treatment**
    - Briefly check for contraindications to the treatment (where relevant)
    - Check patient understanding of condition
    - How treatment works
    - Treatment course and how it's taken
    - Monitoring required
    - Side effects

TIPS

- Let the patient guide the consultation
- Follow cues
- Ask what they want to know and about their worries
- Don't forget **ICE** (**I**deas, **C**oncerns and **E**xpectations)
- Empathise
- Be aware that you may be breaking bad news without realising it! A SPIKES approach can help here (*see notes on breaking bad news p336*).
- Avoid all medical jargon

> **TOP TIP:** practice explaining common conditions without using medical jargon, e.g. multiple sclerosis – compare to wires and insulation

COMMON DRUGS REQUIRING EXPLANATION

Medication	Check for contraindications	How the treatment works	Treatment course and how it's taken	Monitoring required	Side effects
Warfarin	• Pregnancy • Significant risk of major bleeding • Active bleeding	• Thins the blood to treat or prevent blood clots • It does this by blocking vitamin K – the vitamin used by the body to make proteins that cause the blood to clot	• Once daily tablet (usually in the evening) • Usually prescribed for 3 months for a DVT, 6 months for a PE, and lifelong for AF • Dose changes take 2-3 days to take effect	• Started at 5mg each evening • INR on days 3,4 and 5 – warfarin dosing charts tell you how to adjust the dose • Then regular INR checks by anticoagulation clinic – regularity determined by INR stability (patient will be given anticoagulation book)	• Bleeding – seek medical advice if you have a significant head injury, prolonged nose bleeds, unusual headaches, blood in urine/stool/vomit, black stool, unexplained or severe bruising • Also diarrhoea, rash, hair loss, nausea • Many interactions (mostly with P450 cytochrome inducers/inhibitors) – patients should avoid liver, spinach, cranberry juice, alcohol binges, NSAIDs/aspirin
Direct oral anticoagulant (DOAC)	• Significant renal impairment • Significant risk of major bleeding • Active bleeding *Not licensed for metallic heart valves or valvular AF*	• Thins the blood to treat or prevent blood clots • Many proteins are involved in blood clot formation – this medication blocks one of these proteins from working	• Once or twice daily tablet/capsule • Take with full glass of water whilst sitting upright • Usually prescribed for 3 months for a DVT, 6 months for a PE, and lifelong for AF	• None regularly • Check renal function before and annually	• Bleeding – seek medical advice if you have a significant head injury, prolonged nose bleeds, unusual headaches, blood in urine/stool/vomit, black stool, unexplained or severe bruising • GI disturbance • Irreversible if serious bleed occurs (except dabigatran)
Levothyroxine	• None	• A synthetic version of thyroxine, the hormone produced by your thyroid gland • It is given to bring your thyroid activity back up to normal	• Once daily tablet before breakfast • Taken long term • Dose changes take 4-6 weeks to take effect	• TSH test every 2-3 months until stable • When TSH level stable, check annually	• Rare when thyroxine level stable as it's replacing a normal hormone • Hyperthyroid symptoms (vomiting, diarrhoea, headache, palpitations, heat intolerance) may be experienced if dosage is too high; or hypothyroid symptoms (cold intolerance, constipation) if dosage is too low
Statin	• Pregnancy	• Statins stop the liver making cholesterol • High cholesterol causes problems with your arteries, which increases your risk of heart disease, stroke, and kidney disease • It is important to also address other cardiovascular risk factors...	• Once daily tablet in the evening • Taken long term • Decreases risk over many years	• Review in 4 weeks, then every 6-12 months (with lipid profile as required) → dose may be titrated up if target not met • LFTs before starting, at 3 months and at 12 months (statins cause altered LFTs)	• Muscle pains • Headache • Itching • Also nausea, sickness, diarrhoea, abdominal pain • Rhabdomyolysis – tell doctor if you experience unexpected muscle pain • Some statins interact with grapefruit juice
Metformin	• Significant renal impairment • Ketoacidosis • Low BMI	• Increases your response to insulin so your cells take up more glucose from your blood • Also reduces the amount of glucose produced by the liver	• Once, twice or three-times daily tablet with meals • Taken long term	• U&Es before starting, then annually • HbA1C every 3-6 months until stable, then 6 monthly at diabetic check ups	• Nausea, diarrhoea, abdominal pain, weight loss • Lactic acidosis – metformin must not be taken on the day of or for 2 days after having general anaesthetic or X-ray contrast media
Iron tablets	• None	• Replace your body's store of iron, a mineral required to make red blood cells	• 1-3 times daily tablet or syrup (depending on brand) • Works best if taken without food, but most take with meals as iron can irritate the stomach • Takes 3-4 weeks for Hb to normalise, then further 3 months to replenish iron stores	• Haemoglobin in 3-4 weeks to assess response	• GI irritation (nausea, sickness, diarrhoea/constipation, abdominal pain) • Black/green stools • Metallic taste
Selective serotonin reuptake inhibitor (SSRI)	• Suicidal risk • Mania	• Antidepressants alter the balance of some of the chemicals in the brain (neurotransmitters) • SSRI antidepressants affect a neurotransmitter called serotonin. Imbalance of this and other neurotransmitters is thought to play a part in causing depression and other conditions.	• Once daily tablet • May be gradually stopped 6 months after feeling better • Effects in 4-8 weeks	• None	• GI (diarrhoea, nausea, vomiting) • Appetite and weight change • Headaches • Drowsiness (can take at night) • Anxiety for 2 weeks • Withdrawal • May increase risk of suicide in younger patients

Check patient understanding of condition

Medication	Check for contraindications	How the treatment works	Treatment course and how it's taken	Monitoring required	Side effects
Methotrexate	• Pregnancy (including male partner) • Breast-feeding • Hepatic impairment • Active infection • Immunodeficiency	• It is a 'disease-modifying agent' which both reduces inflammation and suppresses the immune system • Early use improves outcome and symptoms	• Once weekly tablet with a folic acid tablet on another day • Same day each week • Dose built up slowly • Taken long-term if effective • Takes 3-12 weeks to work	FBC, LFTs, U&Es • Before starting • Then, every 2 weeks until therapy stabilised • Then, every 2-3 months *Patient should be given monitoring book*	• Alopecia • Headaches • GI disturbance – *advise not to take with NSAIDs/aspirin* • Myelosuppression (infections, unexpected bruising/bleeding, anaemia) – *seek medical advice if you have unexplained bruising/bleeding or have infective symptoms, and get annual flu jab* • Liver and lung toxicity
Lithium	• 1st trimester pregnancy • Breast-feeding • Cardiac insufficiency/rhythm disorder • Significant renal impairment • Addison's disease • Low sodium diets • Untreated hypothyroidism	• Mood stabiliser • Exact mechanism unknown • Thought to interfere with neurotransmitter release and receptors	• Once or twice daily tablet/liquid • Taken long-term if effective • Takes 1-2 weeks to work	• Before starting – FBC, U&Es, TFTs, βHCG, ECG • Check lithium level after 5 days, then every week until stable for 4 weeks, then every 3 months • Check TFTs, U&Es, Ca²⁺ every 6 months	• GI (abdominal pain, nausea) • Metallic taste • Fine tremor • Water symptoms (thirst, polyuria, impaired urinary concentration, weight gain and oedema) • Renal toxicity • Nephrogenic diabetes insipidus • Hypothyroidism **Lithium toxicity symptoms** • GI (anorexia, diarrhoea, vomiting) • Neuromuscular (dysarthria, dizziness, ataxia, impaired coordination, muscle twitching, tremor) • Others (drowsiness, apathy, restlessness)
Atypical antipsychotic	• Hepatic impairment • Phaeochromocytoma	• Schizophrenia thought to be caused by problems with dopamine receptors in your brain • Atypical antipsychotics work by blocking these receptors	• Tablet daily or depot injection every 2-4 weeks • Dose built up over a week or two • Dose adjusted depending on response • Taken long-term if effective (keeps symptoms from returning) • Takes several days or weeks to work	• Before treatment, at 3 months, 12 months, then annually: pulse, BP, weight, waist circumference, ECG, HbA1C, fasting glucose, lipid profile, prolactin • Weight checks weekly for 6 weeks	• Anti-dopaminergic (tardive dyskinesia, tremor, movement disorders) • Anti-cholinergic (constipation, dry mouth) • Anti-histaminergic (weight gain, dizziness, drowsiness) • Anti-adrenergic (hypotension) • Neuroleptic malignant syndrome (high fever and muscle rigidity) • Agranulocytosis (clozapine) • Withdrawal • Hyperglycaemia and diabetes • Hyperprolactinaemia (sexual dysfunction, menstrual disturbance, galactorrhoea etc.) • Prolonged QT • Psychosis • Nausea and vomiting • Dyskinesias • Postural hypotension • Impulsive behaviour • Dizziness
Levodopa	• Glaucoma	• Levodopa is a replacement for some of the dopamine which your brain in no longer able to produce • This will help to reduce your symptoms, particularly your rigidity and slow movements • Given with carbidopa (inhibits peripheral levodopa degeneration)	• Depends on the type of insulin regimens *(see prescribing notes on insulin p295)* • Taken as long as it works effectively – after 5 years most suffer 'on-off'/'wearing off' phenomena (switch between mobility and immobility that occurs before the next dose is due after prolonged levodopa use) • Fast-acting	• None	• Headache • Weight gain • Sharp injuries (pens should be disposed of in sharps bin) • Hypoglycaemia (educate patient about management) • Lipodystrophy at injection sites • 'On-off'/'wearing off' phenomena
Insulin	N/A	• Insulin allows the cells of your body to take up glucose from the blood and use it for energy • This means insulin reduces the blood glucose level • In people with diabetes, insulin may be needed because the body cannot produce it or use it effectively	• 3-4 times daily tablet with food (reduces nausea)	• Capillary glucose monitoring is done before each meal and before bed • It should also be checked if there are any symptoms of a high/low blood sugar (explain)	
Bisphosphonate	• Pregnancy • Dysphagia/abnormalities of oesophagus • Recent peptic ulcer • Significant renal impairment • Unable to sit upright for 30 minutes	• Prevents bone from being broken down and helps to rebuild new bone • Remember lifestyle factors can also help with this, such as exercise, not smoking (we can help), and eating a well-balanced diet	• Once daily or once weekly tablet • Swallow tablet with full glass of water • Take at least 30 minutes before food or anything other than water • Be upright for 30 minutes after swallowing • Taken long term	• Regular dental check-ups (risk of osteonecrosis of jaw)	• Headache • Heartburn, bloating, indigestion • GI (diarrhoea/constipation, abdominal pain) *Seek urgent medical advice if symptoms of…* • Osteonecrosis of the jaw • Dysphagia/odynophagia • Upper GI bleeding/black stools

Check patient understanding of condition

Procedure			Before	During	After	Risks
Bronchoscopy			Oral intake **6 hours** before – clear fluids (sips) only **2 hours** before – NBM Also •Coagulation test •Stop antiplatelets 1 week before (unless high risk, e.g. drug-eluting stent) •Stop warfarin 5 days before (± give LMWH) •Stop direct oral anticoagulants 48 hours before	•Midazolam sedative (→amnesia) •Lidocaine spray/gel to the nose, throat and windpipe	•No eating/drinking 2 hours after as throat still numb •No driving, alcohol, operating machinery, or signing legal documents for 24 hours •Keep someone with you for 24 hours •Arrange follow-up	•**Lung damage/collapse** •**Infection** •**Bleeding** (haemoptysis) •Sore nose/throat •Sedation side effects •Pneumothorax
Gastroscopy			Oral intake **6 hours** before – sips of water only (sips) **2 hours** before – NBM Also •Stop anti-acid medications 2 weeks before	•Lidocaine throat spray or midazolam sedative (→amnesia) •Continuous suction •Air passed through scope (→fullness, belching)	•Arrange follow-up If had throat spray •No eating/drinking 2 hours after as throat still numb If had sedation •No driving, alcohol, operating machinery or signing legal documents for 24 hours •Keep someone with you for 24 hours	•**Perforation** (<0.1%) •**Bleeding** •**Infection** (aspiration pneumonia) •Sore throat •Dental damage •Sedation side effects
Colonoscopy	Explain what procedure is	Explain reason for procedure	Oral intake **2 days** before – low fibre diet (no bran/roughage) **1 day** before – clear fluids only after light breakfast **2 hours** before – NBM Also •Sodium picosulfate sachet afternoon before and morning of the procedure •Stop iron tablets 1 week before, and constipating agents 4 days before (e.g. codeine)	•Midazolam sedative (→amnesia) •Digital rectal examination prior to scope insertion •Air passed through scope (→bloating, you may feel like you need to go to the toilet)	•No driving, alcohol, operating machinery, or signing legal documents for 24 hours •Keep someone with you for 24 hours •Arrange follow-up	•**Perforation** (0.1% with colonoscopy) •**Bleeding** •**Infection** •Abdominal discomfort •Sedation side effects (colonoscopy)
Flexible sigmoidoscopy			Oral intake **2 hours** before – NBM Also •Phosphate enema 2 hours before (can be self-administered at home)	•Digital rectal examination prior to scope insertion •No sedation required	•Arrange follow-up	
Flexible cystoscopy			None	•Anaesthetic jelly •Water passed through scope	•Home after passed urine •Arrange follow-up	•**Bladder damage** (hole) •**Bleeding** (haematuria – normal for a few days) •**Infection** (UTI) •Dysuria •Urethral stricture •Retention •May need temporary catheter afterwards •Anaesthetic side effects (rigid cystoscopy)
Rigid cystoscopy			Oral intake **6 hours** before – clear fluids only **2 hours** before – NBM Also •Normal pre-operative assessment (including stopping anticoagulants/ antiplatelets – *see notes on pre-operative assessment p355*)	•Usually have anaesthetic •Water passed through scope	•Home after recovered from anaesthetic and passed urine •No driving, alcohol, operating machinery, or signing legal documents for 24 hours •Keep someone with you for 24 hours •Arrange follow-up	

DISCUSSION ABOUT SURGERY

INTRODUCTION

- **W**ash hands; **I**ntroduce self; ask **P**atient's name, DOB and what they like to be called; **E**xplain what you propose to do
- Confirm the operation that is planned
- Ask about what they know so far
- Explore concerns and ask about anything specific they want to know

BEFORE THE OPERATION

- Pre-operative **assessment**
  - Aims to assess medical fitness for an operation/anaesthetic; ascertain mobility, independence, who is at home, medications and allergies
  - Involves a history and physical examination
  - Will confirm which medications to stop and when (*see notes on pre-operative assessment p355*)
- Pre-operative **investigations**
  - May include: blood tests, chest x-ray, ECG, echocardiography, cardiopulmonary exercise testing
- There may be **special pre-operative measures** which the patient will be told about if needed, e.g. bowel prep
- The timing of **admission** will be discussed, e.g. whether on the morning of or evening before surgery
- **Consent** will be taken by a surgeon prior to theatre
  - The surgeon will discuss the procedure, the risks and benefits
  - A consent form will need to be signed (but the patient can change their mind at any time)
  - The patient will not be pressured
- The patient should be instructed about **fasting** (when to stop eating and drinking)
  - Usually '2-6 rule' = no food for 6 hours pre-op; can have clear fluids up to 2 hours pre-op; nothing thereafter
- If the operation is on one side (left or right), then the correct side will be '**marked**' with a black arrow

NB: see notes on pre-operative assessment p355 for a more comprehensive summary.

DURING THE OPERATION

- The patient will be taken to the anaesthetic room by a theatre nurse
- Relatives may stay with the patient until this point
- The patient will then meet the anaesthetist who will insert a cannula to give an **anaesthetic**
- If a general anaesthetic is required, the patient will be **intubated**, e.g. 'you will have a tube through your mouth to control breathing during the operation. You will not remember this but you may have a sore throat afterwards. It will be taken out when you are waking up.'
- The **operation** will then be performed – offer details about the specific operation

Types of anaesthetic		
Type	**Detail**	**Examples where it may be used**
General	Medication that is inhaled or injected to induce a reversible loss of consciousness	Many operations
Spinal	Needle is inserted into the lower back and a local anaesthetic is injected into the cerebrospinal fluid (the fluid in the subarachnoid space that surrounds the spinal cord) to numb the lower body	Operations below the umbilicus, e.g. lower limb surgery, pelvic surgery, C-section/childbirth
Epidural	Catheter is inserted into the back and a local anaesthetic is injected as required into the epidural space (the outermost part of the spinal cord) to numb the lower body.	*Epidural is usually performed for longer operations or when analgesia is required post-operatively*
Nerve block	Local anaesthetic injected around the nerve(s) that supplies the area being operated on	Procedures on hands, arms, feet, legs or face
Local	Local anaesthetic injected directly into the area that is being operated on	Minor procedures on small areas

AFTER THE OPERATION

- The patient will wake up in the recovery area
- There may be **tubes** that were inserted in theatre, e.g. catheter, drains
- **Pain control** – there are a variety of options that may be used:
  - Intravenous (patient-controlled analgesia) – 'you will be given a button that you can press whenever you want pain relief'
  - Oral
  - Local wound catheters – 'local anaesthetic may be directly injected into the site by a small tube'
- Depending on the type of surgery, there may be limitations on what the patient is allowed to eat/drink for a period afterwards
- **VTE prophylaxis:** the patient will usually be given a heparin ('a small injection in the skin of your tummy each day') and may be asked to wear compression stockings to prevent blood clots
- **Physiotherapy:** the patient will be seen by physiotherapists to build up their mobility after the operation
- **Occupational therapy:** if required, the patient will be assessed by therapists who will help arrange care or modify their home to help them cope after the operation

RISKS/COMPLICATIONS

These must be explained using lay terms. Try not to scare the patient. Explain most complications are rare and how the risk of complications is minimised.

Generic risks
- Anaesthetic complications (e.g. arrhythmias, hypo-/hypertension, hyperthermia, breathing problems, MI/stroke, allergy, teeth/lip/tongue damage, sore throat)
- Bleeding/haematoma
- Damage to nearby structures/organs
- Infections: local (wound/surgical site) or systemic (chest/UTI/sepsis)
- Venous thromboembolism (DVT/PE)
- Pain
- Fluid collections

Operation-specific complications	
Operation	**Specific complications**
General surgery	
Gastrectomy	Dumping syndrome Malabsorption Anastomotic ulcer Peptic ulcers/gastric cancer Small intestinal bacterial overgrowth Abdominal fullness/gas bloating
Small and large bowel operations	Ileus Anastomotic leaks Stoma retraction Intra-abdominal collections Pre-sacral plexus damage Adhesions/intestinal obstruction Damage to other local structures, e.g. kidneys, ureters, bladder
Cholecystectomy	Common bile duct injury/bile leak
Biliary	Common bile duct injury/bile leak Common bile duct stricture Anastomotic leak Bleeding into biliary tree (results in jaundice) Pancreatitis
Cardiothoracic	
CABG/stenting	Reperfusion arrhythmias Post-operative acute coronary syndrome Inotropes are often needed post-operatively; these may reduce organ perfusion elsewhere
Vascular	
Grafts/stents/bypass procedures	Failure of graft, haemorrhage/haematoma, infection, re-thrombosis, limb or organ ischaemia Arteriovenous fistula Cholesterol embolism (e.g. trash foot) Arteriopaths are at high risk of: ACS, stroke, PE Contrast complications, e.g. anaphylaxis, renal injury
Endocrine	
Thyroidectomy	Airway obstruction secondary to haemorrhage – requires urgent re-opening of thyroidectomy wound Hypocalcaemia (damage to parathyroid glands) Recurrent laryngeal nerve damage
Parotidectomy	Facial nerve damage
Trauma and Orthopaedic	
Any orthopaedic operation	Infection of prosthesis Loss of position/failure of fixation Non-union, malunion, delayed union Neurovascular injury Compartment syndrome
Total hip arthroplasty	Sciatic nerve damage, dislocation, leg length difference, loosening, wear, need for revision surgery
Urology	
Cystoscopy/transurethral resection of the prostate	High risk of UTI Transurethral resection of the prostate syndrome (absorption of irrigation fluid causing hyponatraemia) Impotence/retrograde ejaculation External sphincter damage (incontinence) Urethral stricture
Other	
Endovascular surgery	Retroperitoneal haemorrhage
Lymph node dissection (e.g. axillary nodes in breast cancer surgery)	Lymphoedema
Neck dissection (e.g. branchial cyst excision)	Cranial nerve damage (11, 12)

INHALER TECHNIQUE

INTRODUCTION

- **W**ash hands; **I**ntroduce self; ask **P**atient's name, DOB and what they like to be called; **E**xplain what you propose to do
- Check what patient already knows regarding condition (asthma/COPD), inhaler treatments and technique

Types of inhaler and their use		
Metered dose inhaler/Evohaler		**Dry powder/breath-activated inhaler (Accuhaler, Turbohaler, Clickhaler, Easi-Breathe, Autohaler)**
Salbutamol (reliever)	**Steroid (preventer)**	
Use during an attack to relieve symptoms	Use morning and night to prevent an attack	Use as reliever or preventer as indicated
Use as described below		Technique differs according to type, but typically: click or open to activate, exhale fully, seal mouth around mouthpiece, then breathe in quickly and deeply and hold breath for 10 seconds or as long as possible
Small but some patients find difficult to use		May be easier to use, but not suitable for under 6 years as quick breath required
May be used with a spacer		Cannot be used with a spacer
SEs: tachycardia, tremor	**SEs:** dry mouth, hoarse voice, thrush	**SEs:** depend on constituent drugs

ASTHMA/COPD REVIEW

- Review patient's asthma/COPD control: how often they require salbutamol or experience symptoms; when they use their preventer; number of exacerbations, exercise tolerance; peak flow measurements (for asthma)
- Check understanding of inhalers, technique, and compliance
- Explain type of inhaler, its purpose, and when to use it

INITIAL TECHNIQUE EXPLANATION

- Inhaler contains a set dose of medication
- The aim is to get it into the lungs
- Drug released by pressing canister or twisting/clicking device – demonstrate

STEPS FOR METERED DOSE INHALER USE

1. Check date of **expiration**
2. **Shake** vigorously
3. Remove **cap** and check the inside is clean
4. **Stand** or sit up straight
5. Hold inhaler **upright** with index finger on top and thumb at the bottom
6. **Breathe out** completely
7. **Seal** mouth well around mouthpiece
8. **Press** firmly down on the canister and simultaneously **breathe in slowly** and deeply (aim for back of throat)
9. **Hold breath** for 10 seconds or as long as possible
10. **Breathe out** slowly
11. Replace **cap**
12. **Repeat** after 1 minute if required
13. **Wash** mouth out afterwards (if using steroid inhaler)

DEMONSTRATION AND OBSERVATION

- Demonstrate it yourself
- Clean the mouthpiece of a different placebo inhaler (with an alcohol 70%/chlorhexidine 2% device disinfection wipe)
- Ask the patient to demonstrate how they would use it
- Observe the patient and correct any mistakes
- Get the patient to repeat until they do it correctly

OTHER ADVICE

- Seek emergency help if symptoms are severe or not relieved by inhaler
- See GP or specialist nurse if suffering with side effects or using reliever inhaler more than 3 times per week
- Ask the patient if they have any questions or concerns

USE OF A SPACER DEVICE

- Spacers may be used in children, those experiencing side effects from steroid inhalers, or people having difficulty with inhaler technique
- Usage steps:
    1. Assemble spacer
    2. Shake inhaler and then remove cap
    3. Attach it to the spacer
    4. Breathe out completely
    5. Seal mouth around spacer mouthpiece
    6. Press on the canister to release drug
    7. Breathe in slowly and deeply for 3-5 seconds and then hold for 10 seconds (or, alternatively, take five normal breaths from the spacer in and out through the mouth)
    8. Repeat if required after 1 minute

    NB: if the device whistles they are breathing in too quickly.
- Looking after the spacer
    - Wash spacer with warm water and soap
    - Always leave to drip dry
    - Replace every 6-12 months

CHILDHOOD VACCINATIONS

Immunisation schedule	
2 months:	6 in 1, rotavirus, pneumococcal, meningitis B
3 months:	6 in 1, rotavirus
4 months:	6 in 1, pneumococcal, meningitis B
1 year:	MMR, pneumococcal, meningitis B, *Haemophilus influenzae* type B/meningitis C
Preschool (3 years 4 months):	MMR, 4 in 1 (diphtheria, polio, tetanus, pertussis)
Girls 12-13 years:	HPV (two injections 6-12 months apart)
Teens:	3 in 1 (diphtheria, tetanus, polio), meningitis ACWY

6 in 1 = *diphtheria, tetanus, polio, pertussis,* Haemophilus influenzae *type B, hepatitis B*
MMR = *measles, mumps, rubella*

NB: influenza annual nasal vaccine is also offered to 2-7 year olds

POSSIBLE STATIONS
- Parent wants to find out more about childhood vaccinations
- Parent disagrees with vaccinating their child
- Parent has heard something on the news, e.g. MMR causes autism (it doesn't!)
- Why can't their boy have HPV vaccine

AIMS OF THE STATION
- Empathise and be non-judgemental
- Address the patient's concerns and pick up on their cues
- Explore their beliefs
- Explain how the benefits of getting vaccinated outweigh the risks of the vaccines
- Convey the importance of vaccinations

OVERVIEW OF DISEASES VACCINATED AGAINST

6 in 1
- **Diphtheria**
  - Illness: fever, sore throat, grey membrane on tonsils can narrow lumen
  - Complications: cardiomyopathy, renal failure
- **Tetanus**
  - Illness: muscle spasm in jaw and other muscles (including respiratory muscles)
  - Complications: respiratory muscle impairment
- **Polio**
  - Illness: destruction of nerves resulting in muscle weakness and paralysis
  - Complications: paralysis
- **Pertussis**
  - Illness: whooping cough ('hundred day cough')
  - Complications: pneumonia, convulsions, bronchiectasis
- ***Haemophilus influenzae* type B**
  - Illnesses: can cause epiglottitis, meningitis, pneumonia
- **Hepatitis B**
  - Complications: liver cirrhosis

Rotavirus
- **Rotavirus**
  - Illness: diarrhoea and vomiting
  - Complications: extreme dehydration

Pneumococcal
- **Pneumococcal**
  - Illnesses: meningitis, pneumonia

Meningitis vaccines
- **Meningitis B/C/ACWY**
    - o Illness: different strains of meningitis
    - o Complications: deafness, cerebral oedema, memory difficulty, learning disability

MMR
- **Measles (M)**
    - o Illness: high fever, cough, conjunctivitis, coryza, rash
    - o Complications: encephalitis, corneal ulcer/scar
- **Mumps (M)**
    - o Illness: mild illness with gland swelling and headache
    - o Complications: orchitis (and infertility), unilateral deafness, encephalitis, meningitis
- **Rubella (R)**
    - o Illness: flu-like illness with rash
    - o Complication in pregnant women: congenital rubella syndrome

NB: A paper, published in 1998, linked the MMR vaccine to autism. This research has since been discredited and the author has been struck off the medical register for serious misconduct. Further detailed studies have shown there is no link between the MMR vaccine and autism.

HPV
- **Human papillomavirus (HPV)**
    - o Risks: cervical cancer, oral cancer, anal cancer, vaginal cancer
    - o Given as 2 injections, 6 months apart

RISKS VS. BENEFITS OF VACCINATIONS

- Benefits
    - o Prevent serious diseases with severe consequences
    - o To maintain eradication of diseases that can kill and disable millions of children
    - o It's much safer to have the vaccines than not have them
- Safety
    - o Vaccines are extremely safe
    - o Continually monitored
- Risks
    - o As with all medications, vaccines can have side effects (below)
    - o However, they are rarely serious and generally only last a couple of days

CONTRAINDICATIONS TO VACCINATION

- If your child is ill with a fever, the vaccine should be postponed
- Avoid live vaccines (MMR, BCG, Varicella, nasal flu vaccine) in immunocompromised
- Avoid if known anaphylactic reaction to vaccine or any ingredient
- MMR and flu vaccines contain egg
    - o Egg in MMR is from chick embryos and does not trigger allergy
    - o Flu vaccine may cause reaction in patients allergic to eggs – use egg-free alternative

POSSIBLE SIDE EFFECTS OF VACCINATION

- Local effects: swelling, redness, lump
- Fever
- Allergic reaction and anaphylaxis (can be treated)
- Specific side effects
    - o MMR – fever, swollen glands, rash

CONTRACEPTION COUNSELLING

FIRST ASK A FEW QUESTIONS

'First, I need to ask a few questions about your health and relationships to decide which methods are most appropriate for you...'

- Age
- Relationship (regular partner/multiple partners)
- Menstrual history
- Previous contraception and chance of pregnancy
- Are they post-partum or breast feeding?
- PMHx: current conditions, past history, STIs, past obstetric history/previous ectopic pregnancies
- DHx
- Contraindications to COCP
    - Smoking (+ age >35)
    - Hx/FHx of
        - Venous thromboembolism
        - Breast/cervical cancer
        - Migraine with aura

WHAT THEY LIKE AND WHAT THEY KNOW

- Ask them what they are hoping to get out of the consultation and what they know so far (let the patient lead the consultation)
- Try to determine which type of method will be most appropriate
    - Any preferences
    - Preferred administration method
    - Ability to remember to take pills
    - Tolerance of injections

DESCRIBE A METHOD IN MORE DETAIL

- How it works
- Treatment course
- Side effects/risks (and effects on menstrual cycles)
- Positives vs. negatives

BRIEFLY DISCUSS OTHER OPTIONS

- Mention alternatives

ENDING

- Let the patient think about it and advise them they can return again if they wish to discuss other options
- Summarise
- Give leaflets and recommend websites

Contraceptive methods

Method	Contraindications	How it works	Treatment course	Side effects/risks/effect on cycle	Positives vs. negatives	Comments
Combined oral contraceptive pill 2nd gen (*Microgynon, Rigevidon*), 3rd gen (*Marvelon, Yasmin, Cilest*), 4th gen (*Glaira*) **Combined contraceptive patch *Evra*** **Combined contraceptive vaginal ring *NuvaRing*** >99% effectiveness	Age >50, smoker >35 years, BMI >35, migraine with aura, <21 days postpartum, breast feeding, multiple cardiovascular risks/vascular disease, hypertension, current or past VTE Hx, breast cancer, acute/severe liver disease, enzyme-inducing medications, SLE, AF	•Stops ovulation •↑cervical mucus (i.e. a mechanical barrier to sperm) •Thins endothelium (i.e. reduces chance of implantation)	**Pill:** take daily (3 weeks COCP, 1 week pill-free/placebo) **Patch:** change weekly (one patch-free week per month) **Ring:** leave in for 3 weeks then one ring-free week	Oestrogen and progesterone SEs* Blood clots Increased risk of breast/cervical cancer Periods may become lighter Local irritation from the patch Pain from the ring during intercourse- can be removed if uncomfortable but only for a maximum of 3 hours	+ controls periods, bleeding and pain + reduced risk of endometrial and ovarian cancer	•Start on day 1 of cycle for immediate effect •MISSED PILL→ take ASAP (even with next one). If next taken on time, it's fine. If two missed, take one pill immediately and use condoms for 7 days. Further management depends on week: 1st week of packet: will need emergency contraception if had sex in pill-free interval or 1st week of pill packet 2nd week: no action 3rd week: omit the pill-free week •Use barrier contraception if: having D&V (+7 days after); taking enzyme-inducing drugs (+28 days after stopping)
Progesterone only pill *Cerazette* 99% effectiveness	Breast cancer, undiagnosed PV bleeding, severe decompensated liver cirrhosis, severe arterial disease	•↑cervical mucus •Thins endothelium	Take daily at same time (no breaks)	Progesterone SEs* Periods may stop/become irregular	- must remember to take at an exact time	•Start on day 1 of cycle •Must be taken at same time each day •MISSED PILL → take ASAP (even with next one). But if >3 hours late (or >12 hours late for Cerazette), use condoms for 2 days, and consider emergency contraception if had sex in the 2-3 days before missed pill, or had sex since the missed pill.
Intra-uterine device (IUD) Copper coil >99% effectiveness	Pelvic infection, pelvic inflammatory disease <3months ago, gynaecological cancer, small uterine cavity, undiagnosed	Copper acts as spermicide and also causes intra-uterine inflammation	5-10 years	Coil insertion risks* Periods may be heavier Small increase in risk of ectopic pregnancy if become pregnant on it	+ don't need to remember to take pills or go back regularly - heavy periods	•Check for string monthly •STI check before inserting •Can insert any time if not had sex since period, or within first 5 days of start of period •If fitted >40 years (IUD)/>45 years (IUS), can stay in place until menopause and IUS may be used as progesterone component of HRT
Intra-uterine system (IUS) *Mirena* or *Jaydess* for younger women >99% effectiveness	PV bleeding, fibroids that distort the uterine cavity, long QT, copper allergy (for IUD), ischaemic heart disease (IUS)	•Stops ovulation •↑cervical mucus •Thins endothelium	Lasts for 5 years (3 years for Jaydess)	Coil insertion risks* Spotting in first 6months then periods may become lighter/stop in some women Small increase in risk of ectopic pregnancy if become pregnant on it	+ don't need to remember to take pills or go back regularly + reduces dysmenorrhoea/ menorrhagia - Some continue to have unpredictable spotting	
Progesterone implant *Implanon* >99% effectiveness	Liver/genital/breast cancer, severe decompensated liver cirrhosis, undiagnosed PV bleeding, on enzyme-inducers (implant only), ischaemic heart disease		Lasts for 3 years	Progesterone SEs* Insertion risks (bruising, infection, scarring, expulsion) Periods may become infrequent/ prolonged/stop (⅓ each)	+ don't need to remember to take pills or go back regularly - some continue to have unpredictable spotting	•Placed under skin of inner upper arm (4cm long) under local anaesthetic •Can feel it
Progesterone injection *Depo-Provera* >99% effectiveness			Lasts for 3 months	Progesterone SEs* Periods may stop (most)/become irregular/last longer Fertility may be slow to return Osteoporosis risk (avoid long term use)	- must remember to come back every 3 months - fertility may be slow to return - cannot remove once administered (despite SEs)	
Vasectomy 1 in 2000 fail	May consider children in future	Vas deferens cut and tied via forceps through skin or 2 x 1cm cuts in scrotum. Local anaesthetic. Takes 20 mins.	Single operation	Failure (1 in 2000), bleeding/bruising, infection Swollen scrotum for a few days Sperm granulomas may form if leaks occur Chronic testicular pain (1-3%)	+ long term - consider as irreversible (50%) - surgical risks	•Can take up to 3 months for remaining sperm to be used up so sperm samples are required at 16 weeks and 20 weeks post-vasectomy (both must be -ve prior to having unprotected sex) •Can have sex with a condom while awaiting sperm sample results
Tubal ligation 1 in 200 fail		Fallopian tubes clipped laparoscopically under general anaesthetic	Single operation	Anaesthetic risk, failure (1 in 200), bleeding/bruising, infection		
Condom 98% effectiveness	Allergy to ingredients (latex-free are available)	Physical barrier	New condom every act of intercourse	Small risk of allergy May slip off/break	+ stops STI transmission - interrupts sex	•Only method which stops STI transmission •Oil-based products damage latex

*Oestrogen SEs: menorrhagia, ectropion, breast fullness, migraines, fluid retention, nausea

*Progesterone SEs: scanty menses, breast tenderness, dull headache, premenstrual tension, acne, greasy hair, vaginal dryness, low mood

*Coil insertion risks: infection in first 3 weeks, bleeding, perforation 1 in 1000, expulsion 5%, vasovagal 1 in 10

EMERGENCY CONTRACEPTION

INTRODUCTION
- **W**ash hands; **I**ntroduce self; ask **P**atient's name and what they like to be called; **E**xplain
- Establish patient's age

HISTORY OF PRESENTING COMPLAINT
- **Details of unprotected sexual intercourse:** when, with whom (regular partner, how old are they, check it was consensual)
- **Current contraception:** type (none/barrier/pill), reason for failure (e.g. missed pill, split condom etc.)
- **Menstrual history:** last menstrual period, cycle length, estimated day of ovulation (2 weeks before next menstrual period is due)
  NB: the fertile period is on the day of ovulation and the 5 days before it (but it is possible to conceive at any time).
- Any possibility they could already be pregnant/have they already taken emergency contraception this cycle?

DISCUSSIONS
- **Reasons:** why they want emergency contraception/the impact of pregnancy
- **Emergency contraceptive options**: *see table below*, all must be given ASAP
- **Future contraception options:** hormonal contraception can be started immediately after Levonelle or 5 days after ellaOne – barrier methods should be used until contraception has become effective (after 7 days for COCP; after 2 days for progestogen-only pill)
- **Risk of STIs:** advise screening as appropriate (consider taking a more detailed sexual history)

CONCLUSION
- Pay attention to their concerns (remember ICE – Ideas, Concerns, Expectations)
- Give them a leaflet about the emergency contraception they've taken
- Advise them to come back in 3 weeks for follow-up/to take a pregnancy test

Emergency contraception options			
Type	**Copper intra-uterine device**	**ellaOne®**	**Levonelle®**
	First line	*Second line*	*Third line*
Indication	Within **5 days** of unprotected sex. **But** if sex was >5 days previously, it can still be inserted up to 5 days after the *earliest* estimated day of ovulation (2 weeks before next menstrual period is due, *based on shortest cycle length*)	Within **5 days** of unprotected sex. *But research suggests it is ineffective after ovulation*	Within **3 days** of unprotected sex. *But research suggests it is ineffective after ovulation*
Mechanism	•Inserted vaginally •Inhibits fertilisation and implantation	•Single dose ulipristal acetate 30mg PO (selective progesterone receptor modulator) •Inhibits/delays ovulation	•Single dose levonorgestrel 1.5mg PO (progestogen) – *consider 3mg if >70kg or BMI >26* •Inhibits ovulation
Effectiveness	>99% (most effective method)	98% (more effective than Levonelle)	•95% if <24 hrs •85% if 24-48 hrs •58% if 48-72 hrs
Contraindications	•Pregnancy •Pelvic infection/PID <3 months ago •Gynaecological cancers •Small uterine cavity •Copper allergy	•Pregnancy •<18 years old •Severe asthma or liver disease •May be less effective if taking enzyme-inducing medication	•Pregnancy •Acute porphyria •May be less effective if taking enzyme-inducing medication
Side Effects	•Pain on insertion (give ibuprofen) •Infection •Menorrhagia/dysmenorrhea •Perforation (1 in 1000) •Vasovagal (1 in 10) •Expulsion (1 in 20)	•PV bleeding (immediately, at menses, or later) •Nausea/vomiting •Headache •Breast/pelvic pain	
Extra information	•Can be used as long-term contraception, or removed after 4 weeks •Check-up 6 weeks after insertion	•If vomit within 3 hours, repeat dose with domperidone 10mg PO, or use IUD instead •Can re-start hormonal contraception immediately after Levonelle but should wait 5 days after ellaOne •Use barrier methods until contraception has become effective (7 days for COCP; 2 days for progestogen-only pill) •If next period is >7 days late/light bleeding/concerned, do pregnancy test at 3 weeks post-pill •Levonelle can be taken again in same cycle (unlike ellaOne) but not within 5 days •Research suggests oral emergency contraception is **ineffective if taken after ovulation** (unlike copper IUD)	

BASIC GENETIC COUNSELLING

POSSIBLE STATIONS

- Discuss antenatal screening for genetic abnormalities
- Explain to a newly pregnant mother about the tests for Down's syndrome
- Draw a pedigree chart for a family with an autosomal recessive condition (e.g. cystic fibrosis, sickle cell anaemia) or with an autosomal dominant condition (e.g. Huntington's, myotonic dystrophy) and discuss the risk of the patient having an affected child
- Explain genetic test results and implications, e.g. patient is a carrier for the cystic fibrosis gene

INHERITANCE RISKS

- **Autosomal dominant**: only need one copy of abnormal gene (from either parent) to cause disease
    - If a parent is affected, there is a 1 in 2 chance of the child being affected
- **Autosomal recessive**: need two copies of abnormal gene (one from mother, one from father) to cause disease, and only one copy to be a carrier
    - If one parent (only) is a carrier, there is a 1 in 2 chance of the child being a carrier
    - If one parent (only) is affected, the child will be a carrier
    - If one parent is affected and the other is a carrier, there is a 1 in 2 chance the child will be affected, and a 1 in 2 chance the child will be a carrier
    - If both parents are carriers, there is a 1 in 4 chance of the child being affected, and a 2 in 4 chance of the child being a carrier

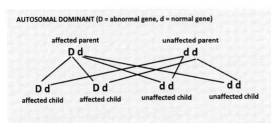
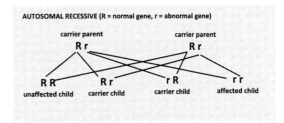

ANTENATAL SCREENING

Conditions of interest

- **Familial (inherited) genetic conditions**
    - Autosomal dominant: Huntington's disease, myotonic dystrophy
    - Autosomal recessive: cystic fibrosis, sickle cell anaemia, thalassaemia, haemochromatosis
    - X-linked recessive: haemophilia
- **Developmental abnormalities** (not genetic), e.g. neural tube defects (spina bifida), other structural developmental defects
- **Chromosomal abnormalities** (caused by cell division error – 'genetic' but not usually inherited), e.g. Down's syndrome – risk increases with age

Parental blood tests

- Genetic testing of mother and father can be performed to determine exact risk of baby being affected by a familial (inherited) genetic condition
- If there is a significant risk to the baby, invasive testing is offered

Down's syndrome risk screening

These tests generate a <u>risk value.</u> If risk > 1 in 150, invasive testing is offered.

- **'Combined test'**: scan + blood test (10-14 weeks) – *used in most cases (better than quadruple test)*
    - Blood test (10-14 weeks): ↓pregnancy-associated plasma protein, ↑βHCG
    - Nuchal translucency scan (11-14 weeks)
- **Quadruple blood test** (14-20 weeks): ↓α-fetoprotein, ↓unconjugated estradiol, ↑βHCG, ↑inhibin A
- **Integrated** (both of above combined)
- **Non-invasive pre-natal testing**, e.g. Harmony/Verifi/NIFTY (≥10 weeks): a maternal blood test that looks at fetal DNA fragments in the maternal blood – >99% accurate but not available on NHS (costs around £400 privately)

NB: very rarely, a parent can have a balanced translocation of chromosome 21 that can cause 'translocation Down's syndrome'. If they've already had a baby with translocation Down's syndrome, the parents should be tested for the abnormality.

Neural tube defect screening

- **Blood test** ↑α-fetoprotein (14-20 weeks) – *gives a risk value. Fetal blood from amniocentesis can also be used and is more accurate.*
- **Anomaly scan** (20 weeks) – *confirms*

Invasive testing for genetic condition diagnosis

Invasive testing is offered if the risk is > 1 in 150.

- **Amniocentesis** (>15 weeks) – 1% miscarriage risk
- **Chorionic villus sampling** (10-14 weeks) – 1-2% miscarriage risk
- These tests give a definite answer to whether the child has a certain genetic condition. Results take 1-2 weeks but rapid tests for chromosome abnormalities can be done in 3 days.
- They can be performed for: babies at high risk of Down's syndrome, familial genetic conditions above
- Termination of pregnancy can be performed at any time if there is confirmed genetic abnormality, but is usually done at <24 weeks

DRAWING A PEDIGREE CHART

Key

- **Sex**
  - Male □
  - Female ○
  - Sex undetermined ◇
  - Pregnancy ◈

- **Conditions**
  - Affected ■ ●
  - Carrier for autosomal recessive condition ◨ ◐
  - Carrier for X-linked recessive condition ◉

- **Matings**
  - Mating □—○
  - Divorced/separated □-//-○
  - Two matings □-//-○—□

- **Patient** ↗ □

- **Siblings**
  - Siblings □ ○
  - Non-identical twins □ ○
  - Identical twins ○ ○

- **Deceased** ⊠ ⊘

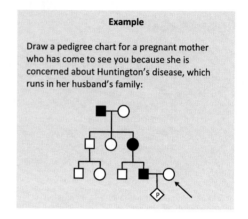

Example

Draw a pedigree chart for a pregnant mother who has come to see you because she is concerned about Huntington's disease, which runs in her husband's family:

BIRTHING OPTIONS

INTRODUCTION
- **W**ash hands; **I**ntroduce self; ask **P**atient's name and what they like to be called; **E**xplain
- Break the ice
  - Congratulate them on their pregnancy
  - Do they know if it's a boy or girl?
  - Do they have a name? (If so, use it when talking about the baby.)
- Find out what they know so far and what they hope to get from the consultation

FIRST ASK A FEW QUESTIONS
'We can talk through a variety of options today to determine which might be best for you and your baby. However, your and your baby's safety is our absolute priority so I just need to ask you a few questions first to determine the most appropriate options...'

Risk factors (if present, recommend hospital birth)
- **Previous births**
  - Previous C-section
  - ≥6 previous children
  - Serious post-partum haemorrhage
- **Current baby**
  - Expecting twins
  - Breech/transverse presentation
  - Placenta praevia
  - Problems with baby
- **Maternal factors**
  - Anaemia
  - Gestational diabetes
  - Pre-eclampsia
  - Age >40 years
  - Obesity (BMI >35)

LOCATIONS
'What options have you heard about so far?'
'Do you have any particular questions or shall we go through the options?'
'Choosing the right place can have a really positive effect on your relationship with your baby.'

Hospital birth
- Birth on the labour ward of the hospital
- Advantages
  - Safest environment – there are obstetricians and paediatricians around if problems arise
  - Can have epidural
- Disadvantages
  - Less personal

Midwife-run birthing centre
- Centres separate from the hospital run by midwives specifically for labour
- Advantages
  - More comfortable and homely
  - More likely to have a midwife you know
- Disadvantages
  - May need to be transferred to hospital if any complications
  - Cannot have epidural

Home birth
- A midwife will come to your home and guide you through labour
- Evidence shows it's as safe as a hospital/birthing centre if it's your second or subsequent baby (slightly higher risk for first babies)
- Advantages
  - Most personal, relaxed environment
  - Privacy
  - You can light candles
  - You can still pay for a birth pool

- Disadvantages
  - May need to be transferred to hospital if any complications – how far is it?
  - Cannot have epidural

MODES OF DELIVERY
- Vaginal
- Caesarean section
  - Recommended if: multiple pregnancy, labour doesn't progress, placenta praevia/accreta, 2 or more previous Caesarean sections, malpresentation (breech/transverse), cephalopelvic disproportion, pelvic cyst/fibroid, maternal infection (*Herpes simplex*/HIV), severe hypertensive disease, fetal distress
  - Disadvantages: major surgery, longer recovery, scar, will be more likely to need it again in the future
  - Patients can request one but, if they don't *need* one, try to find out why – are they worried about pain?

PAIN RELIEF
'Have you thought about pain relief?'
'Pain relief is really important because if you're in control of your pain, you're in control of your labour.'

Treatments
- Natural (none)
- Paracetamol
- Codeine
- Entonox
- Pethidine
- Morphine
- Epidural
- Spinal (for C-section)

WATER BIRTH AND HYPNO BIRTH
- **Water birth**
  - Water birth is available in any environment (although mothers will have to rent one privately if they decide on a home birth)
  - It is a large warm pool
  - It helps with anxiety, pain and muscle relaxation
- **Hypnobirth**
  - Mother can be taught self-hypnosis and controlled breathing by a local practitioner

CONCLUDING
- Summarise
- 'Is there anything else you're concerned about or would like more information on?'
- 'There's no pressure to choose anything now. It's a big decision so take some time to think about what you would prefer and discuss it with your partner.'
- 'You can visit the local birthing centres to help decide.'
- Suggest getting more information and making a birthing plan on the www.nhs.uk website
- Give leaflets and contact details, and book follow-up

HORMONE REPLACEMENT THERAPY

BACKGROUND KNOWLEDGE ON HRT

Indications and contraindications
- **Indications**
  - o Treatment of menopausal symptoms (when benefit outweighs risk)
  - o Treatment of early menopause (until natural menopause age ~ 51 years)
  - o Osteoporotic fracture prophylaxis in women <60 years (when non-oestrogen containing treatments are unsuitable)
- **Contraindications**
  - o Current conditions
    - Undiagnosed PV bleeding
    - Pregnancy/breastfeeding
    - Oestrogen-dependent cancer
    - Acute liver disease
    - Uncontrolled hypertension
  - o Historical conditions
    - History of breast cancer
    - History of venous thromboembolism
    - Recent stroke/MI/angina

Risks and benefits
- **Short-term benefits – relief of:**
  - o Vasomotor symptoms
  - o Psychological symptoms (anxiety, low mood)
  - o Reduced libido
  - o Urogenital atrophy – *use vaginal HRT if symptoms are primarily urogenital*
- **Long-term benefits**
  - o Reduction in osteoporosis (and related fractures)
  - o Reduced risk of colorectal cancer (with combined HRT)
- **Risks**
  - o Venous thromboembolism (no risk with transdermal therapy)
  - o Stroke
  - o Breast cancer (small increase in risk with combined HRT only)
  - o Ovarian cancer (small increase if used >5 years)
  - o Endometrial cancer (only if women with uterus take oestrogen-only HRT – this is why oestrogen-only HRT is only used in women with no uterus)
  - o Coronary heart disease (if started >10 years after menopause)
- **Side effects**
  - o Oestrogen: breast tenderness, leg cramps, nausea/bloating
  - o Progesterone: premenstrual syndrome
  - o Bleeding: PV bleeding occurs towards end of progesterone phase of cyclical HRT

Types of HRT
- **Routes of administration**
  - o **Systemic** (for systemic symptoms, e.g. vasomotor): oral or transdermal (oestrogen/combined patches, oestrogen implant, or oestrogen gel) – *women with a uterus on transdermal oestrogen-only preparations must still take progesterone separately at relevant time*
  - o **Vaginal** oestrogen (for local symptoms, e.g. urogenital atrophy, vaginal dryness): tablet, cream, pessary or vaginal ring
- **Types of systemic therapy**
  - o **No uterus → oestrogen-only HRT** (oral or transdermal)
  - o **Uterus present**
    - **Perimenopausal → cyclical HRT** (oestrogen every day, but oestrogen and progesterone given together for 14 days to cause bleed at the end of every menstrual cycle ('monthly') if still having regular periods; or every 13 weeks ('three-monthly') if having irregular periods)
    - **Post-menopausal (i.e. no periods for >1 year or been on cyclical HRT for >1 year) → continuous HRT** (continuous combined oestrogen and progesterone – no bleed)

Duration of HRT
- No maximum duration – individualise according to risks and benefits for each patient
- Risks increase after age of 65

HRT COUNSELLING

First ask a few questions (screen for contraindications)
'First, I need to ask a few questions to find out if HRT is appropriate for you…'
- Age (menopause usually occurs 45-55 years)
- Confirm menopause if possible
- Discuss their symptoms (and their effect on quality of life)
- PV bleeding
  - Still having periods: ask their regularity
  - No longer having periods: last menstrual period, any post-menopausal/post-coital bleeding
- Relevant past medical history and family history
  - PE/stroke/MI/angina
  - Oestrogen-dependent cancer (breast/endometrial/other)
  - Do they have their uterus? (i.e. no previous hysterectomy)

What they know already
- Find out what they know about HRT
- Ask if there is anything in particular they want to know
- Explain what you would like to do (discuss what HRT is, the risks and benefits, types of HRT, and also talk about contraception if appropriate)

What HRT is and why it is used
- Explain what the menopause is
  - The time when menstrual periods cease and a woman is no longer able to get pregnant
  - It occurs because the ovaries run out of follicles, and this results in reduced production of oestrogen by the ovaries
  - Oestrogen plays a major role in regulating the female reproductive system, but also has many other effects on the body, e.g. mood, libido
  - Symptoms last for 4 years on average (but can be up to 12)
- Explain how HRT treats the symptoms
  - HRT replaces oestrogen ± progesterone
- Benefits of HRT

Risks and benefits
- Discuss both and take care to explore and address patient's concerns
- Outline major side effects

Discuss types of HRT
- Explain how HRT is given
- Explain routes of administration

Briefly mention contraception
- Women are potentially fertile for 1 year after last menstrual period (or 2 years if <50 years)
- Explain HRT is not contraception
- Contraceptive options for women on HRT
  - Barrier methods
  - Progesterone only pill (in addition to HRT)
  - Mirena coil (can be used as progesterone component of HRT)

Discuss alternatives
- Mood: cognitive behavioural therapy, antidepressants
- Vasomotor symptoms: SSRIs, selective serotonin-norepinephrine reuptake inhibitors, and clonidine
- Vaginal dryness: lubricants/moisturisers
- Irregular periods: Mirena coil

Ending
- Summarise
- Let patient think about it and plan follow-up
- Offer leaflets/website links

POSSIBLE STATIONS

- **A patient has a blood-borne disease and does not want this disclosed in a referral letter to the hospital because they know people who work there**
  - You do <u>not</u> have to disclose this (for procedures, every patient should be treated as if they have a blood-borne illness)
  - However, you need to explain why it would be in their best interests for the hospital to know; and how you can help ensure confidentiality
    - Your illness may mean certain drugs will be handled differently by your body and may be dangerous
    - You may be given drugs which interact with your current medications
    - Highlight that every medical professional has a duty of confidentiality, which is taken very seriously
    - Only those directly involved in your care will know
- **A patient thinks their partner (another one of your patients) has an STI and wants to know why they came to see you last week**
  - You cannot give them any information about their partner
  - You can give them a full STI check
- **A patient wants treatment for an STI from the GP surgery but does not want this put on record because their partner knows one of the other GPs**
  - If a treatment is prescribed at the surgery, this <u>must</u> be put in the records
  - Reassure them that all GPs have a duty of confidentiality which is taken very seriously
  - Advise them they can go to the sexual health clinic confidentially, where records are kept separately from GP records
- **A patient has contracted an STI from a prostitute and does not want to tell their partner, with whom they have since had unprotected sex**
  - As a doctor, you can only break confidentiality if the patient has a blood-borne STI and continues to have unprotected sex with their partner. You cannot break confidentiality for non-blood-borne STIs.
  - You have a duty to try to persuade the patient to tell their partner
    - Their partner is at risk
    - If their partner is not treated early, they may suffer irreversible complications (such as infertility for Chlamydia)
    - It is likely to be better to tell their partner now than have them find out later
  - Help with possible ways to tell them
    - They could both come in together and talk to you
    - The sexual health clinic can send an anonymous letter
  - If asked, you can not treat the patient's partner without the partner's consent!
- **An inpatient has become unconscious and unresponsive. The relatives have been told and have come in to see you. They did not know their relative was in hospital and want to know what has happened.**
  - If a patient lacks capacity, you can speak to relatives with regards to their health unless you strongly suspect the patient would object
  - Try to disclose only as much as is necessary
  - You must be sensitive to the relatives' feelings and concerns

AIMS OF THE STATION

- Know the rules surrounding confidentiality and do not breach confidentiality
- Show that you can be firm but also sympathetic, non-judgemental and helpful
- Empathise with the patient and do not attack their motives
- Address their concerns and pick up on cues
- Address confidentiality (what is it; why it is in place; explain why it is in the best interests of all patients)
- Offer what help you can

THE RULES

- You can only breach confidentiality when 'another person is at significant risk of harm' (General Medical Council) – *it is not black and white*
  - You can break confidentiality for blood-borne STIs but not for other STIs
- If a patient's partner is at significant risk, you must take all measures to persuade them to tell their partner before breaching confidentiality (this may require multiple consultations)
- 'You must respect the wishes of any patient who objects to any information being shared with others providing care, except where they would put others at risk of death or significant harm.' (General Medical Council)
- You have a duty to warn patients if their behaviour puts others at risk, and to explain any implications of that risk (e.g. complications of an STI remaining untreated)
- If a patient lacks capacity, you can speak to relatives about their health unless you strongly suspect the patient would object

POSSIBLE STATIONS

- Schizophrenic requires surgery for appendicitis but refuses
- A patient decides to stop all active treatment for metastatic cancer
- A patient wants to self-discharge against medical advice

THE RULES

- The patient has capacity until proven otherwise
- Capacity is decision-dependent (i.e. a patient may lack capacity to make one decision but have capacity to make another)
- If a patient lacks capacity, you must act in their best interests
- If a patient makes a strange or irrational decision, this does not mean they don't have capacity

TWO-STAGE TEST TO ASSESS CAPACITY

The patient only lacks capacity if the answer to both questions is YES:

---

1. **Does the patient have impairment/disturbance of brain function?**
   - If NO, then the patient has capacity (and you do not need to move on to step 2)
2. **If YES, does this mean they are unable to make a decision as a result?**
   - To assess ability to make a decision, you must determine if the patient can:
     - **Understand** information relevant to the decision (e.g. consequences, risks, benefits, alternatives)
     - **Retain** the information (for long enough to make a decision)
     - **Weigh up**/use the information to make a decision (pros and cons)
     - **Communicate** the decision (by any means)

   If the patient can still do all of these, then the patient has capacity.

BEST INTERESTS

If a patient over 18 years old lacks capacity, it is the doctor's duty to make the decision on their behalf, acting in their best interests under the ***Mental Capacity Act***. The relatives/friends have no legal right to make the decision unless they have power of attorney. To decide upon the patient's best interests, you must:

- Try to involve the patient in the decision
- Take into account any of their known beliefs/views
- Consult anyone identified by patient/carers to help determine what is in their best interests (but not make the decision)
- Check for any lasting power of attorney
- Consider if they may regain capacity

NB: if a life-changing decision needs to be made for a patient who lacks capacity and does not have relatives who can be involved, an opinion from an independent mental capacity advocate (IMCA) should be requested.

FORMS AND DOCUMENTATION

- You must clearly document all parts of your capacity assessment, stating why the patient does not have capacity for the decision
- If you are stopping a patient without capacity from **doing** things they may want to (e.g. leaving hospital), you are 'depriving them of their liberties' and must fill in a *Deprivation of Liberty Safeguards* (DoLS) form

MENTAL HEALTH ACT

- Allows detention of a patient with a mental disorder who is **at risk of harm to themselves or others** (nothing to do with capacity)
- Certain sections allow treatment as well as assessment but you can treat only their mental illness without their consent
- However, this can be cautiously extended to treat problems closely related to the mental disorder, e.g. an overdose or self-harm

Sections of the Mental Health Act	
Section 2	28 days for assessment and treatment (by 2 doctors but one must be MHA approved)
Section 3	6 months for treatment (by 2 doctors but one must be MHA approved)
Section 4	72 hours for emergency assessment (by 1 doctor, and an approved mental health practitioner, or the patient's closest relative)
Section 5(2)	72 hours detainment for assessment of patient already in hospital (by doctor in charge of patient's care)
Section 5(4)	6 hours detainment for assessment of patient already in hospital (by approved mental health nurse)

*NB: **common law** may be used in emergencies when there is no opportunity to determine a patient's mental capacity or mental state. It may be used for detention if the patient is at risk to themselves or others; and/or for the minimum treatment of any illness if urgent intervention is required to save the patient's life or to prevent a significant deterioration in their condition. It is used most frequently in the emergency department.*

EXPLAINING THE PROCEDURE

- Explain what it is
- Reason for it
- Explain procedure details (before, during, after)
- Risks and benefits
- Alternatives

THREE THINGS REQUIRED FOR CONSENT TO BE VALID

1. Consent must be <u>informed</u>
2. Consent must be <u>voluntary</u>
3. Patient must have <u>capacity</u>

CONSENT TEST

In order to provide valid consent, the patient must do all four of the following:

Understand	Understand information relevant to the decision (e.g. consequences, risks, benefits, alternatives)
Retain	Retain the information (for long enough to make a decision)
Weigh up	Weigh up and use the information to make a decision (pros and cons)
Communicate	Communicate the decision (by any means)

OTHER POINTS

- A signed consent form is best practice but not a legal requirement
- The person consenting must have a full understanding of the procedure, risks, benefits and alternatives
- The ultimate responsibility for ensuring the patient is consented properly lies with the doctor undertaking the procedure (although they do not have to do this personally)
- You must disclose 'all risks that are material to the patient'

CONSENT RULES FOR CHILDREN

<u>Children 16-18 years old</u>
Children 16-18 years old are presumed to have capacity and generally treated like adults with regard to consent. However, unlike adults, treatment refusal can be overridden in some circumstances (by person with parental responsibility or court).

<u>Gillick competence for children under 16 years old</u>
Children under 16 years old can consent to medical treatment (<u>but not necessarily refuse treatment</u>) 'if they have sufficient maturity and judgement to enable them to fully understand what is proposed' – *i.e. they are 'Gillick competent'*

IF THEY ARE COMPETENT: child can consent to treatment on their own (parents cannot override)
IF THE ARE NOT COMPETENT: parent is responsible for consent (unless it's an emergency and they cannot be contacted)
IF A COMPETENT CHILD REFUSES TREATMENT IN THEIR BEST INTERESTS: settled by the court (emergency court decision can be obtained)
IF A CLINICIAN DISAGREES WITH A PARENT: settled by the court (emergency court decision can be obtained)

<u>Fraser guidelines for prescription of contraceptives</u>
A doctor can prescribe contraception to children under 16 years old if:
- The child understands the advice
- They cannot be persuaded to tell their parents
- They are likely to continue having sex without the contraception
- The child's physical/mental health may suffer without the contraception
- The child's best interests are that they should receive it
NB: bear in mind the age of the partner and risk of sexual abuse.

ADVANCE DECISION TO REFUSE TREATMENT ('LIVING WILL')

WHAT IS IT?

- A legally binding document outlining what medical treatment a patient would <u>not</u> want in the future, if they lacked capacity.

WHAT MAKES IT LEGALLY BINDING?

- Signed
- Witnessed
- It is not felt to have been signed under duress
- There is no doubt about the patient's state of mind at time of signing

ROLE OF RELATIVES

- Relatives have no legal rights to rescind or modify a valid advance decision

LIMITATIONS

- The patient cannot specify which treatments they would want, only those they would not want

LASTING POWER OF ATTORNEY

A third party is appointed (in advance) to make decisions on the patient's behalf should they lose capacity. The third party may be one person or more than one person. If the latter, they can be appointed to act together ('jointly'); or so that each can make decisions alone ('jointly and severally'). The third party may be a relative/friend or legal advocate. There are two types of lasting power of attorney: health and welfare; and property and finance affairs.

HEALTH AND WELFARE

- For decisions regarding health
- Only takes effect if the patient lacks capacity
- The third party can make decisions as if they were the patient. They can decide about the patient's:
  - Daily routine
  - Medical care
  - Moving into a care home
  - Refusing life-saving treatment
- However, the power of attorney only has the right to refuse offered medical treatments, not to choose which treatments to have

PROPERTY AND FINANCE AFFAIRS

- For decisions regarding finances, bills, pensions, and selling property
- Can take effect immediately with patient's consent

HOW TO REGISTER

- There is a fee payable to the Office of the Public Guardian to register a power of attorney, and there will also be legal fees if a solicitor is used
- Application can be made via a solicitor or independently online or by paper forms (www.gov.uk/power-of-attorney)
- Documents will also need to be signed by witnesses

DVLA REPORTING

POSSIBLE STATIONS

- An epileptic patient has agreed not to drive but a nurse saw him parking today before his review
- A heavy goods vehicle driver has had a seizure and you must break the news regarding driving restrictions
- A patient who presented with a seizure is now being discharged: you must speak to them about lifestyle changes
- A relative is concerned about a patient who has an 'alcohol problem' and is driving

PHRASES TO HELP YOU

- 'Safety precautions'
- 'The tablets don't guarantee your safety and the safety of others if you are driving.'
- 'Have you been able to follow the advice given to you with regards to driving?'
- 'If you drive you will be breaking the law and your insurance will not be valid.'

AIMS OF THE STATION

- Show that you can be firm but also sympathetic and non-judgemental
- Address the patient's concerns and pick up on their cues
- Use a 'breaking bad news' approach
- Clearly communicate the importance of not driving
- You may need to be firm with them – how would they feel if they had a seizure at the wheel and harmed/killed their own family or other people?
- Offer solutions to the patient's problems or sources of help if you have any (if not, just listen and empathise)
- Know the DVLA rules

THE DVLA RULES

- The rules differ for normal licences and heavy goods vehicle licences (includes taxis, buses, lorries, large vehicles). Below are some example restrictions but many other conditions also require the patient to inform the DVLA.
- If a patient drives after being advised not to, their insurance is invalid and they are breaking the law

Some important conditions with driving restrictions		
	Normal licence	**Heavy goods vehicle licence**
Diabetes	Must meet certain criteria to drive (depends on hypoglycaemia episodes, hypoglycaemia awareness, glucose monitoring and complications)	
First unprovoked seizure	6 months	5 years
Other seizure	1 year	10 years
Stroke/TIA	1 month*	1 year
Unexplained syncope	6 months	1 year
MI treated with stent	1 week*	6 weeks (but need tests)
Alcohol misuse	6 months (of controlled drinking/abstinence)	1 year (of controlled drinking/abstinence)
Alcohol dependence	1 year (free of alcohol-related problems)	3 years (free of alcohol-related problems)

Do not need to inform DVLA if no residual symptoms (all others need to inform DVLA)

IF THE PATIENT REFUSES TO COMPLY

- It is the doctor's duty to advise the patient that they are not allowed to drive; that if they do they will be breaking the law and their insurance will be invalidated; and advise them they need to inform the DVLA
- If the patient refuses and says they will continue driving, involve senior and have multiple conversations
- If they still insist, you can break confidentiality and inform the DVLA (you must tell the patient you are doing this)

Healthcare professionals have a duty of care towards patients at risk of abuse, harm or neglect (including self-neglect). The correct approach to this varies depending on whether the patient is a child or an adult. If they are an adult, it is also depends upon whether they are vulnerable and if they have capacity to make decisions related to the safeguarding issue.

CHILDREN AND VULNERABLE ADULTS WITHOUT CAPACITY

- Vulnerable adult = an adult who is/may be unable to care for or protect themselves against harm or exploitation
  NB: a vulnerable adult may or may not have capacity; however, if an adult lacks capacity, this will usually make them vulnerable.
- If the risk is posed to a child (<18 years) or a vulnerable adult without capacity, you <u>must break confidentiality</u> (even if they object) and inform social services
- All children at risk must be referred regardless of whether they have capacity or not

ADULTS WITH CAPACITY

- If the person at risk is an adult <u>with</u> capacity, you must explain to them the risks as you perceive them, and what help is available. You must encourage them to accept help from you and/or allow you to refer them on.
- However, if they have capacity and <u>do not</u> give consent, you <u>cannot</u> disclose their situation to anyone else or make a referral

WHO TO REFER TO

- **Children and vulnerable adults**
  - Social services (they will involve other relevant parties)
- **Adults who are not vulnerable**
  - Police
  - Local domestic abuse service
  - Counselling/support services
  - Social services must be informed *if* children or vulnerable adults are involved/at risk

SOURCES OF HELP/ADVICE

- Your seniors
- Safeguarding leads in your hospital/region
  - For adults
  - For vulnerable adults
  - For children (a paediatrician)
- Social services or local domestic abuse service

RECOGNISING A CHILD WITH NON-ACCIDENTAL INJURIES

- **Suggestive factors:** injury incompatible with story; inconsistent stories from child/parents/carers; delay in seeking help; abnormal interaction from child; abnormal affect of parent
- **General indicators:** multiple bruises, black eyes, torn frenulum, bite marks, injuries on non-mobile children
- **Common non-accidental injuries**
  - **Bruises:** on soft tissues, e.g. face, ears, eyes, neck, inner arms, abdomen, groin, buttocks
  - **Fractures:** multiple, ribs, humeral, metaphyseal, spiral
  - **Burns:** hands, buttocks, feet (especially if consistent depth, clear upper limits and symmetrical)
  NB: remember there may be other explanations, e.g. ITP/leukaemia can cause abnormal bruising, and osteogenesis imperfecta can cause multiple fractures.

EXPLAINING SAFEGUARDING CONCERNES TO A CHILD'S PARENTS

- You should tell the parents you are making a referral to social services
- If you feel an urgent social services assessment is required or the child is at immediate risk, then an emergency protection order can be sought if required
- Do not accuse the parents – explain that all children with these types of injuries have to be referred for assessment
- Explain why it is important – 'Some injuries like this are not accidental and it is very difficult for us to tell which, so we have to refer all cases.'
- Explain what it will involve
- Emphasise the rules are there to ensure all children are safe and protected
- Remember you may be met with anger (*see notes on dealing with strong emotions p338*)

DOMESTIC ABUSE STATION

Domestic abuse is very common and can be physical, sexual or emotional. Consequences include traumatic injury and death, and victims are more likely to suffer from chronic illness and mental health problems.

POSSIBLE STATIONS

- A patient comes to see you with recurring headaches which they put down to difficulties at home
- You are asked to speak to a patient who was initially reluctant to be examined but then found to have multiple bruises
- A patient complains that their partner has 'a bit of a temper'

AIMS OF THE STATION

- Be reassuring and non-judgemental
- Don't be afraid to ask about abuse
- Assess risk to patient and their children
- Don't assume the patient wants to leave their partner immediately, just offer advice and support

BEFORE RAISING THE ISSUE

- Develop a good **rapport** with the patient and make them feel comfortable
- Assure them about **privacy, safety and confidentiality**
- Ensure their potential abuser isn't present

WHEN RAISING THE ISSUE

- Use an **open question** to allow them to explain the situation: 'Tell me about things at home', 'Do you feel scared/safe at home?', 'I'm worried someone may have hurt you', 'I'm worried you may not be safe at home', 'Does your partner's behaviour upset you?'
- Establish the details of the abuse
  - **Type(s)** of abuse:
    - **Physical:** 'Has your partner ever hurt you?'
    - **Sexual:** 'Does your partner ever make you do sexual things you don't want to?'
    - **Emotional:** 'How does your partner make you feel? Do they belittle you or try to control you?'
  - **Perpetrator:** Who is it?, What's their relationship?
  - **Pattern:** When does it occur? Are alcohol/drugs involved?
  - **Timeframe:** How long? Has the abuse been escalating?
  - **Coping:** How have they coped? Have they tried anything to stop it/get away?
  - **Who else is involved:** Are any children or vulnerable adults potentially at risk?
- Explore their **social situation/domestic environment**
  - Who do they live with?
  - Are there weapons in the house?
  - Does the patient have an emergency safety plan? If not, consider trying to construct one with them and tell them they can always call the police
  - Do they work?
- Tips
  - Try to be **supportive**, all them **time** to talk and offer tissues if they get upset
  - Be relaxed and compassionate with the patient
  - Don't pressure them into telling you, but they may need to be asked several times before opening up

RISK ASSESSMENT

- **NEVER FORGET RISK!**
  - **To patient:**
    - From partner: Do they currently feel in danger? What would happen if they go home?
    - Risk of self-harm: Has it affected their mood? Have they ever considered harming themselves or taking their own life?
  - **To others:** Are any children or vulnerable adults potentially at risk?
- Abuse risk factor assessment – consider the following if relevant
  - **Victim:** low self-esteem, low income, young
  - **Partner:** pregnancy, alcohol/drug use, psychiatric issues/personality disorders, unemployment, being a victim of poor parenting/abuse/physical discipline, convictions
  - **Relationship:** separation/divorce, poor housing situation

MANAGEMENT

- Be non-judgemental, establish the patient's concerns, and allow them to control the situation and make decisions
- **Acknowledge and reassure**
    - Acknowledge complexity of situation and how difficult it must have been to disclose
    - Reassure patient it is not their fault and that no one should be treated that way
- Explain about sources of **support**
    - Establish if they have any friends/family who could support them
    - Counselling/support and helplines (e.g. national domestic violence helpline, WomensAid.org.uk) – give a leaflet
    - Refuge is available if they cannot go home
- Offer **referrals** (and explain how they can help)
    - Police
    - Local domestic abuse service
    - Counselling/support services
    - Social services <u>must</u> be informed *if* children or vulnerable adults are involved/at risk

    NB: if the victim is an adult with capacity, you can only refer them if they consent (unless a child or vulnerable adult is involved).
- **Encourage** the patient to talk about it and seek help

CONCLUSION

- Again acknowledge how difficult it must be for them
- Formulate a plan together
- Arrange follow-up and advise them they can come to see you at any time

BREAKING BAD NEWS

Breaking bad news requires very delicate communication skills: you must show compassion, sensitivity and tact, while also being clear and straightforward with your patient, avoiding the temptation to play down or obscure painful truths. The **SPIKES protocol** (Baile et al. 2000) is widely used and is a very helpful way to structure the consultation.

SETTING

- Ensure you are in a comfortable and confidential room where you will not be interrupted

PERCEPTION

- Outline events that have led up to the present situation
- Ask them what they already know/expect
- If possible, gently encourage the patient to say what the diagnosis is:

'Could you tell me what's happened so far?'

'Do you have any ideas as to what the problem might be?'

'Is there anything you have been worried about?'

INVITATION

- Check if the patient
    - Wants to know the result now
    - Would like a family member to be present

'I do have the result here today. Would you like me to explain it to you now, or would you prefer to have a family member/friend present?'

KNOWLEDGE

Giving the diagnosis:
- Build up to the result – give a **warning shot**
- **Chunk** the diagnosis (stepped approach)
- After every statement you make, **pause and wait** for the patient to respond (silence is the best thing at this point – there are a million thoughts going around in their head)
- If the silence is very awkward, you can ask a question about what's going through their mind or how they are feeling

Explaining:
- <u>DO NOT</u> launch into explanation – during the **knowledge** stage and afterwards, the patient <u>must</u> lead the consultation – only answer questions they ask (they will not remember anything else you say)
- **Chunk and check** any requested explanations

'As you know, we took a biopsy and, unfortunately, the results are not what we wanted.' <u>PAUSE AND WAIT</u>

'I'm very sorry to tell you it is a cancer.'

EMOTIONS AND EMPATHY

- **Acknowledge and reflect back their emotions** (including body language)
- Don't try to solve their problems or reassure them, just listen and **summarise/bounce back their concerns** and expand on them (it shows you are listening and conveys empathy)
- If there is a lot of silence, you can ask cautiously about their feelings

'I can see this news is a huge shock.' <u>PAUSE AND WAIT</u>

'I imagine this news must be making you very anxious.' <u>PAUSE AND WAIT</u>

'How are you feeling about hearing this news?'

'This must be extremely distressing for you. How are you feeling right now?'

'There must be so much going through your head right now. Would it help to talk about it?'

STRATEGY AND SUMMARY

- Agree on a plan
- Summarise concerns

COMMUNICATING DURING THE CONSULTATION

<u>Breaking the news</u>
- **Stepped approach** (wait for a sign of approval from the patient before moving on from each step):
    - 'I'm afraid it's not good news, Mrs Smith.' <u>PAUSE AND WAIT FOR PATIENT TO ASK</u>
    - 'Unfortunately the lump is a problem.' <u>PAUSE AND WAIT FOR PATIENT TO ASK</u>
    - 'Yes, I'm so sorry to have to tell you, it is a cancer.' <u>PAUSE AND WAIT FOR PATIENT TO ASK</u>
- **Next:** Don't say anything until the patient speaks. This can feel difficult and take a long time but it's the best approach to take from this point onwards in the consultation. But if the silence really is too prolonged, you can try gently moving the discussion forwards to the patient's feelings. (See above under **Emotions and Empathy** stage.)

<u>Responding to cues/questions</u>
- **Cues** can be verbal or non-verbal. They may be subtle and the only manifestations of much stronger feelings – the 'tip of the iceberg'
- **Dealing with a cue**
    - Bounce it back (you <u>must</u> show you have recognised it)
    - Empathise
    - Explore the <u>content</u> of the cue, e.g. 'Would it be OK if I asked more about that?'
    - In general, don't try to solve problems – it may well be that you can't. Concentrate on listening sympathetically and encouraging the patient to open up.

e.g. 'I'm dying, what does it matter?'

'I think I can imagine why you might feel like that. But sometimes it can still be helpful to talk about everything that's going through your head right now.' <u>PAUSE AND WAIT</u>

'I'm so sorry – this news must be devastating for you. I can't imagine how difficult this must be for you right now.' <u>PAUSE AND WAIT FOR PATIENT</u>

<u>Don't start giving information until it is requested</u>
- Patients have such pressing concerns that they can find it difficult to listen to what you're saying. You need to address their concerns out first.
- Prompt if you need to, e.g. 'You must have so much going through your mind right now. Would it help to talk about it?'
- Summarise back and expand on all their concerns

DEALING WITH STRONG EMOTIONS

PROCEDURE FOR DEALING WITH THE EMOTION

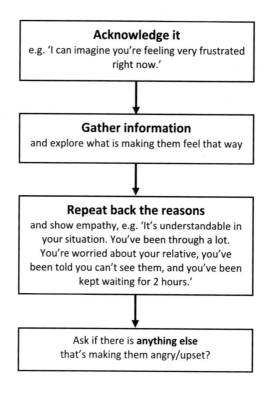

Acknowledge it
e.g. 'I can imagine you're feeling very frustrated right now.'

↓

Gather information
and explore what is making them feel that way

↓

Repeat back the reasons
and show empathy, e.g. 'It's understandable in your situation. You've been through a lot. You're worried about your relative, you've been told you can't see them, and you've been kept waiting for 2 hours.'

↓

Ask if there is **anything else**
that's making them angry/upset?

TIPS

- Avoid saying 'I understand' to an angry patient
- Counter anger with soft, slow speech
- Ensure you are at their eye level
- Don't interrupt an outburst
- Don't take offence personally or become defensive (even if the patient/relative is wrong)
- Demonstrate active listening (eye contact, nodding, verbal acknowledgements, e.g. 'Yes', 'I see', 'Mmm')
- With an upset patient, silence and long pauses are key
- You can say you are sorry to hear something happened, but you should not in general admit guilt or apologise unless you have personally made a mistake
- Try to get the patient seated, ideally with chairs at 90° to each other (not head-on)

RESPONDING TO CUES/QUESTIONS

- **Cues** can be verbal or non-verbal. They may be subtle and the only manifestations of much stronger feelings – the 'tip of the iceberg'
- **Dealing with a cue**
    1. Bounce it back (you <u>must</u> show you have recognised it)
    2. Empathise
    3. Explore the <u>content</u> of the cue, e.g. 'Would it be OK if I asked more about that?'

NB: in general, don't try to solve problems – it may well be that you can't. Concentrate on listening sympathetically and encouraging the patient to open up.

PSYCHOSOCIAL CONCERNS STATION

POSSIBLE STATIONS

<u>With a patient</u>
- Concerned about a test
  - Try to find the underlying reasons for their concern
- Wants a sick note because of problems at work
- Wants to self-discharge because they need to care for a partner at home
- Wants to die
- Wants to lose weight because a relative died recently of obesity-related health problems
- Wants to make a complaint
  - Don't forget to mention the patient advice and liaison service (PALS)
  - You can say you are *sorry they feel that way/went through that* but generally don't apologise/admit guilt
- Feels another doctor examined them inappropriately/didn't offer chaperone

<u>With a patient's relative</u>
- Carer struggling
  - Social services can do a care assessment to provide money/respite/help
  - Charities (e.g. carersuk.org and carerssupport.org.uk) offer help and support groups
  - Health visitor for children
  - Stress they're not alone
- Concerned about social care arrangements for elderly relative
  - Social services can arrange care
  - There are also private care organisations
  - In a crisis, doctors can refer to the rapid response team for short-term care
- Carer says patient has stopped taking their medication and wants to know how to make them take it
- Is concerned their relative may have cancer because they know someone else who had similar symptoms and then died of cancer

<u>With a colleague (e.g. doctor, nurse, midwife, student, secretary, receptionist)</u>
- Another member of the team is not pulling their weight, is always late, makes mistakes, or smells of alcohol etc.
  - Options include speaking to the culprit directly (usually best initially), and then considering speaking to their senior (offer to be present)
  - If patients are/may be at risk, you must take action and inform a senior. You should tell the culprit you are doing so.
- Being bullied by another member of the team
  - Could they approach the perpetrator? Can they speak to their supervisor/senior/human resources? Offer to be present if possible.
  - If they have tried to resolve it but had no success, they may need to make a formal complaint
  - Screen for depression (but remember you are not their doctor and should direct them to their GP if needed)
- Issues at home affecting work
- A colleague who is stressed
- Shaken up by something that has happened (e.g. a patient died)
  - They will need ongoing support – can they speak to their supervisor or occupational health? Offer to be present if possible
- A colleague has made a mistake
  - Have a non-judgemental attitude
  - Emphasise the 'no blame' culture when mistakes are admitted
  - Incident reporting can help everyone learn so the same mistake doesn't happen to others
  - Honesty is the best policy
- A health visitor concerned about a child abuse within a family without any evidence because he/she missed a similar problem previously

AIMS OF THE STATION

- Be non-judgemental
- Empathise
- <u>Listen!</u>
- Pick up on cues and show you have heard them
- Address their ideas, concerns and expectations (ICE)
- Suggest possible solutions

SUGGESTED STRUCTURE:

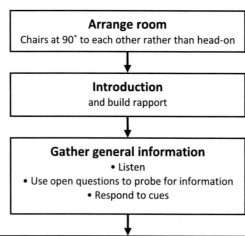

Arrange room
Chairs at 90° to each other rather than head-on

↓

Introduction
and build rapport

↓

Gather general information
• Listen
• Use open questions to probe for information
• Respond to cues

↓

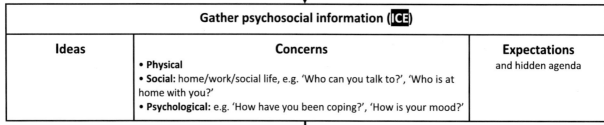

Gather psychosocial information (ICE)		
Ideas	**Concerns** • **Physical** • **Social:** home/work/social life, e.g. 'Who can you talk to?', 'Who is at home with you?' • **Psychological:** e.g. 'How have you been coping?', 'How is your mood?'	**Expectations** and hidden agenda

↓

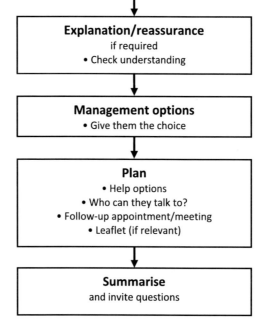

Explanation/reassurance
if required
• Check understanding

↓

Management options
• Give them the choice

↓

Plan
• Help options
• Who can they talk to?
• Follow-up appointment/meeting
• Leaflet (if relevant)

↓

Summarise
and invite questions

TIPS

- Don't be afraid of **silence**
- These stations can be difficult because there isn't a goal like completing a history or explaining a test. Most patients just need a sympathetic ear and some guidance.
- There is often a **hidden agenda** that the patient will only disclose if you probe with 'ICE-type' questions, e.g. they may come in for a sick note but actually they are being bullied at work
- Use the patient's **name** and show **empathy**
- Respond to **cues**! It is important to concentrate on what the patient is saying. Don't distract yourself worrying further questions.
  - Cues may be verbal or non-verbal
  - Comment on it, e.g. 'You look worried.'
  - After recognising a cue, repeat it back to the patient and then ask more about it (e.g. 'You mentioned that sometimes you feel down – can you tell me more about that?')
- Don't treat a colleague like a patient – chat informally if you 'know them' and listen sympathetically. But if there's a medical problem, you cannot treat them – you need to advise them to see their own GP.
- It is not your job to solve their problem – just listen and suggest possible ways to address it. If you don't know of any services that could help them, say you will look into it and arrange to meet them again to discuss further.
- If you need to involve somebody else (e.g. their supervisor/manager), ask the patient/colleague/carer if it would help if you were present too

END OF LIFE AND TREATMENT ESCALATION DISCUSSIONS

Remember: the key to all of these stations is good communication. The conversations should be conducted in an appropriate setting and should not be interrupted by bleeps etc. Find out what the patient/family knows already and try to gauge their level of understanding. Ensure you are empathetic, 'chunk-and-check', and make use of pauses. Don't forget to listen to the patient's/relative's **ideas, concerns and expectations**.

'DO NOT ATTEMPT CARDIOPULMONARY RESUSCITATION' (DNACPR) DISCUSSIONS

Background information
- Decisions regarding CPR are ultimately taken by the patient's **medical team.** A patient can refuse CPR but cannot demand it.
- Success of in-hospital resuscitation is around 20% but this may be much lower if there are comorbidities/reasons why it is less likely to be successful. Of those who survive resuscitation, only around half will make it out of hospital.
- A DNAR form may be completed for one of three reasons:
  - Resuscitation is unlikely to be successful
  - The patient does not want it
  - It may be successful but would result in a length and quality of life that is not in the patient's overall benefit
- If a patient has capacity, they should be informed of the decision (unless it will cause significant physical or psychological harm)
- If a patient does not have capacity, the relatives of the patient should be informed
- All DNAR discussions should be clearly documented
- 'Do Not Resuscitate' does not mean stop treatment
- If the form is signed by a junior doctor, it should be countersigned by a consultant as soon as possible

Approach
- It is usually best brought up during a wider discussion about advance care planning
- Work your way up to it rather than jumping straight in. Try to build rapport and start by discussing current problems and how they are being treated.
- Explain there is always a risk that things might get worse and the patient might deteriorate
- Explain what CPR is and what it involves
- If CPR would not be successful, sensitively explain why your team feels it would not be appropriate. If CPR might be successful, discuss the patient's wishes and feelings. Try to determine whether the benefits would outweigh the risks and burdens; and if the level of recovery would be acceptable to the patient.
- Stress that a DNAR decision does not mean that the patient will not be treated – it is only relevant if their heart stops
- Do not ask the patient or relatives to make the decision
- If the patient/relatives strongly disagree, don't force it – escalate the discussion to your seniors or ask for a second opinion

Phrases to help
- 'One thing that it is important for us to talk about is resuscitation.'
- 'You are very unwell at the moment and we need to talk about what we would do if you were to get worse despite treatment.'
- 'We feel it would be kinder and more appropriate to ensure he is not in any pain or distress in the last moments of his life. If it were to get to the point where his heart stopped, we would not try to restart it.'
- 'We will still give her every treatment available on the ward. The form just means that if she were to become much more unwell and reach the natural end of her life, we would not do chest compressions and shocks to restart it, because this can cause a lot of pain and distress, and prolong suffering.'
- 'His medical condition means that he will eventually get to the natural end of his life and it is important we talk about this before it happens. Trying to restart his heart in this situation would not be the right thing to do.'
- 'We only have one chance with end of life care so it is important to get it right.'
- 'Even if a patient survives resuscitation, they are often more disabled afterwards, and left with a quality of life that they would not want.'

OTHER TREATMENT ESCALATION DECISIONS

- In addition to decisions regarding resuscitation, decisions should also be made about other invasive treatments where appropriate. These should be documented in the patient's notes and on a treatment escalation plan document.
- The patient can only insist upon things they **do not** want
- It is for doctors to decide which treatments are and are not appropriate, e.g. intensive care admission, non-invasive ventilation, parenteral nutrition etc.
- Factors to take into account when considering intensive care admission include:
  - **Diagnosis, severity of illness and prognosis:** to warrant intensive care admission, a patient must have an acute reversible condition and a viable treatment must be available
  - **Age, comorbidities and physiological reserve:** surviving intensive care and invasive treatment requires a good physiological reserve (e.g. there is no point ventilating patients who will not be able to get off the ventilator)
  - **Anticipated quality of life:** there is often a physiological decline after severe illness and it is important to consider if the patient would be left with an acceptable quality of life
  - **Patient wishes:** if a patient does not want invasive treatments, then their choice should be respected. If the patient cannot communicate this, it is important to speak to their family about what their wishes would have been.

EXPLAINING TO RELATIVES THAT A PATIENT IS AT END OF LIFE

Approach
- Use a breaking bad news approach (*see notes on breaking bad news p336*)
- Explain to the family you will involve the palliative care team if required, and offer spiritual support where available, e.g. chaplain
- Ensure you talk about the patient's symptoms and reassure them that they can be managed

Phrases to help
- 'We have tried giving strong antibiotics, fluids and oxygen but he has not made any improvement at all.' – PAUSE
- 'I am afraid, he is not going to recover from this and he is now in the final stages of his life.' – PAUSE
- 'We believe further invasive treatment and tests will prolong his suffering and will not make any difference.'
- 'The most important thing now is for us to concentrate all our efforts on making sure he is comfortable and not in any pain or distress.'

CONSENT FOR POST MORTEM

Background information
- Types and refusal
  - **Coroner's post mortem:** the relatives cannot refuse this (it must be carried out by law)
  - **Consented post mortem** (for educational purposes): written consent required from next of kin
- A consented post mortem is usually performed when the cause of death is already known. The purpose is to learn more about the condition or effects of treatment, and to help better manage other patients in the future.
- It is done in a respectful manner
- Incisions will be hidden by clothes/hair
- All tissue will be replaced inside the body unless required by the coroner or specified on the consent form
- It takes around 3 hours
- It is usually done within 2-3 days so funerals need not be delayed
- The report will be sent whoever requested the post mortem. The relatives will be informed of the cause of death and can request the full report if required for a fee. They can arrange to meet the consultant or GP to discuss the results, which will contain medical terminology.

Approach
- Be respectful and always start by saying you are sorry for their loss
- Ask them how much they know about what happened and what caused the death
- Coroner's post mortem: explain that when it is not clear what has happened, we have to notify the coroner, and that in some circumstances they order a post mortem (remember you may be breaking bad news). Explain why it is important to establish the cause of death.
- Find out what their concerns about post mortem are – they may not understand or have misconceptions about what is involved

BRAINSTEM DEATH

Background information
- Brainstem death = irreversible loss of all brain and brainstem function
- It is confirmed by two qualified specialists who do a series of tests independently to assess brainstem reflexes and breathing

Approach
- Use a breaking bad news approach
- Explain the patient is dead, despite the machine making it look like they are still breathing
- Explain that two senior consultants have done multiple tests to confirm the patient is dead
- Explain that we should now turn off the ventilator

ORGAN DONATION

Background information
- Donation may occur in three ways: after brainstem death, after circulatory death, or as a living donor
- Patients cannot donate if they have HIV, Creutzfeldt-Jakob disease or metastatic cancer
- Consent can be from the patient or relative
- If a patient has clearly consented before death, the relatives do not have the legal right to override the decision
- If a patient has not consented before death, consent from relatives is required

Approach
- Explain what organ donation involves
- Explain the benefits
- Reassure relatives about funerals and the fairness of organ allocation
- If the patient has not expressed a wish to donate, find out what they would have wanted

INTRODUCTIONS

- Initiate introductions

BREAK ICE

- e.g. 'How was your night?'

PATIENTS

- How many to handover?
- Handover each patient separately using **SBAR**:

S **Situation (core details)**
- o Patient details (name, DOB, hospital number)
- o Patient location
- o Major problem at the moment

B **Background (admission and history)**
- o Admission details (if inpatient): date, admission reason, treatments
- o Past medical history
- o ± any other relevant aspects of the history

A **Assessment**
- o Observations
- o Examination findings
- o Investigations received/pending
- o Management so far

R **Recommendations**
- o Diagnosis/differentials
- o Management plan and outstanding jobs

SUMMARISE

- Summarise each patient's details back to your colleague

CLOSING

- Thank the doctor handing over

TIPS FOR RECEIVING A HANDOVER

- Try to get all the important details you normally would get from a patient if you had seen them yourself (including exploring symptoms, risk factors and relevant system reviews). Your colleague won't necessarily remember to hand over all the information without you asking.
- Don't just accept their diagnosis
- Ask if expected management has been done

MAKING A REFERRAL

An **SBAR** approach is a good system to ensure you communicate all details in a systematic way. Think about what the person you are speaking to will want to know, and have the notes, drug and nursing charts available so that you can answer any of their questions.

INTRODUCTION

- Explain your name, role and division
- Explain what you want from them (e.g. see a ward patient, give advice over the phone, take over a patient's care, perform an investigation, or see a patient in clinic)

'Hello, it's Dr Smith here, the FY1 on call for medicine. I am phoning to ask if you could review one of our patients on the ward and consider them for transfer to the intensive care unit.'

S | SITUATION (CORE DETAILS)

- Patient details (name, age, hospital number)
- Patient location
- Major problem at the moment

'The patient is called Alexander Steward, he is a 59 year old man on ward E1 whom I was asked to see because of hypotension.'

B | BACKGROUND (ADMISSION AND HISTORY)

- Admission details (if inpatient): date, admission reason, treatments
- Past medical history
- ± any other relevant aspects of the history, e.g. premorbid state

'He was admitted 3 days ago for community acquired pneumonia, for which he is on amoxicillin and clarithromycin. He is normally fit and well, fully independent, and has a history of mild asthma which is normally well controlled.'

A | ASSESSMENT

- Observations
- Examination findings
- Investigations received/pending
- Management so far

'His blood pressure is currently 85/45, despite 3 litres of IV fluids over the last 2 hours. He has only had 3ml urine output over the last hour. He is oxygenating well and is not pyrexial.
On examination, he is drowsy and confused with cool peripheries and coarse right lower lobe crepitations on auscultation.
I have done an arterial blood gas which shows a lactate of 4.
I have also sent bloods and repeat cultures, although the results are not yet back.'

R | RECOMMENDATION

- Diagnosis/differentials
- Management plan

'I think he has septic shock and wonder whether he needs vasopressors to maintain his blood pressure. I would be grateful for your input as soon as possible.'

WARD ROUND DOCUMENTATION

Date and time (in margin)

Doctor leading ward round, their specialty and role

07.02.16
13.44

Dr Smith Ward Round (Cardiology Consultant)

Δ -Decompensated heart failure
  -New AF
  -Coliform UTI on ward

On day 2 furosemide infusion (10mg/h)
On day 3 trimethoprim

Echo 06/02/16 – poor biventricular function, moderate MR, left atrial dilatation
ECG 07/02/16 – AF @ 102bpm
Bloods 06/02/16 – Hb 102 (stable), WCC 12, CRP 22 (improved), U&Es normal

Pt. feels better today, SOB reduced.
Weight stable at 64kg for last 2 days. 500ml negative fluid balance over last 24 hours.

O/E: Sats 94% (on air), RR 22/min, HR 97bpm,
BP 140/85mmHg, apyrexial. No temp spikes.

Chest clear
JVP 6cm
HS I + II + PSM
Pitting oedema up to knees

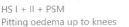

SNT
BS (N)

(P) 1. Continue furosemide infusion x $^3/_7$
2. Add bendroflumethiazide 2.5mg OD
3. Fluid restriction 1L/24h
4. Daily U&Es
5. Daily weights and accurate fluid balance chart

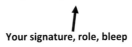

C. Mansbridge
Cardiology FY1 (bleep 6554)

Your signature, role, bleep

SUMMARY
•Summary or problem list or list of diagnoses made so far this admission
•Important management so far
NB: this may not be done everyday.

INVESTIGATIONS
•Investigations results reviewed on ward round

PATIENT ASSESSMENT
•**Questioning:** note anything the patient says
•**Charts:** e.g. fluid balance, weights, bowel chart, glucose chart (for diabetics)
•**Examination:** current observations, how the patient appears (e.g. well/unwell), system exam findings (use diagrams as well as writing findings)

PLAN
•Numerical plan

TIPS!
• Leave enough space for each section and fill in the relevant details as they are covered (often won't be in order!)
• Write down everything said by the consultant/patient
• Different consultants have different preferences about how they like things written down (the above is an example)
• If possible, try to write the first few sections (e.g. time, title, diagnosis and management so far) before the consultant actually gets to the patient to speed things up
• Make a jobs list as well as writing in the notes so you know what you need to do
• Try to get ready everything that the consultant might ask about in advance (results, imaging, drug chart, observations etc.)
• Use medical abbreviations wherever possible to speed things up

COMMON MEDICAL ABBREVIATIONS

<u>Symptoms</u>

BNO	bowels not open
BO	bowels open
SOB	shortness of breath

<u>Examination</u>

AE	air entry
BP	blood pressure
BS	bowel sounds
CN	cranial nerves
ESM	ejection-systolic murmur
HR	heart rate
HS I+II+0	heart sounds one and two with no added sounds
JVP	jugular venous pressure
OBS	observations
O/E	on examination
PSM	pansystolic murmur
RR	respiratory rate
SNT	soft non-tender

<u>Times</u>

$^x/_7$	x days
$^x/_{52}$	x weeks
$^x/_{12}$	x months

<u>Sex</u>

	Male
	Female

<u>Investigations</u>

CXR	chest X-ray
MSU	mid-stream urine

<u>Others</u>

Δ	diagnosis
Ⓝ	normal
Ⓟ	plan
Ⓡ	right
Ⓛ	left
↔	in range
↑	increased
↓	decreased
1°	primary
2°	secondary
+ve	positive
-ve	negative
?	query
#	number
c̄	with
A/W	admitted with
ADL	activities of daily living
c/o	complains of
CA	cancer
mane	in morning
NAD	no abnormality detected
NBM	nil by mouth
Pt	patient
PTOT	physiotherapy and occupational therapy
TTO	to take out (medications)
UTI	urinary tract infection
WB	weight-bearing
WR	ward round

DIAGRAMS

<u>Chest</u>
Clear

Crepitations/crackles

Wheeze

Reduced air entry

Dull to percussion

<u>Abdomen</u>
Tenderness

Hepatomegaly, scar

<u>Other</u>
Erythema

NB: any abbreviations in the front of this book may also be used.

SOAP NOTE

A **SOAP** note is a format that may be used for writing patient notes. It stands for **S**ubjective, **O**bjective, **A**ssessment, **P**lan. It is widely used in the United States, and it is also used in the United Kingdom in general practice and sometimes when reviewing patients on the ward.

Components of a SOAP note		
	Outpatient	**Inpatient**
Subjective *What the patient says*	• Presenting complaint • History of presenting complaint • Systems review • Summary of medical history and medications	• Subjective description of how patient has been since last review • Explore any symptoms
Objective *Anything measured/ examined/tested*	• Patient appearance • Observations • Physical examination (tailor to complaint)	• Patient appearance • Observations (include trend and any temperature spikes) • Other nursing charts, e.g. fluid balance • Physical examination (tailor to complaint) • Test results (lab tests, radiology etc.)
Assessment *Doctor's assessment of what is going on*	• Summary of the clinical problem • Differential diagnosis and clinical reasoning	• Summary (e.g. admission day, antibiotic/ post-op day number) • Diagnosis/diagnoses/problem list
Plan	• Investigations • Management plans • Safety-net (tell the patient when to re-seek medical advice)	• Investigations • Management plans

EXAMPLE

07.02.2014 13.45
GP Patient Review (GPST2 Stewart)

SUBJECTIVE:
38 year old male with tiredness for 3 months. Fatigue throughout the day but worse on exertion. Sleeps well, usually goes to bed at 10pm and wakes at 7am. Still managing to go to the gym and play tennis.
Constipated for 3 months (bowels every 4 days). No blood in stool. Denies any breathlessness, chest pain or abdominal pain. No fever, night sweats or weight loss. Mood is good and he is not under stress.
Medical history: asthma. Medications: salbutamol inhaler PRN. Allergies: none.

OBJECTIVE:
Comfortable at rest.
T 37°C, HR 55, BP 120/80, sats 99% RA, RR 15
Clinically euthyroid with no goitre. No conjunctival pallor. Chest clear with normal heart sounds. Abdomen soft and non-tender. No peripheral oedema. No palpable lymphadenopathy.

ASSESSMENT:
3 month history of tiredness and constipation. Hypothyroidism is possible given his bradycardia and constipation. Anaemia is also possible but there is no clear source of blood loss. Depression is unlikely given the lack of low mood or anhedonia. There are no signs of infection.

PLAN:
1. Full blood count (r/o anaemia)
2. Thyroid function tests (r/o hypothyroidism)
3. Review in 2 weeks with results

CS
C. Stewart
GPST2
GMC number 7112454

VENOUS THROMBOEMBOLISM ASSESSMENT

PHARMACOLOGICAL PROPHYLAXIS

LMWH/fondaparinux or unfractionated heparin are the most commonly used medications for pharmacological VTE prophylaxis.

- Pharmacological prophylaxis is used for most patients (unless contraindicated)
- Assess for **contraindications/cautions**:
  - Not required
    - Patient taking therapeutic anticoagulant (INR>2 if on warfarin)
  - Procedures
    - Invasive procedure scheduled within next 12 hours
    - Invasive procedure performed within previous 4 hours
  - Significant bleeding risk
    - Active bleeding/stroke
    - Thrombocytopenia (platelets <75x10^9/L)
    - Bleeding disorders
    - Acute stroke
    - SBP >230mmHg
- Weigh up the **risks and benefits** of anticoagulation (discuss with senior if unclear)
- If the benefits outweigh the risks, determine **renal function** and **weight**. Each hospital will have a recommended protocol. Example for patients 50-100kg:
  - eGFR >30 – prophylactic-dose LMWH/fondaparinux (e.g. enoxaparin 40mg S/C OD)
  - eGFR <30 – prophylactic-dose unfractionated heparin (e.g. heparin 5000 units S/C BD)

VTE risk factors

- Age >60
- BMI >30
- Dehydration
- Immobility ≥3 days
- Active cancer
- Significant comorbidities
- HRT/oestrogen contraceptives
- Phlebitis/varicose veins
- Surgery taking >90 minutes (or >60 minutes on lower limb/pelvis)
- Pregnancy/<6 weeks post-partum
- Inflammatory condition
- Thrombophilia or PMHx/FHx of VTE
- Obesity
- Critical care admission

MECHANICAL PROPHYLAXIS

Thromboembolic deterrent stockings (TEDs) or foot impulse devices/intermittent pneumatic compression devices (IPCs) may be used for mechanical VTE prophylaxis.

- Mechanical prophylaxis is used for patients unable to take pharmacological prophylaxis, and in addition to pharmacological prophylaxis in surgical patients
- Choice depends on individual patient factors and condition/intervention
- Assess for **contraindications**:
  - Peripheral arterial disease
  - Fragile skin, e.g. 'tissue paper skin', dermatitis, or recent skin graft
  - Severe peripheral oedema
  - Cardiac failure
  - Leg deformity
  - Peripheral neuropathy

TO COMPLETE

- 'I have ensured there are no contraindications, weighed up the risks and benefits, and determined renal function and weight. After obtaining patient consent, I would like to prescribe:
  - LMWH/fondaparinux as per hospital protocol (e.g. enoxaparin 40mg subcutaneously) once every evening
  - And/or thromboembolic deterrent stockings or foot impulse devices/intermittent pneumatic compression devices.'
- 'I would reassess the patient's anticoagulation needs 24 hours after admission.'

DISCHARGE SUMMARY

A discharge summary is an account of the major events of the hospital admission for the patient's GP, so that they can take over the patient's care.

INTRODUCTION

- **Patient**
  - Name
  - Hospital and NHS number
  - DOB
  - Address
  - GP details
- **Hospital stay**
  - Consultant
  - Ward and hospital
  - Admission and discharge date
  - Discharge destination
- **Summary details**
  - Date written
  - Your name and signature

CLINICAL DETAILS

- **Presentation**
  - History
  - Examination
- **Investigations**
  - Important investigation results
  - Any awaited results
- **Diagnosis and patient's comorbidities**
- **Management**
  - How the patient was managed/treated
  - Response/complications

FUTURE MANAGEMENT

- Management plans for after discharge
- Follow-up appointment
- Actions for GP

MEDICATIONS

- Regular medication changes
- Medications to take home (medication, strength, form, directions, quantity)
  - Regular medications
  - Any added medications
  - Any PRN medications still being used (e.g. analgesia, anti-emetics)

NB: out-patient controlled drug prescriptions must be handwritten and must include patient name and address; drug, strength and formulation; dose and frequency. The total quantity must be spelled out as well as written numerically.

Remember: the most important thing for GPs is to know what they need to do and about any medication changes (and why)

DEATH CERTIFICATION

VERIFYING DEATH
- Review the patient's notes, resuscitation status, and recent events with the nursing team – was the death expected/unexpected?
- Wash hands
- Introduce yourself to the family if present, say you are sorry for their loss, and explain what you need to do
- Ask if they want to be present or not
- Confirm the patient's identity on their wristband (name, hospital number, DOB)
- All criteria below must be met and documented:

> - **Pupils** fixed and dilated (with no response to light)
> - No **ventilation observed/breath sounds** on auscultation (1 minute)
> - No **central pulse** palpable (1 minute)
> - No **heart sounds** on auscultation (1 minute)
> - No **response to painful stimulus** (e.g. squeezing trapezius)

- Cover the patient in a dignified manner
- Document the above findings with the date and time at the end of the assessment in the notes (include your full name and role)

WHEN YOU CAN FILL OUT THE DEATH CERTIFICATE
All of the criteria below must be met:
- You must have seen the patient in the last **14 days** before death or after death
- You must have provided care in the last illness before death
- You must be a registered medical practitioner
- You must have 'knowledge and belief' of the cause of death (this should ideally be discussed with the consultant in charge)
- The death must not meet criteria for referral to the coroner (*see box below*)

FILLING OUT A DEATH CERTIFICATE
Demographics
- Name, age, DOB

Details of death
- Place of death
- Date of death and date you last saw the patient alive (format: 'Third *day of* November 2017')
- Whether a post-mortem is required or you have reported the death to the coroner
- Who saw the patient after death (you/another medical practitioner/not seen after death by a medical practitioner)

Cause
- Format:
  - **Ia**: the immediate cause of death
    ↑
  - **Ib**: condition leading to Ia
    ↑
  - **Ic**: condition leading to Ib
  - **II**: other conditions contributing to death (but unrelated to condition in part I)
- Example:
  - Ia: Pulmonary Thromboembolism
  - Ib: Deep Vein Thrombosis
  - II: Metastatic prostate cancer
- Tips:
  - Do not use abbreviations or symbols
  - Give as much information as possible (but you don't need to fill out all sections)
  - Avoid the terms: any organ failure, old age, natural causes

Your details
- Name, role, qualifications, General Medical Council number, signature
- Hospital address
- Consultant in charge

Cases to refer to the coroner
- In hospital <24 hours
- Unknown cause/unexpected
- In custody
- Any suspicious circumstances
- Any drugs involved
- Acute alcohol
- Industrial deaths
- Any blame
- Following accident/fall/violence
- Operation <1 year
- Unknown identity

CHAPTER 9: CLERKING AND REVIEWING PATIENTS

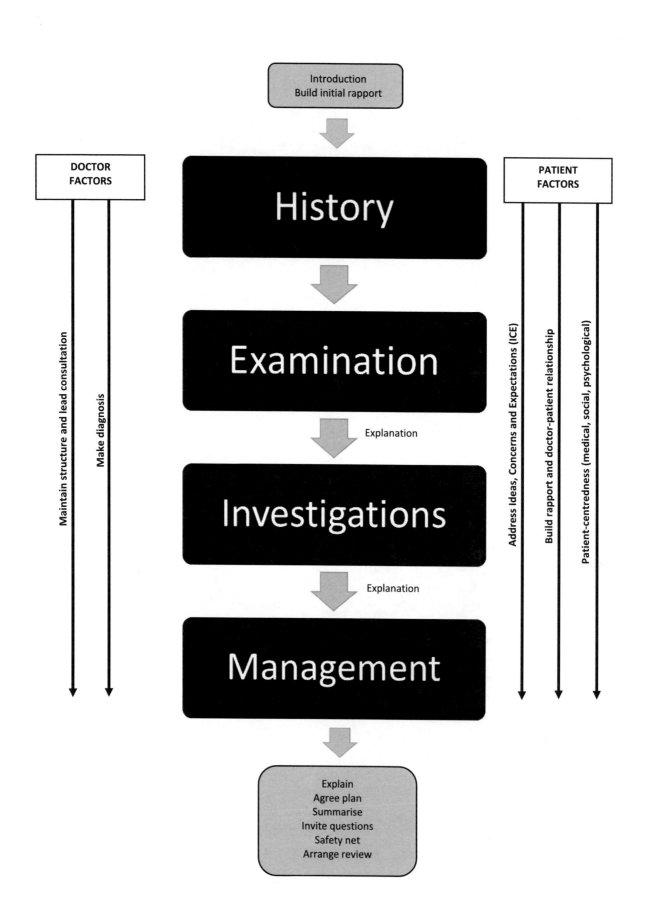

TAKE HISTORY AND EXAMINE PATIENT

- Take a **full history** (*see section on histories p1*)
- **Examine patient** (*see section on examinations p39*)
  - Look at the **observations** chart
  - You should do a basic **multi-system exam** for all new admissions
    - Respiratory: cyanosis, percussion note, lung sounds, calf swelling/tenderness
    - Cardiovascular: capillary refill, pulse (rate/rhythm), JVP, heart sounds, peripheral oedema
    - Abdominal: tenderness, masses/organomegaly, bowel sounds
    - Nervous system: GCS, limb movements, abbreviated mental test score if elderly/confused
  - Examine the **relevant system** in more detail and specifically document the presence/absence of signs of differential diagnoses
- Review any **investigations** that have already been performed (e.g. bloods, X-rays etc.)
- Formulate a **differential diagnosis/impression/problem list** and **plan** investigations/management *based on the above*

DOCUMENT

- **Date and time**
- **Patient age and sex**
- **History**
  - **Presenting complaint**
  - **History of presenting complaint** (e.g. main symptoms as separate major bullet points, with sub-bullet points exploring each symptom, and then relevant system reviews as further major bullet points – include relevant positives <u>and</u> negatives)
    - Symptom A
      - Explore
      - Explore
    - Symptom B
      - Explore
      - Explore
    - Relevant system review A
    - Relevant system review B
  - **PMHx** (supplement with information from computerised records)
  - **DHx** (including allergies)
  - **FHx** (relevant conditions)
  - **SHx** (must be very thorough in elderly patients – get collateral)
- **Examination**
- **Investigation results** so far
- **Differential diagnosis/impression/problem list**
- **Plan**
  - Investigations
  - Management
  - Other considerations
- **Sign** with name, role, bleep

ARRANGE INVESTIGATIONS

- **Perform**
  - Site cannula and take bloods from cannula (consider doing this before taking a history so results are back quicker)
  - Undertake other relevant investigations, e.g. ABG, lumbar puncture, blood cultures
- **Ask nursing staff**
  - Bedside tests, e.g. ECG, urine dip (± MC&S), swabs
- **Order**
  - Relevant imaging
  - Any other tests required

IMPLEMENT MANAGEMENT

- Implement **ABCDE management** as necessary, e.g. oxygen, fluids
- Fill in **drug chart**
  - Disease-specific treatments
  - PRN analgesia ± anti-emetics ± anti-pyretic if required

BOXES approach to investigations

- **Bloods:** venous (e.g. FBC, CRP, U&Es, LFTs ± amylase, G&S, INR), blood cultures (if pyrexial), ABG, capillary glucose
- **Orifice tests:** urine dip, urine/sputum/faeces cultures
- **X-rays/imaging:** CXR, AXR, USS, CT
- **ECG**
- **Special tests:** depending on likely cause

- o Regular medications
- o DVT prophylaxis (e.g. LMWH/fondaparinux ± anti-embolism stockings)
- Order/perform any other disease-specific interventions
- Fill in a **VTE assessment**
- Keep patient NBM if surgery may be required

REVIEW

- Note down the patient's details and which investigations need to be chased (use fill-in boxes – half fill when taken/requested, fully fill when result back and checked)
- Follow-up the results and document them in the notes
- Change/initiate treatments if needed
- Present to seniors (when initial investigation results are back) and implement any additional management plans required

TIPS!

<u>General tips</u>
- You will need to write quickly during the consultation but try to ensure the patient is still the main focus
- Look through all the computerised records (e.g. GP record, discharges, letters, investigation results) for the patient to supplement the past medical/drug history
- In some elderly patients, you may need to call the next of kin or nursing/residential home for collateral history (find out what happened and get more information about past/drug/social history and their baseline)
- Ensure you are leading the consultation – learn how to interrupt patients politely. If the patient is very talkative, use closed, focussed questions.
- Never forget your communication skills – introduce yourself properly, use the patient's name, shake their hand, build rapport, start with open questions and find out their ideas, concerns and expectations

<u>Advancing your clinical practice</u>
- As a medical student, you need to ask about everything and your clerking should be comprehensive. But as your experience grows, your goal is to become more efficient. A senior doctor will ask questions, examine and investigate in a way that stays focussed on the diagnosis and differentials.
- History
  - o You should ask **questions to include/exclude differentials** (e.g. rather than going through the whole of SOCRATES for chest pain, listen to the patient's description and then ask 'Does the pain radiate to the back?' if you need to exclude dissection; or 'Does the pain get worse on exertion?' if angina is a differential)
  - o In addition to an open question about past medical history, you should also ask **specifically about relevant comorbidities and risk factors** (e.g. in suspected MI, ask about diabetes, hypertension, high cholesterol, smoking)
  - o Ask about **relevant family history** and include **travel/sexual histories when relevant**
  - o Social history is always important for older patients, and checking people's occupation can provide key information
- Examination
  - o Quickly determine if the patient is **well or unwell**
    - General: confusion/cognitive change, skin colour, respiratory distress/oxygen requirements
    - Circulation: peripheral pulse rate/volume, capillary refill, peripheral temperature
  - o A simple *baseline* multi-system clinical examination should still be done for everyone on admission but you should focus on **specific signs related to the history** – i.e. signs of the diagnosis/differential, the cause and complications of the condition – you should think about exactly what you are looking for and why
  - o Note the **presence <u>or absence</u> of relevant signs**

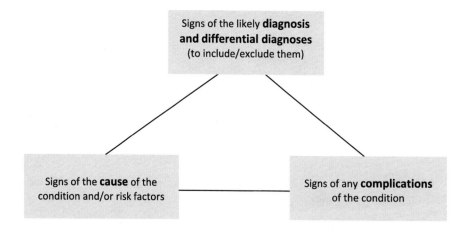

PRE-OPERATIVE ASSESSMENT

SUMMARISE CORE DETAILS
- Patient details
- Operation (and anaesthesia if required)
- Background

NB: look through past notes/e-documents to confirm details.

CURRENT HEALTH
- Recent/current illnesses (within 2 weeks)
- Baseline exercise tolerance (what makes them stop: SOB/chest pain/claudication)
- Symptoms of sleep apnoea (paroxysmal nocturnal dyspnoea, excessive sleepiness, morning headaches)
- Smoking/alcohol

MEDICAL AND DRUG HISTORY
- **Medical conditions**
  - Ask specifically about hypertension, diabetes (should be put first on list), asthma/COPD, cardiovascular disease, IHD, liver disease
  - Determine if conditions are adequately controlled
- **Drug history** (including <u>allergies</u>!)

ANAESTHETIC HISTORY
- Previous anaesthetics and reactions
- Family anaesthetic history

EXAMINATION
- **Anaesthetic assessment**
  - Neck movement limitation/jaw opening limitation/dentures
  - Airway assessment: use Mallampati classification and note BMI
    1. See all soft palate and uvula
    2. See half of uvula
    3. See a small gap at end of soft palate
    4. Can only see hard palate
  - Back examination (if having spinal/epidural): look for skeletal malformations
- **Multi-system examination**
  - General: GCS, limb movements
  - Hands: cyanosis, warm peripheries, cap refill, peripheral pulses
  - Neck: JVP, carotid bruits
  - Chest: heaves/thrills, chest expansion, percussion resonance, lung and heart sounds
  - Abdomen: tenderness, masses/organomegaly, bowel sounds
  - Calves: swelling/tenderness, oedema

INVESTIGATIONS
These tests should be performed for patients having intermediate/major surgery (minimal tests are needed for minor surgery):
- **Routine tests** (NICE have guidelines on exactly who needs what)
  - Bloods within 1 week
    - FBC (*all patients; anaemia increases surgical risk*)
    - U&Es (*all patients; assess risk of AKI post-surgery*)
    - LFTs (*if liver/biliary operation or past liver problems; impairment may delay healing*)
    - Clotting (*if relevant comorbidities or bleeding history*)
    - TFTs (*if taking thyroxine*)
    - Group and save (*all patients*)
  - ECG (*if >65 years or any heart problems*)
- **Other tests** may be necessary – look at the patient's electronic record to see any previous results
  - Echocardiogram (*if murmur/heart failure/cardiac symptoms*)
  - CXR (*only if may need ICU care*)
  - Spirometry (*if significant lung disease*)
  - Pacemaker check (*if have pacemaker*)

PREPARATION

Correct investigation abnormalities

For an immediate pre-operative assessment (day prior to the operation):
- **Correct INR** if abnormal (>1.4)
  - Aggressive correction (if on warfarin for AF): 5-10mg IV vitamin K, then repeat INR in 6 hours – if still high, discuss with haematology regarding giving prothrombin complex concentrate pre-operatively
  - Cautious correction (if on warfarin for artificial heart valve/recent PE): discuss with seniors and haematology – will usually require reversal of warfarin and cover with unfractionated heparin infusion, which will be stopped 4 hours pre-op and restarted after
  - If INR raised due to liver disease: 10mg IV vitamin K, then repeat INR in 6 hours – if still high, discuss with haematology who may advise FFP/cryoprecipitate
- **Blood transfusion** if Hb <9g/dL, or <10g/dL if elderly/cardiovascular/respiratory disease
- Consider **platelet concentrate transfusion** if platelets <50x10⁹/L (discuss with haematology if cause unclear)
- **Correct electrolyte** abnormalities

NB: if there are significant abnormalities, bloods must be repeated again pre-operatively (e.g. at 6am) to show they have been corrected.

For an early pre-operative assessment (>1 week pre-operatively):
- INR may be corrected by stopping warfarin as below
- Anaemia should be investigated and the cause treated – e.g. with iron tablets for iron-deficiency anaemia

NB: if there are <u>any</u> concerns, contact the consultant or an anaesthetist.

Medications

- **IV fluids:** only prescribe fluids overnight (when NBM) if instructed by consultant, or if patient needs variable rate insulin infusion, or is dehydrated
- **New medications**
  - Operation preparation: give drugs required for specific operation (specified in pre-operative checklist), e.g. bowel prep for colorectal
  - VTE prophylaxis: prophylactic LMWH should be given the night before the operation, but omit any doses when the operation is due to start in <12 hours
  - Anti-emetics and analgesia: as required
- **Regular medicines**
  - Vital drugs should be taken on the day of the operation: cardiovascular medications, anti-psychotics, Parkinson's medications, inhalers, glaucoma medications, immunosuppressants, thyroid medications, drugs of dependence (e.g. benzodiazepine)
  - Most other drugs should not be taken on the day of the operation (restarted the day after)
  - Some medications must be stopped/changed pre-operatively:

Medications that should be stopped/changed pre-operatively		
Medication	**Days pre-operatively to stop**	**Details**
Warfarin	5 days	Therapeutic-dose LMWH should be prescribed in interim
Direct oral anticoagulants	24 hours for minor surgery; 48 hours for major surgery	
Therapeutic-dose LMWH	48 hours	May need heparin infusion cover if high risk indication
Unfractionated heparin infusion	4 hours	Restart post-operatively
Aspirin/clopidogrel/dipyridamole	7 days	If patient has had recent stent (<1 year), never stop without liaising with cardiology and seniors
Insulin	Avoid morning dose	Prescribe variable rate insulin infusion with surgical fluid [5% dex/0.45% NaCl/0.15% KCl @ 80ml/h] from midnight the night before (unless minor surgery)
Oral hypoglycaemics	Avoid on day of operation	Prescribe variable rate insulin infusion as above if blood glucose not well controlled. Also avoid metformin for two days after (due to risk of lactic acidosis).
Diuretics/ACE inhibitors	Avoid on day of operation	
Long-term corticosteroids	Change to higher dose hydrocortisone	Liaise with anaesthetist
COCP	4 weeks	Restart 2 weeks after

Forms

- VTE prophylaxis Proforma
- Consent form (complete this only if you have sufficient knowledge, if not call registrar/consultant)

Fasting and admission

- Fasting guidelines
  - '2-6 rule' = NBM for 2 hours pre-operatively; clear fluids only for 6 hours pre-operatively
    NB: if you are unsure of the operation time, prepare the patient for 8am (e.g. say clear fluids only from 2am, NBM from 6am).
- Pre-operative patients only need admission the night before if they are diabetic (and therefore require a variable rate insulin infusion from midnight); or if they need specific medications which must be given overnight; or if INR/Hb/platelets need correction

MEDICAL PATIENT REVIEW

SIPP may be used to remember main sections

•Summarise
•Investigation results review
•Patient assessment
(questioning + charts + exam)
•Plan and medications review

SUMMARISE THE PATIENT'S CASE

- **Demographics:** name, age
- **Patient background:** comorbidities, medical history
- **Admission details:** date of admission, presenting complaint
- **Diagnosis**/diagnoses/differentials so far
- **Management so far**
  - Investigations: results of important investigations the patient has had during this admission
  - Treatments
- **Planned management:** management plan, stage reached, why they are still in hospital

NB: whenever you see a patient you have not previously reviewed yourself, you should go through everything in detail – don't just accept other people's diagnoses/plans. If you have reviewed a patient before and been through the case in detail, a basic diagnosis/problem list every few days will usually suffice.

INVESTIGATION RESULTS REVIEW

- **Latest bloods and trends**, e.g. haemoglobin, inflammatory markers (WCC/CRP), other relevant blood results
- **Other new investigation results**

PATIENT ASSESSMENT

Questioning
- **Current symptoms:** determine current symptoms, explore as usual
- **Changes since last review/coming into hospital**
- **Concerns**
- **Functional assessment:** eating/drinking, bowel habit, mobilisation

Nursing charts
- **Observations:** review current condition and trends on observation chart/temperature spikes
- **If being recorded and relevant**
  - **Stool chart:** check when last opened bowels and stool type
  - **Capillary glucose chart** (if diabetic): check the range of glucose levels
  - **Fluid chart:** check input, output and balance
  - **Food intake chart**

Examination
- **Focussed system examinations** as relevant

PLAN AND MEDICATIONS REVIEW

- Make plan (including further tests/management)
- Review current medications (don't forget about VTE prophylaxis!)

TIPS!

- Reviews must be *patient-centred* (treat the patient, not the disease). Consider:
  - Disease
  - Comorbidities
  - Social factors: home, family, carers (involve nurses and occupational therapists)
  - Occupation (e.g. type of work if epileptic)
  - Mobilisation status (involve physiotherapists)
  - Polypharmacy (involve pharmacist)
  - Strength/habitus and diet (involve dietitian)
- Consider making a problem list
- Ensure you always think about why a patient is still in hospital and think about their case with a view to discharge
- It can be difficult to build and maintain good patient relationships when you are busy and have a long list of jobs to do. Some tips: introduce yourself properly; shake the patient's hand at the start and end; check what they like to be called and use that name throughout the consultation; ensure you check for their concerns/questions at the end.

POST-OPERATIVE GENERAL SURGICAL PATIENT REVIEW

SUMMARISE THE PATIENT'S CASE

- **Demographics:** name and age
- **Operation:** days post-op, type of operation, reason for operation
- **Planned management:** check operation note to ascertain post-operative plan, patient's stage in plan, why they are still in hospital

SIPP may be used to remember main sections

- Summarise
- Investigation results review
- Patient assessment (questioning + charts + exam)
- Plan and medications review

INVESTIGATION RESULTS REVIEW

- **Latest bloods and trends**
  - Inflammatory markers (WCC, CRP) – may rise for first 2 days post-operatively but should fall after that
  - Haemoglobin
  - Electrolytes
  - Other relevant blood results
- **Other new investigation results**

PATIENT ASSESSMENT

Questioning
- **Any symptoms or issues?**
- **Eating and drinking? How much?**
- **Bowels opening? If not, passing flatus?**
- **Pain controlled?**
- **Mobilising?**

Nursing charts
- **Observations:** review current condition and trends on observation chart/temperature spikes
- **Fluid balance chart**
  - **Urine output**
  - **NG/NJ output** (if used for drainage)
  - **Drains output**
- **Stool chart**
- **Food chart** and note current oral intake limitations (see spectrum below)

Examination
- **Tubes in situ**
  - **Drains:** e.g. Wallis drain, Redivac negative pressure drain, Pigtail drain etc. As output decreases, drains are usually 'cut and bagged', then removed when output has decreased to insignificant amounts (e.g. <25ml/d), whereupon the site is covered with a bag. This is later removed and the wound dressed when dry.
  - **Wound catheters:** a local anaesthetic delivery system to provide analgesia – remove when pain controlled
  - **Urinary catheter:** TWOC when fluid balance stable and patient is able to mobilise and control urination
  - **Central line:** remove when no longer needed
  - **NG/NJ tubes or parenteral nutrition lines:** remove when not needed for nutrition or drainage
  - **Patient-controlled analgesia:** remove when oral analgesia is likely to control pain
- **Drain quantity and output** (e.g. serous, bloody, chyle etc.)
- **Wounds** (pain, erythema, discharge, leakiness)
- **Focussed system examinations** as relevant

PLAN AND MEDICATIONS REVIEW

- Make plan (including further tests/management)
- Review current medications (don't forget about VTE prophylaxis!)

TIPS!

- The aim is to get the patient back to normal and then home. Take into consideration:
  - **Oral intake:** may be limited in first few days post-operatively but is increased gradually if there is no distension/vomiting/nausea; if the patient is passing stool/flatus; and if there is no limitation due to bowel anastomosis. Spectrum:
    - NG/NJ with free drainage (i.e. NG/NJ is open-ended and will continually drain stomach contents into bag)
    - Spigotted NG/NJ (where a bung is placed into the end of the NG/NJ) ± '2/4/6 hourly drainage'
    - NBM
    - Sips
    - Clear fluids limited to ml/hour, e.g. '20s' (i.e. 20ml/hour), '40s', '60s', '100s'
    - Clear free fluids, e.g. water, tea without milk etc.
    - Free fluids (anything liquid – includes soup, milk etc.)
    - Light/soft diet
    - Normal diet
  - **Analgesia:** aim to gradually reduce as tolerated (e.g. patient-controlled analgesia → tramadol + paracetamol + Oramorph PRN → paracetamol)
  - **Tubes:** take them out when possible
  - **Fluids and fluid balance:** adjust to achieve good balance; reduce IV fluids when oral intake is adequate
  - **Nutrition:** consider supplementation (e.g. Fortisip drinks and multivitamins) and dietitian input. Consider NG feeding or parenteral nutrition if patient will not be eating within 7 days.
  - Any evidence of infection or other post-surgical complications requiring investigation/intervention
  - Correct electrolyte abnormalities
  - **Mobilise:** patient needs to increase mobility until they are at their pre-morbid level of independence. Consider physiotherapist input.
  - **Medications:** change to oral when possible
  - **Breathing:** ensure patient is breathing properly to prevent post-operative atelectasis/chest infections. Encourage deep breathing, keep pain well controlled (as this limits inspiration), and consider saline nebulisers and chest physiotherapy.
- Do not overuse IV fluids! If the patient can tolerate oral fluids then maintenance bags are rarely required (*see prescribing notes on fluids p281*).
- It can be difficult to build and maintain good patient relationships when you are busy and have a long list of jobs to do. Some tips: introduce yourself properly; shake the patient's hand at the start and end; check what they like to be called and use that name throughout the consultation; ensure you check for their concerns/questions at the end.

FALLS RISK ASSESSMENT

Falls are common in elderly patients and are often multi-factorial. Risk factors must be minimised and all patients who fall frequently need multidisciplinary assessment by doctors/nurses, physiotherapists, occupational therapists and social services (in case more care is required). The differential diagnosis of falls is covered on p182.

FALLS HISTORY

- Age
- Frequency of falls (in past 12 months)
- Reason for falls, e.g. trip, unsteadiness, syncope
- Injuries sustained
- Fear of falling

PAST MEDICAL HISTORY/REVIEW OF SYSTEMS

General	Sensory or visual impairment
Musculoskeletal	Immobility, previous low impact fractures/osteoporosis, arthritis, myopathy
Nervous system	Parkinson's disease, strokes, neuropathy, confusion/dementia/delirium, dizziness, syncope
Cardiovascular	Postural hypotension, syncope, arrhythmias, breathlessness on exertion (aortic stenosis)
Endocrine	Diabetes mellitus (peripheral neuropathy, hypoglycaemia, retinopathy)
Gastrointestinal/genitourinary	Nutrition, incontinence (rushing to toilet), nocturia (may result in patients ambling in the dark)

DRUG HISTORY

- Polypharmacy (*>5 is an independent risk factor for falls*)
- Medications with potentially troublesome side effects: anti-hypertensives (*hypotension*), anti-epileptics (*seizure control*), benzodiazepines (*sedation*), psychotropics (*extrapyramidal side effects*), corticosteroids (*osteoporosis, myopathy*), beta-blockers (*bradycardia*), hypoglycaemics (*hypoglycaemia*), antidepressants (*postural hypotension*), diuretics (*urinary frequency, dehydration*), anticoagulants (*bleeding risk*)
- Bone protection: bisphosphonates, calcium, vitamin D (*reduce fracture risk*)

SOCIAL HISTORY AND ENVIRONMENT

- **Living situation**
  - Residence
  - Any stairs?
  - Who they live with
  - Carers/home support
- **Who performs their daily tasks** (if the patient does them, how well?)
  - Washing
  - Dressing
  - Cooking
  - Cleaning
  - Shopping
- **Mobility:** baseline, mobility aids
- **Alcohol**
- **Footwear:** appropriately fitting?
- **Exercise:** increases muscle strength, reduces frailty and falls risk
- **Home hazards:** rugs, cables, furniture, wet floors, stairs, lighting

EXAMINATION – ADAPT DEPENDING ON RISK FACTORS FROM HISTORY

- **General examination:** frailty, myopathy, sarcopenia
- **Cognitive assessment:** e.g. mini-mental state examination
- **Neurological examination:** including gait, balance and signs of parkinsonism
- **Visual examination**
- **Cardiovascular exam**, postural BPs and ECG

- Specific falls risk tests
    - **Timed 'up and go' test:** request that the patient rise from a chair without the support of their arms, walk 3 metres, then turn round and sit down again. A walking aid can be used if required. Completion of the test without unsteadiness or difficulty suggests a low risk of falling.
    - **'Turn 180°' test:** request that the patient stand up and turn around until they are facing the opposite direction. If more than four steps are required to do this, further assessment is indicated.
- Physiotherapy and occupational therapy assessments

CONCLUSION

- Thank patient
- Summarise your findings and risk factors
- Suggest how risk factors could be mitigated, for example:
    - Strength and balance training
    - Home hazard intervention (occupational therapy assessment)
    - Visual assessment/referral
    - Medication review
    - Alcohol cessation
    - Psychiatric assessment if evidence of cognitive impairment
    - Continence assessment
    - Correct postural hypotension (stop causative medications, keep hydrated, TEDs, fludrocortisone if severe)

DIABETIC CARE REVIEW

Diabetic patients should have a thorough review at least once annually.

HbA1c aim = 48-53mmol/mol

HISTORY

- **Background**
    - Diabetes type
    - Do they monitor capillary glucose?
    - Current treatments
    - Other medical problems (include recurrent infections/abscesses)
    - Medications (include steroid use)
- **Control**
    - Capillary glucose measurements
    - HbA1c readings
    - Any episodes of DKA/hyperosmolar hyperglycaemic state/hypoglycaemia
    - Coping and compliance with regimen (and any side effects)
    - Any changes in regular lifestyle
- **Macrovascular complications**
    - Stroke/TIA
    - MI
    - Claudication
- **Microvascular complications**
    - Eyes
    - Kidneys (note deterioration can reduce excretion of insulin/hypoglycaemic agents and lead to hypoglycaemia)
    - Neuropathy/feet
- **Other cardiovascular risk factors**
    - Smoking
    - Diet
    - Weight
    - Cholesterol
    - Blood pressure
- **Other issues**
    - Planning pregnancy
    - Sexual dysfunction

EXAMINATION

- **Weight, height, BMI**
- **Eyes**
    - Xanthelasma/cataract/ophthalmoplegia
    - Visual acuity
    - Ophthalmoscopy (diabetic retinopathy)
- **Cardiovascular**
    - Pulse
    - Blood pressure
    - Heart sounds
    - Carotid bruits
- **Insulin injection sites** (lipodystrophy)
- **Feet** – *full diabetic foot exam covered on p61*
    - Inspect: shoes, skin (ulcers, infection, pallor, fissures), nails (dystrophy), webspaces (cracking, maceration), deformities (Charcot joints)
    - Arteriopathy: temperature, pulses, capillary refill
    - Neuropathy: 10g monofilament sensation, vibration sense with 128Hz tuning fork, proprioception, ankle jerks

INVESTIGATIONS

- HbA1c
- Lipid profile
- Renal and liver function
- Urinalysis (protein, blood, ketones)
- Urine albumin-creatinine ratio

TREATMENT PLAN

- Review/adjust medication (aim HbA1c 48-53mmol/mol)
- Educate patient about diabetes, monitoring, treatment and complications
- Address other cardiovascular risk factors – consider:

○ Statin	→	If 10-year risk of cardiovascular disease (QRISK2 score) of ≥10% OR if type 1 and >40 years/diabetic >10 years/nephropathy/cardiovascular risk factors
○ Anti-hypertensives	→	aim <135/85mmHg (type 1) or <140/80 (type 2)
○ Aspirin	→	if cardiovascular disease (heart disease, stroke/TIA, peripheral vascular disease)
○ ACE-inhibitor	→	if diabetic nephropathy present
○ Weight loss/exercise/diet		
○ Smoking cessation		

- Refer if needed
    - Ophthalmologist – *patients should have annual retinopathy screens*
    - Dietitian
    - Podiatrist
    - Educational team
- Address any patient worries/concerns

INDEX